Antimicrobial Resistance: Global Challenges and Future Interventions

Antimicrobial Resistance: Global Challenges and Future Interventions

Editor: Steven Blair

AMERICAN
MEDICAL PUBLISHERS
www.americanmedicalpublishers.com

AMERICAN
MEDICAL PUBLISHERS
www.americanmedicalpublishers.com

Cataloging-in-Publication Data

Antimicrobial resistance : global challenges and future interventions / edited by Steven Blair.
p. cm.
Includes bibliographical references and index.
ISBN 978-1-63927-886-2
1. Drug resistance in microorganisms. 2. Drug resistance in microorganisms--Prevention.
3. Anti-infective agents. 4. Communicable Disease--Treatment. 5. Resistance to drugs in microorganisms.
I. Blair, Steven.
QR177 .A58 2023
616.904 1--dc23

American Medical Publishers,
41 Flatbush Avenue,
1st Floor, New York,
NY 11217, USA

ISBN 978-1-63927-886-2 (Hardback)

Contents

Preface

Antimicrobial resistance (AMR) happens when microbes develop mechanisms that guard them against the outcomes of antimicrobials. The agents that kill or stop the growth of microorganisms are called antimicrobials. The classification of antimicrobials is based on their function. For instance, antibiotics are used against bacteria and antifungals are used against fungi. The main causes of rising antimicrobial resistance are the usage of antimicrobials in humans and other animals, and the dissemination of resistant strains between the two. The multifold rise in resistance has also been related to the pharmaceutical sector releasing insufficiently treated effluents in the environment, particularly in nations where bulk medicines are made. Antimicrobials boost selective pressure in microbial populations, leading to the death of vulnerable microorganisms. This results in a rise in the percentage of resistant bacteria that survive. Resistant bacteria usually have a growth advantage and proliferate faster than vulnerable bacteria, even at very low levels of antibiotics. Antimicrobial resistance is becoming more widespread, necessitating the development of alternate treatments. The aim of this book is to present researches that have transformed the study of antimicrobial resistance and aided its advancement. It will help the readers in keeping pace with the rapid changes in this field of study.

This book is a result of research of several months to collate the most relevant data in the field.

When I was approached with the idea of this book and the proposal to edit it, I was overwhelmed. It gave me an opportunity to reach out to all those who share a common interest with me in this field. I had 3 main parameters for editing this text:

1. Accuracy – The data and information provided in this book should be up-to-date and valuable to the readers.

2. Structure – The data must be presented in a structured format for easy understanding and better grasping of the readers.

3. Universal Approach – This book not only targets students but also experts and innovators in the field, thus my aim was to present topics which are of use to all.

Thus, it took me a couple of months to finish the editing of this book.

I would like to make a special mention of my publisher who considered me worthy of this opportunity and also supported me throughout the editing process. I would also like to thank the editing team at the back-end who extended their help whenever required.

Editor

1

Resistance Mutations in *gyrA* and *parC* are Common in *Escherichia* Communities of both Fluoroquinolone-Polluted and Uncontaminated Aquatic Environments

*Anna Johnning[1,2], Erik Kristiansson[2], Jerker Fick[3], Birgitta Weijdegård[1] and D. G. Joakim Larsson[1]**

[1] Department of Infectious Diseases, Institute of Biomedicine, University of Gothenburg, Gothenburg, Sweden, [2] Department of Mathematical Sciences, Chalmers University of Technology, Gothenburg, Sweden, [3] Department of Chemistry, Umeå University, Umeå, Sweden

***Correspondence:**
Joakim Larsson
joakim.larsson@fysiologi.gu.se

Alterations in the target proteins of fluoroquinolones, especially in GyrA and ParC, are known to cause resistance. Here, we investigated environmental *Escherichia* communities to explore the possible link between the abundance of mutations, and the exposure to fluoroquinolones. Sediment samples were collected from a relatively pristine lake, up and downstream from a sewage treatment plant, and from several industrially polluted sites. The quinolone resistance-determining regions of *gyrA* and *parC* were analyzed using amplicon sequencing of metagenomic DNA. Five non-synonymous substitutions were present in all samples, and all of these mutations have been previously linked to fluoroquinolone resistance in *Escherichia coli*. In GyrA, substitutions S83L and D87N were on average detected at frequencies of 86 and 32%, respectively, and 31% of all amplicons encoded both substitutions. In ParC, substitutions S80I, E84G, and E84V were detected in 42, 0.9, and 6.0% of the amplicons, respectively, and 6.5% encoded double substitutions. There was no significant correlation between the level of fluoroquinolone pollution and the relative abundance of resistance mutations, with the exception of the most polluted site, which showed the highest abundance of said substitutions in both genes. Our results demonstrate that resistance mutations can be common in environmental *Escherichia,* even in the absence of a fluoroquinolone selective pressure.

Keywords: antimicrobial agents, mechanisms of resistance, antibiotics, microbial communities, next generation sequencing

INTRODUCTION

Fluoroquinolones are a class of synthetic broad-spectrum antibiotics that target the type II topoisomerases (DNA gyrase and topoisomerase IV) involved in the maintenance of DNA topology. DNA gyrase and topoisomerase IV are both tetrameric enzymes composed of two X and two Y subunits (X_2Y_2). DNA gyrase is encoded by the genes *gyrA* and *gyrB*, and topoisomerase

IV is encoded by *parC* and *parE*. The enzymes are homologues, and there is a considerable sequence similarity between *gyrA* and *parC*, and between *gyrB* and *parE*. One of the main mechanisms of fluoroquinolone resistance is amino acid substitutions in the DNA gyrase and topoisomerase IV proteins, in particular in GyrA and ParC (Ruiz, 2003; Hopkins et al., 2005). Several resistance mutations have been characterized in *Escherichia coli*, and the majority of these are located in the quinolone resistance-determining region (QRDR) defined as codons 67–106 in *gyrA* and 56–108 in *parC* (*E. coli* numbering). Certain single mutations in *gyrA* are sufficient to generate high-level resistance to nalidixic acid, a non-fluorinated first generation quinolone. Additional mutations in *gyrA* or other type II topoisomerase genes are, however, necessary for high-level resistance to later generations of fluoroquinolones, such as ciprofloxacin (Hopkins et al., 2005). Indeed, a study of 58 fluoroquinolone-resistant clinical *E. coli* isolates from two hospitals in Houston, TX, USA, found that all isolates had amino acid substitutions in GyrA and approximately 85% had additional substitutions in ParC (Morgan-Linnell et al., 2009), confirming chromosomal mutations as the main mechanism of clinically relevant fluoroquinolone resistance. The frequency of resistant invasive *E. coli* infections in Europe in 2012 ranged from 9.7% in Iceland to 42.0% in Cyprus (ECDC, 2013). Surveillance outside of Europe is less systematic, but a hospital in India reported that as many as 73% of uropathogenic *E. coli* infections were resistant to ciprofloxacin (Mandal et al., 2012).

Escherichia coli primarily propagate in the intestines of warm blooded animals, but also, to a limited extent, in the environment (Ishii and Sadowsky, 2008). Because fluoroquinolones are strictly synthetic antibiotics, it would be reasonable to assume that resistance mutations are not as common in environmental *E. coli* isolates as they are among clinical isolates. Accordingly, screening of environmental bacteria from an isolated cave for antibiotic resistance showed very few isolates that were resistant to a high concentration of ciprofloxacin (MIC >20 mg/l), whereas resistance to other classes of antibiotics were more common (Bhullar et al., 2012). Similarly, a recent study from our group found that only <1–6% of bacteria isolated from lakes with no documented history of fluoroquinolone pollution, in Sweden and India, were ciprofloxacin-resistant (MIC >2 mg/l) (Flach et al., 2015). A characterization of the QRDR of *gyrA* from 20 environmental *E. coli* isolates showed that there was considerable variability in the amino acid sequence (Waters and Davies, 1997), and a study of 38 highly ciprofloxacin-resistant (MIC 6–128 mg/l) soil-dwelling bacterial isolates of different species showed that nine isolates (24%) contained amino acid substitutions in this region (D'Costa et al., 2006). This suggests that mutations in the QRDR can be present in environmental bacteria even in the absence of fluoroquinolones. The methods used in previous studies have, however, been low throughput, making the estimation of the abundance of mutations unreliable. Previous studies have also been dependent on the culturability of the bacteria, and often focused on phenotypically fluoroquinolone-resistant bacteria (Adachi et al., 2013; Zurfluh et al., 2014). The characteristics and relative abundance of resistance mutations in the QRDRs in environmental bacterial communities, have, thus remained unknown.

Recently, concerns have been raised about the risks of resistance development due to antibiotic contamination of the external environment (Gaze et al., 2013; Pruden et al., 2013; Wellington et al., 2013). Antibiotics, including fluoroquinolones, can enter the environment through, for example, human sewage and use in animal farming (Kümmerer, 2009). The highest concentrations of fluoroquinolones detected in the environment are, however, the result of direct discharge from manufacturing (Larsson et al., 2007; Fick et al., 2009; Kristiansson et al., 2011). It is therefore important to assess the risks of the development and spread of resistant bacteria in contaminated environments. Furthermore, because the discharge of antibiotics may be intermittent and difficult to detect, acquired resistance characteristics of environmental bacteria may, given sufficient evaluation, serve as sentinels and biomarkers for antibiotic exposure. The presence and abundance of *qnr*-genes, a group of mobile fluoroquinolone resistance genes, in microbial communities have been shown previously to correlate with fluoroquinolone contamination of stream sediments (Kristiansson et al., 2011). However, horizontally transferred genes are not ubiquitous and may, therefore, not be optimal as biomarkers. In contrast, chromosomal resistance mutations can appear *de novo* and be enriched in a population under sufficient antibiotic selective pressure. Hence, we hypothesize that resistance mutations in *gyrA* and *parC* could serve as biomarkers for fluoroquinolone exposure in different environments.

The aim of the present study was to assess the abundance of chromosomal fluoroquinolone resistance mutations in environmental *Escherichia* communities and to investigate the potential link to fluoroquinolone pollution. Using massively parallel amplicon sequencing of metagenomic DNA, we determined the full genetic resistance characteristics of the QRDR of *gyrA* and *parC* in *Escherichia* communities without any prior culturing of bacteria. The studied environments included a range of selective pressures for fluoroquinolone resistance from a highly polluted Indian stream, samples taken up and downstream from a Swedish sewage treatment plant, and from a remote small Swedish lake under minimal human impact. This allowed us to investigate a possible correlation between fluoroquinolone pollution and the abundance of resistance mutations. Our analysis showed a high abundance of fluoroquinolone resistance mutations in both *gyrA* and *parC* in all investigated environments, but, interestingly, we did not find any significant correlation with the levels of fluoroquinolones detected.

MATERIALS AND METHODS

Sample Collection

Samples were taken from an Indian stream and a Swedish stream both upstream (two in India, one in Sweden) and downstream (three in India, one in Sweden) of wastewater treatment plants (WWTPs) as described previously (Kristiansson et al., 2011).

The Indian WWTP is situated in Patancheru near Hyderabad, India, and at the time of sampling, it received industrial effluent from approximately 90 pharmaceutical industries. The Swedish WWTP is located in Skövde and receives municipal wastewater, but with no input from pharmaceutical industries. These seven samples have previously been analyzed for the presence of mobile antibiotic resistance genes using metagenomic sequencing (Kristiansson et al., 2011), and *qnr* genes using qPCR (Rutgersson et al., 2014). For this study, three additional sediment samples were collected from an upland Swedish small lake, Valbergs öga, situated far from habitation, roads and farmland and with no apparent inflow of water (2012-07-25, GPS coordinates 57°51′34.2″N 12°04′58.2″E). Although few places on earth could be referred to as completely pristine, very few people, if any, are likely to walk near this small lake in a given year. Thus, it represents an environment at the very low end in terms of human impact. To determine the fluoroquinolone selective pressure at the samplings sites, the concentrations of ciprofloxacin, difloxacin, enoxacin, enrofloxacin, lomefloxacin, ofloxacin, pefloxacin, and norfloxacin were measured in all samples using liquid chromatography coupled to an ion trap mass spectrometer and electro spray interface (LC-ESI-IT-MSMS) described previously by Kristiansson et al. (2011), where the original chemical analysis data of all of the stream sediment samples can be found. The Swedish lake samples were analyzed at a different time point using the same method. Results were expressed per gram organic matter, rather than per total weight as some samples contained a large proportion of inorganic material (gravel). The detection limit was 0.02 μg/g organic matter for each measured substance.

DNA Extraction

The total DNA was extracted from the sediment samples and amplified using uniform whole genome amplification. A PowerSoil® DNA Isolation Kit (MO BIO Laboratories, Inc., Carlsbad, CA, USA) was used for the DNA extraction with the following modification to the manufacturer's protocol: to complete homogenization and cell lysis, the power bead tubes with sediment and solution C1 were incubated at 70°C for 10 min with a brief vortex after 5 and 10 min. The DNA concentration was measured using a NanoDrop (Thermo Fisher Scientific Inc., Waltham, MA, USA), and the samples were stored at −80°C until the whole genome amplification of purified genomic DNA was performed. Uniform whole genome amplification was done using the REPLI-g mini kit (QIAGEN, Hilden, Germany). The DNA (10 ng) was denatured by adding a denaturation buffer and incubating for 3 min at room temperature. The denaturation was interrupted by a neutralization buffer and a master mix containing a reaction buffer, and DNA polymerase was added. All buffers and enzyme mixtures were made according to the protocol. The amplification reaction was performed by incubating the samples at 30°C for 16 h in a thermal cycler, after which the reaction was stopped by heating the sample for 3 min at 65°C. The DNA concentration was measured using a NanoDrop, and the samples were stored at −20°C before the PCR amplification of the target genes.

PCR Amplification of *gyrA* and *parC*

The software Primer3 (Rozen and Skaletsky, 2000) was used through the web interface Primer3Plus (Untergasser et al., 2007) to design PCR primers targeting the regions of *gyrA* and *parC* that include all resistance mutations reported by Ruiz (2003). To avoid placing primers in variable regions, all annotated *gyrA* and *parC* nucleotide sequences belonging to *Escherichia* were downloaded from the Pathosystems Resource Integration Center (PATRIC) (Gillespie et al., 2011) and each gene was aligned using MUSLCE (Edgar, 2004). Because *Shigella* is indistinguishable from *Escherichia* in the targeted gene regions, this genus was also added to the multiple sequence alignment. All variable positions were given as excluded regions in Primer3, and the portions including all resistance mutations were given as the target regions. The product size range was set as 250–350 base pairs (bps) so that the amplicons would, to a large extent, be completely covered by a single 454 sequence read. The top 10 suggested primers were tested experimentally to determine the best primer pair, producing the largest amount of amplicons of the expected length, for each gene. The selected primers, targeted regions, and experimental design are shown in **Table 1**.

All of the samples were amplified using the selected primer pair for each gene and the set-up described in **Table 1**. The following was combined in sterile 0.2 ml tubes: 1xGotaq® Reaction buffer, 0.2 mM dNTP Mix, 0.4 μM forward primer, 0.4 reverse primer, 1.25 μ GoTaq® DNA polymerase (Promega, Madison, WI, USA), 50 ng template, and water up to 25 μl. The PCR amplification used an initial denaturation at 95°C for 2 min, denaturation at 95°C for 10 s, annealing at 57°C for 30 s, extension at 72°C for 1 min, and a final extension for 7 min. Each reaction was run for 40 cycles to maximize the amount of amplicon DNA. The PCR products were separated using 1.5% agarose gel electrophoresis and visualized with ethidium bromide. The DNA fragment of interest was excised from the agarose gel and placed in a microcentrifuge tube, and the GeneJET™ gel extraction kit (Fermentas International Inc., Vilnius, Lithuania) was used according to the enclosed protocol to obtain the DNA amplicons. The purified amplicons were pooled to enable sequencing in a single run, and therefore,

TABLE 1 | Selected primers with target regions and experimental setup.

Gene	Target region	Product size	Forward primer	Reverse primer	Annealing temperature
gyrA	129–439	311 bp	ggtacaccgtcgcgtacttt	caacgaaatcgaccgtctct	57°C
parC	20–306	287 bp	gccttgcgctacatgaattt	accatcaaccagcggataac	57°C

each sample contained amplicons of both *gyrA* and *parC* derived from the same sample site. The amplicons were stored at −20°C before sequencing.

DNA Sequencing and Bioinformatics Analyses

The samples were sent to GATC Biotech (Konstanz, Germany) for multiplexed massively parallel pyrosequencing (Margulies et al., 2005) using titanium chemistry on the GS FLX+ system. The sequencing of the Swedish lake samples was performed on a separate time point. The resulting sequence reads were aligned to their respective reference sequence belonging to *E. coli* K-12 MG1655 (RefSeq locus tags, *gyrA*: b2231; *parC*: b3019) using GS Amplicon Variant Analyzer from 454 (v2.5p1). The aligned reads were exported from the software as one FASTA alignment file per gene and sample site. To limit the risk of interpreting sequence variability between species as resistance mutations, reads too dissimilar to the *Escherichia* and *Shigella* sequences were discarded after matching all reads against all sequences annotated with the gene symbol *gyrA* and *parC*, respectively, in the Comprehensive Microbial Resource (CMR) (Peterson et al., 2001) using BLASTn (Altschul et al., 1990). Only reads with a hit against a *gyrA* or *parC* sequence from either *Escherichia* or *Shigella*, and with an *E*-value lower than 1×10^{-100} were retained in the subsequent analysis. To compensate for the issue of homopolymers, which are common in 454 sequencing, any positions in the multiple sequence alignments with insertions in the reference sequence were removed, and any remaining deletions in the reads were substituted with the reference sequence base of that position. The resulting gapless reads were translated using the EMBOSS tool Transeq (reading frame 1 for *gyrA* and 2 for *parC*) (Rice et al., 2000). The relative abundance of non-synonymous substitutions was recorded. The relative abundance of a certain mutation was defined as the percentage of reads encoding that particular amino acid substitution. The average relative abundance of mutations was defined as the percentage of reads encoding any amino acid substitution averaged over all samples. The computations were done for both individual substitutions, and pairs of substitutions occurring within the same read. The correlation between fluoroquinolone pollution – measured as the total amount of fluoroquinolones detected (log-transformed) – and the abundance of resistance mutations was measured using Pearson's correlation coefficient.

Nucleotide Sequence Accession Number

The raw sequence data have been submitted to the Short Read Archive (SRA) under BioProject accession number PRJNA239415.

RESULTS

The measurements of the fluoroquinolone concentrations present in the sediments confirmed that the sampled environments represented a range of different fluoroquinolone selective pressures (see Supplementary Table S1). Ciprofloxacin, enrofloxacin, and pefloxacin were detected at all Indian sample sites, ofloxacin was detected only upstream from the Indian WWTP, and lomefloxacin and difloxacin were detected only at the Indian downstream sites. None of the analyzed fluoroquinolones were detected in any of the Swedish samples. The highest level of fluoroquinolones was detected in the Indian downstream samples, while the upstream samples contained moderately high levels, as reported previously (Kristiansson et al., 2011).

A total of 35,417 reads aligned to the *gyrA* reference sequence (1,453–6,339 reads per sample), and 51,933 reads aligned to the *parC* reference sequence (537–15,469 reads per sample) (**Table 2**). The filtering of reads dissimilar to known *Escherichia* and *Shigella* sequences retained on average 60% of the *gyrA* reads (45–91% per sample) and 78% of the *parC* reads (72–95% per sample), suggesting that the *parC* primer pair is more specific for the targeted genera in the sampled environments compared to the *gyrA* primers. For *gyrA*, a total of 21,295 reads were used in the subsequent analysis (790–3,104 reads per sample), and 40,521 reads were used for *parC* (509–12,006 reads per sample).

Out of all the non-synonymous substitutions detected, the variability in codon 83 and 87 in *gyrA* and in codon 80 in *parC* was considerably higher than at any other codon (**Figure 1**).

TABLE 2 | Number of reads that aligned and that was retained after quality filtering.

Country	Site	Sample	Aligned reads		Filtered reads	
			GyrA	ParC	GyrA	ParC
India	Downstream	1	3,051	712	2,281	658
		2	1,531	3,759	790	3,425
		3	2,788	537	1,753	509
	Upstream	1	3,409	766	3,104	658
		2	3,057	1,919	1,838	1,664
Sweden	Downstream		1,453	2,079	888	1,831
	Upstream		4,425	2,926	2,773	2,112
	Lake	1	4,672	15,469	2,438	12,006
		2	4,692	12,446	2,609	9,039
		3	6,339	11,320	2,821	8,619
		Sum	35,417	51, 933	21,295	40,521

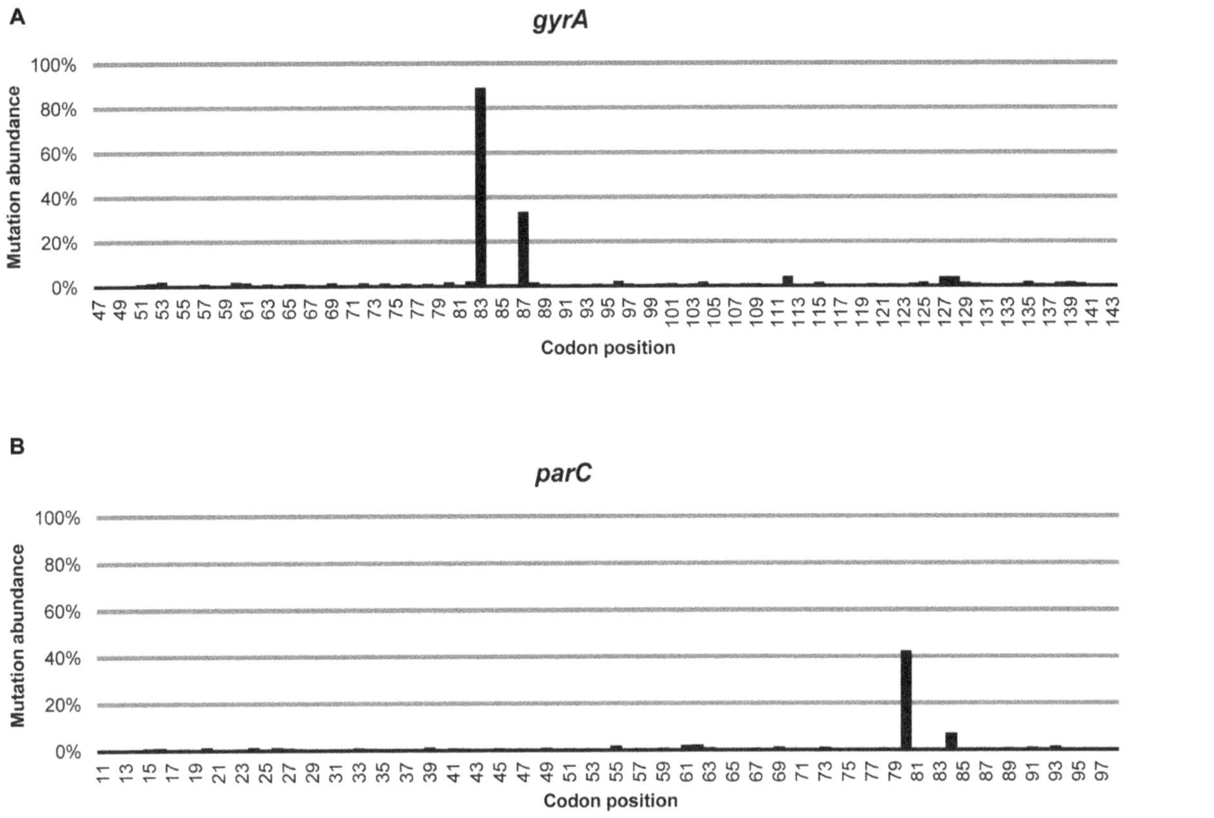

FIGURE 1 | Detected average variability over the amplicon. The average relative abundance of non-synonymous substitutions in each codon of **(A)** the *gyrA* and **(B)** the *parC* amplicons, averaged over all samples.

Three non-synonymous mutations in *gyrA* were detected in all samples and they encode the following amino acid substitutions: S83L, D87N, and D82G (see Supplementary Table S2a). The most common substitution, S83L, was detected in a majority of reads in all samples (61–97%), while D87N was less abundant (1–62%). Almost all of the D87N substitutions (97%) occurred in reads also encoding the S83L substitution. Although the D82G substitution was detected in all samples, it was rare ($\leq$1%), as were other resistance mutations detected in only some of the samples (0–2%). Three non-synonymous mutations in *parC* were detected in all samples and they encode the following amino acid substitutions: S80I, E84G, and E84V (see Supplementary Table S2b). S80I was the most common substitution encoded by the *parC* amplicons, and was detected in 0.4–63% of the reads in each sample. The mutations in codon 84 were far less common, but 98% of all reads carrying substitutions in codon 84 also carried mutations encoding the S80I substitution. Other resistance mutations in *parC*, which were detected in only some of the samples, were rare (0–7%).

The differences in terms of non-synonymous mutations between the environments were small, and there was no obvious link between the abundance of these mutations and the fluoroquinolone selective pressure for either *gyrA* or *parC* (**Figure 2**, also see Supplementary Figures S1 and S2). Pearson's correlation coefficient between the log-transformed detected amounts of total fluoroquinolones (samples with no detected fluoroquinolones were set to the detection limit 0.02 μg/g organic matter) and the abundance of the most commonly detected substitutions were as follows: S83L, −0.058 ($p = 0.87$); D87N, 0.098 ($p = 0.79$); and S83L+D87N in GyrA, 0.088 ($p = 0.81$); S80I, −0.25 ($p = 0.49$); E84G, 0.54 ($p = 0.10$); E84V, 0.28 ($p = 0.42$); and S08I+E84G/V in ParC, 0.34 ($p = 0.26$). However, the sample taken downstream from and closest to the discharge site of the Indian WWTP showed the highest abundance of all said substitutions (**Figure 2**, also see Supplementary Figures S1a and S2a).

DISCUSSION

In this study, we measured the relative abundance of chromosomal fluoroquinolone resistance mutations in *Escherichia* communities residing in both uncontaminated and severely fluoroquinolone polluted aquatic environments. We detected a high abundance of resistance mutations in the chromosomal target genes of fluoroquinolones, *gyrA* and *parC*, in all sampled environments, including environments with no fluoroquinolone pollution or known history thereof. Interestingly, we found no association between the measured concentrations of fluoroquinolones at the samples sites and

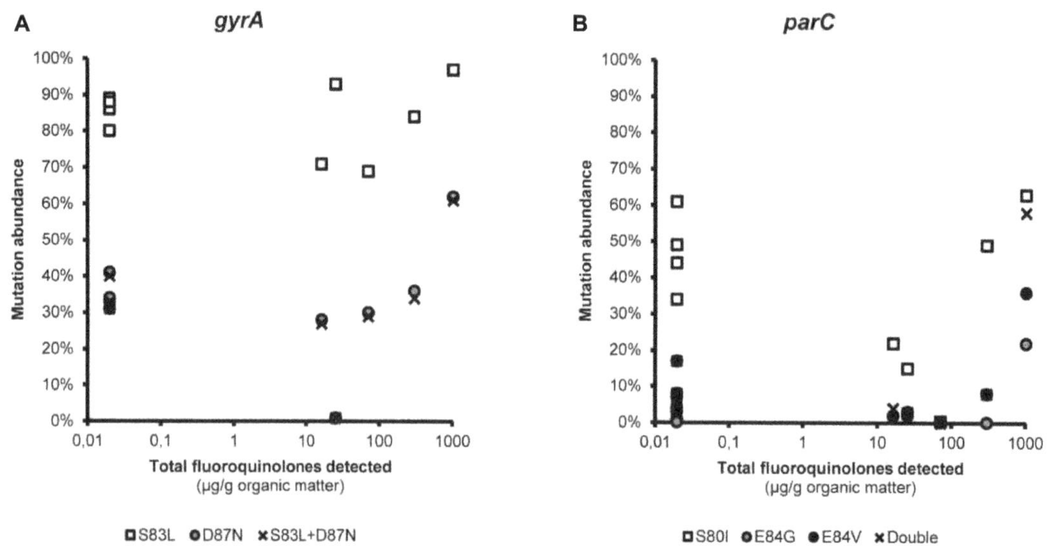

FIGURE 2 | The link between fluoroquinolone pollution and mutations in the quinolone resistance determining region. Correlation between the measured total fluoroquinolone pollution (µg/g organic matter) and the relative abundance of the most commonly detected non-synonymous substitutions in **(A)** *gyrA* and **(B)** *parC*. Samples with no detected fluoroquinolones are indicated in the figure as 0.2 µg/g (i.e., the detection limit).

the abundance of resistance mutations, except for the most polluted site, which showed the highest abundance of the most commonly detected mutations. This suggests that chromosomal mutations conferring fluoroquinolone resistance only could be considered a potential biomarker for detecting very extensive fluoroquinolone pollution. Additionally, the high abundance of mutations previously linked to fluoroquinolone resistance and the low abundance of other mutations indicate that there could be selective advantages to carry the resistance mutations in the sampled environments, even in the absence of fluoroquinolone selective pressure. Note that the levels of fluoroquinolones detected in the sediment cannot be directly compared to those of water solutions, as some fluoroquinolones are known to sorb to soil particles (Girardi et al., 2011). The exact amount of bioavailable antibiotics is, therefore, unknown, but likely lower than the detected levels.

To our best knowledge, the lowest reported minimal selective concentration for any antibiotic and resistance mutation is 0.1 µg/l for ciprofloxacin and the S83L substitution in GyrA (Gullberg et al., 2011). This concentration is just above the ones found in treated Swedish sewage effluents (Lindberg et al., 2005; Fick et al., 2011). However, the concentration was determined through competition experiments in a lab setting, and therefore, comparisons to environmental conditions should be made with some caution. Although no fluoroquinolones were detected downstream from the Swedish sewage treatment plant in this study, bacteria leaving the plant could theoretically have encountered selective concentrations inside the treatment plant. In the investigated Swedish lake, however, there are no plausible sources for fluoroquinolone exposure, indicating that the mutations found here are not present because of a fluoroquinolone selection pressure. Furthermore, since there is little difference in mutation abundance between the severely polluted sites and the remote Swedish lake, the data implies that the mutation abundance is not connected to fluoroquinolone selection pressure, but is largely determined by other, unknown factors.

In *gyrA*, mutations encoding the amino acid substitutions S83L and D87N were detected in all samples, with almost all of the D87N substitutions occurring in reads also encoding the S83L substitution. Both substitutions have been associated with fluoroquinolone resistance for *E. coli* and confer higher levels of resistance than any other substitutions in the QRDR (Yoshida et al., 1991). In fluoroquinolone-resistant clinical *E. coli* isolates, S83 is the most frequently altered amino acid, and, moreover, S83L is the most common substitution (Hopkins et al., 2005). A single substitution at position 83 confers higher resistance than at position 87, but additional mutations in *gyrA* or other genes are necessary for the development of high-level fluoroquinolone resistance. The S83L substitution alone, however, confers the same level of resistance to ciprofloxacin for *E. coli* as the combination of S83L and D87N (increased MIC of ciprofloxacin from 0.016 to 0.38 mg/l), while the D87N substitution alone confers slightly lower resistance (ciprofloxacin MIC = 0.25 mg/l) (Marcusson et al., 2009; Machuca et al., 2014). In *parC*, mutations causing the substitutions S80I, E84G, and E84V were detected in all samples, and these three substitutions have been previously linked to fluoroquinolone resistance in *E. coli*. In fluoroquinolone-resistant clinical isolates, the most commonly altered amino acid in ParC is S80 followed by E84, and, specifically, S80I is the most common substitution (Hopkins et al., 2005). Substitutions in ParC are often, if not always, found together with substitutions in GyrA in fluoroquinolone-resistant isolates (Hopkins et al., 2005; Morgan-Linnell et al., 2009), and substitutions of S80 or E84 alone do not affect the susceptibility to fluoroquinolones unless GyrA is also altered (Bagel et al., 1999). Because of the method used in this study, it is not possible to determine to what extent the detected mutations in *gyrA* and *parC* occur in the same bacterium, but it is worth mentioning that a combination of the substitutions S83L and D87N in GyrA with S80I in ParC confers a very high resistance to ciprofloxacin (ciprofloxacin MIC = 32 mg/l) (Marcusson et al., 2009). To set the MICs into perspective, an Enterobacteriaceae isolate is classified as ciprofloxacin-resistant if its MIC is higher than 1 mg/l according to the EUCAST clinical breakpoints (EUCAST, 2014). Isolates with a MIC lower than 0.5 mg/l are classified as sensitive. It is important to note that fluoroquinolone resistance can be caused by a number of different genetic mechanisms and combinations thereof. To extrapolate a level of resistance solely from mutations in the target genes is associated with a high level of uncertainty, therefore, the MICs given above are only included as a rough reference.

The only sampling site that stood out in terms of high abundance of resistance mutations was the site closest to downstream of the discharge site of the Indian WWTP. Here, we observed the highest abundance of the S83L and D87N substitutions in GyrA, the S80I, E84G, and E84V substitutions in ParC, and, consequently, also the highest abundance of the paired substitutions in both proteins. This is indeed the sample site with the highest total concentration of fluoroquinolones, which would be consistent with the hypothesis that there is a selective advantage for resistance mutations in fluoroquinolone-polluted environments, but only at locations with very high concentrations of fluoroquinolones. However, some reads from the most polluted site did not contain any mutations that resulted in amino acid substitutions in either *gyrA* (1.2%) or *parC* (30%), which suggests that some bacteria thriving there may carry additional resistance factors protecting them. Indeed, we have shown previously that mobile fluoroquinolone-resistance genes (*qnr*) are highly abundant in the stream sediment (Rutgersson et al., 2014). The *qnr* genes provide low to moderate resistance to fluoroquinolones [ciprofloxacin MIC up to 2 mg/l in *E. coli* transconjugants (Robicsek et al., 2006; Flach et al., 2013)]. Given the data presented here, it is possible that the presence of *qnr* genes in aquatic bacterial comminutes constitutes a better marker of fluoroquinolone exposure than chromosomal mutations. Or, there could be other mutations, outside the QRDR sequenced in this study, better suited as markers of exposure. Culturing-based methods will be required to fully elucidate the genetic mechanisms for how bacteria have adapted to survive the high concentrations of fluoroquinolones here.

A contributing factor to the high abundance of fluoroquinolone resistance mutations in the environment could be that there is little to no cost for the bacterium to carry these mutations. It has previously been shown that the substitutions S83L and D87N in GyrA and S80I in ParC occurring alone, or all three in the same organism, do not significantly alter the fitness of *E. coli in vitro*, nor do the pair of S83L in GyrA and S80I in ParC (Marcusson et al., 2009; Machuca et al., 2014). The pair S83L and D87N in GyrA has been shown to confer a fitness cost (measured relative fitness 0.97) when introduced in *E. coli* K-12 MG1655 (Marcusson et al., 2009), while the pair substitution was associated with a fitness gain in *E. coli* ATCC 25922 (relative fitness 1.14) (Machuca et al., 2014). In contrast, the pair of D87N in GyrA together with S80I in ParC introduce a slight fitness gain (measured relative fitness 1.02). Competition experiments with wild type *gyrA* in *E. coli* and mutants encoding either the S83L or the D87N substitution have shown that a ciprofloxacin concentration of 0.1 and 2.5 μg/l, respectively, is sufficient for the mutants to have a selective advantage (Gullberg et al., 2011). Furthermore, competitive *in vivo* studies of other species – i.e., *Neisseria gonorrhoeae* in mice (Kunz et al., 2012) and *Campylobacter jejuni* in chickens (Luo et al., 2005) – have even found a fitness benefit associated with *gyrA* mutations corresponding to codon 83 in *E. coli*. In summary, a lack of fitness cost for these substitutions in the sampled environments could explain why they appear to be very common even in environments without any detectable fluoroquinolone pollutants or any known history thereof. As we do not yet understand the possible advantages these genotypes may have in the absence of fluoroquinolones, and because of the limited number and types of environments investigated in this study, we cannot generalize to the point of claiming that resistance mutations in *gyrA* and *parC* are common in all environmental *Escherichia* communities.

The abundance of resistance mutations in the Swedish samples stands in contrast to the frequency of fluoroquinolone-resistant infections in Sweden. On average, the S83L substitution in GyrA was detected in 87% of the Swedish reads, the combination of S83L and D87N in 33%, and the S80I substitution in ParC in 43%. In Sweden, only 11.6% of the clinical invasive *E. coli* isolates tested with ciprofloxacin were resistant in 2013 (ECDC, 2014). This is far below the abundance of resistance mutations detected in both the Swedish lake samples and the samples taken near a sewage treatment plant. The large difference between the abundance of fluoroquinolone resistance mutations in the environment and the frequency of resistant *E. coli* infections in Sweden is likely due to large differences between the pathogenic *E. coli* strains and the strains residing in the sampled environments. Indeed, the genome of *E. coli* is known to be highly variable (Lukjancenko et al., 2010). Furthermore, competition experiments testing the relative fitness of the resistance mutations is typically performed under optimal growing conditions, unlike environmental conditions. It is possible that there is a selective advantage not linked to fluoroquinolones for these mutations in the sampled environments. Indeed, our finding of how abundant the resistance mutations are even in unpolluted environments suggest that the sequence defined as wild-type for GyrA and ParC, respectively, in *E. coli* is only one of a number of common sequences within the species.

The method presented here proved useful to compare the abundances of mutations occurring within a short genomic region in an entire microbial community. Next generation sequencing techniques provide a cost-effective comprehensive approach to study entire bacterial communities without relying on the cultivation of individual isolates. To distinguish between resistance mutations and inter-species variability, it is important to design the primers as specific for the targeted taxon as possible. If primers are not sufficiently specific, unwanted reads need to be filtered out by matching all reads to the target sequences and discarding reads of low resemblance. However, setting a similarity threshold for such a filtering where you allow for within species variability is not straight-forward. Here, we chose the threshold based on sequence alignments of different *Escherichia* and *Shigella* sequences and closely related genera. Additionally, we propose that amplicon sequencing could also be used to study resistance mutations in the ribosomal rRNA 23S gene that confer resistance to macrolides, lincosamides, and streptogramin B (Vester and Douthwaite, 2001). For future work in finding more suitable markers of fluoroquinolone exposure, we propose a more controlled experimental set up where different environments are dosed with various concentrations of fluoroquinolones for an extended period of time and the effect of the microbiota is studied using metagenomic sequencing.

In this study, we show that there is a significant abundance of fluoroquinolone resistance mutations in environmental *Escherichia* communities residing both in fluoroquinolone-polluted and pristine environments. This suggests that the mutations are not associated with a substantial fitness cost for the bacterium, even where there is no selective pressure for fluoroquinolone resistance. Regardless of whether the detected mutations are sufficient to provide clinically relevant resistance to fluoroquinolones, they are one or two mutations closer to obtaining a high level of resistance.

AUTHOR CONTRIBUTIONS

AJ, EK, and JL conceived of the study and participated in its design. AJ collected samples from the Swedish lakes. JF performed the chemical analyses of the sediments. BW prepared DNA from the samples and did the PCR amplifications. AJ designed the PCR primers, performed all data analyses, and drafted the manuscript. All authors read and approved the final manuscript.

ACKNOWLEDGMENTS

We acknowledge Gamana for help with the sampling in India, and the following funding agencies that supported this study: the Swedish Research Council (K2011-56X-21750-01-6), the Swedish Foundation for Strategic Environmental Research Mistra (2004-147), the Life Science Area of Advance at Chalmers University of Technology, and the Swedish Research Council Formas (244314727).

REFERENCES

Adachi, F., Yamamoto, A., Takakura, K.-I., and Kawahara, R. (2013). Occurrence of fluoroquinolones and fluoroquinolone-resistance genes in the aquatic environment. *Sci. Total Environ.* 444, 508–514. doi: 10.1016/j.scitotenv.2012.11.077

Altschul, S. F., Gish, W., Miller, W., Myers, E. W., and Lipman, D. J. (1990). Basic local alignment search tool. *J. Mol. Biol.* 215, 403–410. doi: 10.1016/S0022-2836(05)80360-2

Bagel, S., Hullen, V., Wiedemann, B., and Heisig, P. (1999). Impact of gyrA and parC mutations on quinolone resistance, doubling time, and supercoiling degree of *Escherichia coli*. *Antimicrob. Agents Chemother.* 43, 868–875.

Bhullar, K., Waglechner, N., Pawlowski, A., Koteva, K., Banks, E. D., Johnston, M. D., et al. (2012). Antibiotic resistance is prevalent in an isolated cave microbiome. *PLoS ONE* 7:e34953. doi: 10.1371/journal.pone.0034953

D'Costa, V. M., Mcgrann, K. M., Hughes, D. W., and Wright, G. D. (2006). Sampling the antibiotic resistome. *Science* 311, 374–377. doi: 10.1126/science.1120800

ECDC (2013). *Antimicrobial Resistance Surveillance in Europe 2012*. Annual Report of the European Antimicrobial Resistance Surveillance Network (EARS-Net). Stockholm: European Centre for Disease Prevention and Control.

ECDC (2014). *Antimicrobial Resistance Surveillance in Europe 2013*. Annual Report of the European Antimicrobial Resistance Surveillance Network (EARS-Net). Stockholm: European Centre for Disease Prevention and Control.

Edgar, R. C. (2004). MUSCLE: multiple sequence alignment with high accuracy and high throughput. *Nucleic Acids Res.* 32, 1792–1797. doi: 10.1093/nar/gkh340

EUCAST. (2014). *Breakpoint Tables for Interpretation of MICs and Zone Diameters. Version 4.0: The European Committee on Antimicrobial Susceptibility Testing*. Available at: http://www.eucast.org

Fick, J., Lindberg, R. H., Kaj, L., and Brorström-Lundén, E. (2011). *Results from the Swedish National Screening Programme 2010. Subreport 3. Pharmaceuticals*. Stockholm: Swedish Environmental Research Institute Ltd.

Fick, J., Soderstrom, H., Lindberg, R. H., Phan, C., Tysklind, M., and Larsson, D. G. J. (2009). Contamination of surface, ground, and drinking water from pharmaceutical production. *Environ. Toxicol. Chem.* 28, 2522–2527. doi: 10.1897/09-073.1

Flach, C.-F., Boulund, F., Kristiansson, E., and Larsson, D. J. (2013). Functional verification of computationally predicted qnr genes. *Ann. Clin. Microbiol. Antimicrob.* 12, 34. doi: 10.1186/1476-0711-12-34

Flach, C. F., Johnning, A., Nilsson, I., Smalla, K., Kristiansson, E., and Larsson, D. G. J. (2015). Isolation of novel IncA/C and IncN fluoroquinolone resistance plasmids from an antibiotic-polluted lake. *J. Antimicrob. Chemother.* 70, 2709–2717. doi: 10.1093/jac/dkv167

Gaze, W. H., Krone, S. M., Larsson, D. G. J., Li, X. Z., Robinson, J. A., Simonet, P., et al. (2013). Influence of humans on evolution and mobilization of environmental antibiotic resistome. *Emerg. Infect. Dis.* 19, e120871. doi: 10.3201/eid1907.120871

Gillespie, J. J., Wattam, A. R., Cammer, S. A., Gabbard, J., Shukla, M. P., Dalay, O., et al. (2011). PATRIC: the comprehensive bacterial bioinformatics resource with a focus on human pathogenic species. *Infect. Immun.* 79, 4286–4298. doi: 10.1128/IAI.00207-11

Girardi, C., Greve, J., Lamshöft, M., Fetzer, I., Miltner, A., Schäffer, A., et al. (2011). Biodegradation of ciprofloxacin in water and soil and its effects on the microbial communities. *J. Hazard. Mater.* 198, 22–30. doi: 10.1016/j.jhazmat.2011.10.004

Gullberg, E., Cao, S., Berg, O. G., Ilbäck, C., Sandegren, L., Hughes, D., et al. (2011). Selection of resistant bacteria at very low antibiotic concentrations. *PLoS Pathog.* 7:e1002158. doi: 10.1371/journal.ppat.1002158

Hopkins, K. L., Davies, R. H., and Threlfall, E. J. (2005). Mechanisms of quinolone resistance in *Escherichia coli* and *Salmonella*: recent developments. *Int. J. Antimicrob. Agents* 25, 358–373. doi: 10.1016/j.ijantimicag.2005.02.006

Ishii, S., and Sadowsky, M. J. (2008). *Escherichia coli* in the environment: implications for water quality and human health. *Microbes Environ.* 23, 101–108. doi: 10.1264/Jsme2.23.101

Kristiansson, E., Fick, J., Janzon, A., Grabic, R., Rutgersson, C., Weijdegård, B., et al. (2011). Pyrosequencing of antibiotic-contaminated river sediments reveals high levels of resistance and gene transfer elements. *PLoS ONE* 6:e17038. doi: 10.1371/journal.pone.0017038

Kümmerer, K. (2009). Antibiotics in the aquatic environment-A review-Part I. *Chemosphere* 75, 417–434. doi: 10.1016/j.chemosphere.2008.11.086

Kunz, A. N., Begum, A. A., Wu, H., D'ambrozio, J. A., Robinson, J. M., Shafer, W. M., et al. (2012). Impact of fluoroquinolone resistance mutations on gonococcal fitness and in vivo selection for compensatory mutations. *J. Infect. Dis.* 205, 1821–1829. doi: 10.1093/infdis/jis277

Larsson, D. G. J., De Pedro, C., and Paxeus, N. (2007). Effluent from drug manufactures contains extremely high levels of pharmaceuticals. *J. Hazard. Mater.* 148, 751–755. doi: 10.1016/j.jhazmat.2007.07.008

Lindberg, R. H., Wennberg, P., Johansson, M. I., Tysklind, M., and Andersson, B. A. (2005). Screening of human antibiotic substances and determination of weekly mass flows in five sewage treatment plants in Sweden. *Environ. Sci. Technol.* 39, 3421–3429. doi: 10.1021/es048143z

Lukjancenko, O., Wassenaar, T. M., and Ussery, D. W. (2010). Comparison of 61 sequenced *Escherichia coli* genomes. *Microb. Ecol.* 60, 708–720. doi: 10.1007/s00248-010-9717-3

Luo, N., Pereira, S., Sahin, O., Lin, J., Huang, S., Michel, L., et al. (2005). Enhanced in vivo fitness of fluoroquinolone-resistant *Campylobacter jejuni* in the absence of antibiotic selection pressure. *Proc. Natl. Acad. Sci. U.S.A.* 102, 541–546. doi: 10.1073/pnas.0408966102

Machuca, J., Briales, A., Labrador, G., Díaz-De-Alba, P., López-Rojas, R., Docobo-Pérez, F., et al. (2014). Interplay between plasmid-mediated and chromosomal-mediated fluoroquinolone resistance and bacterial fitness in *Escherichia coli. J. Antimicrob. Chemother.* 69, 3203–3215. doi: 10.1093/jac/dku308

Mandal, J., Acharya, N. S., Buddhapriya, D., and Parija, S. C. (2012). Antibiotic resistance pattern among common bacterial uropathogens with a special reference to ciprofloxacin resistant *Escherichia coli. Indian J. Med. Res.* 136, 842–849.

Marcusson, L. L., Frimodt-Møller, N., and Hughes, D. (2009). Interplay in the selection of fluoroquinolone resistance and bacterial fitness. *PLoS Pathog.* 5:e1000541. doi: 10.1371/journal.ppat.1000541

Margulies, M., Egholm, M., Altman, W. E., Attiya, S., Bader, J. S., Bemben, L. A., et al. (2005). Genome sequencing in microfabricated high-density picolitre reactors. *Nature* 437, 376–380. doi: 10.1038/nature03959

Morgan-Linnell, S. K., Boyd, L. B., Steffen, D., and Zechiedrich, L. (2009). Mechanisms accounting for fluoroquinolone resistance in *Escherichia coli* clinical isolates. *Antimicrob. Agents Chemother.* 53, 235–241. doi: 10.1128/AAC.00665-08

Peterson, J. D., Umayam, L. A., Dickinson, T., Hickey, E. K., and White, O. (2001). The comprehensive microbial resource. *Nucleic Acids Res.* 29, 123–125. doi: 10.1093/nar/29.1.123

Pruden, A., Larsson, D. G. J., Amézquita, A., Collignon, P., Brandt, K. K., Graham, D. W., et al. (2013). *Management Options for Reducing the Release of Antibiotics and Antibiotic Resistance Genes to the Environment. Environmental Health Perspectives.* Research Triangle Park, NC: National Institute of Environmental Health Sciences (NIEHS).

Rice, P., Longden, I., and Bleasby, A. (2000). EMBOSS: the European molecular biology open software suite. *Trends Genet.* 16, 276–277. doi: 10.1016/S0168-9525(00)02024-2

Robicsek, A., Jacoby, G. A., and Hooper, D. C. (2006). The worldwide emergence of plasmid-mediated quinolone resistance. *Lancet Infect. Dis.* 6, 629–640. doi: 10.1016/S1473-3099(06)70599-0

Rozen, S., and Skaletsky, H. (2000). Primer3 on the WWW for general users and for biologist programmers. *Methods Mol. Biol.* 132, 365–386.

Ruiz, J. (2003). Mechanisms of resistance to quinolones: target alterations, decreased accumulation and DNA gyrase protection. *J. Antimicrob. Chemother.* 51, 1109–1117. doi: 10.1093/jac/dkg222

Rutgersson, C., Fick, J., Marathe, N., Kristiansson, E., Janzon, A., Angelin, M., et al. (2014). Fluoroquinolones and qnr genes in sediment, water, soil, and human fecal flora in an environment polluted by manufacturing discharges. *Environ. Sci. Technol.* 48, 7825–7832. doi: 10.1021/es501452a

Untergasser, A., Nijveen, H., Rao, X., Bisseling, T., Geurts, R., and Leunissen, J. A. M. (2007). Primer3Plus, an enhanced web interface to Primer3. *Nucleic Acids Res.* 35, W71–W74. doi: 10.1093/nar/gkm306

Vester, B., and Douthwaite, S. (2001). Macrolide resistance conferred by base substitutions in 23S rRNA. *Antimicrob. Agents Chemother.* 45, 1–12. doi: 10.1128/AAC.45.1.1-12.2001

Waters, B., and Davies, J. (1997). Amino acid variation in the GyrA subunit of bacteria potentially associated with natural resistance to fluoroquinolone antibiotics. *Antimicrob. Agents Chemother.* 41, 2766–2769.

Wellington, E. M., Boxall, A., Cross, P., Feil, E. J., Gaze, W. H., Hawkey, P. M., et al. (2013). The role of the natural environment in the emergence of antibiotic resistance in Gram-negative bacteria. *Lancet Infect. Dis.* 13, 155–165. doi: 10.1016/S1473-3099(12)70317-1

Yoshida, H., Bogaki, M., Nakamura, M., Yamanaka, L. M., and Nakamura, S. (1991). Quinolone resistance-determining region in the DNA gyrase gyrB gene of *Escherichia coli. Antimicrob. Agents Chemother.* 35, 1647–1650. doi: 10.1128/AAC.35.8.1647

Zurfluh, K., Abgottspon, H., Hächler, H., Nüesch-Inderbinen, M., and Stephan, R. (2014). Quinolone resistance mechanisms among extended-spectrum beta-lactamase (ESBL) producing *Escherichia coli* isolated from rivers and lakes in Switzerland. *PLoS ONE* 9:e95864. doi: 10.1371/journal.pone.0095864

2

Mycoplasma bovis: Mechanisms of Resistance and Trends in Antimicrobial Susceptibility

Inna Lysnyansky[1]* *and Roger D. Ayling*[2]

[1] *Mycoplasma Unit, Division of Avian and Aquatic Diseases, Kimron Veterinary Institute, Beit Dagan, Israel,* [2] *Department of Bacteriology, Animal and Plant Health Agency, Addlestone, UK*

Correspondence:
Inna Lysnyansky
innal@moag.gov.il

Mycoplasma bovis is a cell-wall-less bacterium and belongs to the class *Mollicutes*. It is the most important etiological agent of bovine mycoplasmoses in North America and Europe, causing respiratory disease, mastitis, otitis media, arthritis, and reproductive disease. Clinical disease associated with *M. bovis* is often chronic, debilitating, and poorly responsive to antimicrobial therapy, resulting in significant economic loss, the full extent of which is difficult to estimate. Until *M. bovis* vaccines are universally available, sanitary control measures and antimicrobial treatment are the only approaches that can be used in attempts to control *M. bovis* infections. However, *in vitro* studies show that many of the current *M. bovis* isolates circulating in Europe have high minimum inhibitory concentrations (MIC) for many of the commercially available antimicrobials. In this review we summarize the current MIC trends indicating the development of antimicrobial resistance in *M. bovis* as well as the known molecular mechanisms by which resistance is acquired.

Keywords: *Mycoplasma bovis*, minimum inhibitory concentrations, tetracyclines, macrolides, aminoglycosides, fluoroquinolones, chloramphenicols, pleuromutilins

INTRODUCTION

Mycoplasma bovis is a cell-wall-less bacterium and belongs to the class *Mollicutes* (Razin, 1978). It is the most important etiological agent of bovine mycoplasmosis in North America and Europe, causing respiratory disease, mastitis, otitis media, arthritis, and reproductive disease (Nicholas and Ayling, 2003). Until *M. bovis* vaccines are universally available, sanitary control measures and antimicrobial treatment are the only approaches that can be used in attempts to control *M. bovis* infections. However, *M. bovis* is refractory to ß-lactams and to all antimicrobials that target the cell wall. In addition, mycoplasmas are also naturally resistant to polymyxins, sulfonamides, trimethoprim, nalidixic acid, and rifampin (Taylor-Robinson and Bebear, 1997). Antimicrobials that are mycoplasmastatic provide an opportunity for the host's immune response to develop and counteract infection, but *M. bovis* has defense mechanisms that include an ability to vary its surface proteins (Lysnyansky et al., 1996) and form biofilms (McAuliffe et al., 2006).

The potential effectiveness of antimicrobials *in vivo* can be assessed by *in vitro* susceptibility testing to determine the minimum inhibition concentration (MIC). Guidelines for *in vitro* testing of veterinary mycoplasma species have been published (Hannan, 2000). However, the data produced are subject to interpretation as there are currently no *in vitro* testing standards and interpretive breakpoints have not been determined. Standards for testing *Mollicutes* that cause clinical infections in humans *Mycoplasma pneumoniae*, *Mycoplasma hominis*, and *Ureaplasma urealyticum* have been published (Waites et al., 2012). However, the growth requirements of these species differ from those of *M. bovis*. In addition, the authors are not aware of specific published *M. bovis* pharmacokinetics (PK)/pharmacodynamics (PD) studies which can influence the interpretation of *in vitro* antimicrobial sensitivity.

Herein, we review *in vitro* MIC data that indicate that *M. bovis* is developing antimicrobial resistance, which is increasingly being supported by molecular evidence of genetic mutations consistent with antimicrobial resistance and by reports of treatment failure.

ANTIMICROBIAL CLASSES ACTIVE AGAINST *M. BOVIS*

Control of *M. bovis* infection requires early identification and treatment with antimicrobials including the tetracyclines, macrolides and some fluoroquinolones. However, few are specifically approved for treating *M. bovis* in cattle and with the exception of the fluoroquinolones, which are mycoplasmacidal, and the aminoglycosides, which are mycoplasmacidal at high concentrations, the remaining antimicrobials are mycoplasmastatic, and generally work by inhibiting protein synthesis. The typical tetracyclines, chlortetracyline and doxycycline which are polycyclic structures of the perhydronaphthacene carboxamide inhibit protein synthesis in the ribosome by binding to the 30S ribosomal subunit and blocking an attachment of aminoacyl-tRNA to the A site (Bryskier, 2005a). Other plasmid related resistance, or efflux mechanisms present in some *Mycoplasma* species have not been described in *M. bovis*.

The macrolides which are known to be good for treating respiratory infections have been shown to have a preferential distribution *in vivo*, concentrating in diseased lungs, up to three times the concentration detected in healthy lungs (Reeve-Johnson, 1999). Macrolides are hydrophobic molecules that have a central 12-16-membered-ring lactone with few or no double bonds. They inhibit protein synthesis possibly by preventing peptidyltransferase from adding the growing peptide attached to tRNA to the next amino acid as well as inhibiting ribosomal translation. Another potential mechanism is premature dissociation of the peptidyl-tRNA from the ribosome. Macrolides can penetrate phagocytic cells thereby allowing treatment of intracellular infections. Lincosamides consist of an amino acid and a sugar connected by an amide bond. They act on the 50S subunit of the ribosome, preventing transpeptidation by inhibiting peptidyl-transferase.

The fluoroquinolones are synthetic antimicrobials and all have a pyridine-ß-carboxylic nucleus. Their activity depends on several factors: the aromatic system associated with the pyridine-ß-carboxylic acid nucleus, the substituents, and their spatial disposition. These substituents produce greater affinity for the target enzymes (DNA gyrase and topoisomerase IV) but also allow penetration of the bacterial outer membrane (Bryskier, 2005b). The activity of these antimicrobials can be affected by pH, magnesium and calcium ions.

The aminoglycosides are amino sugars and fall into two broad groups based on their chemical structures: streptomycin and its derivatives and deoxystreptamines. The ribosome is the prime target of their action, but other actions on membranes and modifications of RNA synthesis have been observed. They are considered mycoplasmacidal, but that is concentration dependent.

The phenicols are derived from dichloroacetic acid with an aromatic nucleus and an alkyl group and an aminopropanediol chain. The fluoro derivative of chloramphenicol, florfenicol, is commonly used in the veterinary field. It inhibits protein synthesis by binding to the 50S ribosomal subunit inhibiting the peptidation reaction and the translation of bacterial mRNA.

Pleuromutilins, such as tiamulin and valnemulin are semisynthetic derivatives that have a tricyclic diterpenoid structure with different side chains. They have been used in veterinary medicine; they bind to the peptidyl transferase component of the 50S ribosomal subunit to inhibit protein synthesis (Long et al., 2006). Tiamulin was the first pleuromutilin compound to be approved for veterinary use in 1979, followed by valnemulin in 1999 (Novak and Shlaes, 2010).

M. BOVIS IN VITRO SUSCEPTIBILITY PROFILES AND TRENDS

M. bovis treatment failures are increasingly being associated with antimicrobial resistance. However, different research groups report variations in the proportion of *M. bovis* isolates with decreased susceptibility. This may be related to geographical origin, year of isolation, type of livestock production system, clinical presentation, or site of isolation of the strains tested. However, this may also indicate differences among the countries in regulatory practices for use of antimicrobials. Not all studies included epidemiology or typing of *M. bovis* isolates, but those which did, reported that in some countries the acquisition of resistance to antimicrobials in *M. bovis* was attributed to the emergence and spread of a single clone (Becker et al., 2015) while in other the genetic heterogeneity of *M. bovis* isolates with decreased susceptibility was identified (Lysnyansky et al., 2009).

M. bovis susceptibility testing has a role in epidemiological monitoring of acquired resistance and can guide the veterinarian in the selection of the most likely effective antimicrobial treatment, but published MIC data requires some interpretation, as there is no agreed standard method or controls for susceptibility testing of *M. bovis*. Although guidelines were produced by Hannan (2000), variations in the growth and approaches to determining the endpoint by different laboratories are reported and make it hard to compare results from different laboratories. However, these differences do not detract from the trends observed, which are now being supported by genetic evidence of resistance correlated with high MIC values (Lysnyansky et al., 2009; Sato et al., 2013; Lerner et al., 2014; Amram et al., 2015; Khalil et al., 2015). Nevertheless, standardized methods, controls and breakpoint interpretations would be highly beneficial for future epidemiology assessment of antimicrobial sensitivities and treatment guidance. In **Table 1** we

TABLE 1 | Minimal inhibitory concentration ranges (μg/ml) and MIC_{50} and MIC_{90} ranges for various antimicrobials against *M. bovis*[a].

Antimicrobials	MIC[b] Range	MIC_{50} Range	MIC_{90} Range
Tetracyclines			
Tetracycline	<0.03–>64	1–8	4–64
Oxytetracycline	0.05–128	2–128	4–128
Chlortetracycline	0.25–256	2–128	2–256
Doxycycline	≤0.03–1	0.5	1
MLSK Group			
Erythromycin	4–>512	>3.2–512	32–512
Tylosin	0.2–>256	1–>128	6.25–>128
Tilmicosin	≤0.5–>512	2–512	4–>512
Gamithromycin	128–>128	128	128
Tildipirosin	128–>128	128	128
Tulathromycin	≤0.063–>128	0.25–128	8–>64
Kitasamycin	1–128	4	64
Josamycin	0.78–12.5	1.56	6.25
Spiramycin	0.39–>100	3.12	25
Lincomycin	0.06–>256	0.78–>64	3.12–>64
Clindamycin	0.03–>256	0.5–8	>32
Pirlimycin	<0.125–0.5	0.25	0.5
Pleuromutilins			
Tiamulin	<0.03–2	0.06–0.2	0.78–1
Valnemulin	<0.03	<0.03	<0.03
Fluoroquinolones			
Enrofloxacin	0.025–>32	0.12–1	0.12–32
Danofloxacin	0.078–32	0.156–0.5	0.312–8
Marbofloxacin	0.25–>32	0.625–1.25	0.625–32
Flumequine	16–128	64	128
Ciprofloxacin	0.125–1	0.5	1
Aminoglycosides			
Gentamycin	2–>64	8	32
Kanamycin	8–>128	32–64	64–>128
Aminocyclitol			
Spectinomycin	0.03–>256	1–>256	2–>256
Chloramphenicols/Phenicols			
Chloramphenicol	0.25–>32	2–8	2–32
Thiamphenicol	3.12–>512	6.25–>512	12.5–>512
Florfenicol	0.06–64	1–8	2–32

[a] *The data are compiled from multiple published studies (Ayling et al., 2000; Hirose et al., 2003; Thomas et al., 2003; Rosenbusch et al., 2005; Godinho, 2008; Gerchman et al., 2009; Uemura et al., 2010; Soehnlen et al., 2011; Kroemer et al., 2012; Hendrick et al., 2013; Ayling et al., 2014; Gautier-Bouchardon et al., 2014; Kawai et al., 2014; Sulyok et al., 2014; Kong et al., 2016) in which different methodologies (microbroth and agar dilution, but not E-test) and different antimicrobial concentrations were used (adapted from Bebear and Kempf, 2005; Waites et al., 2014).*

[b] *Only MIC data obtained for M. bovis isolated after 1990 were included.*

present the susceptibility profiles (ranges of MICs, MIC_{50}, and MIC_{90}), obtained by microdilution and agar dilution methods, of *M. bovis* isolated in different countries since 1990. Both the MIC_{50} and MIC_{90} may indicate shifts in the susceptibility of bacterial populations to antimicrobials since MIC_{50} values show the general potency of an antimicrobial against a specific type of bacteria, while the MIC_{90} values indicates the potential and first stages of specific bacteria developing resistance to an antimicrobial.

Tetracyclines

In vitro susceptibility data from all over the world reveal heterogeneity in the susceptibility pattern to tetracyclines with MIC_{50} values for oxytetracycline ranging from 2 to <8 μg/ml for isolates from Belgium, North America and Israel (Thomas et al., 2003; Rosenbusch et al., 2005; Gerchman et al., 2009; Soehnlen et al., 2011; Hendrick et al., 2013); while the MIC_{50} of isolates from the UK, the Netherlands, France, Hungry and Japan (Ayling et al., 2000, 2014; Hirose et al., 2003; Uemura et al., 2010; Gautier-Bouchardon et al., 2014; Kawai et al., 2014; Sulyok et al., 2014) was reported to be ≥8 μg/ml. Notably, when susceptibility to tetracyclines was tested in two cohorts of respiratory *M. bovis* isolates isolated in the UK in 2004 and 2009, a significant increase in the MIC_{50} from 1 to 32 μg/ml was identified (Ayling et al., 2014). In contrast, in France, the group of archived isolates (1978–1979) already demonstrated high MIC_{50} to oxytetracycline (32 μg/ml), which increased to ≥32 μg/ml in recent isolates (2010–2012) (Gautier-Bouchardon et al., 2014). The authors suggested that less susceptible *M. bovis* isolates had developed by 1978–1979.

Macrolides and Lincosamides

Acquired resistance to macrolides in *M. bovis* is a widely known phenomenon and isolates with high MICs are frequently identified (**Table 1**). For example, MIC_{50} values of ≥32 μg/ml for tilmicosin alone or for tylosin and tilmicosin were identified in recent British and Hungarian isolates (Ayling et al., 2014; Sulyok et al., 2014) as well as in isolates from western Canada, Japan and the USA (Rosenbusch et al., 2005; Uemura et al., 2010; Hendrick et al., 2013; Kawai et al., 2014). All recent French isolates had MICs of ≥64 μg/ml for tylosin and tilmicosin (Gautier-Bouchardon et al., 2014). Gerchman et al. (2009) reported marked differences in susceptibility profiles to tylosin and tilmicosin in isolates from different geographical regions. Israeli isolates were significantly more resistant to macrolides than isolates from calves imported from Hungary (2005–2007). However, recent Hungarian isolates (2010–2013) are more resistant to these antimicrobials (MIC_{50} and MIC_{90} ≥128 μg/ml) (Sulyok et al., 2014). Such data emphasize the requirement for periodic antimicrobial susceptibility testing on a regional basis.

Both archived and recent French isolates possessed high MICs for the new-generation macrolides, gamithromycin and tildipirosin. In addition, all tested French isolates and 27% of British tested isolates had MIC values of ≥128 μg/ml to tulathromycin, a relatively new semi-synthetic macrolide (Ayling et al., 2014; Gautier-Bouchardon et al., 2014). Interestingly, results of a susceptibility study comparing MICs for tulathromycin in *M. bovis* respiratory isolates isolated in Europe prior to 2002 and between 2004 and 2006 showed an increase in MIC_{50} (from 0.25 to 4 μg/ml) without a change in the MIC_{90} (>64 μg/ml) (Godinho, 2008). The authors suggested that a high MIC does not necessarily reflect a lack of clinical efficacy of tulathromycin since an isolate with an MIC >64 μg

/ml was effectively treated in an experimental trial (Godinho et al., 2005; Godinho, 2008).

The MIC_{50} for lincomycin ranged from 0.78 to ≥64 µg/ml in several studies (Hirose et al., 2003; Thomas et al., 2003; Uemura et al., 2010; Ayling et al., 2014; Sulyok et al., 2014) and MIC_{50} of 0.19 µg/ml (but with MIC_{90} of >256 µg/ml; tested by *E*-test) for clindamycin were reported from Canada (Francoz et al., 2005). Interestingly, Ayling et al. (2014) reported decreased MIC_{50} values for lincomycin (from 8 to 1 µg/ml) and clindamycin (from ≥32 to 0.25 µg/ml) in *M. bovis* isolates isolated in the UK in 2004 and 2009. Low MIC_{50} and MIC_{90} of 0.25 and 0.5 µg/ml, respectively for pirlimycin (**Table 1**) were reported in one study from Japan (Kawai et al., 2014).

Fluoroquinolones

In contrast to acquired resistance to macrolides which has been reported for a long time, the resistance to veterinary fluoroquinolones is a relatively new phenomenon. For example, only a single fold increase in MIC_{50} and MIC_{90} (in both cases from 0.25 to 0.5 µg/ml for enrofloxacin and danofloxacin; and from 0.5 to 1 µg/ml for marbofloxacin) was reported between 1978–1979 and 2010–2012 for French isolates (Gautier-Bouchardon et al., 2014). The same increase in the MIC_{50} was also found in UK isolates isolated between 2004–2005 and during 2007–2009. However, their MIC_{90} values differed considerably (0.5−1 vs. 8− >32 µg/ml) (Ayling et al., 2014). Relatively low enrofloxacin MIC_{50} values of 0.12 to 0.5 µg/ml were reported in North America, Japan and some European countries (Hirose et al., 2003; Thomas et al., 2003; Rosenbusch et al., 2005; Uemura et al., 2010; Soehnlen et al., 2011; Hendrick et al., 2013; Gautier-Bouchardon et al., 2014; Kawai et al., 2014; Sulyok et al., 2014). This may reflect differences in therapeutic use of antimicrobials in different countries.

Aminocyclitol and Aminoglycosides

Several studies have demonstrated relatively low MIC_{50} and MIC_{90} values for spectinomycin (up to 8 µg/ml) (Rosenbusch et al., 2005; Uemura et al., 2010; Hendrick et al., 2013), while others reported that the difference between the MIC_{50} (1–8 µg/ml) and MIC_{90} (>32 µg/ml) was high (Ayling et al., 2000, 2014; Thomas et al., 2003; Soehnlen et al., 2011; Sulyok et al., 2014). In addition high MIC_{50} and high MIC_{90} (≥256 µg/ml) values for spectinomycin were also reported (Ayling et al., 2000, 2014; Thomas et al., 2003; Soehnlen et al., 2011; Sulyok et al., 2014). Interestingly, higher spectinomycin MIC values have been reported for isolates from milk. Rosenbusch et al. (2005) reported that 6 out of 14 USA milk isolates had MIC values >16 µg/ml while Soehnlen et al. (2011) reported a significant difference between MIC_{50} of milk (>256 µg/ml) and lung (8 µg/ml) isolates. MIC values for gentamycin ranged from 2 to >64 µg/ml (Thomas et al., 2003; Sulyok et al., 2014) and kanamycin from 8 to >128 µg/ml (Uemura et al., 2010; Kawai et al., 2014).

Chloramphenicols

The MIC_{50} values for florfenicol ranging from 1 to 8 µg/ml were identified in North America, Europe and China (Rosenbusch et al., 2005; Soehnlen et al., 2011; Hendrick et al., 2013; Kong et al., 2016). In addition, *M. bovis* isolates from Japan gave MIC_{50} values of 6.25-8 µg/ml and 6.25->512 µg/ml to chloramphenicol and thiamphenicol, respectively (Hirose et al., 2003; Uemura et al., 2010). Due to the potential toxicity of phenicols and chloramphenicols (not florfenicol), their use is now illegal in food animals in many countries (Papich and Riviere, 2013).

Pleuromutilins

The few MIC studies on tiamulin and valnemulin showed low MIC values for both antimicrobials (**Table 1**; Thomas et al., 2003; Gautier-Bouchardon et al., 2014). The efficacy of valnemulin against *M. bovis* infection was also demonstrated *in vivo* (Stipkovits et al., 2001, 2005).

MOLECULAR MECHANISMS OF *IN VIVO* ACQUIRED RESISTANCE BY *M. BOVIS*

In general, until now, the only mechanisms of acquired *in vivo* resistance described in *Mollicutes* are target modification and ribosome protection by the *tet*(M) determinant (Bebear and Kempf, 2005).

Tetracyclines

The genetic background for decreased tetracycline susceptibility has been elucidated in greater detail in mycoplasmas of human origin than in *M. bovis* (reviewed by Waites et al., 2014). Ribosomal protection by *tet*(M) determinants in *M. hominis* and *Ureaplasma* spp. tetracycline-resistant isolates was identified (Roberts et al., 1985, 1986) while target modification with point mutation(s) in the 16S rRNA genes was described for *in vitro* obtained mutants of *M. pneumoniae* with MICs of ≤2 µg/ml (Degrange et al., 2008). Recent correlation between decreased susceptibility to tetracycline hydrochloride in *M. bovis* isolates and mutations identified in the primary binding pocket for tetracycline (Tet-1 site) located in 16S rRNA-encoding genes (*rrs3* and *rrs4* alleles) was shown (Amram et al., 2015). An increase in MICs to tetracycline (MICs ≥2 µg/ml) was correlated with the number of mutated nucleotide positions within the Tet-1 site. Indeed, decreased susceptibilities to tetracycline were associated with mutations present at two (A965 and A967; *E. coli* numbering) or three positions (A965, A967, and G1058) in the two *rrs* alleles. No *tet*(M), *tet*(O), or *tet*(L) determinants were identified in any of the 70 *M. bovis* isolates tested. Notably, no *M. bovis* isolates with high MICs (≥32 µg/ml) to tetracycline were available and tested in this study.

Macrolides and Lincosamides

Macrolide resistance in mollicutes, which have 1–3 ribosomal operons, is caused by point mutations of the macrolide-binding site located in the 23S rRNA genes or in the genes encoding ribosomal proteins L4 and L22 (reviewed by Waites et al., 2014). Recently, *M. bovis* decreased susceptibility to tylosin and tilmicosin was attributed to any one of the point mutations G748A, C752T, A2058G, A2059G, or A2059C (*E. coli* numbering) identified in one or both alleles of the 23S rRNAs (Lerner et al., 2014). The data revealed that a combination of mutations in two domains (II and V of 23S rRNA) was necessary to achieve higher MICs (≥128 µg/ml) to tylosin, while a single mutation in one of the domains could be sufficient to cause a decrease in susceptibility to this antimicrobial. In that study, amino acid (aa) substitution L22-Q90H (*E. coli* numbering) was also identified in 24 of 32 representative *M. bovis* isolates with different MICs, but no clear correlation between this mutation and decreased MICs to tylosin and tilmicosin was found. In addition, multiple aa substitutions were identified in the L4 protein, including at positions 185–186 (positions 64 and 65 in *E. coli*), which are adjacent to the macrolide-binding site (Lerner et al., 2014). However, the actual impact of L4 aa substitutions is hard to define since they were identified in isolates with various MICs, some of which also possessed nt substitution/s within the macrolide binding site of 23S rRNA gene/s. Clarification of the role of mutations at positions 90-L22 and 64/or 64-65-L4 in decreased macrolide susceptibility by *M. bovis* is required.

Fluoroquinolones

The only mechanism of acquired fluoroquinolone resistance described in *Mollicutes* is alterations within the quinolone resistance-determining regions (QRDRs) of DNA gyrase subunits GyrA and GyrB and/or topoisomerase IV subunits ParC and ParE. However, an active efflux mechanism has also been demonstrated *in vitro* (Raherison et al., 2002). Amino acid substitution in the QRDR of GyrA (Ser83Phe) alone or with concurrent mutation Asn84Asp in ParC was found in *M. bovis* isolates with MICs to enrofloxacin ranging from 0.32–1.25 to 2.5–5 µg/ml, respectively (Lysnyansky et al., 2009). In another study, mutation Ser83Leu in GyrA was identified in 32 isolates with MICs of 0.25–2 µg/ml to enrofloxacin, orbifloxacin and danofloxacin; mutations in Ser83Leu of GyrA and Ser81Pro of ParC were present in three isolates (4–16 µg/ml) while mutations Ser83Phe in GyrA and Ser80Ile in ParC were found in four isolates (8–16 µg/ml) (Sato et al., 2013). The mutations Ser83Phe in GyrA and Ser80Ile in ParC were also identified in a Chinese *M. bovis* isolate with MICs ≥16 µg/ml to ciprofloxacin, levofloxacin, lomefloxacin and norfloxacin (Mustafa et al., 2013). In addition, Sato et al. (2013) showed that laboratory-derived fluoroquinolone-resistant mutants selected from two isolates with Ser83Leu in GyrA possessed an aa substitution Ser80Ile or Ser81Tyr in ParC. Results of both studies (Lysnyansky et al., 2009; Sato et al., 2013) suggest a cumulative effect of the mutations in GyrA and ParC on fluoroquinolone resistance. Previously, *in vivo* acquired resistance by veterinary mycoplasmas to the fluoroquinolones has been attributed to aa changes at positions 80 or 84 in the ParC as well as positions 83 in the GyrA (Hirose et al., 2004; Le Carrou et al., 2006; Vicca et al., 2007).

Aminoglycosides

No enzymes responsible for chemical modification of aminoglycosides have been identified in the *M. bovis* genome. However, decreased susceptibility to streptomycin in *M. bovis* was associated with nt T at position 912 (*E. coli* numbering) in the 16S rRNA genes (Konigsson et al., 2002), a position converting to resistance in *E. coli* (Frattali et al., 1990).

In an aminocyclitol antimicrobials, spectinomycin, isolates with high MIC (>512 µg/ml) were found to exhibit a C to A transition at position 1192 (*E. coli* numbering) either in *rrs3* or in both *rrs* alleles (C. Schnee et al., abstract, IOM 2014, p. 60) as has been previously shown for spectinomycin-resistant *E. coli* (Sigmund et al., 1984).

Chloramphenicols and Pleuromutilins

To the best of our knowledge, no investigations of the phenicols /chloramphenicols and pleuromutilins resistance mechanisms for *M. bovis* have been published.

SUMMARY

Control of *M. bovis* infections in cattle is inherently difficult. The resulting clinical signs and disease are increasingly recognized as having a significant adverse impact on animal welfare and the economy of cattle farming around the world. Other than sanitary preventative measures, treatment with antimicrobials is the only approach for disease treatment. However, as emphasized herein, the number of potentially effective antimicrobials is limited as *M. bovis* lacks a cell wall. Among the few antimicrobials licensed for treatment of *M. bovis*, there is increasing evidence for resistance. Based on MIC levels and genetic analysis, antimicrobial resistance by *M. bovis* to the tetracyclines, macrolides, lincosamides, aminoglycosides, chloramphenicols, and fluoroquinolones has been reported and appears to be increasing. The mechanisms of *M. bovis* antimicrobial resistance have largely been based on genetic point mutations; few studies have examined efflux mechanisms and no plasmids have so far been detected in *M. bovis*.

This review highlights the necessity to agree a standardized method and controls for animal mycoplasma antimicrobial susceptibility testing. In addition breakpoints should be determined and the use of molecular resistance markers could be used to define them.

AUTHOR CONTRIBUTIONS

IL, RA designed the study and analyzed and interpreted data. IL, RA drafted the manuscript. All authors read and approved the final version of the manuscript.

REFERENCES

Amram, E., Mikula, I., Schnee, C., Ayling, R. D., Nicholas, R. A. J., Rosales, R. S., et al. (2015). 16S rRNA gene mutations associated with decreased susceptibility to tetracycline in *Mycoplasma bovis*. *Antimicrob. Agents Chemother.* 59, 796–802. doi: 10.1128/AAC.03876-14

Ayling, R. D., Baker, S. E., Peek, M. L., Simon, A. J., and Nicholas, R. A. (2000). Comparison of *in vitro* activity of danofloxacin, florfenicol, oxytetracycline, spectinomycin and tilmicosin against recent field isolates of *Mycoplasma bovis*. *Vet. Rec.* 146, 745–747. doi: 10.1136/vr.146.26.745

Ayling, R. D., Rosales, R. S., Barden, G., and Gosney, F. L. (2014). Changes in antimicrobial susceptibility of *Mycoplasma bovis* isolates from Great Britain. *Vet Rec*, 175, 486. doi: 10.1136/vr.102303

Bebear, C. M., and Kempf, I. (2005). "Antimicrobial therapy and antimicrobial resistance," in *Mycoplasmas: Molecular Biology, Pathogenicity and Strategies for Control*, eds A. Blanchard and G. F. Browning (Norwich: Horizon Bioscience), 535–568.

Becker, C. A., Thibault, F. M., Arcangioli, M. A., and Tardy, F. (2015). Loss of diversity within *Mycoplasma bovis* isolates collected in France from bovines with respiratory diseases over the last 35 years. *Infect Genet. Evol.* 33, 118–126. doi: 10.1016/j.meegid.2015.04.019

Bryskier, A. (2005a). "Tetracyclines," in *Antimicrobial Agents, Antibacterials and Antifungals*, ed A. Bryskier (Washington, DC: ASM Press), 642–651.

Bryskier, A. (2005b). "Fluoroquinolones," in *Antimicrobial Agents, Antibacterials and Antifungals*, ed A. Bryskier (Washington, DC: ASM Press), 668–788.

Degrange, S., Renaudin, H., Charron, A., Pereyre, S., Bebear, C., and Bebear, C. M. (2008). Reduced susceptibility to tetracyclines is associated *in vitro* with the presence of 16S rRNA mutations in *Mycoplasma hominis* and *Mycoplasma pneumoniae*. *J. Antimicrob. Chemother.* 61, 1390–1392. doi: 10.1093/jac/dkn118

Francoz, D., Fortin, M., Fecteau, G., and Messier, S. (2005). Determination of *Mycoplasma bovis* susceptibilities against six antimicrobial agents using the E test method. *Vet. Microbiol.* 105, 57–64. doi: 10.1016/j.vetmic.2004.10.006

Frattali, A. L., Flynn, M. K., De Stasio, E. A., and Dahlberg, A. E. (1990). Effects of mutagenesis of C912 in the streptomycin binding region of *Escherichia coli* 16S ribosomal RNA. *Biochim. Biophys. Acta* 1050, 27–33. doi: 10.1016/0167-4781(90)90136-P

Gautier-Bouchardon, A. V., Ferre, S., Le Grand, D., Paoli, A., Gay, E., and Poumarat, F. (2014). Overall decrease in the susceptibility of *Mycoplasma bovis* to antimicrobials over the past 30 years in France. *PLoS ONE* 9:e87672. doi: 10.1371/journal.pone.0087672

Gerchman, I., Levisohn, S., Mikula, I., and Lysnyansky, I. (2009). *In vitro* antimicrobial susceptibility of *Mycoplasma bovis* isolated in Israel from local and imported cattle. *Vet. Microbiol.* 137, 268–275. doi: 10.1016/j.vetmic.2009.01.028

Godinho, K. S. (2008). Susceptibility testing of tulathromycin: interpretative breakpoints and susceptibility of field isolates. *Vet. Microbiol.* 129, 426–432. doi: 10.1016/j.vetmic.2007.11.033

Godinho, K. S., Rae, A., Windsor, G. D., Tilt, N., Rowan, T. G., and Sunderland, S. J. (2005). Efficacy of tulathromycin in the treatment of bovine respiratory disease associated with induced *Mycoplasma bovis* infections in young dairy calves. *Vet. Ther.* 6, 96–112.

Hannan, P. C. (2000). Guidelines and recommendations for antimicrobial minimum inhibitory concentration (MIC) testing against veterinary mycoplasma species. *Vet. Res.* 31, 373–395. doi: 10.1051/vetres:2000100

Hendrick, S. H., Bateman, K. G., and Rosengren, L. B. (2013). The effect of antimicrobial treatment and preventive strategies on bovine respiratory disease and genetic relatedness and antimicrobial resistance of *Mycoplasma bovis* isolates in a western Canadian feedlot. *Can. Vet. J.* 54, 1146–1156.

Hirose, K., Kawasaki, Y., Kotani, K., Abiko, K., and Sato, H. (2004). Characterization of a point mutation in the *parC* gene of *Mycoplasma bovirhinis* associated with fluoroquinolone resistance. *J. Vet. Med. B* 51, 169–175. doi: 10.1111/j.1439-0450.2004.00748.x

Hirose, K., Kobayashi, H., Ito, N., Kawasaki, Y., Zako, M., Kotani, K., et al. (2003). Isolation of mycoplasmas from nasal swabs of calves affected with respiratory diseases and antimicrobial susceptibility of their isolates. *J. Vet. Med. B* 50, 347–351. doi: 10.1046/j.1439-0450.2003.00681.x

Kawai, K., Higuchi, H., Iwano, H., Iwakuma, A., Onda, K., Sato, R., et al. (2014). Antimicrobial susceptibilities of Mycoplasma isolated from bovine mastitis in Japan. *Anim. Sci. J.* 85, 96–99. doi: 10.1111/asj.12144

Khalil, D., Becker, C. A., and Tardy, F. (2015). Alterations in the quinolone resistance-determining regions and fluoroquinolone resistance in clinical isolates and laboratory-derived mutants of *Mycoplasma bovis*: not all genotypes may be equal. *Appl. Environ. Microbiol.* 82, 1060–1068. doi: 10.1128/AEM.03280-15

Kong, L. C., Gao, D., Jia, B. Y., Wang, Z., Gao, Y. H., Pei, Z. H., et al. (2016). Antimicrobial susceptibility and molecular characterization of macrolide resistance of *Mycoplasma bovis* isolates from multiple provinces in China. *J. Vet. Med. Sci.* 78, 293–296. doi: 10.1292/jvms.15-0304

Konigsson, M. H., Bolske, G., and Johansson, K. E. (2002). Intraspecific variation in the 16S rRNA gene sequences of *Mycoplasma agalactiae* and *Mycoplasma bovis* strains. *Vet. Microbiol.* 85, 209–220. doi: 10.1016/S0378-1135(01)00517-X

Kroemer, S., Galland, D., Guerin-Faublee, V., Giboin, H., and Woehrle-Fontaine, F. (2012). Survey of marbofloxacin susceptibility of bacteria isolated from cattle with respiratory disease and mastitis in Europe. *Vet. Rec.* 170, 53. doi: 10.1136/vr.100246

Le Carrou, J., Laurentie, M., Kobisch, M., and Gautier-Bouchardon, A. V. (2006). Persistence of *Mycoplasma hyopneumoniae* in experimentally infected pigs after marbofloxacin treatment and detection of mutations in the *parC* gene. *Antimicrob. Agents Chemother.* 50, 1959–1966. doi: 10.1128/AAC.01527-05

Lerner, U., Amram, E., Ayling, R. D., Mikula, I., Gerchman, I., Harrus, S., et al. (2014). Acquired resistance to the 16-membered macrolides tylosin and tilmicosin by *Mycoplasma bovis*. *Vet. Microbiol.* 168, 365–371. doi: 10.1016/j.vetmic.2013.11.033

Long, K. S., Hansen, L. H., Jakobsen, L., and Vester, B. (2006). Interaction of pleuromutilin derivatives with the ribosomal peptidyl transferase center. *Antimicrob. Agents Chemother.* 50, 1458–1462. doi: 10.1128/AAC.50.4.1458-1462.2006

Lysnyansky, I., Mikula, I., Gerchman, I., and Levisohn, S. (2009). Rapid detection of a point mutation in the *parC* gene associated with decreased susceptibility to fluoroquinolones in *Mycoplasma bovis*. *Antimicrob. Agents Chemother.* 53, 4911–4914. doi: 10.1128/AAC.00703-09

Lysnyansky, I., Rosengarten, R., and Yogev, D. (1996). Phenotypic switching of variable surface lipoproteins in *Mycoplasma bovis* involves high-frequency chromosomal rearrangements. *J. Bacteriol.* 178, 5395–5401.

McAuliffe, L., Ellis, R. J., Miles, K., Ayling, R. D., and Nicholas, R. A. J. (2006). Biofilm formation by mycoplasma species and its role in environmental persistence and survival. *Microbiology* 152, 913–922. doi: 10.1099/mic.0.28604-0

Mustafa, R., Qi, J., Ba, X., Chen, Y., Hu, C., Liu, X., et al. (2013). *In vitro* quinolones susceptibility analysis of Chinese *Mycoplasma bovis* isolates and their phylogenetic scenarios based upon QRDRs of DNA topoisomerases revealing a unique transition in ParC. *Pak. Vet. J.* 33, 364–369.

Nicholas, R. A., and Ayling, R. D. (2003). *Mycoplasma bovis*: disease, diagnosis, and control. *Res. Vet. Sci.* 74, 105–112. doi: 10.1016/S0034-5288(02)00155-8

Novak, R., and Shlaes, D. M. (2010). The pleuromutilin antibiotics: a new class for human use. *Curr Opin Investig Drugs*, 11, 182–191.

Papich, M. G., and Riviere, J. E. (2013). "Chloramphenicol and derivatives, macrolides, lincosamides, and miscellaneous antimicrobials," in *Veterinary Pharmacology and Therapeutics*, eds J. E. Riviere and M. G. Papich (Iowa, IA: Wiley-Blackwell), 945–982.

Raherison, S., Gonzalez, P., Renaudin, H., Charron, A., Bebear, C., and Bebear, C. M. (2002). Evidence of active efflux in resistance to ciprofloxacin and to ethidium bromide by *Mycoplasma hominis*. *Antimicrob. Agents Chemother.* 46, 672–679. doi: 10.1128/AAC.46.3.672-679.2002

Razin, S. (1978). The mycoplasmas. *Microbiol. Rev.* 42, 414–470.

Reeve-Johnson, L. (1999). "The impact of mycoplasma infections in respiratory diseases of cattle in Europe," in *Mycoplasma of Ruminants: Pathogenicity, Diagnostics, Epidemiology and Molecular Genetics*, eds L. Stipkovits, R. Rosengarten, and J. Frey (Brussels: European Commision Press), 18–31.

Roberts, M. C., Hillier, S. L., Hale, J., Holmes, K. K., and Kenny, G. E. (1986). Tetracycline resistance and *tetM* in pathogenic urogenital bacteria. *Antimicrob. Agents Chemother.* 30, 810–812. doi: 10.1128/AAC.30.5.810

Roberts, M. C., Koutsky, L. A., Holmes, K. K., LeBlanc, D. J., and Kenny, G. E. (1985). Tetracycline-resistant *Mycoplasma hominis* strains contain streptococcal *tetM* sequences. *Antimicrob. Agents Chemother.* 28, 141–143. doi: 10.1128/AAC.28.1.141

Rosenbusch, R. F., Kinyon, J. M., Apley, M., Funk, N. D., Smith, S. C., and Hoffman, L. J. (2005). *In vitro* antimicrobial inhibition profiles of *Mycoplasma bovis* isolates recovered from various regions of the United States from 2002 to 2003. *J. Vet. Diagn. Invest.* 17, 436–441. doi: 10.1177/104063870501700505

Sato, T., Okubo, T., Usui, M., Higuchi, H., and Tamura, Y. (2013). Amino acid substitutions in GyrA and ParC are associated with fluoroquinolone resistance in *Mycoplasma bovis* isolates from Japanese dairy calves. *J. Vet. Med. Sci.* 75, 1063–1065. doi: 10.1292/jvms.12-0508

Sigmund, C. D., Ettayebi, M., and Morgan, E. A. (1984). Antibiotic resistance mutations in 16S and 23S ribosomal RNA genes of *Escherichia coli*. *Nucleic Acids Res.* 12, 4653–4663. doi: 10.1093/nar/12.11.4653

Soehnlen, M. K., Kunze, M. E., Karunathilake, K. E., Henwood, B. M., Kariyawasam, S., Wolfgang, D. R., et al. (2011). *In vitro* antimicrobial inhibition of *Mycoplasma bovis* isolates submitted to the Pennsylvania Animal Diagnostic Laboratory using flow cytometry and a broth microdilution method. *J. Vet. Diagn. Invest.* 23, 547–551. doi: 10.1177/1040638711404155

Stipkovits, L., Ripley, P. H., Tenk, M., Glavits, R., Molnar, T., and Fodor, L. (2005). The efficacy of valnemulin (EconorR) in the control of disease caused by experimental infection of calves with *Mycoplasma bovis*. *Res. Vet. Sci.* 78, 207–215. doi: 10.1016/j.rvsc.2004.09.005

Stipkovits, L., Ripley, P. H., Varga, J., and Palfi, V. (2001). Use of valnemulin in the control of *Mycoplasma bovis* infection under field conditions. *Vet. Rec.* 148, 399–402. doi: 10.1136/vr.148.13.399

Sulyok, M., Kreizinger, Z., Fekete, L., Hrivnak, V., Magyar, T., Janosi, S., et al. (2014). Antibiotic susceptibility profiles of *Mycoplasma bovis* strains isolated from cattle in Hungary, Central Europe. *BMC Vet. Res.* 10:256. doi: 10.1186/s12917-014-0256-x

Taylor-Robinson, D., and Bebear, C. (1997). Antibiotic susceptibilities of mycoplasmas and treatment of mycoplasmal infections. *J. Antimicrob. Chemother.* 40, 622–630. doi: 10.1093/jac/40.5.622

Thomas, A., Nicolas, C., Dizier, I., Mainil, J., and Linden, A. (2003). Antibiotic susceptibilities of recent isolates of *Mycoplasma bovis* in Belgium. *Vet. Rec.* 153, 428–431. doi: 10.1136/vr.153.14.428

Uemura, R., Sueyoshi, M., and Nagatomo, H. (2010). Antimicrobial susceptibilities of four species of mycoplasma isolated in 2008 and 2009 from cattle in Japan. *J. Vet. Med. Sci.* 72, 1661–1663. doi: 10.1292/jvms.10-0165

Vicca, J., Maes, D., Stakenborg, T., Butaye, P., Minion, F., Peeters, J., et al. (2007). Resistance mechanism against fluoroquinolones in *Mycoplasma hyopneumoniae* field isolates. *Microb. Drug Resist.* 13, 166–170. doi: 10.1089/mdr.2007.716

Waites, K. B., Duffy, L. B., Bebear, C. M., Matlow, A., Talkington, D. F., Kenny, G. E., et al. (2012). Standardized methods and quality control limits for agar and broth microdilution susceptibility testing of *Mycoplasma pneumoniae*, *Mycoplasma hominis*, and *Ureaplasma urealyticum*. *J. Clin. Microbiol.* 50, 3542–3547. doi: 10.1128/JCM.01439-12

Waites, K. B., Lysnyansky, I., and Bébéar, C. M. (2014). "Emerging antimicrobial resistance in mycoplasmas of humans and animals," in *Mollicutes: Molecular Biology and Pathogenesis*, eds G. F. Browning and C. Citti (Norfolk,VA: Caister Academic Press), 289–322.

3

High Genetic Similarity of Ciprofloxacin-Resistant *Campylobacter jejuni* in Central Europe

*Jasna Kovač[1†], Neža Čadež[1], Beatrix Stessl[2], Kerstin Stingl[3], Igor Gruntar[4], Matjaž Ocepek[4], Marija Trkov[5], Martin Wagner[2] and Sonja Smole Možina[1]**

[1] Department of Food Science and Technology, Biotechnical Faculty, University of Ljubljana, Ljubljana, Slovenia, [2] Department for Farm Animals and Veterinary Public Health, Institute of Milk Hygiene, Milk Technology and Food Science, University of Veterinary Medicine, Vienna, Austria, [3] National Reference Laboratory for Campylobacter, Department of Biological Safety, Federal Institute for Risk Assessment, Berlin, Germany, [4] Institute of Microbiology and Parasitology, Veterinary Faculty, University of Ljubljana, Ljubljana, Slovenia, [5] Department for Public Health Microbiology Ljubljana, Centre for Medical Microbiology, National Laboratory of Health, Environment and Food, Ljubljana, Slovenia

***Correspondence:**
Sonja Smole Možina
sonja.smole@bf.uni-lj.si

†Present address:
Jasna Kovač,
Department of Food Science, Cornell University, Ithaca, NY, USA

Campylobacteriosis is the leading zoonosis in the European Union with the majority of cases attributed to *Campylobacter jejuni*. Although the disease is usually self-limiting, some severe cases need to be treated with antibiotics, primarily macrolides and quinolones. However, the resistance to the latter is reaching alarming levels in most of the EU countries. To shed light on the expansion of antibiotic resistance in central Europe, we have investigated genetic similarity across 178 ciprofloxacin-resistant *C. jejuni* mostly isolated in Slovenia, Austria and Germany. We performed comparative genetic similarity analyses using allelic types of seven multilocus sequence typing housekeeping genes, and single nucleotide polymorphisms of a quinolone resistance determining region located within the DNA gyrase subunit A gene. This analysis revealed high genetic similarity of isolates from clonal complex ST-21 that carry *gyrA* allelic type 1 in all three of these central-European countries, suggesting these ciprofloxacin resistant isolates arose from a recent common ancestor and are spread clonally.

Keywords: *Campylobacter jejuni*, ciprofloxacin resistance, multilocus sequence typing, *gyrA*, QRDR, resistance expansion

INTRODUCTION

Campylobacteriosis is the leading zoonosis in the European Union (EU), with the majority of cases attributed to *Campylobacter jejuni* (EFSA, 2015). Severe or prolonged cases of campylobacteriosis are conventionally treated with antibiotics from the macrolide (erythromycin) and quinolone (ciprofloxacin) classes. While macrolide resistance is successfully retained at low levels (human isolates EU average, 1.5%), some EU Member States report up to 91.5% prevalence of quinolone resistance (EFSA, 2015). The resistance prevalence among *C. jejuni* from humans was 64.1 and 63.0% in Slovenia and Austria in 2013, respectively (EFSA, 2015). The main mechanism that confers high-level resistance to ciprofloxacin in *Campylobacter* is the occurrence of the Thre86Ile point mutation in the quinolone-resistance-determining region (QRDR) of the gene that encodes DNA gyrase subunit A (*gyrA*), although other mutations within *gyrA*, as well as enhanced efflux activity can contribute to development of ciprofloxacin resistance (Wieczorek and Osek, 2013). The Thre86Ile resistant mutants have also been demonstrated to have increased chicken colonization fitness (Luo et al., 2005) in certain genetic backgrounds, giving them an advantage over susceptible strains. In other genetic backgrounds, the advantage was not observed (Zeitouni and Kempf, 2011). The resistance to quinolones is especially problematic due to their therapeutic use in human and veterinary medicine, including in food production animals, which allows for transmission of antibiotic resistance along the food-production chain to humans (EMA/ESVAC, 2011).

Several studies have reported the resistance and genotype data that demonstrated increased prevalence of resistance in certain genotypes in different geographical regions (Kinana et al., 2006: D'lima et al., 2007; Gu et al., 2009; Habib et al., 2009; Wirz et al., 2010; Stone et al., 2013; Wu et al., 2014; Jonas et al., 2015). Furthermore, associations of particular multilocus sequence typing (MLST) clonal complexes with resistance were suggestive of clonal expansion of ciprofloxacin resistance in Slovenia, the UK and Switzerland (Cody et al., 2012; Kittl et al., 2013; Wimalarathna et al., 2013; Kovač et al., 2014).

To provide better insight into the epidemiology of *C. jejuni* antibiotic resistance in central Europe, we performed a comparative genetic similarity analysis of 178 ciprofloxacin-resistant *C. jejuni* strains isolated in Slovenia, Austria and Germany. We used standard MLST coupled with single nucleotide polymorphism (SNP) analysis of the QRDR of *gyrA* to investigate the genetic relatedness of ciprofloxacin resistant *C. jejuni* isolates and shed light on the nature of their expansion in these three central-European countries.

MATERIALS AND METHODS

Bacterial Strains

The 178 ciprofloxacin resistant *C. jejuni* strains included in this study were isolated from poultry, cattle, chicken meat, cow milk, surface water, dog, strawberry, a zoo animal, and human stools in central Europe (Slovenia, Austria, Germany); two isolates were obtained from the southern Balkan region (Serbia, Bosnia, and Herzegovina) (**Supplementary Table S1**). The strains were isolated between 2001 and 2013 according to ISO10272, as part of national monitoring of retail meat and production animals, human clinical cases, and from other national and EU research projects.

Bacterial Growth Conditions and DNA Extraction

Stocks of *C. jejuni* isolates were stored at −80°C and grown on selective Karmali agar (Oxoid, Hampsire, UK) for 24 h at 42°C under microaerobic conditions (5% O_2, 10% CO_2, in N_2). DNA used for molecular species confirmation and MLST typing was extracted with PrepMan Ultra Sample Preparation Reagent (Applied Biosystems, Foster City, CA, USA), according to the manufacturer protocol. DNA was used for *C. jejuni* species confirmation according to Wang et al. (2002), and amplification of MLST housekeeping genes and *gyrA* QRDR. All primers used in this study are listed in **Supplementary Table S2**.

Antibiotic Resistance

Resistances to ciprofloxacin (0.06–4 mg/l), chloramphenicol (2–32 mg/l), erythromycin (0.5–32 mg/l), gentamicin (0.12–16 mg/l), streptomycin (1–16 mg/l) and tetracycline (0.25–16 mg/l) were determined by broth microdilution using Eucamp microtitre plates (Sensititre, Thermo Fischer Scientific) by following manufacturers' instructions. The reference strain ATCC 33560, which is susceptible to all seven tested antibiotics was used as a quality control. The minimum inhibitory concentration (MIC) cut-offs as recommended by EFSA (2015) were used to identify the resistant phenotypes. Briefly, isolates with MICs of ciprofloxacin >0.5 mg/l, chloramphenicol >16 mg/l, erythromycin >4 mg/l, gentamicin >2 mg/l, streptomycin >4 mg/l, and tetracycline >1 mg/l were identified as resistant. The MICs and resistance breakpoints are available in **Supplementary Table S1**.

Multilocus Sequence Typing

Multilocus sequence typing was carried out according to the established *C. jejuni* MLST scheme, with primers listed in **Supplementary Table S2** (Dingle et al., 2001). Sequences (Sanger sequencing; Macrogen, South Korea) were used for the identification of MLST profiles using Bionumerics 7.1 with the MLST plugin (Applied Maths NV, Sint-Martens-Latem, Belgium). The MLST profiles identified in this study have been deposited in the PubMLST database http://pubmlst.org/campylobacter (Jolley and Maiden, 2010). The PubMLST IDs are available in **Supplementary Table S1**. The minimum-spanning tree (**Figure 1**) demonstrating the genetic similarity among strains was built using MLST allele variants in Bionumerics version 7.1 (Applied Maths).

Quinolone-Resistance-Determining Region

The QRDR of *gyrA* of 178 ciprofloxacin-resistant *C. jejuni* isolates was amplified using primers GZgyrA5 and GZgyrA6 in a single PCR, and Sanger sequenced using primers GZgyrA7 and GZgyrA8 (Zirnstein et al., 1999; **Supplementary Table S2**). The 389-bp-long QRDR sequences spanning from nucleotide positions 92 to 481 within *gyrA* were aligned in MEGA V6.0 (Tamura et al., 2013) to identify the unique variants of *gyrA*. Every sequence with new SNP (synonymous or non-synonymous) observed was designated a new *gyrA* allelic type number. The conserved region of *gyrA* outside of QRDR was previously used by others for epidemiological investigation of *C. jejuni* and *C. coli* host specificity (Ragimbeau et al., 2014). Here we have investigated the QRDR region, as its sequence diversity is directly associated with ciprofloxacin resistance.

Statistical Analysis

Statistical associations between *gyrA* types and MLST clonal complexes, and between *gyrA*+MLST types and multidrug

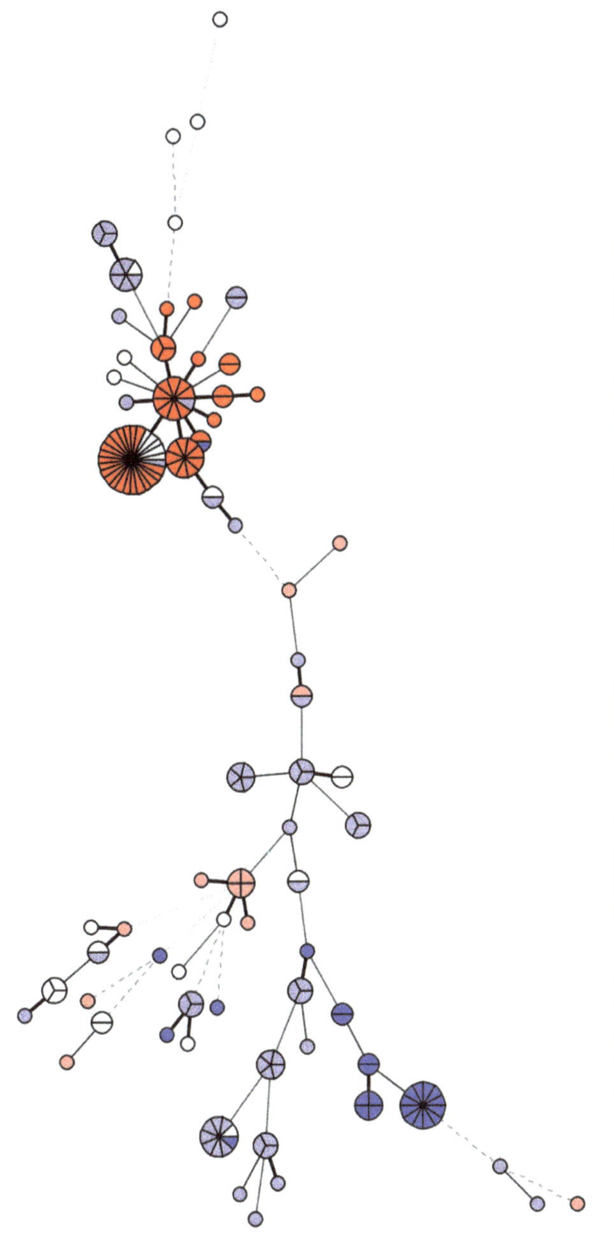

FIGURE 1 | Genetic similarity of the 178 analyzed *Campylobacter jejuni* isolates. The minimum spanning tree was constructed based on the multilocus sequence typing (MLST) allelic profiles using Bionumerics, version 7.1. The genotype specific for clonal complex ST-21 + *gyrA* 1 is presented in dark red and for *gyrA* 1 in combination with a clonal complex other than ST-21 is in light red; the genotype for clonal complex ST-353 + *gyrA* 13 is in dark blue; and for *gyrA* 13 in combination with a clonal complex other than ST-353 is in light blue. The figure demonstrates higher similarity of isolates carrying *gyrA* allelic type 1, which cluster within clonal complex ST-21 (dark red), compared to isolates carrying *gyrA* 13, which are found within clonal complex ST-353 (dark blue), but are also dispersed among other clonal complexes (light blue).

resistance were carried out using Fischer's exact tests in R, version 3.1.2, with the statistical relevance cut-off set at $p < 0.01$ (R Core Team, 2014).

RESULTS

Analyses of antibiotic co-resistance (multidrug resistance) were carried out on the isolates, with the MICs determined for all seven of the antibiotics tested ($n = 163$). The MICs of ciprofloxacin-resistant isolates ranged from 2 to over 4 mg/l, confirming a high-level resistance in all of them (resistance MIC cut-off is >0.5 mg/l). Among them, 76 (46.6%) isolates were either resistant to ciprofloxacin only ($n = 4$) or were cross-resistant to nalidixic acid ($n = 72$). The MICs of nalidixic acid ranged from 32 to over 46 mg/ml. Seventy-six isolates (46.6%) were co-resistant to ciprofloxacin and another antibiotic from a different class, which was exclusively tetracycline. MICs of tetracycline were ranging from 2 to over 16 mg/l, however most of the isolates ($n = 61$; 80.3%) were resistant to concentrations 16 mg/l or higher. Seven of the ciprofloxacin-resistant isolates (4.3%) were additionally resistant to either streptomycin and erythromycin, or streptomycin and tetracycline. Three isolates (1.8%) were resistant to antibiotics from four different classes, and a single isolate (0.6%) was resistant to antibiotics from five different classes (**Supplementary Table S1**). As demonstrated in **Figure 2**, higher proportion of resistance only to quinolone (1R) antibiotics was observed among isolates from poultry source ($n = 50$; 34.9%, $p < 0.001$), compared to isolates of bovine origin, where resistance to two classes of antibiotics (quinolones and tetracyclines - 2R) was prevailing ($n = 20$; 74.0%; $p = 0.003$). However, these differences arise mostly due to the high proportion of 1R among Slovenian poultry isolates ($n = 33$; 55%), compared to Austrian ($n = 8$; 17.4%) and German ($n = 9$; 33.3%), suggesting divergent antibiotic treatment practices in Slovenia, Austria, and Germany.

We identified 67 different MLST sequence types (STs) that were distributed among 21 clonal complexes (**Table 1**). Twenty isolates could not be assigned to any of the existing clonal complexes. Novel variants of alleles *aspA* (*aspA 387*), *glyA*

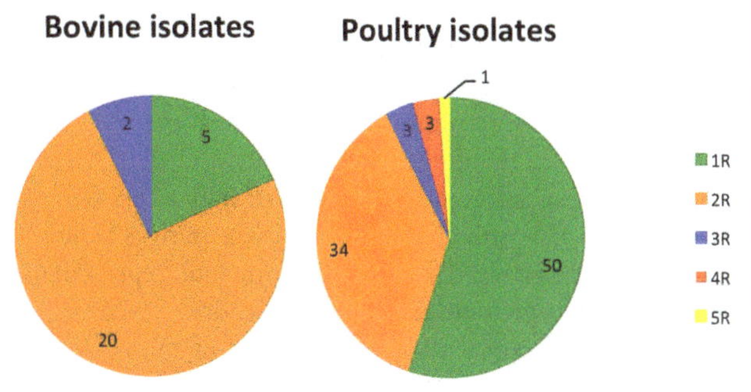

FIGURE 2 | Co-existence of quinolone resistance with resistances to other classes of antibiotics among isolates from bovine ($n = 27$) and poultry ($n = 91$) source. 1R, 2R, 3R, 4R, 5R, resistance to quinolone alone (1R), and to antibiotics from one, two (exclusively quinolone and tetracycline), three, four and five other classes, respectively. Only isolates with resistance determined for all seven antibiotics tested ($n = 163$) were included in the analysis.

TABLE 1 | The distribution of ciprofloxacin-resistant *Campylobacter jejuni* isolates, originating from different countries among MLST clonal complexes.

	Austria	Germany	Slovenia	Serbia	Bosnia and Herzegovina	SUM
ST-21 complex	22	15	24			61
ST-353 complex	7	3	15		1	26
UA	10	1	9			20
ST-354 complex	2		8			10
ST-206 complex	5	1	3			9
ST-464 complex	6	1	1			8
ST-257 complex	4	1	1			6
ST-45 complex		4	2			6
ST-443 complex	4		1			5
ST-48 complex	2	1	2			5
ST-52 complex	1		4			5
ST-574 complex	4					4
ST-22 complex	1		1			2
ST-607 complex	1			1		2
ST-658 complex			2			2
ST-1034 complex		1				1
ST-283 complex			1			1
ST-362 complex			1			1
ST-42 complex		1				1
ST-49 complex	1					1
ST-692 complex		1				1
ST-828 complex			1			1
SUM	70	30	76	1	1	178

(599), *tkt* (578), and *uncA* (458) were identified, along with the definition of their novel corresponding STs: ST 7514, ST 7517, ST 7516, and ST 7515, respectively. One new ST, ST 7506, was identified as a novel combination of previously reported allele types, according to the information in the PubMLST database.

Sequence type 50 (clonal complex ST-21) was the most prevalent ST that was common to all three countries, Austria ($n = 12$), Slovenia ($n = 12$) and Germany ($n = 3$). The second-most frequent ST among the Slovenian isolates was ST 5205 (clonal complex ST-353) ($n = 11$), which was identified for the first time in our previous study (Kovač et al., 2014) and has been so far reported only for Slovenian ($n = 11$) and Austrian ($n = 1$) isolates, according to the PubMLST database (accessed on 20 June 2015). The most-prevalent clonal complex in all three of these countries was ST-21, with 24 representatives in Slovenia, 22 in Austria, and 15 in Germany, followed by ST-353, with 15 and seven representatives in Slovenia and Austria, respectively, and ST-45, with four representatives in Germany (**Supplementary Table S1**). Both, ST-21 and ST-353 were highly represented by chicken and human isolates, but no bovine isolate was assigned to ST-353. The 64.5% ($n = 20$; $p < 0.001$) of bovine isolates carried *gyrA* type 1, while 59.8% ($n = 49$, $p < 0.001$) of chicken isolates carried *gyrA* type 13.

The comparative analysis of the 389-bp-long QRDR sequences revealed 15 different *gyrA* allelic types with variations on 25 nucleotide sites (**Supplementary Table S1**; GenBank KP794628-KP794805). The sequences were checked for presence of previously reported resistance-conferring mutations on nucleotide positions 210, 255, 258, 270, and 312 (according to full-length *gyrA*), which corresponded to amino acids Ala70, Asp85, Thr86, Asp90, and Pro104 (Wieczorek and Osek, 2013). A total of 171 isolates carried the main resistance-conferring mutation Thr86Ile. This mutation was not detected in seven isolates, which still exhibited high level resistance to ciprofloxacin (MICs 2 to over 4 mg/l), possibly due to enhanced efflux activity. The *gyrA* types identified in isolates lacking the Thr86Ile mutation were *gyrA* 7, 8, 9, and 10. None of the isolates analyzed carried the alternative resistance-conferring mutations at amino-acid positions 70, 85, or 90, however five of the isolates had the Pro104Thr mutation. Pro104Thr is a newly identified mutation, as only Pro104Ser has been reported so far (Wieczorek and Osek, 2013). Pro104Thr was found in four strains that were isolated in Austria (08/000367, MRC-09/00280, MRC-10/00374, MRC-11/00224), and in a single strain isolated in Germany (Bfr-CA-10467) (**Supplementary Table S1**). All of the isolates with Pro104Thr mutation possessed the *gyrA* type 6.

The most prevalent *gyrA* STs were *gyrA* type 13 ($n = 86$) and *gyrA* type 1 ($n = 65$), with the remaining *gyrA* STs represented by only up to five isolates. The isolates with *gyrA* type 13 were distributed among 14 clonal complexes, and 26.7% of these isolates were assigned to ST-353 (ST-353 + *gyrA* 13; $p < 0.001$). On the other hand, isolates with *gyrA* type 1 were distributed among eight different clonal complexes, with 80.0% of these isolates clustering in ST-21 (ST-21 + *gyrA* 1; $p < 0.001$). Sequence analysis revealed closer relationships between isolates carrying *gyrA* type 1, which mostly belonged to clonal complex 21 (ST-21 + *gyrA* type 1), compared to isolates carrying *gyrA* type 13 (**Figure 1**). Both of these *gyrA* types were found in isolates from Slovenia, Austria, and Germany.

Isolates with genotype ST-353 + *gyrA* 13 were in most cases ($n = 13$; 61.9%; $p < 0.001$) resistant only to ciprofloxacin or to ciprofloxacin and nalidixic acid. Similar numbers, but lower proportions, of solely ciprofloxacin resistant isolates ($n = 18$; 39.1%; $p = 0.2244$) were observed also for genotype ST-21 + *gyrA* 1. A higher proportion of isolates with genotype ST-21 + *gyrA* 1 were resistant to two classes of antibiotics ($n = 25$; 54.3%; $p = 0.222$), than of isolates with genotype ST-353 + *gyrA* 13 ($n = 5$; 23.8%, $p = 0.035$). The proportions of isolates resistant to three antibiotics from different classes were low, both for ST-353 + *gyrA* 13 ($n = 3$; 14.3%) and for ST-21 + *gyrA* 1 ($n = 1$; 2.2%). Isolates that showed resistance to four and five antibiotics were represented only by genotype ST-21 + *gyrA* 1.

DISCUSSION

The current antibiotic-resistance problem among zoonotic agents demonstrates the need for improvements to resistance management policy. The EU ban on antibiotic use for growth promotion in animal husbandry was a step forward (European Commission, 2011). However, the extensive amounts of clinically important antibiotics that are applied for treatment and control of pathogens in food-production animals still support the spread and persistence of resistant bacterial populations in the food production chain, and therefore compromise efficient treatment of human infections (EMA/ESVAC, 2014).

Although the ban on the use of antibiotics in food animals may not produce the immediate targeted effects, studies from several countries that have established such policies have provided evidence for its sustainability, in terms of decreasing the prevalence of antibiotic resistance (Norström et al., 2006; Nelson et al., 2007; Skjøt-Rasmussen et al., 2009). Nevertheless, the implications of such policies and risk analyses for the expansion of antibiotic resistance through the international trade in chicken meat have not been evaluated to date, although such investigations are urgently needed.

Here, we have investigated the genetic similarity of ciprofloxacin-resistant strains isolated from the environment, animals, food and human in three central-European countries over the last 12 years to gain knowledge about their distribution among different genotypes that could potentially explain the mechanisms driving the increase in ciprofloxacin resistance prevalence in *C. jejuni*. We have found that resistance to ciprofloxacin alone (1R) is more frequently observed among poultry isolates, compared to bovine isolates where resistance to ciprofloxacin and tetracycline (2R) is more common. Although the associations were statistically significant according to Fischer's exact test, the observations are biased, as substantially higher proportion of 1R isolates originates from Slovenia, compared to Austria and Germany. According to an opinion of Slovenian veterinary expert familiar with the field use of antibiotics in poultry, this can be explained with preferential use of enrofloxacin, rather than tetracyclines for poultry treatment in Slovenia. Main reason for that is the shorter withdrawal period and less problems with antibiotic precipitation in water.

Ciprofloxacin-resistant isolates clustered in two groups of high genetic similarity, as inferred based on MLST and SNP analyses of the QRDR. These two groups comprised isolates from MLST clonal complex ST-353 with *gyrA* type 13 and isolates from clonal complex ST-21 with *gyrA* type 1. While isolates from both of these MLST clonal complexes were significantly associated with their corresponding *gyrA* types, the sequence similarity analysis revealed closer relationships between isolates carrying *gyrA* type 1. Isolates with *gyrA* type 13 were widely dispersed also in clonal complexes other than ST-353, while isolates with *gyrA* type 1 belonged almost exclusively to MLST clonal complex 21, indicating they have expanded from a recent common ancestor. Furthermore, strains isolated from all three countries over several different years can be found within the group.

We have found 17 STs appearing between animal, as well as human isolates. Five of those (STs 50, 21, 104, 5205, and 572) were found more than once among human isolates. Of those, ST 50, 21, and 104 belong to clonal complex ST-21, ST 5205 to clonal complex ST-353, while 572 was unassigned. These findings suggest epidemiological linkage between animal and human isolates from clonal complexes ST-21 and ST-353, which also had the highest accumulation of ciprofloxacin resistant isolates.

The ST-21, and in particular ST 50 were highly represented among our set of ciprofloxacin resistant isolates, nevertheless previous studies in other geographical regions had not found significant associations between this genotype and quinolone resistance or susceptibility (Cody et al., 2012; Kittl et al., 2013). On the other hand, they have found ST 464 and ST 45 to be significantly associated with quinolone resistance, and susceptibility, respectively (Cody et al., 2012; Kittl et al., 2013). These two STs, however, were not identified frequently enough among our ciprofloxacin resistant isolates, to draw statistically relevant conclusions.

It is becoming increasingly evident that the global escalation of quinolone resistance in *Campylobacter* is associated with spreading of certain resistant genotypes (Cody et al., 2012; Kittl et al., 2013; Wimalarathna et al., 2013; Kovač et al., 2014), which may be driven by globalization in the poultry trade (AVEC, 2014) and/or of travel. Our findings suggest that the ciprofloxacin resistance is expanding with widespread *C. jejuni* clonal complex ST-21 in central Europe. Further research focused on identifying the genetic traits other than antibiotic resistance determinants that may facilitate this process is needed, in order to better understand the antibiotic resistance epidemiology, and implement successful resistance control measures.

ACKNOWLEDGMENTS

This study was funded by project PROMISE (FP7-265877) and the Slovenian Research Agency (CRP V4-1110). The authors thank to Dr. Sandra Jelovcan from AGES and Dr. Marija Lušicky from NLZOH for providing *C. jejuni* strains, and Eva Sobočan Zajc and Diletta DiMarco for technical assistance.

SUPPLEMENTARY MATERIAL

TABLE S1 | Isolates used in this study. The source of isolates, their antibiotic resistance profiles, MLST types and *gyrA* QRDR types.

TABLE S2 | Primers used in this study.

REFERENCES

AVEC (2014). *Association of Poultry Processors and Poultry Trade in the EU Countries Annual Report.* Available at: http://www.avec-poultry.eu/system/files/archive/new-structure/avec/AnnualReport/2014/Version%20Finale.pdf

Cody, A. J., McCarthy, N. M., Wimalarathna, H. L., Colles, F. M., Clark, L., Bowler, I. C., et al. (2012). A longitudinal 6-year study of the molecular epidemiology of clinical *Campylobacter* isolates in Oxfordshire, United Kingdom. *J. Clin. Microbiol.* 50, 3193–3201. doi: 10.1128/JCM.01086-12

Dingle, K. E., Colles, F. M., Wareing, D. R., Ure, R., Fox, A. J., Bolton, F. E., et al. (2001). Multilocus sequence typing system for *Campylobacter jejuni. J. Clin. Microbiol.* 39, 14–23. doi: 10.1128/JCM.39.1.14-23.2001

D'lima, C. B., Miller, W. G., Mandrell, R. E., Wright, S. L., Siletzky, R. M., Carver, D. K., et al. (2007). Clonal population structure and specific genotypes of multidrug-resistant *Campylobacter coli* from turkeys. *Appl. Environ. Microbiol.* 73, 2156–2164. doi: 10.1128/AEM.02346-06

EFSA (2015). The European union summary report on antimicrobial resistance in zoonotic and indicator bacteria from humans, animals and food in 2013. *EFSA J.* 13:4036. doi: 10.2903/j.efsa.2015.4036

EMA/ESVAC (2011). *European Medicines Agency, European Surveillance of Veterinary Antimicrobial Consumption (ESVC). Trends in Sales of Veterinary Antimicrobial Agents in European Countires. Reporting Period 2005-2009.* Available at: http://www.ema.europa.eu/docs/enGB/documentlibrary/Report/2014/10/WC500175671.pdf [accessed April 13, 2015].

EMA/ESVAC (2014). *European Medicines Agency, European Surveillance of Veterinary Antimicrobial Consumption, 2014. Sales of Veterinary Antimicrobial Agents in 26 EU/EEA Countries in 2012.* Available at : http://www.ema.europa.eu/docs/en_GB/document_library/Report/2014/10/WC500175671.pdf [accessed October 13, 2015].

European Commission (2011). *Communication from the Commission to the European Parliament and the Council Action Plan Against the Rising Threats from Antimicrobial Resistance.* Available at: http://ec.europa.eu/dgs/health food-safety/docs/communicationamr2011748en.pdf

Gu, W., Siletzky, R. M., Wright, S., Islam, M., and Kathariou, S. (2009). Antimicrobial susceptibility profiles and strain type diversity of *Campylobacter jejuni* isolates from turkeys in eastern North Carolina. *Appl. Environ. Microbiol.* 75, 474–482. doi: 10.1128/AEM.02012-08

Habib, I., Miller, W. G., Uyttendaele, M., Houf, K., and De Zutter, L. (2009). Clonal population structure and antimicrobial resistance of *Campylobacter jejuni* in chicken meat from Belgium. *Appl. Environ. Microbiol.* 75, 4264–4272. doi: 10.1128/AEM.00168-09

Jolley, K. A., and Maiden, M. C. (2010). BIGSdb: scalable analysis of bacterial genome variation at the population level. *BMC Bioinformatics* 11:595. doi: 10.1186/1471-2105-11-595

Jonas, R., Kittl, S., Overesch, G., and Kuhnert, P. (2015). Genotypes and antibiotic resistance of bovine *Campylobacter* and their contribution to human Campylobacteriosis. *Epidemiol. Infect.* 143, 2373–2380. doi: 10.1017/S0950268814003410

Kinana, A. D., Cardinale, E., Tall, F., Bahsoun, I., Sire, J. M., Garin, B., et al. (2006). Genetic diversity and quinolone resistance in *Campylobacter jejuni* isolates from poultry in senegal. *Appl. Environ. Microbiol.* 72, 3309–3313. doi: 10.1128/AEM.72.5.3309-3313.2006

Kittl, S., Heckel, G., Korczak, B. M., and Kuhnert, P. (2013). Source attribution of human *Campylobacter* isolates by MLST and fla-typing and association of genotypes with quinolone resistance. *PLoS ONE* 14:e81796. doi: 10.1371/journal.pone.0081796

Kovač, J., Čadež, N., Lušicky, M., Nielsen, E. M., Ocepek, M., Raspor, P., et al. (2014). The evidence for clonal spreading of quinolone resistance with a particular clonal complex of *Campylobacter jejuni. Epidemiol. Infect.* 42, 2595–2603. doi: 10.1017/S0950268813003245

Luo, N., Pereira, S., Sahin, O., Lin, J., Huang, S., Michel, L., et al. (2005). Enhanced in vivo fitness of fluoroquinolone-resistant *Campylobacter jejuni* in the absence of antibiotic selection pressure. *Proc. Natl. Acad. Sci. U.S.A.* 102, 541–546. doi: 10.1073/pnas.0408966102

Nelson, J. M., Chiller, T. M., Powers, J. H., and Angulo, F. J. (2007). Fluoroquinolone-resistant *Campylobacter* species and the withdrawal of fluoroquinolones from use in poultry: a public health success story. *Clin. Infect. Dis.* 44, 977–980. doi: 10.1086/512369

Norström, M., Hofshagen, M., Stavnes, T., Schau, J., Lassen, J., and Kruse, H. (2006). Antimicrobial resistance in *Campylobacter jejuni* from humans and broilers in Norway. *Epidemiol. Infect.* 134, 127–130. doi: 10.1017/S0950268805004814

R Core Team (2014). *R: A Language and Environment for Statistical Computing.* Vienna, R Foundation for Statistical Computing. Avialble at: http://www.R-project.org/

Ragimbeau, C., Colin, S., Devaux, A., Decruyenaere, F., Cauchie, H., Losch, S., et al. (2014). Investigating the host specificity of *Campylobacter jejuni* and *Campylobacter coli* by sequencing gyrase subunit A. *BMC Microbiol.* 14:205. doi: 10.1186/s12866-014-0205-7

Skjøt-Rasmussen, L., Ethelberg, S., Emborg, H., Agersø, Y., Larsen, L. S., Nordentoft, S., et al. (2009). Trends in occurrence of antimicrobial resistance in *Campylobacter jejuni* isolates from broiler chickens, broiler chicken meat, and human domestically acquired cases and travel associated cases in Denmark. *Int. J. Food. Microbiol.* 131, 277–279. doi: 10.1016/j.ijfoodmicro.2009.03.006

Stone, D., Davis, M., Baker, K., Besser, T., Roopnarine, R., and Sharma, R. (2013). MLST genotypes and antibiotic resistance of *Campylobacter* spp. isolated from poultry in Grenada. *Biomed. Res. Internat.* 2013:794643. doi: 10.1155/2013/794643

Tamura, K., Stecher, G., Peterson, D., Filipski, A., and Kumar, S. (2013). MEGA6: molecular evolutionary genetics analysis version 6.0. *Mol. Biol. Evol.* 30, 2725–2729. doi: 10.1093/molbev/mst197

Wang, G., Clark, C. G., Taylor, T. M., Pucknell, C., Barton, C., Price, L., et al. (2002). Colony multiplex PCR assay for identification and differentiation of *Campylobacter jejuni, C. coli, C. lari, C. upsaliensis,* and *C. fetus* subsp. fetus. *J. Clin. Microbiol.* 40, 4744–4747. doi: 10.1128/JCM.40.12.4744-4747.2002

Wieczorek, K., and Osek, J. (2013). Antimicrobial resistance mechanisms among *Campylobacter. Biomed. Res. Int.* 2013:340605. doi: 10.1155/2013/340605

Wimalarathna, H. M., Richardson, J. F., Lawson, A. J., Elson, R., Meldrum, R., Little, C. L., et al. (2013). Widespread acquisition of antimicrobial resistance among *Campylobacter* isolates from UK retail poultry and evidence for clonal expansion of resistant lineages. *BMC Microbiol.* 5:160. doi: 10.1186/1471-2180-13-160

Wirz, S. E., Overesch, G., Kuhnert, P., and Korczak, B. M. (2010). Genotype and antibiotic resistance analyses of *Campylobacter* isolates from ceca and carcasses of slaughtered broiler flocks. *Appl. Environ. Microbiol.* 76, 6377–6386. doi: 10.1128/AEM.00813-10

Wu, Z., Sippy, R., Sahin, O., Plummer, P., Vidal, A., Newell, D., et al. (2014). Genetic diversity and antimicrobial susceptibility of *Campylobacter jejuni* isolates associated with sheep abortion in the united states and Great Britain. *J. Clin. Microbiol.* 52, 1853–1861. doi: 10.1128/JCM.00355-14

Zeitouni, S., and Kempf, I. (2011). Fitness Cost of fluoroquinolone resistance in *Campylobacter coli* and *Campylobacter jejuni*. *Microb. Drug Resist.* 17, 171–179. doi: 10.1089/mdr.2010.0139

Zirnstein, G., Li, Y., Swaminathan, B., and Angulo, F. (1999). Ciprofloxacin resistance in *Campylobacter jejuni* isolates: detection of gyrA resistance mutations by mismatch amplification mutation assay PCR and DNA sequence analysis. *J. Clin. Microbiol.* 37, 3276–3280.

4

Correlation of PK/PD Indices with Resistance Selection for Cefquinome against *Staphylococcus aureus* in an *In Vitro* Model

*Yafei Li[1†], Baoyi Feng[1†], Xiaoyan Gu[2], Dawei Yang[3], Zhenling Zeng[1], Bingxu Zhang[1] and Huanzhong Ding[1]**

[1] Laboratory of Veterinary Pharmacology, College of Veterinary Medicine, South China Agricultural University, Guangzhou, China, [2] Centre for Veterinary Drug Residues, College of Veterinary Medicine, South China Agricultural University, Guangzhou, China, [3] China Institute of Veterinary Drug Control, Beijing, China

***Correspondence:**
Huanzhong Ding
hzding@scau.edu.cn

† These authors have contributed equally to this work.

Cefquinome is a fourth-generation Cephalosporin approved for use in animals exclusively. The objective of this study was to explore the relationship of cefquinome pharmacokinetic/pharmacodynamic (PK/PD) indices with resistance selection of *Staphylococcus aureus* ATCC25923 in an *in vitro* model. Six dosing regiments of cefquinome at an interval of 24 h for three consecutive times were simulated, resulting in maximum concentrations (C_{max}) from 1/2 to 16MIC and terminal half-lives ($t_{1/2\beta}$) of 3 and 6 h, respectively. The *in vitro* sensitivity of *S. aureus* was monitored by bacterial susceptibility and dynamic time-kill curve experiments over the six cefquinome concentrations. The correlation between changes in bacterial susceptibility (MIC_{72}/MIC_0) and the percentage of time within mutant selection window versus dosing interval (T_{MSW} %) was subjected to the Gaussian function and regression analysis. Our results favored the consensus that time above MIC (T > MIC) was recognized as an important PK/PD parameter of cephalosporins for antibacterial efficiency. Cefquinome reached the maximum killing effect when T > MIC% attained approximately 40~60%. The subsequent correlation analysis demonstrated that resistant *S. aureus* ATCC25923 was easy to occur when T_{MSW}% attained an index of about 20% with $t_{1/2\beta}$ of 3 h after multiple dosing, and 40% with $t_{1/2\beta}$ of 6 h after multiple dosing, respectively.

Keywords: cefquinome, *Staphylococcus aureus*, PK/PD, MPC, *in vitro* model

INTRODUCTION

Staphylococcus aureus is a major pathogen for animals and humans, which contributes to a variety of severe infections, including bacteremia, meningitis, endocarditis, skin and wood infection or other diseases for animals and humans (Archer, 1998; Lowy, 1998; Azizoglu et al., 2013). More importantly, *S. aureus* plays an important role in the food contamination by foodborne pathogens. Food poisoning caused by staphylococcal enterotoxin (SE) is a pressing worldwide health problem (Tauxe, 2002; Le Loir et al., 2003). In spite of the progress in antimicrobial therapy, treatment of *S. aureus* infection has become more and more challenging because drug-resistance of *S. aureus* has increased globally over the past decade. The methicillin-resistant *S. aureus* (MRSA) and vancomycin-resistant *S. aureus* (VRSA) were particularly reported and well documented (Harris et al., 2010; Mohammed Fayaz et al., 2011).

In veterinary medicine, cefquinome (CEQ) has been licensed in European countries by virtue of its broad antibacterial spectrums and remarkable antibacterial activities. Despite of this, the cephalosporins should be in prudent use considering the escalating antimicrobial resistance. Evidence has showed that different animal species may harbor the same resistance determinant and are recognized as possible reservoirs of antimicrobial-resistant bacteria (Guardabassi et al., 2004). It has been also observed that cefquinome exerted a selective effect on bla_{CTX-M} producing *Escherichia coli* strains (Cavaco et al., 2008). Therefore, further information concerning the ability of cefquinome to prevent occurring of resistant strains seems to be investigated.

Since mutant prevention concentration (MPC) of antibiotics was first described by Dong et al. (1999), it has been successfully applied to evaluate the ability of antibiotics that restrict the selection of resistant strains (Allen et al., 2004; Allen and Hankins, 2009; Wang et al., 2010; Blondeau et al., 2012) and optimize the current dosing regimens of antibiotics to slow the emergence of resistant strains. MPC was taken as the lowest doubling dilution drug concentration that prevented a population of 10^{10} colony forming unit (CFU)/mL or even more microorganisms from first-step mutation. Zone of the drug concentrations between minimum inhibitory concentration (MIC) and MPC was defined as the mutant selection window (MSW). MPC and MSW concepts, representing the ability of antibiotics to select resistant strains, have been tested in various *in vitro* studies(Allen et al., 2004; Croisier et al., 2004b; Ferran et al., 2007), in *ex vivo* pharmacodynamic studies (Bronner et al., 2002) and in *in vivo* studies (Croisier et al., 2004a; Cui et al., 2006). Here, we developed an *in vitro* kinetic model to investigate the relationship between pharmacokinetic/pharmacodynamic (PK/PD) indices of cefquinome with terminal half-lives ($t_{1/2\beta}$) of 3 or 6 h and resistance development of *S. aureus* ATCC25923.

MATERIALS AND METHODS

Antimicrobial Agents, Medium, and Bacterial Strains

Raw material of cefquinome (purity of 84.1%) was obtained from Hebei yuanzheng Pharmaceutical Enterprise, Co., Ltd. Mueller-Hinton broth (MHB) and agar were purchased from Guangzhou huankai Comapany. *S. aureus* ATCC 25923 was purchased from the China Institute of Veterinary Drug Control (Beijing, China).

In Vitro Susceptibility Testing

The MIC of CEQ against *S. aureus* with an inoculum of 5×10^5 CFU/mL was determined by standard agar dilution method established by the Clinical and Laboratory Standards Institute (CLSI).

Measurement of MIC_{99}, Mutant Prevention Concentration (MPC) and Selection Index (SI)

The MIC_{99} was defined as the drug concentration that inhibited 99% of bacteria colony formation. MPC was reckoned as the lowest cefquinome concentration blocking $\geq 10^{10}$ CFU/mL inoculants growth. The measurements of MIC_{99} and MPC were mainly based on the method reported by Zhao and Drlica (2002) with slight modification. For MIC_{99}, agar plates containing a series of cefquinome (concentrations ranging from 0.5 to 0.164 μg/mL) at 20% per sequential decrease were prepared. 3×10^7 CFU/mL *S. aureus* suspension in logarithmic phase of growth was then subjected to serial 10-fold dilutions with MHB to 3×10^2 CFU/mL bacteria. Again, 100 μL of each dilution was plated onto the agar plates containing the series of CEQ concentrations mentioned above and incubated at 37°C overnight. Bacterial colonies that recovered growth in each dilution were counted. Drug concentrations versus the percentages of colony recovery were plotted and the interpolation method was adopted to calculate the cefquinome concentration blocking 99% bacteria growth.

The determination of MPC was similar to that of MIC_{99}. Instead, 100 μL of 10^{10} CFU/mL inoculants was spread on agar plates containing a series of antimicrobial concentrations. The lowest antimicrobial concentration preventing bacterial colony formation at 72 h after incubation was measured as provisional mutant prevention concentration (MPC_{pr}). A second determination that utilized linear MPC_{pr} decreases (about 20% per sequential decrease) was performed. MPC was the lowest CEQ concentration preventing 100% growth of *S. aureus* colony.

The calculated ratio of MPC/MIC_{99} for *S. aureus* was defined as selection index (SI) of cefquinome.

In Vitro Dynamic PK/PD Model Simulation

A previous described dynamic model (Grasso et al., 1978) with modification was developed in this study. One-compartment open model with first-order absorption of pharmacokinetics for cefquinome was simulated. The schematic representation of *in vitro* PK/PD model used is depicted in **Figure 1**. Briefly, the system was mainly composed of three sealed containers

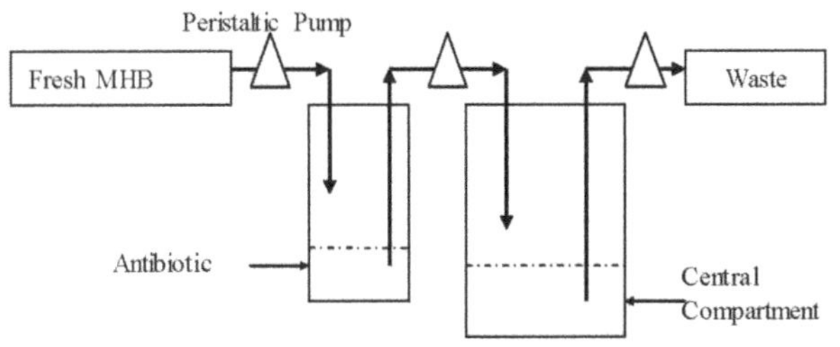

FIGURE 1 | Scheme of the *in vitro* dynamic model for bactericidal kinetics.

(compartments) and they were connected with peristaltic pumps in line, each containing sterile MHB and a magnetic stirrer to ensure adequate mixing. One 500 mL sealed compartment containing 300 mL MHB, provided with either a bacterial culture alone (control growth experiments) or a bacterial culture plus antibiotic (killing/re-growth experiments), acted as the central chamber. Another 100 mL sealed container charged with 60 mL of sterile MHB, acted as the absorption chamber, with desired calculated drug concentrations. The third one was used to provide fresh MHB. Waste was also collected. Peristaltic pumps circulated fresh broth to central and absorption compartments at the desired flow rate. The flow rate of the pump was set on the basis of the terminal half-life being simulated. A series of dosage regimens were designed to generate different CEQ concentration profiles with terminal half-lives of 3 and 6 h for three consecutive administrations in this apparatus.

In Vitro PK/PD Model and CEQ Dosing Regimens

The apparatus ran under 37°C. The elimination terminal half-lives of cefquinome reported in the literature varied from 0.5 to 10 h (Limbert et al., 1991; Li et al., 2008; Al-Taher, 2010; Tohamy, 2011; Yuan et al., 2011; Zonca et al., 2011; Dumka et al., 2013), therefore, 3 and 6 h were selected in our study. Peristaltic pumps circulated fresh MHB medium to and from the central compartment at a flow rate of 15.75 r/min for $t_{1/2\beta}$ of 3 h or 7.86 r/min for $t_{1/2\beta}$ of 6 h, respectively. 3 mL bacterial suspensions (10^8 CFU/mL) at the logarithmic phase were injected into the central compartment container. The bacteria were incubated in the model for 2 h to result in exponentially growing cultures before addition of cefquinome. Antibiotic doses were calculated to generate CEQ initial concentrations of 1/2MIC, MIC, 2MIC, 4MIC, 8MIC, and 16MIC levels, respectively. The *in vitro* pharmacokinetics of cefquinome for all doses after three consecutive administrations with 24 h interval for terminal half-lives of 3 and 6 h were simulated.

Quantification of Cefquinome in MHB

Samples were collected from the central compartment immediately before and at 0.5, 1.0, 2.0, 3.0, 4.0, 6.0, 8.0, 10.0, 12.0, and 24.0 h after the first and second administration, and 0.5, 1.0, 2.0, 3.0, 4.0, 6.0, 8.0, 10.0, 12.0, 24.0, 30.0, 36.0, and 48.0 h after the third administration. These samples were stored at −20°C until analysis.

1.5 mL of MHB was extracted for the determination of cefquinome. The concentrations of cefquinome in MHB were analyzed by high-performance liquid chromatography-MS/MS (HPLC-MS/MS) with an assay range of 0.005–0.5 μg/mL. The protein in MHB sample (1 mL) was precipitated by 2 mL acetonitrile, and the supernatant was directly injected into HPLC-MS/MS after high speed centrifugation. Analysis of quality control (QC) samples at three levels (0.01, 0.05, 0.2 μg/mL) showed that the recoveries of the method were above 70%; the intra-day and inter-day coefficients of variation were within 15%. The pharmacokinetic parameters were calculated by a WinNonlin software (version 5.2.1; Pharsight Corporation, USA).

In Vitro Time-Kill Experiments and Susceptibility Testing of *S. aureus*

To measure the antimicrobial effect of cefquinome with different terminal half-lives against *S. aureus*, the colony count and susceptibility of bacteria in each time point were performed after treatment. Half of each sample was subjected to time-kill kinetic assays. Samples (100 μL) in series of 10-fold dilution with sterile saline (0.9% NaCl) were spread onto Mueller-Hinton agar to determine the number of total or resistant cells. The $\log_{10}$ of surviving *S. aureus* cells (CFU/mL) was plotted against each time point. The other half of each sample was used for the susceptibility test. MIC values of bacteria post-exposed in each time point was conducted using tube dilution method according to the criteria established by the Clinical Laboratory Standards Institute [CLSI] (2013).

Pharmacokinetic/Pharmacodynamic (PK/PD) Integration Analysis

By using the individual pharmacokinetic result from each *in vitro* dosage regimen, the following PK/PD parameters were obtained: ratio of area under the curve of cefquinome concentration versus time to MIC ($AUC_{0-\infty}$/MIC) or ($AUC_{0-24\ h}$/MIC), ratio of area under the curve of cefquinome concentration exceeding MIC to MIC ($AUC_{C\ >\ MIC}$/MIC), time of concentration above MIC (T > MIC) or MPC (T > MPC), time of concentration within MPC and MIC (T_{MSW}) or expressed as percentage (T_{MSW}%), ratio of MIC_{72} to $MIC_{initial}$ ($MIC_{72}/MIC_{initial}$).

Gaussian function was used to simulate the correlation of $MIC_{72\ h}/MIC_{initial}$ with T_{MSW}% (percentage of the time during which cefquinome concentrations were inside the MSW). The formula was as follows:

$$y = y_0 + \frac{A}{\sqrt{2\pi}\sigma} e^{-\frac{(x-x_0)^2}{2\sigma^2}}$$

where A was the area under curve and upper baseline; x_0 was the minimum value of T_{MSW}% which resulted in the maximum $MIC_{72\ h}/MIC_{initial}$.

RESULTS

MIC_{99} and MPC

The MIC_{99} and MPC of cefquinome against *S. aureus* ATCC 25923 were 0.4 and 4.096 μg/mL, respectively. So the SI was 10.24 (MPC/MIC_{99}).

In Vitro Simulated Pharmacokinetics

The *in vitro* simulated time-concentration curves for cefquinome with terminal half-lives of 3 and 6 h are shown in **Figure 2**. This study used time-concentration curves of the unbound fractions of cefquinome in Mueller-Hinton broth. The maximum concentrations were approximately equal to 1/2MIC to 16-fold MIC of cefquinome against *S. aureus* ATCC 25923 after three

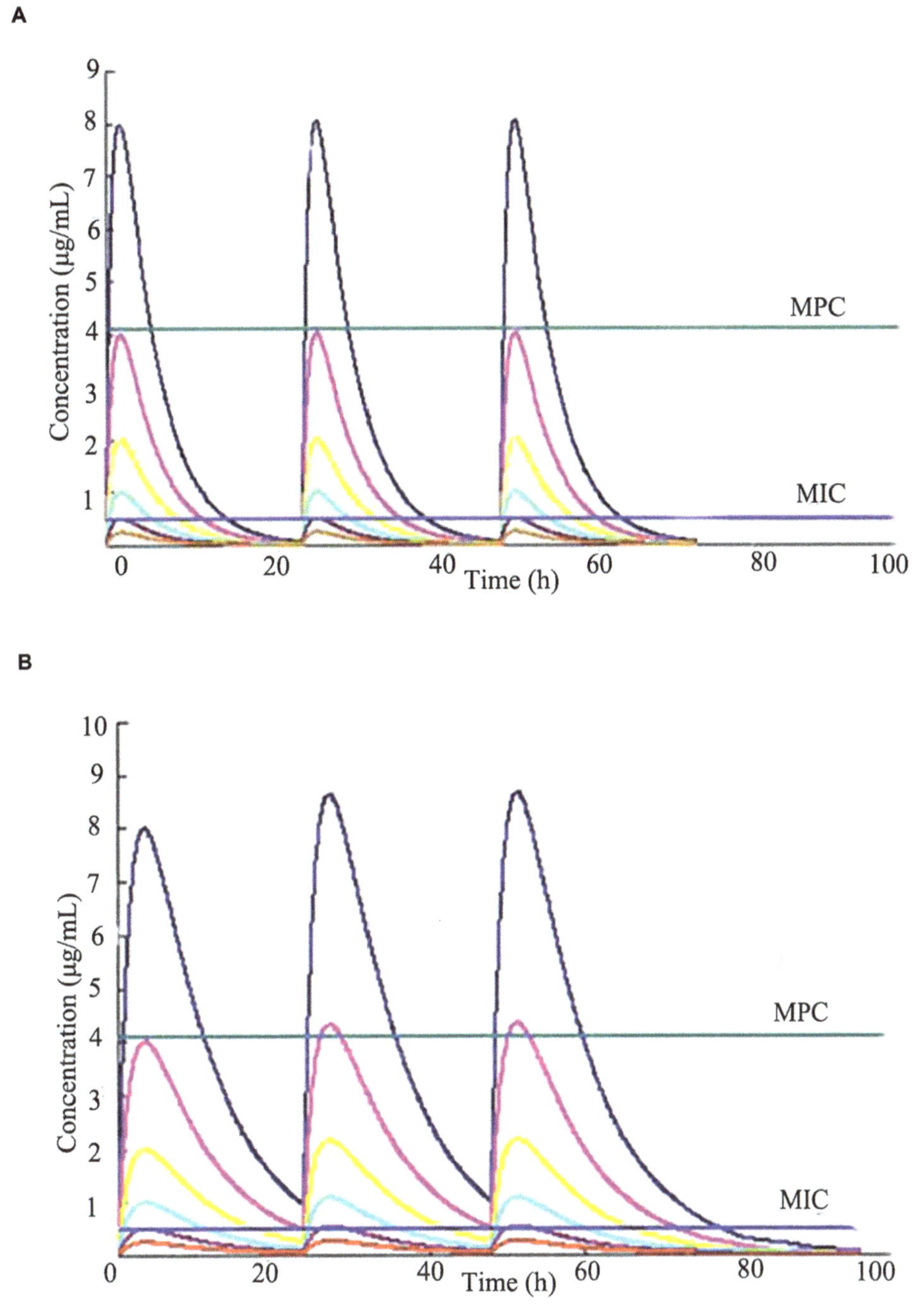

FIGURE 2 | Concentration-time curves of cefquinome in the *in vitro* pharmacokinetics model of two terminal half-lives ($t_{1/2\beta}$). The horizontal lines indicate the MPC (4.096 µg/mL) and MIC (0.4 µg/mL) for *Staphylococcus aureus* ATCC 25923, respectively. **(A)** $t_{1/2\beta} = 3$ h, **(B)** $t_{1/2\beta} = 6$ h.

consecutive administrations. The MPC and MIC levels were also indicated in the simulated time-concentration curves.

The Bacteria Killing Curves in *In Vitro* Models

Time-killing curves of *S. aureus* ATCC 25923 in the *in vitro* model under different dosing regimens are shown in the following **Figure 3**. For a $t_{1/2\beta}$ of 3 h multiple dosages, bacteriostatic or bactericidal action was observed when maximum cefquinome concentrations were equal to MIC or over MIC levels (dosages ranged from 0.672 to 10.767 mg). For a $t_{1/2\beta}$ of 6 h multiple dosages, continuous bactericidal action was observed when maximum cefquinome concentrations were at 4MIC, 8MIC, 16MIC (dose ranged from 2.691 to 10.767 mg), and the continuous time of bactericidal action at 16MIC was the longest among three concentrations.

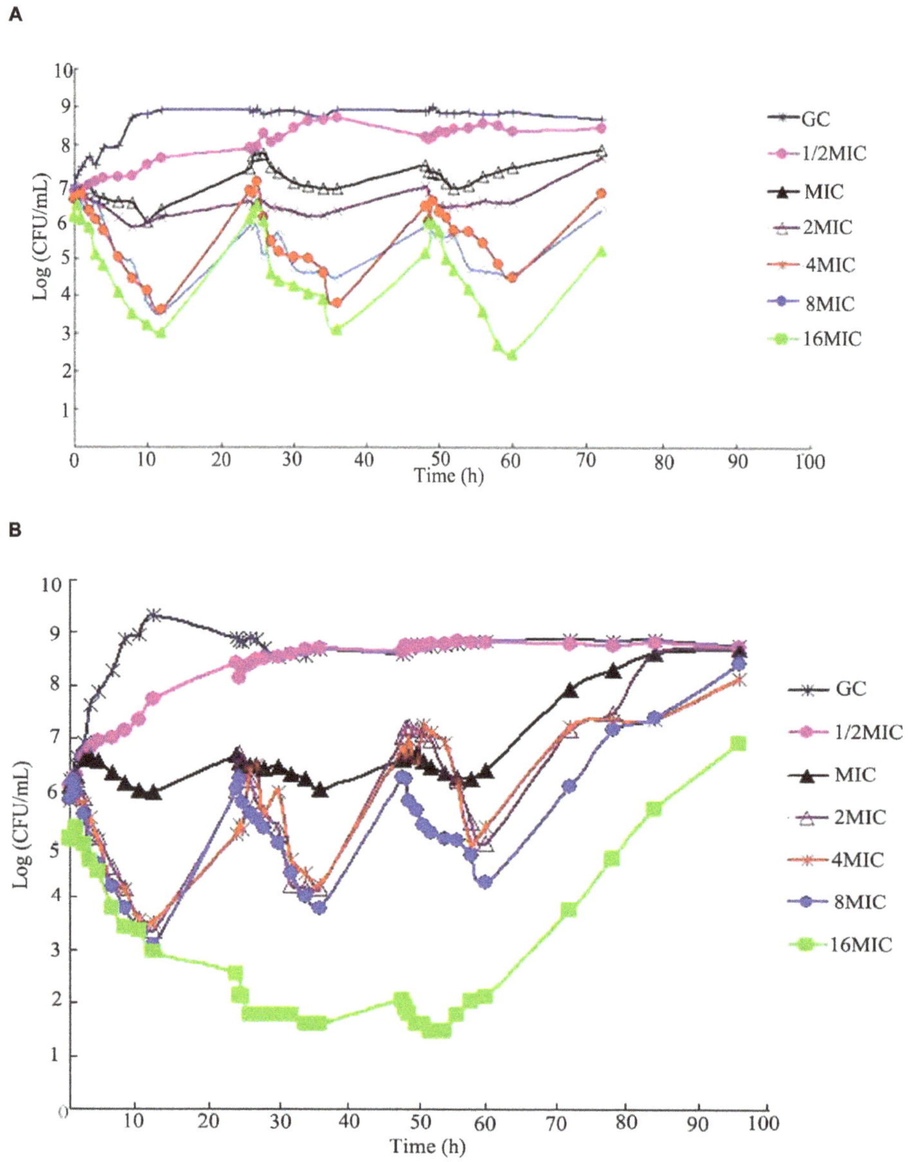

FIGURE 3 | Viable counts of *S. aureus* ATCCC 25923 in time-kill assays with cefquinome in different terminal half-lives ($t_{1/2\beta}$) at cefquinome concentrations from a half to 16-fold the minimum inhibitory concentration (MIC), in comparison with a cefquinome-free control. (A) $t_{1/2\beta} = 3$ h, **(B)** $t_{1/2\beta} = 6$ h.

Loss of Susceptibility to Cefquinome

Compared to drug-free group, loss of susceptibility was observed in MIC, 2MIC, and 4MIC concentration groups after administrations, as shown in **Figure 4**. For multiple dosages with $t_{1/2\beta}$ of 3 h, the bacterial MICs after administration increased to 4.0, 8.0, and 1.0 μg/mL for MIC, 2MIC, and 4MIC groups, respectively. For multiple dosages with $t_{1/2\beta}$ of 6 h, the bacterial MICs after administration increased to 2.0, 4.0, and 0.8 μg/mL for MIC, and 2MIC, and 4MIC concentration administrations, respectively. The MIC values did not change through the whole experiment period in 8MIC and 16MIC administration groups with two different terminal half-lives.

Correlation of PK/PD Indices with Resistance Selection

Pharmacokinetic/pharmacodynamic indices, such as $AUC_{24\ h}$/MIC (where AUC_{24h} is the area under the drug concentration time curve in a 24 h interval) and time above the MIC, provide an empirical way to relate antimicrobial dose to favor the treatment effect of bactericidal agents. Relationships between PK/PD indices and loss of susceptibility are shown in **Table 1**. For cephalosporin, T > MIC was the index most commonly associated with restricting susceptible cell growth. When T > MIC attained 17.14 h or T > MIC% attained 24%, the MIC value of cefquinome against *S. aureus* increased to

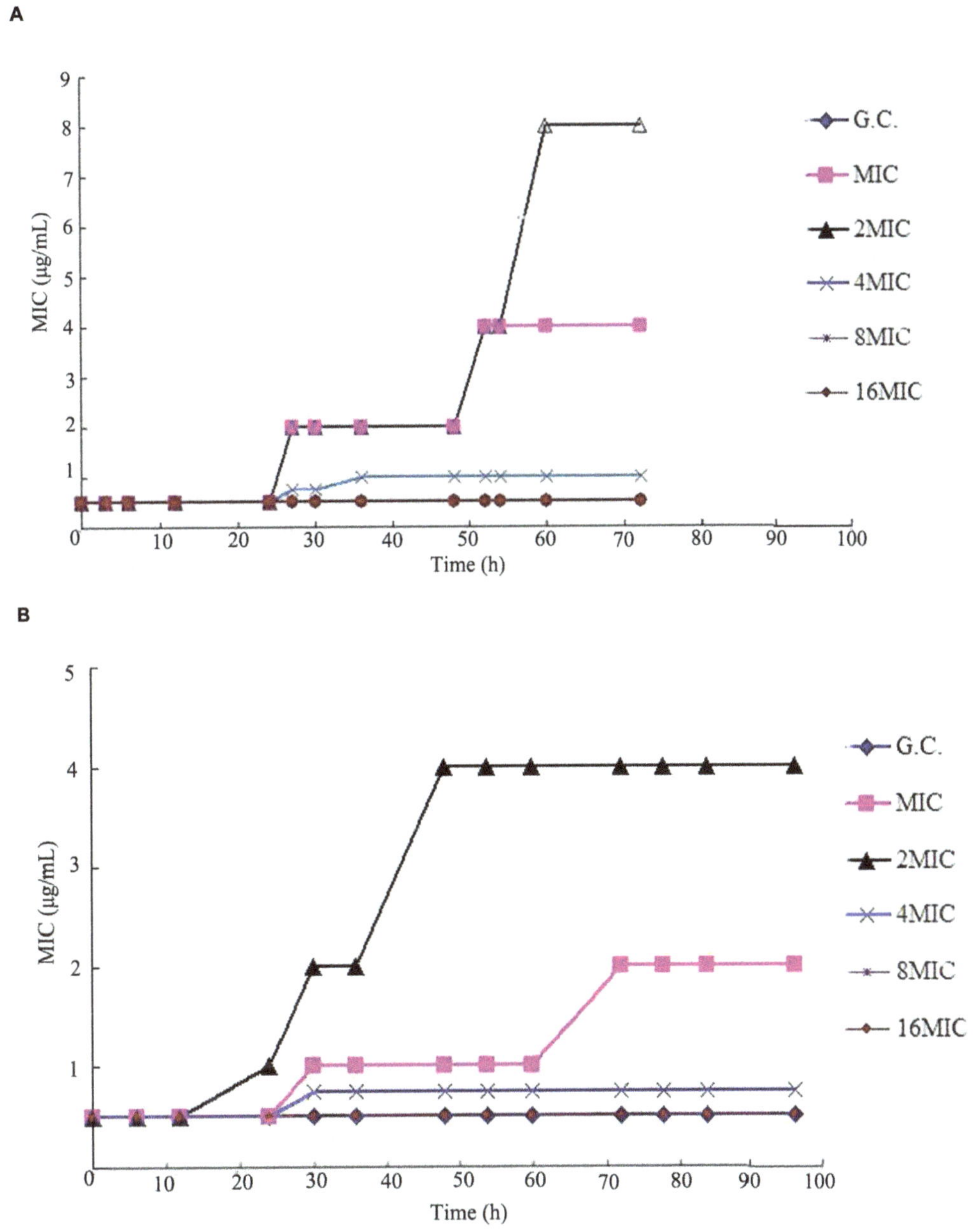

FIGURE 4 | Typical susceptibility responses of *S. aureus* ATCCC 25923 observed in the *in vitro* PK/PD model simulating the pharmacokinetics of cefquinome with different terminal half-lives ($t_{1/2\beta}$). (A) $t_{1/2\beta} = 3$ h, **(B)** $t_{1/2\beta} = 6$ h.

16-fold of initial value at 72 h after multiple administrations in groups with $t_{1/2\beta}$ of 3 h. Similarly, in groups with $t_{1/2\beta}$ of 6 h, when T > MIC = 34.28 h or T > MIC% = 48%, the value of cefquinome MIC increased to eightfold of initial value after multiple dosages.

Other PK/PD indices also showed correlation with the selection of resistance (**Table 1**). When T_{MSW} and T_{MSW}% were 17.14 h and 24%, the MIC increased to 16-fold of initial value in groups with $t_{1/2\beta}$ of 3 h after multiple dosages, and the MIC increased to eightfold of initial value When T_{MSW} and T_{MSW}% were 34.28 h and 48% with $t_{1/2\beta}$ of 6 h after multiple dosages, respectively.

Correlation Analysis of MIC Increase with T_{MSW}%

According to Gaussian function and regression analysis results, the bacteria was prone to develop resistance when T_{MSW}% was about 20% (x_0 = 0.2027) in groups with $t_{1/2\beta}$ of 3 h after multiple dosages (R^2 = 0.9989), and T_{MSW}% was

TABLE 1 | Pharmacokinetic/pharmacodynamic (PK/PD) indices of antimicrobial efficacy and risk of resistance selection amongst *Staphylococcus aureus* ATCC 25923 over the complete dosing interval following PK simulations of three consecutive administrations of cefquinome in $t_{1/2\beta}$ of 3 and 6 h.

$t_{1/2\beta}$(h)	D (mg)	$\frac{AUC_{C\geq MIC}}{MIC}$ (h)	$\frac{AUC_{24}}{MIC}$ (h)	T > MIC (h)	T > MPC (h)	T_{MSW} (h)	T_{MSW}%	T > MIC%	$\frac{MIC_{72}}{MIC_{initial}}$
3	1/2MIC	0	3.22	0	0	0	0	0	1
	MIC	6.41	6.43	8.11	0	8.11	11	11	8
	2MIC	25.89	12.89	17.14	0	17.14	24	24	16
	4MIC	64.68	25.76	26.13	0	26.13	36	36	2
	8MIC	142.34	51.52	35.13	7.81	27.32	38	49	1
	16MIC	297.75	103.07	44.14	16.82	27.32	38	61	1
6	1/2MIC	0	5.96	0	0	0	0	0	1
	MIC	12.81	11.92	16.21	0	16.21	23	23	4
	2MIC	51.77	23.89	34.28	0	34.28	48	48	8
	4MIC	129.35	47.73	52.26	0	52.26	73	73	1.5
	8MIC	284.68	95.45	70.26	15.63	54.64	76	98	1
	16MIC	595.50	190.96	88.28	33.64	54.64	76	123	1

about 40% (x_0 = 0.4102) in groups with $t_{1/2\beta}$ of 6 h after multiple dosages (R^2 = 0.9986), respectively, as shown in **Figure 5**. Those results were consistent with the data from **Table 1**.

DISCUSSION

Antimicrobial resistance has been a global problem and a great number of strategies have been proposed to slow the emergence of resistance (Stratton, 2003; Levy and Marshall, 2004). *In vivo* or *in vitro* PK/PD models have previously been applied to optimize the dosage regimen of various antibiotics in the literature (Croisier et al., 2004b; Ferran et al., 2009; Andraud et al., 2011; Gebru et al., 2012). However, PK/PD model has been renewably used to investigate relationship of bacterial resistance with AUC/MIC, C_{max}/MIC and T > MIC, recently. In the present study, we simulated the cefquinome pharmacokinetic profiles with different terminal half-lives using this dynamic model and tried to predict the selection of resistant *S. aureus* with some indices, such as T > MIC and T_{MSW}%.

It is believed that integration of drug pharmacokinetics, mutant prevention concentration is helpful in slowing the emergence of resistance. In this experiment, the MPC and MSW of cefquinome against *S. aureus* ATCC25923 were determined. The SI, ratio of MPC to MIC_{99}, is the ability of a drug to select resistant mutants (Zhao and Drlica, 2001). In other word, the bigger the SI is, the easier the drug is to induce resistance. The SI of cefquinome against *S. aureus* ATCC25923 was 10.24 in our study, which suggested that cefquinome could induce *S. aureus* resistant mutation easily and effectively.

T > MIC was regarded as a promising predictor for the efficacy of cephalosporins. Previous pharmacodynamic studies have addressed separate issues around the relationships between T > MIC and efficacy for cephalosporins. Craig (1995) has reviewed the data of efficacy for cephalosporins against *Enterbacteriaceae*, *streptococci* and *S. aureus* in several animal infection models and found that the time above MIC required for a bacteriostatic effect against strains of *Enterbacteriaceae*, *Streptococci* were generally 60–70%, and 40–50% for *S. aureus*, respectively. In our study, the value of T > MIC for maximal killing was 40~60% for cefquinome against *S. aureus* reference strain. In consistent with the widespread idea that antibacterial efficacy of β-lactams depend on T > MIC, the effect of cefquinome against *S. aureus* in our study exhibited similar correlation. As observed in **Figure 3**, killing curves of *S. aureus* exposed to each dose of cefquinome showed the typical pattern of time-dependent bactericidal action. The similar observation was also reported for other β-lactam drugs in previous studies (Lindecrona et al., 2000; Burgess and Hall, 2004). Considering that the T > MIC was one of the most important parameters for optimal dosage regimen, T > MIC was selected as a parameter to evaluate resistant mutation in this article. In the present study, the values of T > MIC ranging from 8.11 to 17.14 h were dangerous zones for inducing resistant mutation in groups with $t_{1/2\beta}$ of 3 h after multiple dosages, and values ranging from 16.21 to 34.28 h were dangerous zones for inducing resistant mutation in groups with $t_{1/2\beta}$ of 6 h multiple dosages. Compared these values with previously reported study data that T > MIC value ranged from 42 to 54 h for cefquinome in dairy cows (Zonca et al., 2011), the prevention of selecting resistant *S. aureus* strains seems to be achieved by the present dosage regimens approved by the European Medicines Agency (EMA) for the treatment of dairy cow mastitis.

T_{MSW} is another important parameter used for evaluating resistant mutation. A previous study conducted in a rabbit lung infection model with *Streptococcus pneumonia* showed that the selection of resistant bacteria occurred systematically when concentrations of gatifloxacin were within the MSW (T_{MSW}) for more than 45% of the treatment duration (Croisier et al., 2004b). Another experiment in rabbits infected by *S. aureus* also showed that time in the MSW > 33% was preferable to select mutants (Cui et al., 2006). When the abilities of the indices T_{MSW}, $AUC_{24\ h}$/MIC, C_{max}/MIC to predict the selection of resistant bacteria were compared, only T_{MSW} appeared to be a good predictor of the prevention of resistance (Ferran et al., 2009). In this study, T_{MSW} was also used to predict selection of

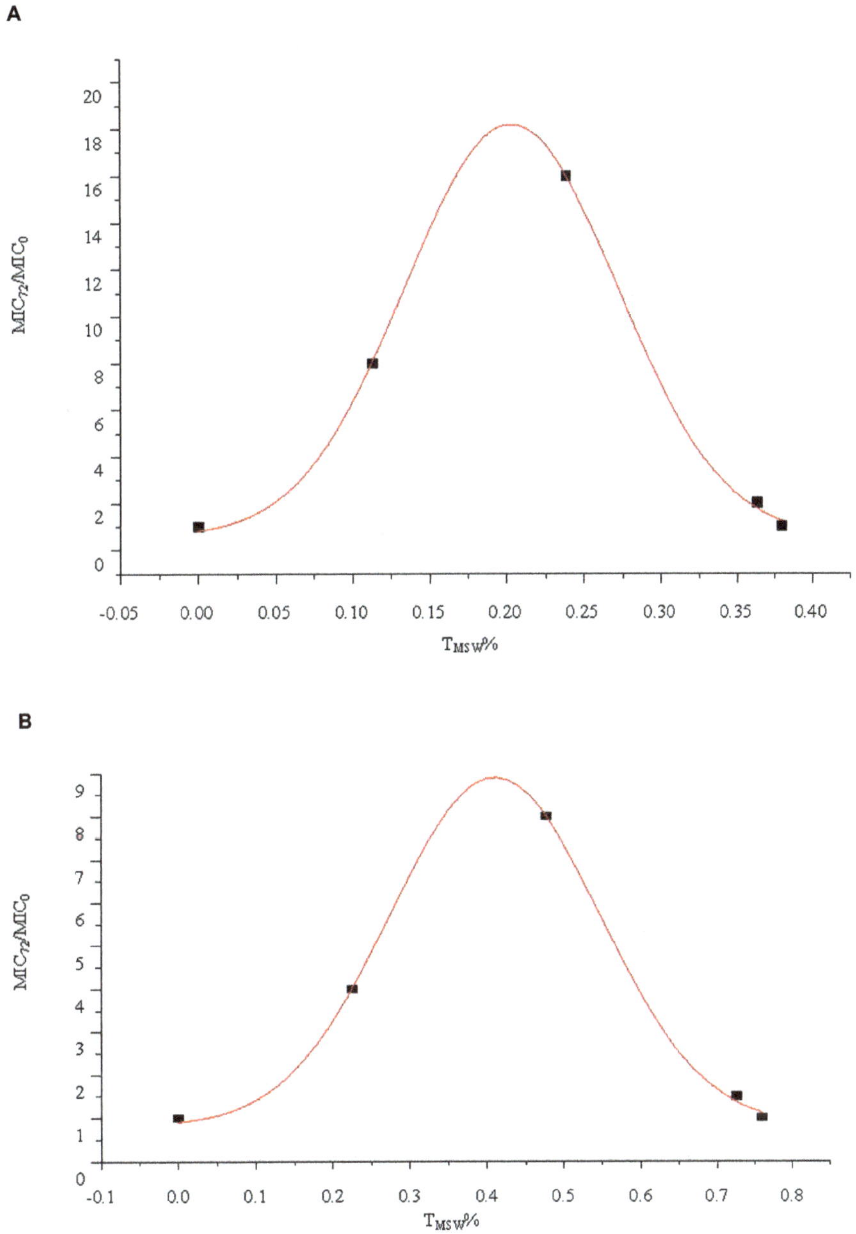

FIGURE 5 | Relationship between the $T_{MSW}\%$ and MIC_{72}/MIC_0 for *S. aureus* ATCC 25293 exposed to cefquinome in the *in vitro* model with two terminal half-lives ($t_{1/2\beta}$). (A) $t_{1/2\beta} = 3$ h, **(B)** $t_{1/2\beta} = 6$ h.

resistant *S. aureus* against cefquinome. It was clearly determined that when T_{MSW} was above 36% in groups with $t_{1/2\beta}$ of 3 h after multiple dosages or above 73% in groups with $t_{1/2\beta}$ of 6 h after multiple dosages, cefquinome could restrict the resistant mutation.

In the present investigation, the bacterial resistant mutation was affected by different terminal half-lives and dosages. Within the group of the same terminal half-life (3 or 6 h), the bacterial resistant mutation happened under the condition of relative low dosage (maximum concentrations were 2MIC and 4MIC). When the maximum concentration was over 8MIC, resistant mutation was prevented. In the same dosages (maximum concentration was 2MIC or 4MIC), the $MIC_{72\ h}$ increased from 8- to 16-fold in groups with $t_{1/2\beta}$ of 3 h after multiple dosages and increased from 4- to 8-fold in groups with $t_{1/2\beta}$ of 6 h after multiple dosages, respectively. Those results suggested that the bacterial resistant mutation might happen at a low concentration. In high dosages or long terminal half-lives, the drug concentrations might exceed the MPC value, the upper boundary of MSW, and the resistant mutation could be inhibited. The conclusion from this study was consistent with other similar studies (Cui et al., 2006; Ferran et al., 2009; Zhu et al., 2012).

The limitation of the study was that only one reference strain was used to simulate the efficacy of cefquinome in this *in vitro* model; however, the multi-resistance is becoming an urgent trend all over the world. It may be reasonable that more clinical isolates of *S. aureus* could be used for further study. Firsov et al. (2008) used two methicillin-resistant strains of *S. aureus*, ATCC 6538 and ATCC 43300, to study the enrichment of ciprofloxacin resistant mutation in an *in vitro* dynamic model. Liang et al. (2011), chose three clinical isolates of *S. aureus*, SA99, RN450 and RN450-A1, to analyze the enrichment of levofloxacin resistant mutation with *in vitro* dynamic model. From the results obtained in the dynamic model, more clinical isolates could be used to study resistant mutation easily based on the substantial method. Moreover, to our knowledge, evaluation of antimicrobial activity for cefquinome with different terminal half-lives is scarce. Considering the fact that cefquinome is the time-dependent drug, it is positive to study the correlation resistant mutation with different terminal half-life conditions. Another limitation of the current study was the absence of resistance mechanisms of *S. aureus* observed *in vitro*. Therefore, the pattern of *S. aureus* resistant to cefquinome, such as production of β-lactamases, alteration of drug targets, porin-mediated resistance, and/or efflux-mediated resistance, needs confirmation in the further study.

CONCLUSION

The present study of resistant mutation with *S aureus* ATCC 25923 exposed to cefquinome with two different terminal half-lives in *in vitro* dynamic models supports the MSW hypothesis and provides some useful parameters to predict the resistant mutation, especially T > MIC and T_{MSW}%. Further study will concentrate on more clinical isolates which could be used for verification of these results and resistance patterns of *S. aureus* resistant to cefquinome.

AUTHOR CONTRIBUTIONS

All authors listed, have made substantial, direct and intellectual contribution to the work, and approved it for publication.

ACKNOWLEDGMENTS

The authors would like to thank the financial support by the Natural Science Foundation of China (grant number 31172366) and 973 program (grant number 2013CB127200/ 2013CB127203).

REFERENCES

Allen, G. P., and Hankins, C. D. (2009). Evaluation of the mutant selection window for fluoroquinolones against *Neisseria gonorrhoeae. J. Antimicrob. Chemother.* 64, 359–363. doi: 10.1093/jac/dkp172

Allen, G. P., Kaatz, G. W., and Rybak, M. J. (2004). In vitro activities of mutant prevention concentration-targeted concentrations of fluoroquinolones against *Staphylococcus aureus* in a pharmacodynamic model. *Int. J. Antimicrob. Agents* 24, 150–160. doi: 10.1016/j.ijantimicag.2004.03.011

Al-Taher, A. (2010). Pharmacokinetics of cefquinome in camels. *J. Animal Vet. Adv.* 9, 848–852. doi: 10.3923/javaa.2010.848.852

Andraud, M., Chauvin, C., Sanders, P., and Laurentie, M. (2011). Pharmacodynamic modeling of in vitro activity of marbofloxacin against *Escherichia coli* strains. *Antimicrob. Agents Chemother.* 55, 756–761. doi: 10.1128/AAC.00865-10

Archer, G. L. (1998). *Staphylococcus aureus*: a well-armed pathogen. *Clin. Infect. Dis.* 26, 1179–1181. doi: 10.1086/520289

Azizoglu, R. O., Lyman, R., and Anderson, K. L. (2013). Bovine *Staphylococcus aureus*: dose response to iodine and chlorhexidine and effect of iodine challenge on antibiotic susceptibility. *J. Dairy Sci.* 96, 993–999. doi: 10.3168/jds.2012-5857

Blondeau, J., Borsos, S., Blondeau, L., Blondeau, B., and Hesje, C. (2012). Comparative minimum inhibitory and mutant prevention drug concentrations of enrofloxacin, ceftiofur, florfenicol, tilmicosin and tulathromycin against bovine clinical isolates of *Mannheimia haemolytica. Vet. Microbiol.* 160, 85–90. doi: 10.1016/j.vetmic.2012.05.006

Bronner, S., Murbach, V., Peter, J.-D., Levêque, D., Elkhaïli, H., Salmon, Y., et al. (2002). Ex vivo pharmacodynamics of amoxicillin-clavulanate against β-lactamase-producing *Escherichia coli* in a *Yucatan miniature* pig model that mimics human pharmacokinetics. *Antimicrob. Agents Chemother.* 46, 3782–3789. doi: 10.1128/AAC.46.12.3782-3789.2002

Burgess, D. S., and Hall, R. G. II, (2004). In vitro killing of parenteral beta-lactams against standard and high inocula of extended-spectrum beta-lactamase and non-esbl producing *Klebsiella pneumoniae. Diagn. Microbiol. Infect. Dis.* 49, 41–46. doi: 10.1016/j.diagmicrobio.2003.11.007

Cavaco, L., Abatih, E., Aarestrup, F. M., and Guardabassi, L. (2008). Selection and persistence of CTX-M-producing *Escherichia coli* in the intestinal flora of pigs treated with amoxicillin, ceftiofur, or cefquinome. *Antimicrob. Agents Chemother.* 52, 3612–3616. doi: 10.1128/AAC.00354-08

Clinical Laboratory Standards Institute (CLSI) (2013). *Performance Standards for Antimicrobial Disk, and Dilution Susceptibility Tests for Bacteria Isolated From Animals*, Approved Standard-Fourth Edn. Wayne, PA: Clinical Laboratory Standards Institute.

Craig, W. A. (1995). Interrelationship between pharmacokinetics and pharmacodynamics in determining dosage regimens for broad-spectrum cephalosporins. *Diagn. Microbiol. Infect. Dis.* 22, 89–96. doi: 10.1016/0732-8893(95)00053-D

Croisier, D., Etienne, M., Bergoin, E., Charles, P.-E., Lequeu, C., Piroth, L., et al. (2004a). Mutant selection window in levofloxacin and moxifloxacin treatments of experimental pneumococcal pneumonia in a rabbit model of human therapy. *Antimicrob. Agents Chemother.* 48, 1699–1707. doi: 10.1128/AAC.48.5.1699-1707.2004

Croisier, D., Etienne, M., Piroth, L., Bergoin, E., Lequeu, C., Portier, H., et al. (2004b). In vivo pharmacodynamic efficacy of gatifloxacin against *Streptococcus pneumoniae* in an experimental model of pneumonia: impact of the low levels of fluoroquinolone resistance on the enrichment of resistant mutants. *J. Antimicrob. Chemother.* 54, 640–647. doi: 10.1093/jac/dkh393

Cui, J., Liu, Y., Wang, R., Tong, W., Drlica, K., and Zhao, X. (2006). The mutant selection window in rabbits infected with *Staphylococcus aureus. J. Infect. Dis.* 194, 1601–1608. doi: 10.1086/508752

Dong, Y., Zhao, X., Domagala, J., and Drlica, K. (1999). Effect of fluoroquinolone concentration on selection of resistant mutants of *Mycobacterium bovis* BCG and *Staphylococcus aureus. Antimicrob. Agents Chemother.* 43, 1756–1758.

Dumka, V. K., Dinakaran, V., Ranjan, B., and Rampal, S. (2013). Comparative pharmacokinetics of cefquinome following intravenous and intramuscular administration in goats. *Small Ruminant Res.* 113, 273–277. doi: 10.1016/j.smallrumres.2013.02.010

Ferran, A., Dupouy, V., Toutain, P.-L., and Bousquet-Mélou, A. (2007). Influence of inoculum size on the selection of resistant mutants of *Escherichia coli* in relation to mutant prevention concentrations of marbofloxacin. *Antimicrob. Agents Chemother.* 51, 4163–4166. doi: 10.1128/AAC.00156-07

Ferran, A. A., Kesteman, A.-S., Toutain, P.-L., and Bousquet-Mélou, A. (2009). Pharmacokinetic/pharmacodynamic analysis of the influence of inoculum size on the selection of resistance in *Escherichia coli* by a quinolone in a mouse thigh bacterial infection model. *Antimicrob. Agents Chemother.* 53, 3384–3390. doi: 10.1128/AAC.01347-08

Firsov, A. A., Lubenko, I. Y., Smirnova, M. V., Strukova, E. N., and Zinner, S. H. (2008). Enrichment of fluoroquinolone-resistant *Staphylococcus aureus*: oscillating ciprofloxacin concentrations simulated at the upper and lower portions of the mutant selection window. *Antimicrob. Agents Chemother.* 52, 1924–1928. doi: 10.1128/AAC.01371-07

Gebru, E., Damte, D., Choi, M.-J., Lee, S.-J., Kim, Y.-H., and Park, S. C. (2012). Mutant prevention concentration and phenotypic and molecular basis of fluoroquinolone resistance in clinical isolates and in vitro-selected mutants of *Escherichia coli* from dogs. *Vet. Microbiol.* 154, 384–394. doi: 10.1016/j.vetmic.2011.07.033

Grasso, S., Meinardi, G., De Carneri, I., and Tamassia, V. (1978). New in vitro model to study the effect of antibiotic concentration and rate of elimination on antibacterial activity. *Antimicrob. Agents Chemother.* 13, 570–576. doi: 10.1128/AAC.13.4.570

Guardabassi, L., Schwarz, S., and Lloyd, D. H. (2004). Pet animals as reservoirs of antimicrobial-resistant bacteria review. *J. Antimicrob. Chemother.* 54, 321–332. doi: 10.1093/jac/dkh332

Harris, S. R., Feil, E. J., Holden, M. T., Quail, M. A., Nickerson, E. K., Chantratita, N., et al. (2010). Evolution of MRSA during hospital transmission and intercontinental spread. *Science* 327, 469–474. doi: 10.1126/science.1182395

Le Loir, Y., Baron, F., and Gautier, M. (2003). *Staphylococcus aureus* and food poisoning. *Genet. Mol. Res.* 2, 63–76.

Levy, S. B., and Marshall, B. (2004). Antibacterial resistance worldwide: causes, challenges and responses. *Nat. Med.* 10, S122–S129. doi: 10.1038/nm1145

Li, X., Wu, W., Su, D., Wang, Z., Jiang, H., and Shen, J. (2008). Pharmacokinetics and bioavailability of cefquinome in healthy piglets. *J. Vet. Pharmacol. Ther.* 31, 523–527. doi: 10.1111/j.1365-2885.2008.00989.x

Liang, B., Bai, N., Cai, Y., Wang, R., Drlica, K., and Zhao, X. (2011). Mutant prevention concentration-based pharmacokinetic/pharmacodynamic indices as dosing targets for suppressing the enrichment of levofloxacin-resistant subpopulations of *Staphylococcus aureus*. *Antimicrob. Agents Chemother.* 55, 2409–2412. doi: 10.1128/AAC.00975-10

Limbert, M., Isert, D., Klesel, N., Markus, A., Seeger, K., Seibert, G., et al. (1991). Antibacterial activities in vitro and in vivo and pharmacokinetics of cefquinome (HR 111V), a new broad-spectrum cephalosporin. *Antimicrob. Agents Chemother.* 35, 14–19. doi: 10.1128/AAC.35.1.14

Lindecrona, R., Friis, C., and Aarestrup, F. M. (2000). The pharmacodynamic effect of amoxicillin and danofloxacin against *Salmonella typhimurium* in an in-vitro pharmacodynamic model. *Res. Vet. Sci.* 68, 261–264. doi: 10.1053/rvsc.2000.0374

Lowy, F. D. (1998). *Staphylococcus aureus* infections. *New Engl. J. Med.* 339, 520–532. doi: 10.1056/NEJM199808203390806

Mohammed Fayaz, A., Girilal, M., Mahdy, S. A., Somsundar, S., Venkatesan, R., and Kalaichelvan, P. (2011). Vancomycin bound biogenic gold nanoparticles: a different perspective for development of anti VRSA agents. *Process Biochem.* 46, 636–641. doi: 10.1016/j.procbio.2010.11.001

Stratton, C. W. (2003). Dead bugs don't mutate: susceptibility issues in the emergence of bacterial resistance. *Emerg. Infect. Dis.* 9:10. doi: 10.3201/eid0901.020172

Tauxe, R. V. (2002). Emerging foodborne pathogens. *Int. J. Food Microbiol.* 78, 31–41. doi: 10.1016/S0168-1605(02)00232-5

Tohamy, M. (2011). Age-related intramuscular pharmacokinetics of cefquinome in sheep. *Small Ruminant Res.* 99, 72–76. doi: 10.1016/j.smallrumres.2011.03.004

Wang, L., Yuanshu, Z., Yuhan, Z., and Yingxia, L. (2010). Mutant prevention concentrations of fluoroquinolones against *Campylobacter jejuni* isolated from chicken. *Vet. Microbiol.* 144, 409–414. doi: 10.1016/j.vetmic.2010.02.020

Yuan, L., Sun, J., Wang, R., Sun, L., Zhu, L., Luo, X., et al. (2011). Pharmacokinetics and bioavailability of cefquinome in healthy ducks. *Am. J. Vet. Res.* 72, 122–126. doi: 10.2460/ajvr.72.1.122

Zhao, X., and Drlica, K. (2001). Restricting the selection of antibiotic-resistant mutants: a general strategy derived from fluoroquinolone studies. *Clin. Infect. Dis.* 33, S147–S156. doi: 10.1086/321841

Zhao, X., and Drlica, K. (2002). Restricting the selection of antibiotic-resistant mutant bacteria: measurement and potential use of the mutant selection window. *J. Infect. Dis.* 185, 561–565. doi: 10.1086/338571

Zhu, Y.-L., Hu, L.-F., Mei, Q., Cheng, J., Liu, Y.-Y., Ye, Y., et al. (2012). Testing the mutant selection window in rabbits infected with methicillin-resistant *Staphylococcus aureus* exposed to vancomycin. *J. Antimicrob. Chemother.* 67, 2700–2706. doi: 10.1093/jac/dks280

Zonca, A., Gallo, M., Locatelli, C., Carli, S., Moroni, P., Villa, R., et al. (2011). Cefquinome sulfate behavior after intramammary administration in healthy and infected cows. *J. Dairy Sci.* 94, 3455–3461. doi: 10.3168/jds.2010-4109

5

A Decade-Long Commitment to Antimicrobial Resistance Surveillance in Portugal

*Catarina M. Marinho[1,2†], Tiago Santos[1,2†], Alexandre Gonçalves[1,2], Patrícia Poeta[3,4] and Gilberto Igrejas[1,2,4]**

[1] Department of Genetics and Biotechnology, School of Life and Environment Sciences, University of Trás-os-Montes and Alto Douro, Vila Real, Portugal, [2] Functional Genomics and Proteomics Unit, University of Trás-os-Montes and Alto Douro, Vila Real, Portugal, [3] Veterinary Science Department, University of Trás-os-Montes and Alto Douro, Vila Real, Portugal, [4] UCIBIO-REQUIMTE, Faculty of Science and Technology, University Nova of Lisbon, Lisbon, Portugal

***Correspondence:**
Gilberto Igrejas
gigrejas@utad.pt

† These authors have contributed equally to this work and should be considered as first authors.

Antimicrobial resistance (AMR) is a worldwide problem with serious health and economic repercussions. Since the 1940s, underuse, overuse, and misuse of antibiotics have had a significant environmental downside. Large amounts of antibiotics not fully metabolized after use in human and veterinary medicine, and other applications, are annually released into the environment. The result has been the development and dissemination of antibiotic-resistant bacteria due to many years of selective pressure. Surveillance of AMR provides important information that helps in monitoring and understanding how resistance mechanisms develop and disseminate within different environments. Surveillance data is needed to inform clinical therapy decisions, to guide policy proposals, and to assess the impact of action plans to fight AMR. The Functional Genomics and Proteomics Unit, based at the University of Trás-os-Montes and Alto Douro in Vila Real, Portugal, has recently completed 10 years of research surveying AMR in bacteria, mainly commensal indicator bacteria such as enterococci and *Escherichia coli* from the microbiota of different animals. Samples from more than 75 different sources have been accessed, from humans to food-producing animals, pets, and wild animals. The typical microbiological workflow involved phenotypic studies followed by molecular approaches. Throughout the decade, 4,017 samples were collected and over 5,000 bacterial isolates obtained. High levels of AMR to several antimicrobial classes have been reported, including to β-lactams, glycopeptides, tetracyclines, aminoglycosides, sulphonamides, and quinolones. Multi-resistant strains, some relevant to human and veterinary medicine like extended-spectrum β-lactamase-producing *E. coli* and vancomycin-resistant enterococci, have been repeatedly isolated even in non-synanthropic animal species. Of particular relevance are reports of AMR bacteria in wildlife from natural reserves and endangered species. Future work awaits as this threatening yet unsolved problem persists.

Keywords: antimicrobial resistance, surveillance, molecular microbiology, enterococci, *Escherichia coli*, wildlife

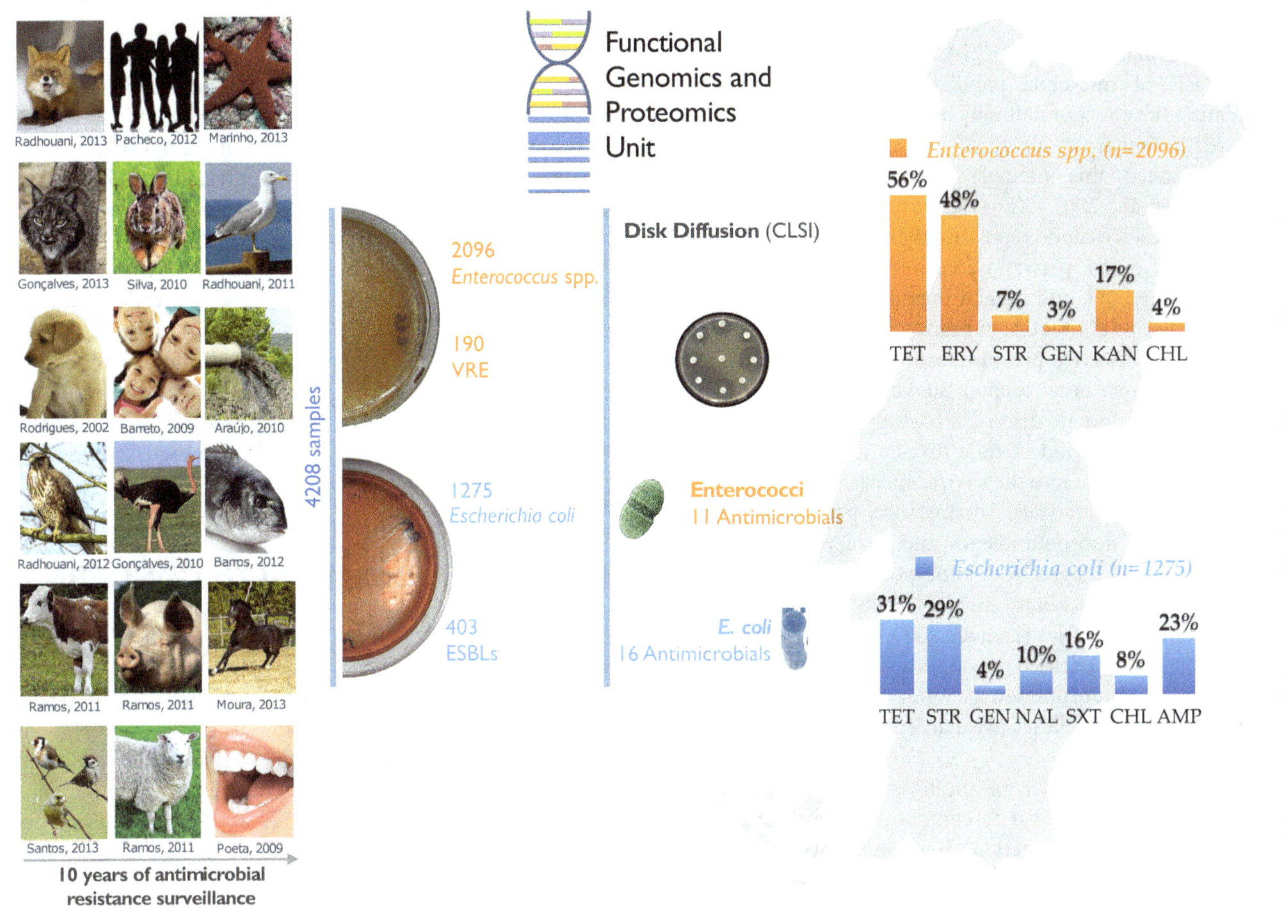

Graphical Abstract | Summary diagram of the antimicrobial resistance surveillance work developed by the UTAD Functional Genomics and Proteomics Unit.

INTRODUCTION

The early XX century witnessed the beginning of the modern antibiotic era with the first true antibiotic treatment, an asfernamina (Salvarsan) discovered by Paul Ehrlich that was successfully used to treat Syphilis (Elsner, 1910; Aminov, 2010). The reign of antibiotics in clinical practice is commonly associated with the discovery of penicillin produced by the fungus *Penicillium notatum* by Fleming (2001). However, the first wide use of antibiotics was with a sulfanamide antibiotic powder carried by Second World War soldiers with effectiveness against a wide range of infections (Davenport, 2012). The use of antibiotics to treat bacterial infections became one of the main scientific accomplishments; leading many scientists to believe that the threat of infectious diseases had ended (Jones, 1999). However, this golden age has come to an end in recent decades as we have become aware of the evolution of antibiotic resistance in bacterial strains, particularly in pathogens developing resistance to an extensive range of antibiotics (Davies and Davies, 2010).

Antibiotics are small secondary metabolites, either naturally produced by microorganisms or chemically synthetized, to mediate competition among bacterial populations and communities (Allen et al., 2010; Cordero et al., 2012). Antibiotics are commonly found in the environment in sub-inhibitory concentrations diminishing the growth rate of competing populations rather than killing them. Natural or synthetic antibiotics can also act as signal molecules regulating expression of a large number of transcripts in different bacteria. Moreover, antimicrobial compounds might target self-regulation of growth, virulence, sporulation, motility, mutagenesis, stress response, phage induction, transformation, lateral gene transfer, intrachromosomal recombination, or biofilm formation (Goh et al., 2002; Yim et al., 2007; Baquero et al., 2013).

Currently, antibiotics available for consumption are produced either by microbial fermentation, semi- or full synthetically manufactured. Antibiotics cause bacterial death or inhibit growth by different mechanisms of action: (a) disrupting cell walls, e.g., β-lactam and glycopeptides; (b) targeting the protein synthetic machinery, e.g., macrolides, chloramphenicol, tetracycline, linezolid, and aminoglycosides; (c) affecting the synthesis of nucleic acids, e.g., fluoroquinolones and rifampin; (d) inhibiting metabolic pathways, e.g., sulphonamides and folic acid analogs; or (e) disrupting the membrane structure, e.g., polymyxins and daptomycin (Sengupta et al., 2013).

Antimicrobial resistance (AMR) contributes to the homeostasis of microbial populations and communities by modulating the effect of naturally produced antibiotics (Cordero et al., 2012; Baquero et al., 2013). Human misuse of antibiotics has unbalanced this natural genetic system of resistance (Osterblad et al., 2001; Xi et al., 2009). In some developed countries, livestock alone represent about 50–80% of antibiotics consumption; crops, pets and aquaculture collectively account for an estimated 5%, and human therapy the remainder (Cully, 2014). The use of antibiotics in human and veterinary medicine exerts a major selective pressure leading to the emergence and spread of resistance because about 30–90% of antibiotics used are not metabolized and are discarded basically unchanged (Sarmah et al., 2006). The period of time that an antibiotic takes to be degraded after release into the environment might influence how it spreads and accumulates. For instance, penicillins are easily degraded, while fluoroquinolones and tetracyclines persist for longer. Direct discharges from antibiotics industries into water effluents can be shockingly high, a reality in both developed and developing countries (Li et al., 2009; Joakim Larsson, 2014). Antibiotics are also released into the environment via agricultural application of manure and sewage water as fertilizers, and leakage from waste storage facilities (Sarmah et al., 2006; Le-Minh et al., 2010; Barrett, 2012).

The high concentration of antibiotics used prophylactically by humans might have led to contamination of human waste streams and exerted selection pressure on commensal and pathogenic bacteria. It is not surprising that non-metabolized antibiotics, resistance genes and mobile genetic elements are frequently detected in wastewaters and sewage treatment plants (Pellegrini et al., 2011). Often these compounds are not removed during sewage treatment to the extent that incidences of resistance genes are used as indicators of human impact on aquatic ecosystems (Zuccato et al., 2000; Araujo et al., 2010). Although antibiotics might be considered simply as chemical pollutants, genetic mobile elements are capable of self-replication and can be transmitted horizontally even between phylogenetically distant bacteria (Gillings and Stokes, 2012). Consequently, increased concentration of antibiotics in the environment raises the diversity and the abundance of resistance genes.

The consequences of antibiotic pollution are being actively examined, and there is an imperative need for novel strategies to curtail the release of antibiotics and bacteria from human sources (Baquero et al., 2013). Furthermore, the long-term consequences of spreading antibiotics and resistance genes cannot be predicted without quantitative analysis over suitable timescales (Chee-Sanford et al., 2009). The spread of AMR into the environment occurs not only through the contamination of natural resources but also through the food chain and direct contact between human and animals.

Currently, AMR has been reported for all antibiotic classes used both in human or veterinary medicine. An association between antibiotic use and clinical AMR proliferation has also been described (Skurnik et al., 2006; Pallecchi et al., 2008). AMR is now considered a major challenge requiring urgent action in the present to prevent a worldwide catastrophe in the future.

Portugal boasts some of the most diverse fauna and flora in Europe, and in relation to its size is considered one of the 25 biodiversity hotspots of the world (Pereira et al., 2004). Its farming systems are also numerous and varied. However, Portugal is at high risk of losing this diversity. With the mission of long-term surveillance of AMR in bacteria from different sources, the Functional Genomics and Proteomics Unit, based at the University of Trás-os-Montes and Alto Douro (Vila Real, Portugal), has recently completed a decade of unceasing research. Over the years, we have investigated the resistomes of several bacteria, mainly commensal indicator bacteria such as enterococci and *Escherichia coli* sampled from the microbiota of different animals or from other sources. Here, we present an overview of the resistance profiles of these bacteria in relation to where they were found.

AMR AS A PUBLIC HEALTH CONCERN

Antimicrobial resistance has become recognized as a major clinical and public health problem (Gillings, 2013). Every year about 25,000 patients perish in the European Union (EU) because of hospital-acquired resistant bacterial infection (ECDC, 2011). Likewise, in the United States of America (USA), infections caused by antibiotic resistant bacteria are more common among the population than cancer, with at least 2 million people infected every year, at least 23,000 of whom die (CDC, 2013). Besides the clinical consequences of AMR, there are also large societal costs. The number of new antibiotics coming to the market over the past three decades has dramatically declined as several pharmaceutical companies stopped searching for antibiotics in favor of other antimicrobial drugs (Spellberg et al., 2004; Walsh, 2013). When antimicrobial drugs are discovered and developed, it is imperative to understand and predict how resistance mechanisms might evolve in order to find a method to control dissemination (Walsh, 2013). Genome-scale research may offer insight into unknown mechanisms of AMR (Tenover, 2006; Rossolini and Thaller, 2010). This will then inform decisions on appropriate policies, surveillance, and control strategies. The ideal AMR surveillance system should be able to track long-term antibiotic resistance trends, regularly alert healthcare professionals to novel resistance profiles, identify emerging resistance patterns, and create an easy-access database for physicians and scientists (Jones, 1999). To avoid a crisis, governments must recognize the importance of this valuable resource and implement a wiser and more careful use of antibiotics, raising everyone's awareness of this issue.

Investigating the zoonotic AMR problem in its full complexity requires the collection of many types of data. Identifying the most efficient points at which intervention can control AMR mainly depends on quality collaboration between all the stakeholders involved (Wegener, 2012). The One Health concept is a universal strategy for improving connections between stakeholders in all aspects of health for humans, animals and the environment. The aim is that the synergism achieved between interdisciplinary collaborations will push forward healthcare, accelerate biomedical research breakthroughs, increase the effectiveness of public health, extend scientific knowledge and improve clinical care. When properly implemented, millions of lives can be protected and saved in the near future (Pappaioanou and Spencer, 2008). The One Health initiative is therefore an ideal framework for addressing zoonotic transmission of AMR bacteria by monitoring and managing agricultural activities, food safety professionals, human and animal clinicians, environment and wildlife experts, while maintaining a global vision of the problem.

RESISTOME

The antibiotic resistome defines the pool of genes that contribute to an antibiotic resistance phenotype (D'Costa et al., 2006). Bacterial populations have exquisite mechanisms to transfer antibiotic resistance genes by horizontal transfer, mainly in densely populated microbial ecosystems. The human gut, for instance, offers ample opportunities for bacteria of different provenance to share genetic material, including the many antibiotic resistance genes harbored by gut microflora (van Schaik, 2015).

Currently, there is urgent focus on the natural resistome. A resistome database was set up in Liu and Pop (2009) and contains information on about 20,000 genes reported so far. Conclusions from several metagenomics approaches are that those 20,000 genes are just a small portion of all resistomes, since other genes with different purposes not directly related to antibiotic resistance may be implicated (Gillings, 2013). Recently, a new bioinformatics platform has been developed, the comprehensive antibiotic research database (CARD), which integrates molecular and sequence data allowing a fast identification of putative antibiotic resistance genes in newly annotated genome sequences (McArthur et al., 2013). Environmental and human associated microbial communities have been shown to harbor distinct resistomes, suggesting that antibiotic resistance functions are mainly constrained by ecology (Gibson et al., 2015). However, to date, studies investigating the roles of antibiotics and AMR outside of the clinical environment are scarce. To know more about resistome composition and the dynamics among AMR genes, new studies should be performed on AMR communities in the environment.

AMR SURVEILLANCE IN INDICATOR BACTERIA

Living organisms are defined by the genes they possess, while the control of expression of this gene set, both temporally and in response to the environment, determines whether an organism can survive changing conditions and compete for the resources it needs to reproduce. Changes to a bacterial genome are likely to threaten the microbe's ability to survive, but acquisition of new genes may enhance its chances of thriving by allowing growth in a formerly hostile environment. If a pathogenic bacteria gains resistance genes it is more likely to survive in the presence of antimicrobials that would otherwise eradicate it, thus compromising clinical treatments. Bacterial genomes are dynamic entities evolving through several processes, including intrachromosome genetic rearrangements, gene duplication, gene loss and gene gain by lateral gene transfer, and several other chemical and genetic factors can trigger changes by locally altering nucleotide sequences (Lawrence, 2005). AMR strains emerge and spread as a combined result of intensive antibiotics use and bacterial genetic transfer, and the incidences of resistant bacteria from diverse habitats have been increasing (Coque et al., 2008).

Recently, several pathogens have been reported as being multidrug-resistant (MDR) and believed to be 'unbeatable' (Grundmann et al., 2006). Incidences of MDR strains of *Staphylococcus aureus*, *E. coli*, *Salmonella*, and *Enterococcus* are of international concern and have been reported thoroughly by global health organizations (ECDC, 2013; WHO, 2014). Methicillin-resistant *Staphylococcus aureus* (MRSA) is one of the main causes of AMR associated clinical infections. Resistant isolates are still being reported at a high rate, as in Portugal where MRSA is recovered from more than 50% of isolates from humans (ECDC, 2013). In 2011, the percentage of *E. coli* isolates resistant to third-generation cephalosporins, through production of extended-spectrum beta-lactamases (ESBLs), ranged from 3 to 36% in Europe. Over the last 4 years, MDR in *E. coli* has been reported to be on the increase (ECDC, 2013). Also on European territory, enterococci resistant to high-level aminoglycosides (25–50% of recovered isolates) and vancomycin (VRE) (less than 5% of isolates) have been reported with some countries noting an increase (ECDC, 2013). *Salmonella* are considered potential sources of zoonosis. MDR *Salmonella* strains are often recovered from human and animal isolates in Europe, with high incidence in children (ECDC, 2013).

Human and animal commensal gastrointestinal bacteria are continuously subject to diverse antimicrobial pressures (Levy and Marshall, 2004). Resistant strains may act as reservoirs of resistance genes that can easily be spread to pathogenic strains (Allen et al., 2013). The potential pathogens *E. coli* and enterococci are commonly used as indicators of the selection pressure and AMR evolution through the environment (Radhouani et al., 2014).

Escherichia coli are facultative anaerobic Gram-negative bacteria belonging to the *Enterobacteriaceae* family. As a commensal bacterium *E. coli* colonizes the gastrointestinal tract of humans and animals, but it is found ubiquitously in soil, plants, vegetables and water (van den Bogaard and Stobberingh, 2000). *E. coli* is a potential pathogen and the leading cause of human urinary tract infection, bacteraemia and gastroenteritis, among many other infections that require therapeutic intervention (Fluit et al., 2001; Kaper et al., 2004). *E. coli* has an outstanding capacity to acquire and transfer antibiotic resistance genes from or to other bacteria, which can later be disseminated from humans to animals and to the natural environment, and vice versa (Teuber, 1999). AMR *E. coli* strains, particularly those resistant to important antibiotics, have been increasing (Collignon, 2009).

Likewise, *Enterococcus* are commensal bacteria from the intestinal flora of humans and animals, and are frequently monitored as indicators of fecal contamination of food products (Teuber and Perreten, 2000; Ramos et al., 2012). Enterococci are facultative anaerobes capable of persisting in extreme conditions caused by temperature and pH variations, dehydration, and oxidative stress. In the last two decades they have become dangerous nosocomial pathogens, persisting in hospital environments where selective pressure from the presence of antibiotics improves their resistome (Franz et al., 2011; Arias and Murray, 2012). Enterococci can cause urinary tract, wound and intra-abdominal infections, endocarditis, and bacteraemia. *Enterococcus faecalis* and *Enterococcus faecium* are the major species responsible for enterococci infections. Enterococci are intrinsically resistant to some antibiotics (β-lactams and aminoglycosides) and some species have specific AMR, such as *E. faecalis* to lincosamides and streptogramins A, and *Enterococcus gallinarum* and *E. casseliflavus* to vancomycin. They can also easily exchange resistance genes with other bacteria. Use of avoparcin, a glycopeptide antibiotic chemically similar to vancomycin, as an animal feed additive in Europe, and of high amounts of vancomycin in USA hospitals has led to the spread of VRE in animals, humans, food, and the environment (Kirst et al., 1998; Wegener, 1998). However, banning avoparcin in 2006 has not been sufficient to eradicate the AMR mechanisms present in bacteria and some VRE still persist in animals and the environment (Poeta et al., 2007b; Araujo et al., 2010; Ramos et al., 2012).

COMPILATION OF UTAD AMR SURVEILLANCE DATA

Antibiotic prescribing practices in the EU differ widely, and the introduction of standardization would be one way to monitor use more closely and possibly reduce the emergence of resistant bacteria. The antimicrobials market has been increasing with an average annual growth of 6.6% between 2005 and 2011. Worldwide demand for antibiotics is conjectured to reach about €34.1 billion in 2016. Currently, the market is dominated by aminoglycosides, which account for 79% of demand, while penicillins account for 8%, erythromycin 7%, tetracyclines 4%, and chloramphenicol 1%. Market expansion is expected to slow down to 4.6% in coming years (GR & DS, 2012). Between 2000 and 2010, consumption of antibiotic drugs increased by 36% (from 54 billion standard units to 73 billion standard units). The greatest increase was in low- and middle-income countries, but in general, high-income countries still use more antibiotics per capita (Van Boeckel et al., 2014). Portugal is in the top 10 European countries with the greatest consumption of antibiotics, at around 21–25 doses per 1,000 habitants each year (Hede, 2014). Nonetheless, exposure to antibiotics it is not only of antibiotic consumption through prescribed human treatments but also by their use in animal production. The antibiotic environmental contamination can contribute further to the increased emergence of resistance in pathogenic and environmental bacteria. The antibiotics used in animal production may be excreted directly into the environment, or accumulate in manure which could later be spread on land as fertilizer (Almeida et al., 2014). The global total consumption of antibiotics in livestock was estimated in 2010 to be around 63,151 tons and it is project to rise 67% by 2030. Increase driven by the growth in consumer demand for livestock products in middle-income countries and a shift to large-scale farms where antimicrobials are used routinely (Van Boeckel et al., 2014).

The Portuguese annual amount of antibiotics used in human and animal consumption was discussed in a report with data from 2010 to 2011. A first comparison of the antibiotic usage in human and veterinary medicine in Portugal indicates that two-thirds of the consumed antibiotics are used in veterinary medicine whereas the rest one-third in human medicine. For human medicine antibiotic prescription increased 4.5 tons (81.4–85.9 tons). In these two registered years, the annual amount of the different antibiotic groups was markedly larger for penicillins, which alone accounted for more than 65.0%, followed by quinolones (13.0%), macrolides (7.0%), cephalosporins (6.0%), and sulfonamides (5.0%). In veterinary medicine the annual amount of antibiotics sold was 179 tons in 2010 and 163 tons in 2011. Tetracyclines and penicillins were the most sold therapeutic solutions for the both years (Almeida et al., 2014).

Although it has been registered a decrease in the use of antibiotics in Portugal, their consumption and use is still high. Surveying AMR trends among bacteria is necessary to inform risk analyses and guide public policy. Over one decade at University of Trás-os-Montes and Alto Douro (UTAD), the antimicrobial profiles of indicator bacteria *E. coli* (**Table 1**) and enterococci (**Table 2**) have been studied in samples isolated from more than 75 different sources in Portugal. **Figure 1** summarizes the data according to the four groups of sources from which samples were collected: humans, pets, food-producing animals, and wild animals.

The fecal samples used in all studies, either from Human or animal origin, were obtained following similar guidelines. The fecal samples (one per animal) were recovered from patients (in the case of human studies) and directly from the intestinal tract in the animal studies. Samples were transported in Cary-Blair medium from the place of recovery to the Centre of Studies of Animal and Veterinary Sciences (CECAV) facilities for processing. For *E. coli* selection, fecal samples were seeded onto Levine agar plates and incubated for 24 h at 37°C. One colony per sample with typical *E. coli* morphology was selected and identified by classical biochemical methods (Gram-staining, catalase, oxidase, indol, Methyl-Red, Voges-Proskauer, citrate, urease, and triple sugar iron), and by the API 20E system (BioMerieux, La Balme Les Grottes, France). As for the enterococcal isolation, fecal samples were sampled onto Slanetz-Bartley agar plates and incubated at 37°C for 24 h. One colony with typical enterococcal morphology were identified to the genus level by cultural characteristics, Gram staining, catalase test, and bile-aesculin reaction. Antibiotic susceptibility tests were made by the disk diffusion method following CLSI recommendations. 16 antibiotics were tested against *E. coli* isolates: ampicillin (10 mg), amoxicillin + clavulanic acid (20 mg + 10 mg), cefoxitin (30 mg), cefotaxime (30 mg), ceftazidime (30 mg), aztreonam (30 mg), imipenem (10 mg), gentamicin (10 mg), amikacin (30 mg), tobramycin (10 mg),

TABLE 1 | Description of all sources of *Escherichia coli* isolates analyzed in a decade of antimicrobial resistance (AMR) surveillance in Portugal by the UTAD Functional Genomics and Proteomics Unit.

Sampling group	Sample source	Recovered samples (n = 1,841)	Recovered isolates (n = 1,275)	Reference
Pets	Dogs and cats	75	144	Costa et al., 2008
Humans	Children	118	92	Barreto et al., 2009
	Oral hygiene patients	46	2	Poeta et al., 2009
Food-producing animals	Pigs, cattle, and sheep	198	192	Ramos et al., 2012
Wild animals	Diarrheic rabbits	52	52	Poeta et al., 2010
	Wild rabbits	77	44	Silva et al., 2010
	Buzzards	42	36	Radhouani et al., 2012
	Red foxes	52	22	Radhouani et al., 2013
	Several wild animals	72	56	Costa et al., 2006
	Seagulls	53	53	Radhouani et al., 2009
	Lusitano horses	90	71	Moura et al., 2010
	Iberian wolf	237	195	Goncalves et al., 2013a
	Iberian lynx	27	18	Goncalves et al., 2012
	Iberian lynx	98	96	Goncalves et al., 2013b
	Echinoderms	250	10	Marinho et al., 2013
	Wild birds	218	115	Santos et al., 2013
	Wild rabbits	136	77	Silva et al., 2010

TABLE 2 | Description of all sources of *Enterococcus* spp. isolates analyzed in a decade of AMR surveillance in Portugal by the UTAD Functional Genomics and Proteomics Unit.

Sampling group	Sample source	Recovered samples (n = 2,730)	Recovered isolates (n = 2,287)	Reference
Pets	Dogs and cats	104	104	Rodrigues et al., 2001
	Dogs and cats	220	142	Poeta et al., 2005a
Humans	Humans	220	146	Poeta et al., 2005a
	Children	118	101	Barreto et al., 2009
	Oral hygiene patients	46	8	Poeta et al., 2009
Food-producing animals	Poultry	220	152	Poeta et al., 2005a
	Pigs, cattle, and sheep	198	194	Ramos et al., 2012
Wild animals	Wild animals	77	140	Poeta et al., 2005b
	Wild boars	67	134	Poeta et al., 2007b; Silva et al., 2010
	Wild rabbit	77	64	Silva et al., 2010
	Gilthead seabream	118	73	Barros et al., 2011
	Seagulls	57	54	Radhouani et al., 2011
	Buzzards	42	31	Radhouani et al., 2012
	Iberian wolf	237	227	Goncalves et al., 2013a
	Iberian lynx	30	27	Goncalves et al., 2011
	Iberian lynx	98	96	Goncalves et al., 2013b
	Echinoderms	250	144	Marinho et al., 2013
	Lusitano horses	90	71	Moura et al., 2010
	Red foxes	52	50	Radhouani et al., 2013; Santos et al., 2013
	Wild birds	218	138	Santos et al., 2013

streptomycin (10 mg), nalidixic acid (30 mg), ciprofloxacin (5 mg), sulfamethoxazole-trimethoprim (1.25 mg + 23.75 mg), tetracycline (30 mg), and chloramphenicol (30 mg). The identification of phylogenetic groups was performed as described by Clermont *E. coli* phylo-typing method (Clermont et al., 2000). In the case of enterococci, the isolates were tested for 11 antibiotics: [vancomycin (30 μg), teicoplanin (30 μg), Ampicillin (10 μg), streptomycin (300 μg), gentamicin (120 μg), kanamycin (120 μg), chloramphenicol (30 μg), tetracycline (30 μg), erythromycin (15 μg), quinupristin-dalfopristin (15 μg), and ciprofloxacin (5 μg)], also by the disk diffusion method. Species identification was confirmed by polymerase chain reaction (PCR) using primers and conditions for the different enterococcal species. *E. coli* and enterococci isolates with resistance to one or more antibiotics were selected for the characterization of antibiotic-resistance genes. Their DNA was extracted and tested

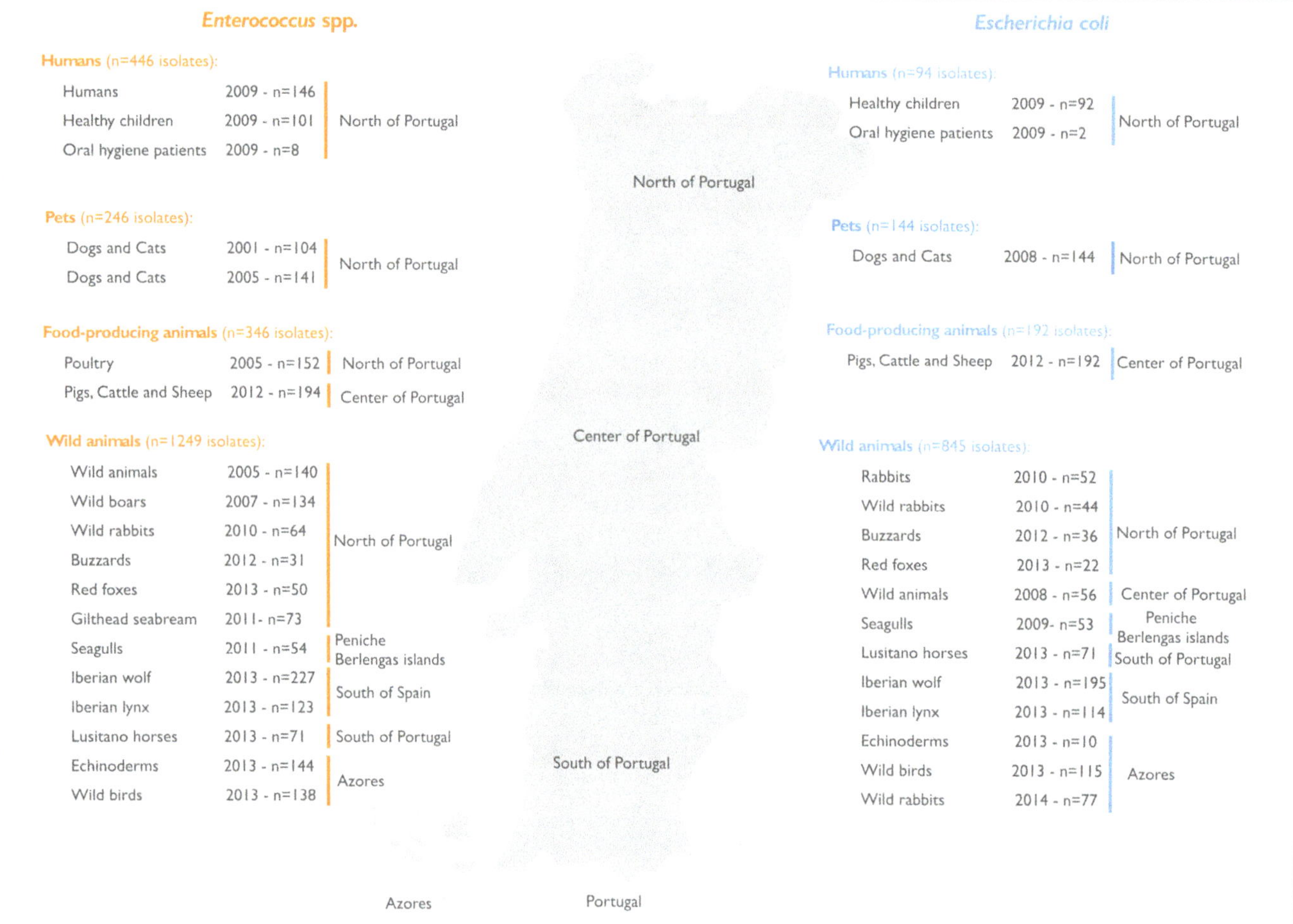
Enterococcus spp.
Humans (n=446 isolates):
Humans 2009 - n=146
Healthy children 2009 - n=101
Oral hygiene patients 2009 - n=8
North of Portugal
Pets (n=246 isolates):
Dogs and Cats 2001 - n=104
Dogs and Cats 2005 - n=141
North of Portugal
Food-producing animals (n=346 isolates):
Poultry 2005 - n=152
North of Portugal
Pigs, Cattle and Sheep 2012 - n=194
Center of Portugal
Wild animals (n=1249 isolates):
Wild animals 2005 - n=140
Wild boars 2007 - n=134
Wild rabbits 2010 - n=64
Buzzards 2012 - n=31
Red foxes 2013 - n=50
Gilthead seabream 2011- n=73
North of Portugal
Seagulls 2011 - n=54
Peniche
Berlengas islands
Iberian wolf 2013 - n=227
Iberian lynx 2013 - n=123
South of Spain
Lusitano horses 2013 - n=71
South of Portugal
Echinoderms 2013 - n=144
Wild birds 2013 - n=138
Azores
North of Portugal
Center of Portugal
South of Portugal
Azores
Portugal
Escherichia coli
Humans (n=94 isolates):
Healthy children 2009 - n=92
Oral hygiene patients 2009 - n=2
North of Portugal
Pets (n=144 isolates):
Dogs and Cats 2008 - n=144
North of Portugal
Food-producing animals (n=192 isolates):
Pigs, Cattle and Sheep 2012 - n=192
Center of Portugal
Wild animals (n=845 isolates):
Rabbits 2010 - n=52
Wild rabbits 2010 - n=44
Buzzards 2012 - n=36
Red foxes 2013 - n=22
North of Portugal
Wild animals 2008 - n=56
Center of Portugal
Seagulls 2009- n=53
Peniche
Berlengas islands
Lusitano horses 2013 - n=71
South of Portugal
Iberian wolf 2013 - n=195
Iberian lynx 2013 - n=114
South of Spain
Echinoderms 2013 - n=10
Wild birds 2013 - n=115
Wild rabbits 2014 - n=77
Azores

FIGURE 1 | Geographical distribution in Portugal showing the sources of samples containing bacterial isolates. The number and provenance of samples containing enterococci (orange) and *Escherichia coli* (blue) are shown. Both types of bacteria were frequently isolated from several samples from humans, pets, food-producing animals, and wild animals.

by PCR with specific primers already published. *E. coli* resistant isolates were screened for the following resistance genes: *bla*TEM and *bla*SHV (in ampicillin-resistant isolates); *tet*A and *tet*B (in tetracycline resistant isolates); *aad*A, *aad*A5, *str*A, and *str*B (in streptomycin-resistant isolates); and *sul*1, *sul*2, and *sul*3 (in sulfa-methoxazoletrimethoprim-resistant isolates). Also, the presence of *int*I, *int*I2 and *qac*ED + *sul*1 genes was analyzed by PCR in all sulfamethoxazole-trimethoprim-resistant isolates. On the other hand, enterococci resistant isolates were tested by PCR for detection of the following resistance genes: *erm*(B) and *erm*(C) (in erythromycin-resistant isolates), *tet*(M) and *tet*(L) (in tetracycline-resistant isolates), *aph*(3′)-IIIA (in kanamycin-resistant isolates), *aac*(6′)-aph(2′′) (in gentamicin-resistant isolates), *ant*(6)-Ia (in streptomycin-resistant isolates), *vat*(D) and *vat*(E) (in quinupristin/dalfopristin-resistant isolates), and *van*(A) (in vancomycin-resistant isolates). Positive and negative controls were used in all PCR reactions, from the strain collection of the University of Trás-os-Montes and Alto Douro (Portugal).

In this collation of data, a total of 1,841 samples were collected and screened for *E. coli*. The overall *E. coli* recovery rate was 69.26% (**Table 1**), but rates were different among the different sampling groups, ranging from 96.97% in fecal samples from food-producing animals down to 52.08% in fecal samples from pets. These are higher percentages than the *E. coli* recovery rate (51%) from humans, domestic and food-producing animal feces, or sewage and surface water in the USA (Sayah et al., 2005). A total of 2,539 samples were screened for enterococci, and a total of 2,096 enterococci isolates were obtained giving a recovery rate of 78.1% (**Table 2**). Rates of recovery from the four sampling groups were similar (75.93% for pet fecal samples, 66% for human samples, 82.78% for fecal samples from food-producing animals; and 88.39% for fecal samples from wild animals). These rates are very similar to previously reported rates (77%) of enterococci recovery from human, animal and environmental samples in several European countries (Kuhn et al., 2003).

Escherichia coli DATA DESCRIPTION

Phenotypic and genotypic studies were used to assess the AMR profile of the isolates. **Figures 2** and **3** summarize the results of tests for antibiotic resistance and identification of

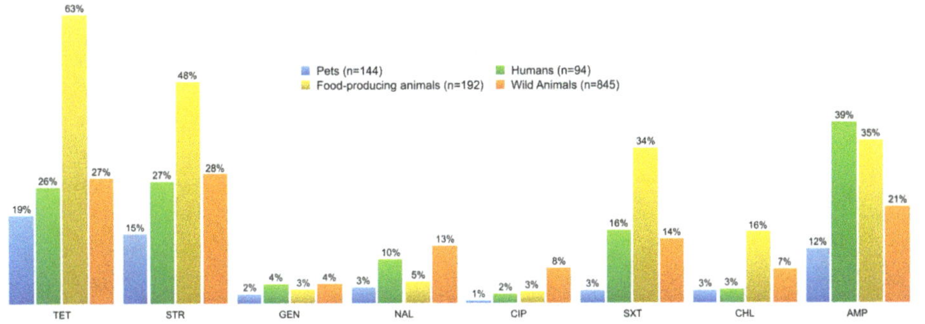

FIGURE 2 | Percentage of phenotypic antibiotic resistance detected in enterococci and *E. coli* isolates from each of the four sampling groups. The resistance profile of enterococci from food-producing animals is distinct from those of the other sampling groups, showing the highest resistance to tetracycline, streptomycin, trimethoprim-sulfamethoxazole, and chloramphenicol. Enterococci from pets displayed the lowest resistance profile to all tested antibiotics. TET, tetracycline; STR, streptomycin; GEN, gentamicin; NAL, nalidixic acid; CIP, ciproflaxin; SXT, trimethoprim-sulfamethoxazole; CHL, chloramphenicol; AMP, ampicillin.

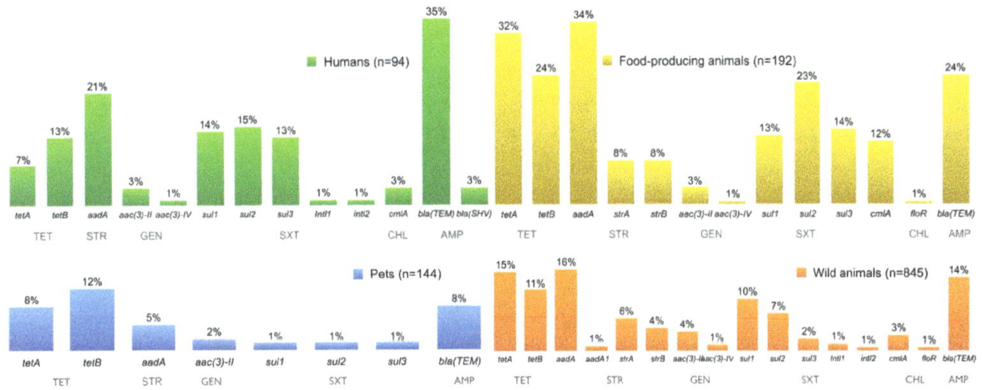

FIGURE 3 | Percentage of antimicrobial resistance (AMR) genes detected in *E. coli* resistant isolates from all sources over a decade.

associated resistance genes in *E. coli* isolates, comparing the four different sample groups described in **Table 1**. Resistance to all the antibiotics tested was found among the samples. Remarkably, *E. coli* from food-producing animals showed higher rates of resistance to tetracycline, streptomycin, trimethoprim-sulfamethoxazole, and chloramphenicol than *E. coli* from humans (**Figure 2**). Indeed fecal *E. coli* isolates recovered from food-producing animals all across Europe have shown a high prevalence of resistance to these antimicrobial agents (Guerra et al., 2003; Enne et al., 2008; Lapierre et al., 2008). Despite the ban on chloramphenicol use in farming in Europe since 1994, food-producing animals still carry resistant strains. Regular and multipurpose use of antibiotics, dissemination of resistant bacteria via fecal contamination and intensive animal production have turned husbandry facilities into important reservoirs of AMR bacteria (van den Bogaard and Stobberingh, 2000). High levels of resistance to tetracycline and streptomycin have been found in bacteria from wild animals. The high prevalence of tetracycline resistance in either *E. coli* or enterococci found in different wild animal species might be related to the recurrent use of this antibiotic in veterinary medicine. The same may be true of the prevalence of resistance to erythromycin, ampicillin, aminoglycosides, and quinolones. One of the main routes of transmission of resistant strains and resistant genes has been shown to be through the food chain (Aarestrup et al., 2008). Antibiotics can be administered to animals to treat (therapy) or prevent (prophylaxis or metaphylaxis) illness and in the past were also used to promote animal growth. Several classes of antimicrobial agents are frequently used in veterinary medicine. A 2013 report showed that in 2011 in 25 countries from the EU/European Economic Area, tetracyclines (37%) were the most sold antimicrobial class for administering to food-producing species, followed by penicillins (23%), sulfonamides (11%), macrolides (8%), lincosamides (2.9%), aminoglycosides (2%), trimethoprim (1.6%), and fluoroquinolones (1.6%) (European Medicines Agency, 2013). Antimicrobial use in veterinary medicine and AMR in commensal *E. coli* from various food-producing animals has indeed been correlated (Chantziaras et al., 2014). Ampicillin is a β-lactam used as a farm animal growth promoter (Sayah et al., 2005). *E. coli* from human samples differ from *E. coli* from other sampling groups in terms of their ampicillin resistance, which is of particular importance considering that ampicillin is a first-line antibiotic commonly effective against a broad spectrum of pathogens.

Comparing AMR *E. coli* from independent sources, several genes conferring AMR were found in resistant isolates (**Figure 3**).

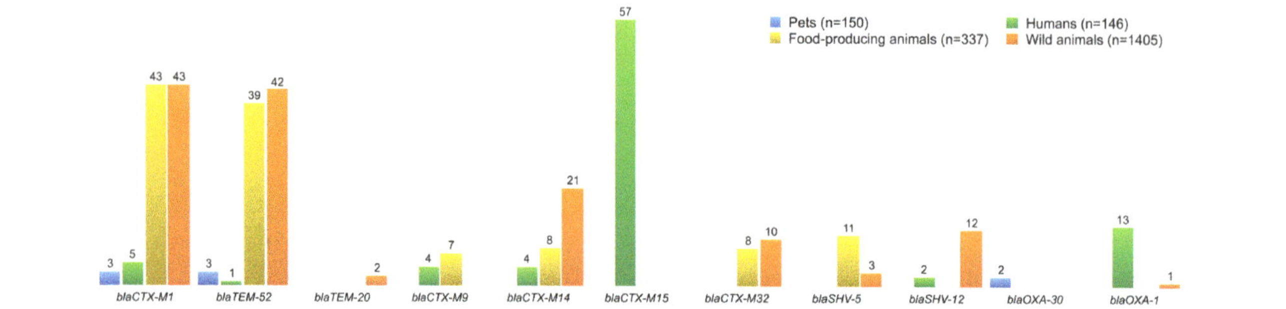

FIGURE 4 | Number of ESBL-producing *E. coli* and resistance genes present in all isolates from different groups. blaCTX-M15 was the most frequent ESBL gene recovered from *E. coli*, followed by blaCTX-M-1 and blaTEM-52. Otherwise, blaTEM-20, blaOXA-30, and blaCTX-M-9 genes were found in a few ESBL-producing *E. coli*.

Fourteen different *tet* genes have been reported in Gram-negative bacteria, encoding proteins active in the three mechanisms of tetracycline resistance, namely an efflux pump, ribosomal protection, or direct enzymatic inactivation of the antibiotic. The resistance genes *tet*A and *tet*B confer resistance to tetracycline, and were found at similar frequencies in all different sources of resistant *E. coli*. However, *tet*A and *tet*B are more likely to be associated with tetracycline resistance in *E. coli* isolated from human and animal samples (Bryan et al., 2004).

The streptomycin resistance genes *aad*A, *str*A, *str*B, and *aad*A1 were found, in descending order of frequency, in resistant *E. coli*. The *str*A and *str*B genes encode streptomycin-inactivating enzymes which confer streptomycin resistance in many Gram-negative bacteria distributed worldwide. The *aad*A gene encodes an adenylylation enzyme that modifies streptomycin and, in the *aad*A1 gene cassette, is often found in streptomycin-resistant *E. coli* strains from human, animal, and food samples (Saenz et al., 2004).

Gentamicin resistance genes *aac*(3)-II and *aac*(3)-IV were present in resistant *E. coli* isolates. Trimethoprim-sulfamethoxazole-resistant *E. coli* isolates had *sul*1, *sul*2 and/or *sul*3 genes, and the integrons *intI*1 and *intI*2 genes, encoding class 1 and class 2 integrases, respectively. The *sul1*, *sul2,* and *sul3* genes each encode dihydropteroate synthases to confer plasmid-mediated resistance to sulphonamides (Perreten and Boerlin, 2003; Skold, 2010). The *sul1* gene is frequently found linked to other resistance genes in class 1 integrons, while *sul2* is normally located on small plasmids of the *inc*Q incompatibility group, or other small plasmids represented by pBP1 (Skold, 2010). The *sul1* and *sul2* genes have been regularly found at similar frequencies among sulphonamide resistant Gram-negative clinical isolates. However, an increase in prevalence of the *sul2* gene has been observed. The association between *sul2* and multiresistance plasmids, which may be co-selected through the use of other antimicrobial agents, might explain the increased prevalence (Blahna et al., 2006; Frank et al., 2007).

Chloramphenicol resistant *E. coli* isolates have the resistance genes *cml*A and *flo*R, both coding efflux pumps that reduce the intracellular concentration of antibiotics by exporting different molecules (Saenz et al., 2004). Some infections are difficult to treat because of bacterial expression of multidrug efflux systems causing resistance. ESBLs confer resistance to penicillins and most cephalosporins, including third-generation cephalosporins, and more than 700 different ESBLs have now been described (van Duijn et al., 2011). A total of 403 isolates of ESBL-producing *E. coli* were obtained from all four sampling groups: humans (n = 138), pets (n = 8), food-producing animals (n = 116), and wild animals (n = 141). **Figure 4** shows all genes encoding ESBLs that were detected in these isolates. The most prevalent ESBL genes were $bla_{\text{CTX-M-1}}$ (n = 94) and $bla_{\text{TEM-52}}$ (n = 85), specifically isolated from *E. coli* from food-producing and wild animals, followed by the $bla_{\text{CTX-}M\text{-32}}$ (n = 57) gene found in isolates from human samples. The mechanisms of resistance against one antibiotic might not be exclusive, and activity may be exhibited against other similar compounds. For instance, it has been proven that mutations in the genes encoding penicillin-inactivating enzymes (e.g., TEM and SHV) can also confer resistance to third-generation cephalosporins or β-lactamase inhibitors (Martinez et al., 2007).

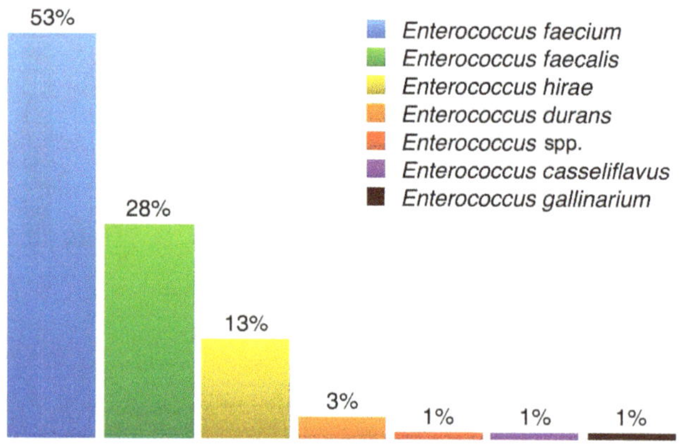

FIGURE 5 | Percentages of enterococci species isolated from samples. *Enterococcus faecium* is the most frequently isolated enterococci species among all recovered samples and *Enterococcus gallinarum* the least.

ENTEROCOCCI DATA DESCRIPTION

Several species of enterococci were recovered from different environments, with some being more common than others depending on the source of the sample. **Figure 5** summarizes all data on enterococci species prevalence reported in the publications listed in **Table 2**. *E. faecalis* is the most common enterococcal species in human stools and the most frequent cause of clinical infection. The natural resistance of this species to penicillin, cephalosporins, and quinolones has contributed to its emergence as a cause of nosocomial infection. However, *E. faecium* is inherently more antibiotic-resistant and has also gradually become a major hospital pathogen (French, 2010; Radimersky et al., 2010). Overall from all the enterococci species we isolated, *E. faecium* was by far the most frequently recovered (52.9%), followed by *E. faecalis*, *E. hirae*, *E. durans*, *E. casseliflavus*, and *E. gallinarum* (**Figure 5**).

Figures 6 and **7** show the collated antibiotic resistance data of enterococci isolates from the different sources listed in **Table 2**. Remarkably, more enterococci from the group of food-producing animals were resistant to tetracycline and erythromycin than from the human group (**Figure 6**). Many enterococci resistant to tetracycline and erythromycin were also found in the wild animals group. Enterococci resistant to kanamycin and chloramphenicol were more frequent in samples from humans than from other sources.

The distribution of AMR genes in the different sampling groups is illustrated in **Figure 7**. The *tet*M and *tet*L genes are associated with the tetracycline-resistance phenotype in enterococci. Tetracycline resistance due to TetL efflux proteins has been becoming more frequently reported among Gram-positive bacteria from animal sources (Figueiredo et al., 2009; Radhouani et al., 2010).

Erythromycin-resistance in enterococci is usually associated with the presence of the *erm*B gene. The *erm*B and *tet*M genes have been frequently identified together in the same isolate, probably because of they both occur in the mobile conjugative transposon *Tn1545*, prevalent in clinically important Gram-positive bacteria (De Leener et al., 2004). The resistance genes *ant*(6)-Ia, *aac*(6′)-*aph*(2′), *aph*(3′)-IIIA and *cat*A were present in enterococci isolates resistant to streptomycin, gentamicin,

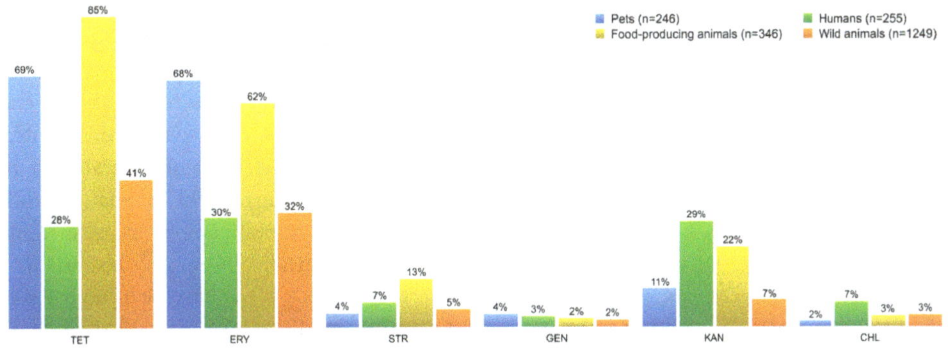

FIGURE 6 | Percentage of phenotypic antibiotic resistance detected in *Enterococcus* spp. isolates from each of the four sampling groups. Enterococci isolates showed high resistance levels to tetracycline and erythromycin, regardless of the source. However, food-producing animals and pets stand out from the other sampling groups. Streptomycin, kanamycin, and chloramphenicol-resistant enterococci are more frequent in samples from humans than from other sources. TET, tetracycline; ERY, erythromycin; STR, streptomycin; GEN, gentamicin, KAN, kanamycin; CHL, chloramphenicol.

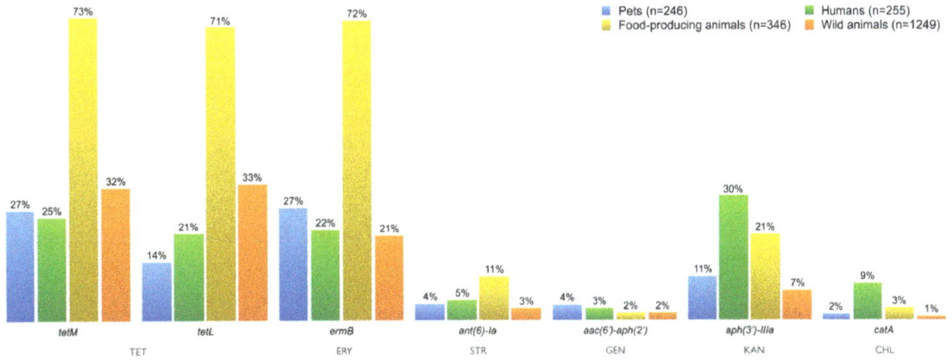

FIGURE 7 | Percentage of AMR genes detected in resistant Enterococci isolates from all sources over a decade. Resistance genes tet(M)/tet(L), erm(B), ant(6)-Ia, aac(6′)-aph(2′), aph(3′)-IIIA, and catA were present in enterococci isolates resistant to tetracycline, erythromycin, streptomycin, gentamicin, kanamycin, and chloramphenicol, respectively. TET, tetracycline; ERY, erythromycin; STR, streptomycin; GEN, gentamicin; KAN, kanamycin, CHL, chloramphenicol.

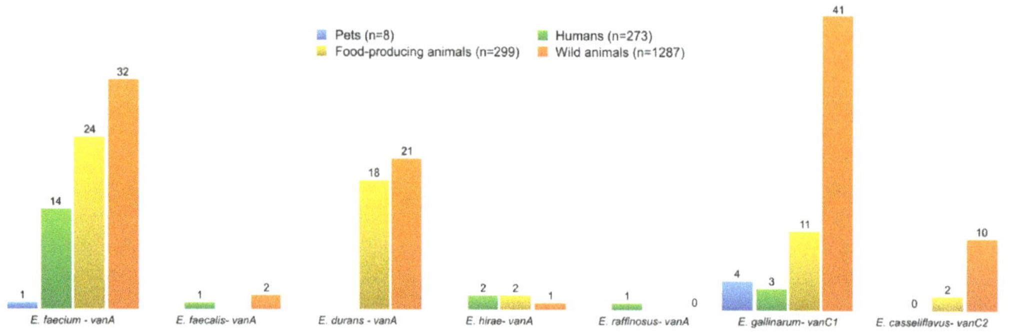

FIGURE 8 | Number of vancomycin-resistant enterococci species, and resistance genes present in all isolates from different groups. *E. gallinarum* and *E. casseliflavus* are intrinsically resistant to vancomycin, and harbor the genes vanC1 and vanC2, respectively, in their genome.

kanamycin, and chloramphenicol, respectively. Resistance to all tested antibiotics has been showed in isolates from all groups.

The presence of VRE isolates was noted in all four groups (**Figure 8**): humans ($n = 21$), pets ($n = 5$), food-producing animals ($n = 57$), and wild animals ($n = 107$). The presence of VRE isolates in diverse samples from Portugal is likely to be related to the use of avoparcin to promote growth of food animals in Europe since the 1970s until its prohibition in 2006. VRE was first characterized in Uttley et al. (1988), and has been repeatedly isolated since then from several sources. Many antimicrobials used in food animals belong to the same classes as those used in humans, leading to concerns about cross-resistance (Furuya and Lowy, 2006). For instance, vancomycin is still the most widely used antibiotic to treat serious infections like MRSA. Vancomycin resistance has emerged in *S. aureus* through acquisition of the *vanA* gene from VRE (Chang et al., 2003). It is important therefore to highlight the higher number of vancomycin resistant determinants found in wild animals compared to humans. In Europe, spread from animals to humans appears to have occurred outside hospital facilities, which explains why VRE is more commonly found in the environment than in the community (Furuya and Lowy, 2006).

CONCLUSION

Generalized use of antibiotics by humans is a recent addition to the natural and ancient process of antibiotic production and resistance evolution that still occurs on a global scale in the soil (Woolhouse et al., 2015). The main attributed cause of the rise and spread of AMR is the extensive clinical use of antibiotics in both human and veterinary medicine (Levy, 2001). However, antibiotic use in veterinary medicine alone does not explain the spread and persistence of AMR bacteria in animal populations in which the antibiotic use is discontinued or else is very sporadic or limited like in wildlife. AMR does not have borders, so it can freely cross through several populations, and homologous resistance genes have been reported in bacteria from pathogens, normal flora and soil. Farm animals are a significant factor in this system and they are still exposed to large amounts of antibiotics and act as reservoirs of many resistance genes. Other risk factors such as antibiotic residues in the environment and AMR gene dissemination in different human and animal populations also have an impact on the AMR levels (Alali et al., 2009). We are currently facing the potential loss of antimicrobial therapy, so it is essential to continue tracking AMR.

FUTURE PERSPECTIVES

Human use of antibiotics for medicine and agriculture may have consequences far beyond their intended applications. The environment is a major reservoir of resistant organisms and antibiotic drugs freely circulating; though not much is known about the antibiotic resistome, shading their hypothetical impact on clinically important bacteria (Allen et al., 2010). Several resistance genes have been reported in distinct bacterial species, from diverse sources (Poeta et al., 2007a; Pallecchi et al., 2008; Gillings and Stokes, 2012). Nonetheless, more studies using standardized methods are required to recognize roles and patterns of antibiotic resistance genes in microbial communities. In the meantime, it is important to moderate the use of antimicrobials and restrain the rise and dissemination of AMR bacteria, so the management of emerging zoonotic diseases and their impacts might be forecasted (Allen et al., 2010). The foreseen decline in antibiotics effectiveness and the current lack of new antimicrobials on the horizon to replace those that become ineffective brings added urgency to the protection of the efficacy of existing drugs (Carlet, 2012; WHO, 2014). Meanwhile, omics approaches to generate molecular data on AMR mechanisms will continue to be the foundation of our work at the Functional Genomics and Proteomics Unit at UTAD.

AUTHOR CONTRIBUTIONS

CM and TS wrote the manuscript. AG, PP, and GI helped interpret compiled data. GI conceived the review. All the authors reviewed and contributed to the manuscript.

REFERENCES

Aarestrup, F. M., Wegener, H. C., and Collignon, P. (2008). Resistance in bacteria of the food chain: epidemiology and control strategies. *Expert Rev. Anti Infect. Ther.* 6, 733–750. doi: 10.1586/14787210.6.5.733

Alali, W. Q., Scott, H. M., Christian, K. L., Fajt, V. R., Harvey, R. B., and Lawhorn, D. B. (2009). Relationship between level of antibiotic use and resistance among *Escherichia coli* isolates from integrated multi-site cohorts of humans and swine. *Prev. Vet. Med.* 90, 160–167. doi: 10.1016/j.prevetmed.2009.05.018

Allen, H. K., Donato, J., Wang, H. H., Cloud-Hansen, K. A., Davies, J., and Handelsman, J. (2010). Call of the wild: antibiotic resistance genes in natural environments. *Nat. Rev. Microbiol.* 8, 251–259. doi: 10.1038/nrmicro2312

Allen, S. E., Janecko, N., Pearl, D. L., Boerlin, P., Reid-Smith, R. J., and Jardine, C. M. (2013). Comparison of *Escherichia coli* recovery and antimicrobial resistance in cecal, colon, and fecal samples collected from wild house mice (*Mus musculus*). *J. Wildl. Dis.* 49, 432–436. doi: 10.7589/2012-05-142

Almeida, A., Duarte, S., Nunes, R., Rocha, H., Pena, A., and Meisel, L. (2014). Human and veterinary antibiotics used in Portugal—a ranking for ecosurveillance. *Toxics* 2, 188–225. doi: 10.3390/toxics2020188

Aminov, R. I. (2010). A brief history of the antibiotic era: lessons learned and challenges for the future. *Front. Microbiol.* 1:134. doi: 10.3389/fmicb.2010.00134

Araujo, C., Torres, C., Silva, N., Carneiro, C., Goncalves, A., Radhouani, H., et al. (2010). Vancomycin-resistant enterococci from Portuguese wastewater treatment plants. *J. Basic Microbiol.* 50, 605–609. doi: 10.1002/jobm.201000102

Arias, C. A., and Murray, B. E. (2012). The rise of the *Enterococcus*: beyond vancomycin resistance. *Nat. Rev. Microbiol.* 10, 266–278. doi: 10.1038/nrmicro2761

Baquero, F., Tedim, A. P., and Coque, T. M. (2013). Antibiotic resistance shaping multi-level population biology of bacteria. *Front. Microbiol.* 4:15. doi: 10.3389/fmicb.2013.00015

Barreto, A., Guimaraes, B., Radhouani, H., Araujo, C., Goncalves, A., Gaspar, E., et al. (2009). Detection of antibiotic resistant *E. coli* and *Enterococcus* spp in stool of healthy growing children in Portugal. *J. Basic Microbiol.* 49, 503–512. doi: 10.1002/jobm.200900124

Barrett, J. R. (2012). Preventing antibiotic resistance in the wild: a new end point for environmental risk assessment. *Environ. Health Perspect.* 120, a321. doi: 10.1289/ehp.120-a321a

Barros, J., Igrejas, G., Andrade, M., Radhouani, H., Lopez, M., Torres, C., et al. (2011). Gilthead seabream (*Sparus aurata*) carrying antibiotic resistant enterococci. A potential bioindicator of marine contamination? *Mar. Pollut. Bull.* 62, 1245–1248. doi: 10.1016/j.marpolbul.2011.03.021

Blahna, M. T., Zalewski, C. A., Reuer, J., Kahlmeter, G., Foxman, B., and Marrs, C. F. (2006). The role of horizontal gene transfer in the spread of trimethoprim-sulfamethoxazole resistance among uropathogenic *Escherichia coli* in Europe and Canada. *J. Antimicrob. Chemother.* 57, 666–672. doi: 10.1093/jac/dkl020

Bryan, A., Shapir, N., and Sadowsky, M. J. (2004). Frequency and distribution of tetracycline resistance genes in genetically diverse, nonselected, and nonclinical *Escherichia coli* strains isolated from diverse human and animal sources. *Appl. Environ. Microbiol.* 70, 2503–2507. doi: 10.1128/AEM.70.4.2503-2507.2004

Carlet, J. (2012). World Alliance against antibiotic resistance (WAAR): safeguarding antibiotics. *Intensive Care Med.* 38, 1723–1724. doi: 10.1007/s00134-012-2643-8

CDC (ed.). (2013). *Antibiotic Resistance Threats in the United States, 2013.* Atlanta, GA: Centers for Disease Control and Prevention.

Chang, S., Sievert, D. M., Hageman, J. C., Boulton, M. L., Tenover, F. C., Downes, F. P., et al. (2003). Infection with vancomycin-resistant *Staphylococcus aureus* containing the vanA resistance gene. *N. Engl. J. Med.* 348, 1342–1347. doi: 10.1056/NEJMoa025025

Chantziaras, I., Boyen, F., Callens, B., and Dewulf, J. (2014). Correlation between veterinary antimicrobial use and antimicrobial resistance in food-producing animals: a report on seven countries. *J. Antimicrob Chemother.* 69, 827–834. doi: 10.1093/jac/dkt443

Chee-Sanford, J. C., Mackie, R. I., Koike, S., Krapac, I. G., Lin, Y. F., Yannarell, A. C., et al. (2009). Fate and transport of antibiotic residues and antibiotic resistance genes following land application of manure waste. *J. Environ. Qual.* 38, 1086–1108. doi: 10.2134/jeq2008.0128

Clermont, O., Bonacorsi, S., and Bingen, E. (2000). Rapid and simple determination of the *Escherichia coli* phylogenetic group. *Appl. Environ. Microbiol.* 66, 4555–4558. doi: 10.1128/AEM.66.10.4555-4558.2000

Collignon, P. (2009). Resistant *Escherichia coli*–we are what we eat. *Clin. Infect. Dis.* 49, 202–204. doi: 10.1086/599831

Coque, T. M., Novais, A., Carattoli, A., Poirel, L., Pitout, J., Peixe, L., et al. (2008). Dissemination of clonally related *Escherichia coli* strains expressing extended-spectrum beta-lactamase CTX-M-15. *Emerg. Infect. Dis.* 14, 195–200. doi: 10.3201/eid1402.070350

Cordero, O. X., Wildschutte, H., Kirkup, B., Proehl, S., Ngo, L., Hussain, F., et al. (2012). Ecological populations of bacteria act as socially cohesive units of antibiotic production and resistance. *Science* 337, 1228–1231. doi: 10.1126/science.1219385

Costa, D., Poeta, P., Saenz, Y., Coelho, A. C., Matos, M., Vinue, L., et al. (2008). Prevalence of antimicrobial resistance and resistance genes in faecal *Escherichia coli* isolates recovered from healthy pets. *Vet. Microbiol.* 127, 97–105. doi: 10.1016/j.vetmic.2007.08.004

Costa, D., Poeta, P., Saenz, Y., Vinue, L., Rojo-Bezares, B., Jouini, A., et al. (2006). Detection of *Escherichia coli* harbouring extended-spectrum beta-lactamases of the CTX-M, TEM and SHV classes in faecal samples of wild animals in Portugal. *J. Antimicrob. Chemother.* 58, 1311–1312. doi: 10.1093/jac/dkl415

Cully, M. (2014). Public health: the politics of antibiotics. *Nature* 509, S16–S17. doi: 10.1038/509S16a

Davenport, D. (2012). The war against bacteria: how were sulphonamide drugs used by Britain during World War II? *Med. Humanit.* 38, 55–58. doi: 10.1136/medhum-2011-010024

Davies, J., and Davies, D. (2010). Origins and evolution of antibiotic resistance. *Microbiol. Mol. Biol. Rev.* 74, 417–433. doi: 10.1128/MMBR.00016-10

D'Costa, V. M., Mcgrann, K. M., Hughes, D. W., and Wright, G. D. (2006). Sampling the antibiotic resistome. *Science* 311, 374–377. doi: 10.1126/science.1120800

De Leener, E., Martel, A., Decostere, A., and Haesebrouck, F. (2004). Distribution of the erm (B) gene, tetracycline resistance genes, and Tn1545-like transposons in macrolide- and lincosamide-resistant enterococci from pigs and humans. *Microb. Drug Resist.* 10, 341–345. doi: 10.1089/mdr.2004.10.341

ECDC (ed.) (2011). *Antimicrobial Resistance Surveillance in Europe.* Stockholm: European Centre for Disease Prevention and Control.

ECDC (ed.) (2013). *Surveillance Report: Anual Epidemiological Report 2013.* Stockholm: Centre for Disease Prevention and Control.

Elsner, H. (1910). The new treatment of syphilis (ehrlich-hata): observations and results. *J. Am. Med. Assoc.* 55, 2052–2057.

Enne, V. I., Cassar, C., Sprigings, K., Woodward, M. J., and Bennett, P. M. (2008). A high prevalence of antimicrobial resistant *Escherichia coli* isolated from pigs and a low prevalence of antimicrobial resistant *E. coli* from cattle and sheep in Great Britain at slaughter. *FEMS Microbiol. Lett.* 278, 193–199. doi: 10.1111/j.1574-6968.2007.00991.x

European Medicines Agency (2013). *Sales of Veterinary Antimicrobial Agents in 25 EU/EEA Countries in 2011.* Report EMA/236501/2013. London: European Medicines Agency.

Figueiredo, N., Radhouani, H., Goncalves, A., Rodrigues, J., Carvalho, C., Igrejas, G., et al. (2009). Genetic characterization of vancomycin-resistant enterococci isolates from wild rabbits. *J. Basic Microbiol.* 49, 491–494. doi: 10.1002/jobm.200800387

Fleming, A. (2001). On the antibacterial action of cultures of a penicillium, with special reference to their use in the isolation of *B. influenzae*, 1929. *Bull. World Health Organ.* 79, 780–790.

Fluit, A. C., Schmitz, F. J., Verhoef, J., and European, S. P. G. (2001). Frequency of isolation of pathogens from bloodstream, nosocomial pneumonia, skin and soft tissue, and urinary tract infections occurring in European patients. *Eur. J. Clin. Microbiol. Infect. Dis.* 20, 188–191. doi: 10.1007/s10096-001-8078-8

Frank, T., Gautier, V., Talarmin, A., Bercion, R., and Arlet, G. (2007). Characterization of sulphonamide resistance genes and class 1 integron gene cassettes in Enterobacteriaceae, Central African Republic (CAR). *J. Antimicrob. Chemother.* 59, 742–745. doi: 10.1093/jac/dkl538

Franz, C. M., Huch, M., Abriouel, H., Holzapfel, W., and Galvez, A. (2011). Enterococci as probiotics and their implications in food safety. *Int. J. Food Microbiol.* 151, 125–140. doi: 10.1016/j.ijfoodmicro.2011.08.014

French, G. L. (2010). The continuing crisis in antibiotic resistance. *Int. J. Antimicrob. Agents* 36(Suppl. 3), S3–S7. doi: 10.1016/S0924-8579(10)70003-0

Furuya, E. Y., and Lowy, F. D. (2006). Antimicrobial-resistant bacteria in the community setting. *Nat. Rev. Microbiol.* 4, 36–45. doi: 10.1038/nrmicro1325

Gibson, M. K., Forsberg, K. J., and Dantas, G. (2015). Improved annotation of antibiotic resistance determinants reveals microbial resistomes cluster by ecology. *ISME J.* 9, 207–216. doi: 10.1038/ismej.2014.106

Gillings, M. R. (2013). Evolutionary consequences of antibiotic use for the resistome, mobilome and microbial pangenome. *Front. Microbiol.* 4:4. doi: 10.3389/fmicb.2013.00004

Gillings, M. R., and Stokes, H. W. (2012). Are humans increasing bacterial evolvability? *Trends Ecol. Evol.* 27, 346–352. doi: 10.1016/j.tree.2012.02.006

Goh, E. B., Yim, G., Tsui, W., Mcclure, J., Surette, M. G., and Davies, J. (2002). Transcriptional modulation of bacterial gene expression by subinhibitory concentrations of antibiotics. *Proc. Natl. Acad. Sci. U.S.A.* 99, 17025–17030. doi: 10.1073/pnas.252607699

Goncalves, A., Igrejas, G., Radhouani, H., Correia, S., Pacheco, R., Santos, T., et al. (2013a). Antimicrobial resistance in faecal enterococci and *Escherichia coli* isolates recovered from Iberian wolf. *Lett. Appl. Microbiol.* 56, 268–274. doi: 10.1111/lam.12044

Goncalves, A., Igrejas, G., Radhouani, H., Estepa, V., Alcaide, E., Zorrilla, I., et al. (2012). Detection of extended-spectrum beta-lactamase-producing *Escherichia coli* isolates in faecal samples of Iberian lynx. *Lett. Appl. Microbiol.* 54, 73–77. doi: 10.1111/j.1472-765X.2011.03173.x

Goncalves, A., Igrejas, G., Radhouani, H., Lopez, M., Guerra, A., Petrucci-Fonseca, F., et al. (2011). Detection of vancomycin-resistant enterococci from faecal samples of Iberian wolf and Iberian lynx, including *Enterococcus faecium* strains of CC17 and the new singleton ST573. *Sci. Total Environ.* 41, 266–268. doi: 10.1016/j.scitotenv.2011.09.074

Goncalves, A., Igrejas, G., Radhouani, H., Santos, T., Monteiro, R., Pacheco, R., et al. (2013b). Detection of antibiotic resistant enterococci and *Escherichia coli* in free range Iberian *Lynx* (*Lynx pardinus*). *Sci. Total Environ.* 45, 115–119. doi: 10.1016/j.scitotenv.2013.03.073

GR & DS (ed.) (2012). *Global Antibiotics Market to 2016.* Lahti: GlobalResearch & Data Services.

Grundmann, H., Aires-De-Sousa, M., Boyce, J., and Tiemersma, E. (2006). Emergence and resurgence of meticillin-resistant *Staphylococcus aureus* as a public-health threat. *Lancet* 368, 874–885. doi: 10.1016/S0140-6736(06) 68853-3

Guerra, B., Junker, E., Schroeter, A., Malorny, B., Lehmann, S., and Helmuth, R. (2003). Phenotypic and genotypic characterization of antimicrobial resistance in German *Escherichia coli* isolates from cattle, swine and poultry. *J. Antimicrob. Chemother.* 52, 489–492. doi: 10.1093/jac/dkg362

Hede, K. (2014). Antibiotic resistance: an infectious arms race. *Nature* 509, S2–S3. doi: 10.1038/509S2a

Joakim Larsson, D. G. (2014). Pollution from drug manufacturing: review and perspectives. *Philos. Trans. R. Soc. B Biol. Sci.* 369:20130571. doi: 10.1098/rstb.2013.0571

Jones, M. E. (1999). Towards better surveillance of bacterial antibiotic resistance. *Clin. Microbiol. Infect.* 5, 61–63. doi: 10.1111/j.1469-0691.1999.tb00103.x

Kaper, J. B., Nataro, J. P., and Mobley, H. L. (2004). Pathogenic *Escherichia coli*. *Nat. Rev. Microbiol.* 2, 123–140. doi: 10.1038/nrmicro818

Kirst, H. A., Thompson, D. G., and Nicas, T. I. (1998). Historical yearly usage of vancomycin. *Antimicrob. Agents Chemother.* 42, 1303–1304.

Kuhn, I., Iversen, A., Burman, L. G., Olsson-Liljequist, B., Franklin, A., Finn, M., et al. (2003). Comparison of enterococcal populations in animals, humans, and the environment–a European study. *Int. J. Food Microbiol.* 88, 133–145. doi: 10.1016/S0168-1605(03)00176-4

Lapierre, L., Cornejo, J., Borie, C., Toro, C., and San Martin, B. (2008). Genetic characterization of antibiotic resistance genes linked to class 1 and class 2 integrons in commensal strains of *Escherichia coli* isolated from poultry and swine. *Microb. Drug Resist.* 14, 265–272. doi: 10.1089/mdr.2008. 0810

Lawrence, J. G. (2005). "The dynamic bacterial genome," in *The Bacterial Chromosome*, ed. N. Higgins (Washington, DC: ASM Press).

Le-Minh, N., Khan, S. J., Drewes, J. E., and Stuetz, R. M. (2010). Fate of antibiotics during municipal water recycling treatment processes. *Water Res.* 44, 4295–4323. doi: 10.1016/j.watres.2010.06.020

Levy, S. B. (2001). Antibiotic resistance: consequences of inaction. *Clin. Infect. Dis* 33(Suppl. 3), S124–S129. doi: 10.1086/321837

Levy, S. B., and Marshall, B. (2004). Antibacterial resistance worldwide: causes, challenges and responses. *Nat. Med.* 10, S122–S129. doi: 10.1038/nm1145

Li, D., Yang, M., Hu, J., Zhang, J., Liu, R., Gu, X., et al. (2009). Antibiotic-resistance profile in environmental bacteria isolated from penicillin production wastewater treatment plant and the receiving river. *Environ. Microbiol.* 11, 1506–1517. doi: 10.1111/j.1462-2920.2009.01878.x

Liu, B., and Pop, M. (2009). ARDB–antibiotic resistance genes database. *Nucleic Acids Res.* 37, D443–D447. doi: 10.1093/nar/gkn656

Marinho, C., Silva, N., Pombo, S., Santos, T., Monteiro, R., Goncalves, A., et al. (2013). Echinoderms from Azores islands: an unexpected source of antibiotic resistant *Enterococcus* spp. and *Escherichia coli* isolates. *Mar. pollut. Bull.* 69, 122–127. doi: 10.1016/j.marpolbul.2013.01.017

Martinez, J. L., Baquero, F., and Andersson, D. I. (2007). Predicting antibiotic resistance. *Nat. Rev. Microbiol.* 5, 958–965. doi: 10.1038/nrmicro1796

McArthur, A. G., Waglechner, N., Nizam, F., Yan, A., Azad, M. A., Baylay, A. J., et al. (2013). The comprehensive antibiotic resistance database. *Antimicrob. Agents Chemother.* 57, 3348–3357. doi: 10.1128/AAC.00419-13

Moura, I., Radhouani, H., Torres, C., Poeta, P., and Igrejas, G. (2010). Detection and genetic characterisation of vanA-containing *Enterococcus* strains in healthy Lusitano horses. *Equine Vet. J.* 42, 181–183. doi: 10.2746/042516409X480386

Osterblad, M., Norrdahl, K., Korpimaki, E., and Huovinen, P. (2001). Antibiotic resistance. How wild are wild mammals? *Nature* 409, 37–38.

Pallecchi, L., Bartoloni, A., Paradisi, F., and Rossolini, G. M. (2008). Antibiotic resistance in the absence of antimicrobial use: mechanisms and implications. *Expert Rev. Anti Infect. Ther.* 6, 725–732. doi: 10.1586/14787210.6.5.725

Pappaioanou, M., and Spencer, H. (2008). "One Health" initiative and ASPH. *Public Health Rep.* 123:261.

Pellegrini, C., Celenza, G., Segatore, B., Bellio, P., Setacci, D., Amicosante, G., et al. (2011). Occurrence of class 1 and 2 integrons in resistant *Enterobacteriaceae* collected from a urban wastewater treatment plant: first report from central Italy. *Microb. Drug Resist.* 17, 229–234. doi: 10.1089/mdr.2010.0117

Pereira, H. M., Domingos, T., and Vicente, L. (eds). (2004). *Portugal Millennium Ecosystem Assessment: State of the Assessment Report.* Lisbon: Faculdade de Ciências da Universidade de Lisboa.

Perreten, V., and Boerlin, P. (2003). A new sulfonamide resistance gene (sul3) in *Escherichia coli* is widespread in the pig population of Switzerland. *Antimicrob. Agents Chemother.* 47, 1169–1172. doi: 10.1128/AAC.47.3.1169-1172.2003

Poeta, P., Costa, D., Igrejas, G., Rodrigues, J., and Torres, C. (2007a). Phenotypic and genotypic characterization of antimicrobial resistance in faecal enterococci from wild boars (*Sus scrofa*). *Vet. Microbiol.* 125, 368–374. doi: 10.1016/j.vetmic.2007.06.003

Poeta, P., Costa, D., Igrejas, G., Rojo-Bezares, B., Saenz, Y., Zarazaga, M., et al. (2007b). Characterization of vanA-containing *Enterococcus faecium* isolates carrying Tn5397-like and Tn916/Tn1545-like transposons in wild boars (*Sus Scrofa*). *Microb. Drug Resist.* 13, 151–156. doi: 10.1089/mdr.2007.759

Poeta, P., Costa, D., Rodrigues, J., and Torres, C. (2005a). Study of faecal colonization by vanA-containing *Enterococcus* strains in healthy humans, pets, poultry and wild animals in Portugal. *J. Antimicrob. Chemother.* 55, 278–280. doi: 10.1093/jac/dkh549

Poeta, P., Costa, D., Saenz, Y., Klibi, N., Ruiz-Larrea, F., Rodrigues, J., et al. (2005b). Characterization of antibiotic resistance genes and virulence factors in faecal enterococci of wild animals in Portugal. *J. Vet. Med. B Infect. Dis. Vet. Public Health* 52, 396–402. doi: 10.1111/j.1439-0450.2005.00881.x

Poeta, P., Igrejas, G., Goncalves, A., Martins, E., Araujo, C., Carvalho, C., et al. (2009). Influence of oral hygiene in patients with fixed appliances in the oral carriage of antimicrobial-resistant *Escherichia coli* and *Enterococcus* isolates. *Oral Surg. Oral Med. Oral Pathol. Oral Radiol. Endod.* 108, 557–564. doi: 10.1016/j.tripleo.2009.06.002

Poeta, P., Radhouani, H., Goncalves, A., Figueiredo, N., Carvalho, C., Rodrigues, J., et al. (2010). Genetic characterization of antibiotic resistance in enteropathogenic *Escherichia coli* carrying extended-spectrum beta-lactamases recovered from diarrhoeic rabbits. *Zoonoses Public Health* 57, 162–170. doi: 10.1111/j.1863-2378.2008.01221.x

Radhouani, H., Igrejas, G., Goncalves, A., Pacheco, R., Monteiro, R., Sargo, R., et al. (2013). Antimicrobial resistance and virulence genes in *Escherichia coli* and enterococci from red foxes (*Vulpes vulpes*). *Anaerobe* 23, 82–86. doi: 10.1016/j.anaerobe.2013.06.013

Radhouani, H., Igrejas, G., Pinto, L., Goncalves, A., Coelho, C., Rodrigues, J., et al. (2011). Molecular characterization of antibiotic resistance in enterococci recovered from seagulls (*Larus cachinnans*) representing an environmental health problem. *J. Environ. Monit.* 13, 2227–2233. doi: 10.1039/c0em00682c

Radhouani, H., Pinto, L., Coelho, C., Sargo, R., Araujo, C., Lopez, M., et al. (2010). MLST and a genetic study of antibiotic resistance and virulence factors in vanA-containing *Enterococcus* from buzzards (*Buteo buteo*). *Lett. Appl. Microbiol.* 50, 537–541. doi: 10.1111/j.1472-765X.2010.02807.x

Radhouani, H., Poeta, P., Goncalves, A., Pacheco, R., Sargo, R., and Igrejas, G. (2012). Wild birds as biological indicators of environmental pollution: antimicrobial resistance patterns of *Escherichia coli* and enterococci isolated from common buzzards (*Buteo buteo*). *J. Med. Microbiol.* 61, 837–843. doi: 10.1099/jmm.0.038364-0

Radhouani, H., Poeta, P., Igrejas, G., Goncalves, A., Vinue, L., and Torres, C. (2009). Antimicrobial resistance and phylogenetic groups in isolates of *Escherichia coli* from seagulls at the Berlengas nature reserve. *Vet. Rec.* 165, 138–142. doi: 10.1136/vr.165.5.138

Radhouani, H., Silva, N., Poeta, P., Torres, C., Correia, S., and Igrejas, G. (2014). Potential impact of antimicrobial resistance in wildlife, environment and human health. *Front. Microbiol.* 5:23. doi: 10.3389/fmicb.2014.00023

Radimersky, T., Frolkova, P., Janoszowska, D., Dolejska, M., Svec, P., Roubalova, E., et al. (2010). Antibiotic resistance in faecal bacteria (*Escherichia coli. Enterococcus* spp.) in feral pigeons. *J. Appl. Microbiol.* 109, 1687–1695. doi: 10.1111/j.1365-2672.2010.04797.x

Ramos, S., Igrejas, G., Rodrigues, J., Capelo-Martinez, J. L., and Poeta, P. (2012). Genetic characterisation of antibiotic resistance and virulence factors in vanA-containing enterococci from cattle, sheep and pigs subsequent to the discontinuation of the use of avoparcin. *Vet. J.* 193, 301–303. doi: 10.1016/j.tvjl.2011.12.007

Rodrigues, J., Poeta, P., Martins, A., and Costa, D. (2001). The importance of pets as reservoirs of resistant *Enterococcus* strains, with special reference to vancomycin. *J. Vet. Med.* 49, 278–280. doi: 10.1046/j.1439-0450.2002.00561.x

Rossolini, G. M., and Thaller, M. C. (2010). Coping with antibiotic resistance: contributions from genomics. *Genome Med.* 2:15. doi: 10.1186/gm136

Saenz, Y., Brinas, L., Dominguez, E., Ruiz, J., Zarazaga, M., Vila, J., et al. (2004). Mechanisms of resistance in multiple-antibiotic-resistant *Escherichia coli* strains of human, animal, and food origins. *Antimicrob. Agents Chemother.* 48, 3996–4001. doi: 10.1128/AAC.48.10.3996-4001.2004

Santos, T., Silva, N., Igrejas, G., Rodrigues, P., Micael, J., Rodrigues, T., et al. (2013). Dissemination of antibiotic resistant *Enterococcus* spp. and *Escherichia coli* from wild birds of Azores Archipelago. *Anaerobe* 24, 25–31. doi: 10.1016/j.anaerobe.2013.09.004

Sarmah, A. K., Meyer, M. T., and Boxall, A. B. (2006). A global perspective on the use, sales, exposure pathways, occurrence, fate and effects of veterinary antibiotics (VAs) in the environment. *Chemosphere* 65, 725–759. doi: 10.1016/j.chemosphere.2006.03.026

Sayah, R. S., Kaneene, J. B., Johnson, Y., and Miller, R. (2005). Patterns of antimicrobial resistance observed in *Escherichia coli* isolates obtained from domestic- and wild-animal fecal samples, human septage, and surface water. *Appl. Environ. Microbiol.* 71, 1394–1404. doi: 10.1128/AEM.71.3.1394-1404.2005

Sengupta, S., Chattopadhyay, M. K., and Grossart, H. P. (2013). The multifaceted roles of antibiotics and antibiotic resistance in nature. *Front. Microbiol.* 4:47. doi: 10.3389/fmicb.2013.00047

Silva, N., Igrejas, G., Figueiredo, N., Goncalves, A., Radhouani, H., Rodrigues, J., et al. (2010). Molecular characterization of antimicrobial resistance in enterococci and *Escherichia coli* isolates from European wild rabbit (*Oryctolagus cuniculus*). *Sci. Total Environ.* 408, 4871–4876. doi: 10.1016/j.scitotenv.2010.06.046

Skold, O. (2010). Sulfonamides and trimethoprim. *Expert Rev. Anti Infect. Ther.* 8, 1–6. doi: 10.1586/eri.09.117

Skurnik, D., Ruimy, R., Andremont, A., Amorin, C., Rouquet, P., Picard, B., et al. (2006). Effect of human vicinity on antimicrobial resistance and integrons in animal faecal *Escherichia coli. J. Antimicrob. Chemother.* 57, 1215–1219. doi: 10.1093/jac/dkl122

Spellberg, B., Powers, J. H., Brass, E. P., Miller, L. G., and Edwards, J. E. Jr. (2004). Trends in antimicrobial drug development: implications for the future. *Clin. Infect. Dis.* 38, 1279–1286. doi: 10.1086/420937

Tenover, F. C. (2006). Mechanisms of antimicrobial resistance in bacteria. *Am. J. Infect. Control* 34, S3–S10. doi: 10.1016/j.ajic.2006.05.219

Teuber, M. (1999). Spread of antibiotic resistance with food-borne pathogens. *Cell Mol. Life Sci.* 56, 755–763. doi: 10.1007/s000180050022

Teuber, M., and Perreten, V. (2000). Role of milk and meat products as vehicles for antibiotic-resistant bacteria. *Acta Vet. Scand. Suppl.* 93, 75–87;discussion 111–117.

Uttley, A. H., Collins, C. H., Naidoo, J., and George, R. C. (1988). Vancomycin-resistant enterococci. *Lancet* 1, 57–58. doi: 10.1016/S0140-6736(88)91037-9

Van Boeckel, T. P., Gandra, S., Ashok, A., Caudron, Q., Grenfell, B. T., Levin, S. A., et al. (2014). Global antibiotic consumption 2000 to 2010: an analysis of national pharmaceutical sales data. *Lancet Infect. Dis.* 14, 742–750. doi: 10.1016/S1473-3099(14)70780-7

van den Bogaard, A. E., and Stobberingh, E. E. (2000). Epidemiology of resistance to antibiotics. Links between animals and humans. *Int. J. Antimicrob. Agents* 14, 327–335. doi: 10.1016/S0924-8579(00)00145-X

van Duijn, P. J., Dautzenberg, M. J., and Oostdijk, E. A. (2011). Recent trends in antibiotic resistance in European ICUs. *Curr. Opin. Crit. Care* 17, 658–665. doi: 10.1097/MCC.0b013e32834c9d87

van Schaik, W. (2015). The human gut resistome. *Philos. Trans. R. Soc. Lond. B Biol. Sci.* 370, 20140087. doi: 10.1098/rstb.2014.0087

Walsh, F. (2013). The multiple roles of antibiotics and antibiotic resistance in nature. *Front. Microbiol.* 4:255. doi: 10.3389/fmicb.2013.00255

Wegener, H. (2012). "Antibiotic resistance - linking human and animal health," in *Improving Food Safety Through a One Health Approach: Workshop Summary*, ed. Institute of Medicine. (Washington, DC: National Acedemies Press).

Wegener, H. C. (1998). Historical yearly usage of glycopeptides for animals and humans: the American-European paradox revisited. *Antimicrob. Agents Chemother.* 42, 3049.

WHO (ed.) (2014). *Antimicrobial Resistance: Global Report in Surveillance*. Geneva: World Health Organization.

Woolhouse, M., Ward, M., Van Bunnik, B., and Farrar, J. (2015). Antimicrobial resistance in humans, livestock and the wider environment. *Philos. Trans. R. Soc. Lond. B Biol. Sci.* 370, 20140083. doi: 10.1098/rstb.2014.0083

Xi, C., Zhang, Y., Marrs, C. F., Ye, W., Simon, C., Foxman, B., et al. (2009). Prevalence of antibiotic resistance in drinking water treatment and distribution systems. *Appl. Environ. Microbiol.* 75, 5714–5718. doi: 10.1128/AEM.00382-09

Yim, G., Wang, H. H., and Davies, J. (2007). Antibiotics as signalling molecules. *Philos. Trans. R. Soc. Lond. B Biol. Sci.* 362, 1195–1200. doi: 10.1098/rstb.2007.2044

Zuccato, E., Calamari, D., Natangelo, M., and Fanelli, R. (2000). Presence of therapeutic drugs in the environment. *Lancet* 355, 1789–1790. doi: 10.1016/S0140-6736(00)02270-4

6

Drug Resistance Mechanisms in Bacteria Causing Sexually Transmitted Diseases and Associated with Vaginosis

Boris Shaskolskiy[1], *Ekaterina Dementieva*[1*], *Arvo Leinsoo*[1], *Anastassia Runina*[2], *Denis Vorobyev*[2], *Xenia Plakhova*[2], *Alexey Kubanov*[2], *Dmitrii Deryabin*[2] and *Dmitry Gryadunov*[1*]

[1] Laboratory for Molecular Diagnostics Technologies, Engelhardt Institute of Molecular Biology, Russian Academy of Sciences, Moscow, Russia, [2] State Research Center of Dermatovenerology and Cosmetology of the Russian Ministry of Health, Moscow, Russia

***Correspondence:**
Ekaterina Dementieva
kdem@biochip.ru;
Dmitry Gryadunov
grad@biochip.ru

Here, we review sexually transmitted diseases (STDs) caused by pathogenic bacteria and vaginal infections which result from an overgrowth of opportunistic bacterial microflora. First, we describe the STDs, the corresponding pathogens and the antimicrobials used for their treatment. In addition to the well-known diseases caused by single pathogens (i.e., syphilis, gonococcal infections, and chlamydiosis), we consider polymicrobial reproductive tract infections (especially those that are difficult to effectively clinically manage). Then, we summarize the biochemical mechanisms that lead to antimicrobial resistance and the most recent data on the emergence of drug resistance in STD pathogens and bacteria associated with vaginosis. A large amount of research performed in the last 10–15 years has shed light on the enormous diversity of mechanisms of resistance developed by bacteria. A detailed understanding of the mechanisms of antimicrobials action and the emergence of resistance is necessary to modify existing drugs and to develop new ones directed against new targets.

Keywords: human reproductive system, sexually transmitted diseases, bacterial vaginosis, antimicrobials, antimicrobial resistance

INTRODUCTION

The infections of human reproductive system include the sexually transmitted diseases (STDs) that are defined as infections that spread primarily through person-to-person sexual contact, and non-STDs which are endogenous infections of the genital organs such as bacterial vaginosis (BV). Both STDs and non-STDs are the major concern for public health systems worldwide.

According to the WHO, each year there are approximately half a billion new cases of STDs worldwide (WHO, 2014a), of which 105.7 million are chlamydial infections, 106.1 million are gonorrhea, and 10.6 million are syphilis (WHO, 2013). STDs lead to a decrease in fertility and are harmful to the offspring. Up to 40% of women with untreated gonococcal and chlamydial infections develop inflammatory diseases of the pelvic organs that lead to infertility in 25% of cases; pregnancy in women with the untreated early forms of syphilis results in stillbirth in 25% of cases and neonatal death in 14% (CDC, 2015). Obviously, the timely detection of STDs and adequate antimicrobial therapy are crucial for the successful treatment and prevention of the spread of the disease.

STDs are often polymicrobial and are caused not only by obligate pathogens (*Neisseria gonorrhoeae, Chlamydia trachomatis, Treponema pallidum,* and *Mycoplasma genitalium*) but also by a variety of opportunistic microorganisms which are mostly not sexually transmitted and can occur without sexual relationship. The polymicrobial nature of the reproductive tract pathologies modifies the clinical pattern of the disease, aggravates the inflammatory process, and reduces the efficacy of the determination of their etiologies, which can result in inadequate treatment (Josey and Schwebke, 2008).

A major worldwide problem is the increase in drug resistance of pathogens, which makes it difficult to select proper treatments. In April 2014, the WHO published the report "Antimicrobial resistance: A global report on epidemiological surveillance" (WHO, 2014b). The report emphasized the threat of an increase in the resistance of many pathogens. The greatest concern in addition to tuberculosis, malaria, and staphylococcal infection is the emergence of *N. gonorrhoeae* strains with reduced susceptibility to third-generation cephalosporins. Thus, elucidating the etiology of infections and the concurrent inflammatory processes of the urogenital tract and developing successful therapies require the detection of the primary infectious agents in clinical specimens, the simultaneous identification of a large number of other opportunistic pathogens and an analysis of their susceptibility to common antimicrobial drugs.

This review focuses on the characterization of the most common sexually transmitted bacterial pathogens (excluding viral, fungal, and parasitic infections) and non-STD infections which result from an overgrowth of opportunistic bacterial microflora, and discusses the mechanisms and molecular determinants of their drug resistance.

BRIEF DESCRIPTION OF THE MOST COMMON BACTERIAL INFECTION OF THE HUMAN REPRODUCTIVE SYSTEM AND THE DRUGS USED TO TREAT THEM

Syphilis

This disease is caused by the sexually transmitted, Gram-negative, spirochetal bacterium *T. pallidum* and is characterized by lesions of the skin, mucous membranes, nervous system, internal organs, and musculoskeletal system. Syphilis can cause intrauterine infections of the fetus. The disease can occur in both symptomatic and latent forms. Despite significant achievements in the fight against this disease, syphilis remains a challenge for treatment and public health care due to the variations in the course of the disease and the diversity of its clinical manifestations. Syphilis is treated with benzathine penicillin G, tetracycline and its derivative doxycycline, macrolides (e.g., erythromycin and azithromycin), and cephalosporins (e.g., the third generation drug ceftriaxone). The main drug of choice for syphilis treatment in the 2015 CDC recommendations is benzathine penicillin G (Workowski and Bolan, 2015). Patients allergic to penicillin are treated with the other antibiotics mentioned above. In clinical trials, some antibiotics (e.g., azithromycin) proved to be more effective than penicillin G for the treatment of early syphilis (Bai et al., 2008).

Gonococcal Infection

Gonorrhea is one of the most common STDs and is caused by the Gram-negative diplococci *N. gonorrhoeae*. Health complications resulting from the gonococcus disease occur mainly in women and are largely attributed to the predominately asymptomatic nature of lower genital tract, i.e., cervical, infection. Untreated, subclinical infection of the cervix can lead to upper genital tract involvement (e.g., salpingitis) and, potentially, to infertility. The infection primarily affects the genitals, including the cylindrical and glandular epithelium. Although gonococcal vaginitis develops in female children in which menarche has not yet occurred, keratinization occurring with menarche prevents gonococcal vaginitis in the adult female (Edwards and Butler, 2011).

Gonococcal infection is usually treated with ciprofloxacin, ofloxacin, spectinomycin, and β-lactam antibiotics; currently, the most effective recommended drugs are ceftriaxone and azithromycin (Workowski and Bolan, 2015). The widespread occurrence of penicillin-resistant gonorrhea has led to a decrease in the use of first and second generation β-lactams, protected penicillins (clavulanate-potentiated amoxicillin or ticarcillin-clavulanate), and cephalosporins in clinical practice. Ceftriaxone belonging to cephalosporin drugs, that are more resistant to β-lactamases, remains widely used.

Spectinomycin, from the aminocyclitol class of drugs closely related to the aminoglycosides, since 1960s was used for specific treatment of gonorrhea. It was useful in an alternative therapy for gonorrhea resistant to antibiotics of the other groups or in patients allergic to β-lactams. After 10–20 years of treatment, spectinomycin-resistant gonococcal strains were reported in Netherlands, South Korea, United Kingdom, and USA (Unemo and Shafer, 2014). There is a consistent trend of increasing resistance of gonococci to spectinomycin in Russia (up to 15% in 2010) (Kubanova et al., 2010, 2014). Spectinomycin is not used now as a first-line drug for gonorrhea therapy in many countries.

Chlamydiosis

The infection is caused by the Gram-negative intracellular bacterium *C. trachomatis*. There are 15 identified serovars of *C. trachomatis*. Serotypes Ab, B, Ba, and C are pathogens that cause trachoma, serovars D, E, F, G, H, I, J, and K cause urogenital chlamydiosis, urethritis, prostatitis, vaginitis, and chlamydial cervicitis, and serovars L1, L2, and L3 cause lymphogranuloma venereum and genital ulcers (Workowski and Bolan, 2015). The socio-economic significance of urogenital chlamydial infection is due not only to the high rate of disease but also to a significant percentage of complications, especially the development of secondary infertility in men and women (Vasilevsky et al., 2014).

The drugs of choice for the treatment of chlamydial infections are tetracyclines (doxycycline) and macrolides (josamycin and azithromycin); alternatively, fluoroquinolones (levofloxacin and ofloxacin) can be used (Workowski and Bolan, 2015). Despite the availability of a whole range of drugs against chlamydia, its treatment is not always successful due to the presence of co-infections with the causative agent of urogenital ureaplasmosis (*Ureaplasma urealyticum*). Thus, adequate therapy requires the accurate identification of additional microorganisms associated with the chlamydia infection and the simultaneous treatment of opportunistic infections.

Mycoplasmosis and Ureaplasmosis

The diseases are caused by opportunistic microorganisms of the genus *Mycoplasma* (*M. genitalium* and *Mycoplasma hominis*) and *Ureaplasma*. The latter is classified in a separate genus due to its ability to break down urea. Researchers have identified two species of *Ureaplasma* (*U. parvum* and *U. urealyticum*) that are further classified into 14 serovars. Mycoplasma and ureaplasma are detected in more than 40% of patients with inflammatory diseases of the urogenital system; three species have the highest clinical significance (*M. genitalium, U. urealyticum,* and *M. hominis*). Mycoplasma and ureaplasma can cause urethritis in both sexes and probably cervicitis, cystitis, and pregnancy complications including post-partum period and post-abortion complications (Larsen and Hwang, 2010). The drugs of choice for the treatment of infections are macrolides (azithromycin and josamycin) and tetracyclines (doxycycline). Alternative medications are fluoroquinolones (levofloxacin and ofloxacin) (Workowski and Bolan, 2015).

Bacterial Vaginosis (BV)

BV is an infectious non-inflammatory disease of a polymicrobial nature that is predominantly detected in women of reproductive age. The disease is not immediately life-threatening, but it is a risk factor for pregnancy complications and pelvic inflammatory diseases. Moreover, BV is associated with increased risk for acquiring sexually transmitted infections (Martin, 2012). For example, BV can increase a woman's risk of acquiring *N. gonorrhoeae* (gonococcal infection hazard ratio: 1.7; 95% CI: 1.1–2.6), *C. trachomatis* (chlamydial infection odds ratio: 3.4; 95% CI: 1.5–7.8), and *Trichomonas* (trichomonal genital infection hazard ratio: 1.8; 95% CI: 1.3–2.4) (Margolis and Fredricks, 2015).

BV occurs as the result of a drastic imbalance in the normal vaginal microflora rather than as an invasion of a foreign pathogen. In this case, the normal protective lactobacilli are replaced by high quantities of anaerobes (Turovskiy et al., 2012; Margolis and Fredricks, 2015). Among the most commonly detected causative agents of the disease are the microaerophilic bacteria *Gardnerella vaginalis*, obligate anaerobic Gram-positive bacteria (*Mobiluncus* spp. and *Peptostreptococcus* spp.), and the facultative anaerobic bacteria *Atopobium vaginae*. Additionally, the obligate anaerobic Gram-negative bacteria *Prevotella* spp., *Bacteroides* spp., and *Fusobacterium* spp. are sometimes present in clinical samples (Verhelst et al., 2004; Menard, 2011). The list of bacteria that have been shown to be associated with vaginosis is constantly widening (i.e., *Dialiester, Prevotella,* and *Megasphaera*) (Margolis and Fredricks, 2015).

G. vaginalis bacteria are commonly detected at moderately high concentrations in BV-positive women but their presence alone is not specific for BV (Kalra et al., 2007). The frequent detection of genital mycoplasmas together with anaerobic microflora is due to the ability of *G. vaginalis* to secrete succinic acid, which is used by other microorganisms. In turn, ureaplasma and mycoplasma, which actively consume oxygen during their metabolism, stimulate the proliferation of anaerobic bacteria (Africa et al., 2014). Agents active against *G. vaginalis* include metronidazole and clindamycin.

The proportion of *A. vaginae* (another causative agent of vaginitis) ranges from 50 to 95%. This Gram-positive anaerobic bacillus from the *Coriobacteriaceae* family produces organic acids and can be found together with *G. vaginalis* within the layer of microorganisms on the surface of the vaginal mucosa in bacterial vaginosis patients (Verhelst et al., 2004). The dominant growth of *A. vaginae* is also treated with metronidazole and clindamycin.

Mobiluncus is a motile anaerobic microorganism belonging to the family *Actinomycetaceae*. Two species of the genus *Mobiluncus* are usually found in the human genitourinary tract (*M. curtisii* and *M. mulieris*). Both bacteria are susceptible to β-lactam antibiotics, glycopeptide drugs, clindamycin, chloramphenicol, and rifampicin and are primarily resistant to metronidazole (Spiegel, 1987). Currently, infections caused by *Mobiluncus* spp. are commonly treated with clindamycin (Verstraelen and Verhelst, 2009).

Bacteroides fragilis is a Gram-negative anaerobic bacterium that is a constituent of the normal microflora of the vagina and vulva. *B. fragilis* may cause pyelonephritis, cystitis, urethritis, prostatitis, and other infectious diseases of the genitourinary system in both sexes. The main drug for the treatment of infections caused by *B. fragilis* is metronidazole (Löfmark et al., 2010); alternative treatments include β-lactam antibiotics in combination with β-lactamase inhibitors, clindamycin and chloramphenicol.

Taking into account the leading role of obligate anaerobic bacteria in BV, the drugs of choice for BV treatment are those with anti-anaerobic activity (e.g., clindamycin and 5-nitroimidazole derivatives). Notably, effective BV treatment must be based on a differential diagnosis with other urogenital diseases caused by pathogens (*N. gonorrhoeae, C. trachomatis, Trichomonas vaginalis,* and *M. genitalium*) (Menard, 2011; Workowski and Bolan, 2015).

DRUG RESISTANCE OF STD PATHOGENS

The continuously increasing resistance of STD pathogens to antimicrobial agents is a worldwide problem. Antibiotics that have lost their effectiveness are replaced by new drugs, but new strains appear with new determinants of resistance; this issue applies to all classes of drugs. The increase in the resistance and diversity of the drugs used in clinical practice leads to the emergence of bacteria with multidrug resistance (MDR). Some strains with MDR have the ability to spread rapidly (so-called high-risk clones). Some pathogens acquire simultaneous resistance to most drugs developed for their treatment (extensively drug-resistant pathogens) or even to all drugs (pandrug resistance) (Unemo and Nicholas, 2012;

Rossolini et al., 2014). Currently, multidrug-resistant isolates have been identified for both Gram-positive and Gram-negative species, including *N. gonorrhoeae*.

T. pallidum

Although diagnostic tests for syphilis and antibiotic therapy are now available, the disease remains endemic in many developing countries. Widespread syphilis epidemics occurred in Russia in the 1990s (Stamm, 2010) and more recently in China (Tucker and Cohen, 2011). A recent increase in syphilis rates in women and infants in the USA has also been described (CDC, 2015).

Although penicillins have been used for the treatment of syphilis for 70 years, no natural penicillin-resistant forms have been found. To date, no clinically proven cases of treatment failure using penicillin-related drugs have been described in patients with syphilis. However, the possibility of the emergence of acquired resistance is still discussable (Stamm, 2010). Recent analysis of *T. pallidum* resistance to antibiotics in the Russian Federation revealed no resistance to β-lactam antibiotics. Specifically, no meaningful mutations were found in the *tp47* and *tromp* genes encoding the targets of β-lactams (Kubanova et al., 2013).

Currently, there is no documented resistance of *T. pallidum* to the tetracyclines. Clinically significant resistance of *T. pallidum* to macrolides (a second-line alternative to penicillin) has been demonstrated by many authors, and macrolide-resistant strains are now prevalent in several developed countries (Stamm, 2010). Clinical cases of *T. pallidum* resistance to macrolides (particularly erythromycin; Stamm and Bergen, 2000), azithromycin (Katz and Klausner, 2008; Stamm, 2010), clarithromycin (Stamm, 2010), and spiramycin (Matějková et al., 2009) have been reported. There was a report concerning treatment failure with clindamycin but these data were not confirmed and *T. pallidum* appeared to have intrinsic resistance to this drug (Stamm, 2010).

The first strain resistant to erythromycin and azithromycin was isolated in 1977 (Street strain 14) (Stamm, 2012). Sequencing of the *T. pallidum* genome has shown that it lacks the genetic elements responsible for horizontal gene transfer (plasmids and transposons); thus, it was concluded that the resistance to macrolides in Street strain 14 emerged endogenously by a spontaneous chromosomal mutation in the 23S rRNA gene. The mutations responsible for macrolide resistance were shown to be A2058G and A2059G (23S rRNA). Mutation A2058G was reported in several areas of the USA, Canada, Europe, and China (Stamm, 2012), whereas the replacement of A2059G was less common but was not geographically isolated (Matějková et al., 2009; Cruz et al., 2013). There were reports concerning patients with *T. pallidum* bearing the A2059G mutation in the Czech Republic (Matějková et al., 2009), Columbia (Cruz et al., 2013), and the UK (Tipple et al., 2011). The proportion of isolates resistant to macrolides has been growing, indicating a need for further drug development and surveillance for resistance in *T. pallidum* (Tipple et al., 2011).

N. gonorrhoeae

The pathogen *N. gonorrhoeae* is characterized by an extraordinary ability to develop resistance to clinically used antimicrobial drugs within 10–20 years (Unemo and Nicholas, 2012). *N. gonorrhoeae* is able to quickly accumulate mutations and acquire resistance to drugs, including multiple drug resistance. There are now strains of *N. gonorrhoeae* that are resistant to all major drugs used to treat gonorrhea, including β-lactams, fluoroquinolones, macrolides, tetracyclines, spectinomycin, cephalosporins, and azithromycin. The spread of super-resistant forms of the gonorrhea pathogen is a major concern and requires the strengthening of control on a global scale (WHO, 2014b). Given the rate of increase of *N. gonorrhoeae* resistance to other drugs, some cases of gonorrhea may become incurable by 2021 because no vaccines or new drugs are being developed (Unemo, 2015). Unemo and his coworkers in Sweden and the WHO report have repeatedly stressed that the situation with drug-resistant gonorrhea can spiral out of control; thus, it is extremely urgent to develop rapid genetic analysis methods to monitor the resistance patterns of the pathogen worldwide and to apply these data to the treatment of patients (Unemo et al., 2014; WHO, 2014b).

Gonococci use most of the known mechanisms to acquire resistance: the inactivation of the antibiotic, alteration of the drug binding sites, reduction of membrane permeability, and increased drug efflux (**Figure 1**). The bacteria acquire these new characteristics via chromosomal mutations, plasmids carrying the determinants of resistance (i.e., *TEM-1, TEM-135*-encoding plasmids for resistance to penicillins, *TetM*-encoding plasmids for tetracycline resistance), and horizontal gene transfer from other species, especially from other species of *Neisseria*. Mutations altering the membrane permeability and increasing the activity of the efflux pumps are particularly efficient in the emergence of in *N. gonorrhoeae* because both mechanisms affect a wide variety of drugs.

When the penicillin treatment regimen was initiated in the 1940s, this drug was highly effective against gonococci. However, within the next 10–15 years a gradual decrease in penicillin susceptibility was observed; this decrease was mainly due to the sequential accumulation of chromosomal mutations in the bacteria. As the result, strains with MIC for penicillin as high as 4.0 mg/L were formed. Over the next few years, the same process was repeated with erythromycin, tetracycline, and azithromycin (Unemo and Shafer, 2014).

There are several mechanisms that explain the resistance of *N. gonorrhoeae* to β-lactam antibiotics. First, the bacteria produce TEM β-lactamases using a plasmid gene (*N. gonorrhoeae* does not produce chromosomally-encoded beta-lactamases). Because the gonococcal β-lactamase encoded by the plasmid gene bla_{TEM-1} is not able to destroy cephalosporins, these antibiotics have taken a leading role in the treatment of gonorrhea (Klausner and Kerndt, 2013). Mutations that decrease the affinity of the corresponding penicillin-binding proteins PBP1 and PBP2 to penicillins have been identified in the chromosomal genes *ponA* and *penA*. The main mutation in the *ponA* gene leading to the development of resistant phenotype is L421P (Lindberg et al., 2007; Endimiani et al., 2014), whereas an insertion in the *penA* gene leads to the appearance of D345 (Lindberg et al., 2007; Jeverica et al., 2014). The insertion of an extra codon for D345 in the wild-type

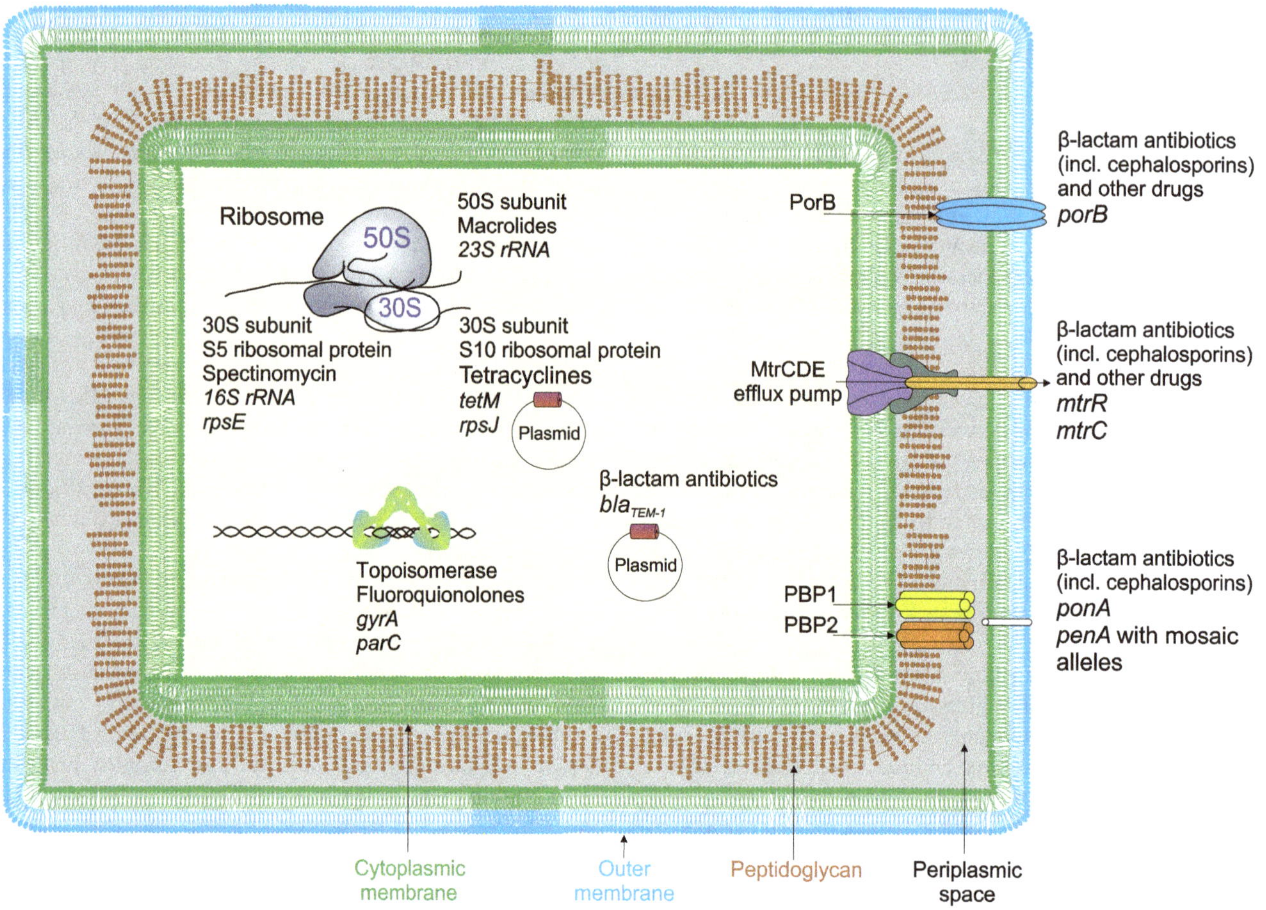

FIGURE 1 | Resistance determinans in *N. gonorrhoeae* for widely used antimicrobial drugs (a general scheme). Resistance to **β-lactam antibiotics** (penicillins) appears due to the presence of bla_{TEM-1} plasmid, encoding β-lactamase, and mutations in penicillin-binding proteins PBP1 and PBP2 (*penA* and *ponA* genes); **cephalosporins**, mutations in plasmid genes encoding β-lactamase and *penA* gene involving appearance of mosaic *penA* alleles with up to 70 amino acid alterations; **fluoroquinolones**, mutations in *gyrA* and *parC* genes encoding DNA gyrase and topoisomerase; **tetracyclines**, the presence of *tetM*-encoding plasmids and mutations in *rpsJ* gene encoding S10 ribosomal protein (ribosome 30S subunit); **macrolides**, mutations in 23S RNA genes encoding peptidyltransferases, rRNA-methylases; **spectinomycin**, mutations in *rpsE* gene encoding S5 ribosomal protein (23S rRNA); **various classes of drugs**, structural changes in major outer membrane porin protein (PorB) resulting in reducing of membrane permeability; and also mutations in efflux pump genes, particularly, in *mtrR* genes in the promoter or coding region, causing increased efflux.

penA gene results in a four-fold reduction in the susceptibility of gonococci to penicillin (Spratt, 1988).

In addition to the various mechanisms of penicillin resistance of *N. gonorrhoeae* described above, a mutation in the *pilQ2* gene (E666K) was found to increase resistance to penicillin *in vitro*. E666K works in combination with mutations in the *penA*, *mtrR*, and *penB* genes (Zhao et al., 2005; Helm et al., 2007). Because mutations in the *pilQ2* gene disrupt the formation of pili, which are required for the pathogenicity of gonococci, it is unlikely that similar genotypes could be found in clinical specimens.

During the past few years, the rate of gonococcal strains resistant to penicillin in the Russian Federation has varied between 9.6 and 13.2% (Kubanova A. et al., 2014). Globally, the proportion of resistant *N. gonorrhoeae* strains has widely varied: 81% in China, 85% in Switzerland, 79% in Hungary, 27% in Poland, and 9.9% in Belarus in 2009 (Unemo, 2015). At present, strains have been isolated that exhibit resistance to extended-spectrum cephalosporins (including ceftriaxone), which are the last drugs available for gonorrhea monotherapy. The detections of isolates with decreased susceptibility to cephalosporins (especially ceftriaxone) has been reported from all over the world (Unemo and Shafer, 2014). On average, the proportion of strains with reduced susceptibility to cefixime (MIC > 0.125 mg/L) in the European Union is approximately 8% (Unemo, 2015).

The reduced susceptibility mechanism is dependent on the mosaic organization of the *penA* gene, which may result from genetic recombination between the *N. gonorrhoeae, N. cinera*, and *N. perflava* species (Ohnishi et al., 2011). The resistance of *N. gonorrhoeae* (especially broad drug resistance to penicillins and cephalosporins) is associated with the emergence of mosaic alleles of *penA* and non-mosaic alleles carrying the A501 mutation. Mosaic alleles contain up to 70 amino acid substitutions compared to the wild-type protein. The mutations

G545S, I312M, and V316T were found in strains resistant to broad spectrum cephalosporins. Their resistance can be explained by modification of the β-lactam binding site (Unemo et al., 2012; Lewis et al., 2013; Golparian et al., 2014). Notably, the introduction of these three mutations in the wild-type PBP2 has almost no effect on the resistance of the pathogen *N. gonorrhoeae*; these mutations enhance pathogen resistance only in the presence of other mosaic alleles in the *penA* gene. It is possible that this effect is due to epistasis (the suppression of a non-allelic gene) (Tomberg et al., 2010).

Reduced susceptibility of the gonorrhea pathogen to ceftriaxone is also associated with mutations of codon 501 in non-mosaic alleles of *penA* (most often A501V but sometimes A501T). The A501 mutation is assumed to be specific for *N. gonorrhoeae* because it is not found among other *Neisseria*; this mutation possibly appeared spontaneously in gonococci under selective antibiotic pressure and was not acquired from another species (Unemo et al., 2012). A detailed study of mutations in the *penA* gene of *N. gonorrhoeae* leading to its resistance to third generation cephalosporins (cefixime and ceftriaxone) was published by Kubanova et al. (Kubanova et al., 2014). Increased resistance to ceftriaxone was observed in the presence of mutations at positions 346, 505, 511, 517, 543, 567, 575, and 576 of PBP2. The replacement of glycine with serine at position 543 results in a manifold increase in resistance to ceftriaxone.

The first highly resistant strain to ceftriaxone (H041; NG-MAST ST4220) was a sporadic case in Japan. Another strain with a similar level of resistance (F89; NG-MAST ST1407; and MLST ST7363) was first described in France and now has spread throughout the world. These strains cause unsuccessful attempts of patient treatment with cefixime and ceftriaxone (Unemo and Nicholas, 2012; Morita-Ishihara et al., 2014). The *N. gonorrhoeae* H041 and F89 strains are highly resistant to third generation cephalosporins with a minimal inhibitory concentration (MIC) of 2–4 mg/L. An investigation of the *N. gonorrhoeae* strain H041 revealed 13 additional amino acid substitutions in a mosaic allele X *penA* compared to the mosaic *penA* gene from the strain with intermediate-level cephalosporin resistance (specifically, the mutations A311V and T316S located near the β-lactam-binding pocket close to the active-site nucleophile Ser310 and the mutation Thr483 that may interact with the carboxylate of the β-lactam antibiotic) (Tomberg et al., 2013). Two cases of extended-spectrum cephalosporin-resistant *N. gonorrhoeae* were recently isolated from patients in South Africa. These strains were shown to belong to a multidrug-resistant gonococcal clone (MLST ST1901) that was associated with several cefixime treatment failures in Europe and North America (Lewis et al., 2013).

The resistance of *N. gonorrhoeae* to macrolides (azithromycin) is caused by the presence of the *erm* (erythromycin ribosome methylation) and *mef* (associated with the active efflux of antibiotics) genes. The substitution C2611T (Ng et al., 2002) in the 23S rRNA gene (the *rrl* gene) leads to the emergence of strains with moderate resistance, whereas A2059G (Katz et al., 2012; Unemo et al., 2014) leads to the emergence of highly resistant strains. In addition to the nucleotide substitutions themselves, resistance depends on the number of mutant alleles. Unemo et al. (2014) demonstrated that the presence of the C2611T substitution in all four alleles resulted in a high level of resistance, whereas strains with one mutant allele did not differ from the wild type.

N. gonorrhoeae becomes resistant to tetracycline either of the expression of a plasmid-encoded TetM protein or by a combination of three gene mutations: (i) the *mtrR* mutation, which results in overexpression of an nonspecific efflux pump (MtrC-MtrD-MtrE) that promotes the efflux of a range of hydrophobic agents and detergents; (ii) the *penB* determinant, which is a mutated porin IB that decreases the influx of tetracycline into the cell, and (iii) and mutations in the *rpsJ* gene that result in the amino acid substitution V57M in the ribosomal protein S10 (Nguyen et al., 2014). Although the combination of these mutations does not confer a level of tetracycline resistance as high as that observed with tetracycline-specific efflux pumps or the TetM determinant, the *mtrR-penB-rpsJ1* gene triad is highly effective and provides levels of resistance above those clinically achievable at the site of infection. In the same time, the *rpsJ* allele acts independently of other resistance factors and increases the MIC of tetracycline between three- and four-fold (Hu et al., 2005).

There are several determinants of *N. gonorrhoeae* resistance to spectinomycin that binds to the 30S ribosomal subunit and inhibits translation during elongation by blocking the EF-G-catalyzed translocation of peptidyl-tRNA from the A site to the P site. One of these determinants affects the segment formation of the spectinomycin binding site (*rrs* gene) by introducing one mutation in the 16S rRNA (G1064C, G1058C, or C1192U) (Galimand et al., 2000). A high-level spectinomycin-resistant (MIC > 1 mg/L) *N. gonorrhoeae* strain was isolated in Norway. The resistance determinant was a deletion of codon 27 (valine) and a K28E alteration in the ribosomal protein S5 (Unemo et al., 2013). Mutation T24P in the *rpsE* gene leading to spectinomycin resistance has also been described (Ilina et al., 2013). Generally, there are few examples of MIC-verified stains of *N. gonorrhoeae* with high-level resistance to spectinomycin (Kirkcaldy et al., 2013; Unemo, 2015). However, in Russia the proportion of spectinomycin-resistant isolates increased from 0.9 to 11.6% in a short period between 2009 and 2012 (Kubanova A. et al., 2014).

At the end of 80's, since the introduction of quinolones (fluoroquinolones) for the primary treatment of uncomplicated gonorrhea, most of the isolates of gonococci were found to be extremely susceptible to fluoroquinolones. Since the importance of antimicrobial susceptibility studies was understood, data concerning fluoroquinolone-resistant *N. gonorrhoeae* strains became available from all parts of the world (Knapp et al., 1997). In these studies, it was evident that the resistance toward fluoroquinolones, which is chromosomally mediated, develops in an incremental manner. The initial isolates which were less susceptible toward ciprofloxacin were found to have MIC values of 0.06 mg/L, which gradually increased to 1 mg/L (such strains being referred to as intermediate resistant) and later to as high as 16 mg/L (classified as resistant isolates). Strains with MIC > 4 mg/L were considered as high level resistance strains.

The main mechanism of resistance to fluoroquinolones is the decrease in the affinity of the drug for the DNA-enzyme complex. This decrease is caused by mutations in the *gyrA*, *gyrB*, *parC*, and *parE* genes in the topoisomerase polypeptide chains that form the "quinolone pocket." The resistance of *N. gonorrhoeae* to fluoroquinolones is associated with mutations S91F and D95N/G in *gyrA* gene and D86N, S88P, and E91K in *parC* gene (Vereshchagin et al., 2004). Mutations in *parC* at positions 87, 104, and 131 have also been described. Isolates with high level resistance may carry several mutations in the *gyrA* and *parC* genes (Vereshchagin et al., 2004; Pottumarthy et al., 2006). The more recent (fourth generation) fluoquinolones are more active against strains with altered ParC, but are less effective against GyrA mutants, thus, these compounds will in theory, be active against some, but not all, ciprofloxacin-resistant gonococci (Patel et al., 2011).

Resistance of *N. gonorrhoeae* to different antibiotics also arises as the result of modifications in the protein that transports antibiotics across the outer membrane (the porin PorB). In *N. gonorrhoeae,* porins are encoded by the *porB* gene and have a molecular mass ranging from 34 to 38 kDa in different strains (Zeth et al., 2013). Protein molecules form three-dimensional structures that puncture the outer membrane. Analysis of the penicillin- and tetracycline-resistant strains of *N. gonorrhoeae* revealed the G120D, A121D, and G121K mutations in the porin protein. Further studies demonstrated that these mutations were important for the diffusion of antibiotics (Olesky et al., 2006). In the same work, Olesky et al. described the G120K, G120D, and A121D mutations in the gene encoding *N. gonorrhoeae* porins. These mutations in the porin genes are widely spread and have been reported in Russia (Ilina et al., 2008), Switzerland (Endimiani et al., 2014), and Canada (Thakur et al., 2014). Notably, mutations in the *porB* gene do not increase the resistance of *N. gonorrhoeae* to β-lactams in the absence of mutations in the *mtrR* gene (a transcriptional repressor of the *mtrCDE* operon). Thus, the increase in resistance is caused by combined effort of the MtrC-MtrD-MtrE pump and PorB1b, which decreases the concentration of the antibiotic in the periplasm of the microorganism (Veal et al., 2002; Olesky et al., 2006).

Four efflux pump systems (MtrCDE, MacAB, NorM, and FarAB) have been found in gonococci belonging the RND, ABC, MATE, and MFS superfamilies (Alvarez-Ortega et al., 2013; Sun et al., 2014; Li et al., 2015; Sharkey et al., 2016), respectively (**Figure 2**). The most studied efflux pump from *N. gonorrhoeae* (MtrC-MtrD-MtrE from the RND superfamily) is responsible for the efflux of β-lactam antibiotics, macrolides, rifampin, detergents, fatty acids, steroid hormones, and cationic peptides (Veal et al., 2002). The efflux system involves a linker (MFP), a transporter, and a protein that forms a channel across the outer membrane (OMP protein). Inactivation of the MtrCDE pump in clinical isolates displaying high levels of MDR leads to significant decrease in the resistance to azithromycin, penicillin, and tetracycline (Golparian et al., 2014). Mutations in *mtrR* gene lead to the emergence of penicillin-resistant strains by increasing the expression of the MtrC-MtrD-MtrE efflux pump. Some of these mutations are located in the coding region and cause the amino acid substitutions A39T, R44H, G45D, and L47P (Ilina et al., 2008; Endimiani et al., 2014); others affect the promoter region (e.g., the insertions insTT at position −10 and deletion

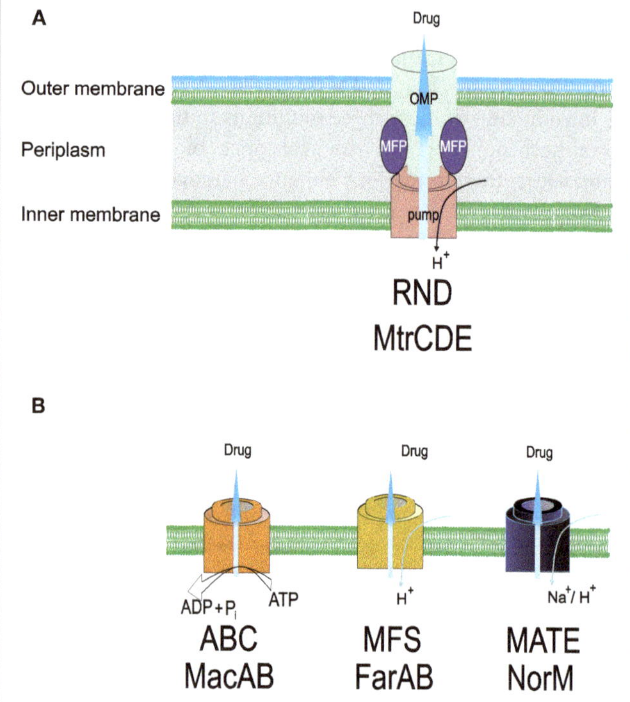

FIGURE 2 | Schematic representation of efflux systems found in *N. gonorrhoeae*. (A) MtrCDE, ternary efflux system crossing inner and outer membranes (RND superfamily). OMP, outer membrane channel protein; MFP, membrane fusion protein. Specific mutations in the promoter and/or coding sequence of *mtrR*—transcriptional repressor of the *mtrCDE* operon increase expression of the MtrCDE pump resulting in the increase in drug resistance, particularly, to ceftriaxone (*mtrR* mutations can also activate the *penB* resistance determinant). **(B)** Single-component transporters (ABC, MFS, MATE superfamilies). NorM is responsible for the efflux of fluoroquinolones, aminoglycosides, tetracyclines, FarAB—efflux of hydrophobic substances including macrolides. Overexpression of MacAB pump increases, mainly, MIC of macrolides. For the removal of antimicrobials ABC transporters use ATP as an energy source, other transporters employ an electrochemical gradient of cations, usually, protons.

delA at position −35) (Lindberg et al., 2007; Ilina et al., 2008; Endimiani et al., 2014). The most common mutations are the deletion delA in the promoter region and the substitution G45D in the coding region of the gene. Other rarer mutations also exist, such as the insertion of 153 bp between the *mtrR/mtrC* promoter and the *mtrC* gene. The resistance of *N. gonorrhoeae* to fluoroquinolones is greatly increased by the G45D or −35 delA mutations (Zarantonelli et al., 1999).

The *macA* and *macB* genes for MacAB system are organized as an operon. A SNP in the promoter region increases the transcription of *macAB* and results in an increased resistance to macrolides (Rouquette-Loughlin et al., 2005). The Na/cation antiporter NorM belonging to MATE superfamily in *N. gonorrhoeae* removes fluoroquinolones, aminoglycosides, and cationic dyes. Inactivation of NorM results in an to eight-fold decrease in the MIC for tetracycline (Golparian et al., 2014). Mutation of the promoter region of the *norM* gene has been shown to reduce susceptibility to the fluoroquinolones ciprofloxacin and norfloxacin (Rouquette-Loughlin et al., 2003).

In addition, the *mef*-encoded efflux pump protein, which is located on a conjugative transposon has been also found in *N. gonorrhoeae* strains. The protein exports macrolides out of the cell, thus, its overexpression results in resistance to macrolides (Luna et al., 2000). There is a synergistic interaction between the change in membrane permeability and the activity of efflux pumps. For example, simultaneous mutations in the porin protein and efflux pump from the RND superfamily in *N. gonorrhoeae* result in a significant increase in pathogen resistance to penicillin and ceftriaxone (Shafer and Folster, 2006).

As mentioned above, a multidrug-resistant strain from South Africa (Lewis et al., 2013) was resistant to cefixime, ciprofloxacin, penicillin, and tetracycline, exhibited intermediate resistance to azithromycin and was susceptible to ceftriaxone and the aminoglycosides, gentamicin and spectinomycin. The pathogen carried determinants of resistance for several antibiotics: mutations in the promoter region of *mtrR* gene (deletion A) resulting in overexpression of the MtrC-MtrD-MtrE efflux pump; G101K and A102N in *porB1b* encoding loop 3 of PorB1b, which decreases the influx of antibacterial drugs into the cell; mutation L421P in the *ponA1* gene that encodes the second penicillin target PBP1, thereby reducing the penicillin acylation of PBP1; and mosaic allele *penA*, type XXXIV, encoding the penicillin-binding protein PBP2.

Thus, *N. gonorrhoeae* has developed resistance to all antimicrobials introduced for first-line therapy during the last 70–80 years, and, probably, for more sustainable future treatment. To overcome this problem it is necessary to focus not only on derivatives of previously developed antimicrobials but also on the development and investigation of new targets, compounds, and approaches for treatment. As an example of such developments, the topoisomerase II inhibitor ETX0914 (also known as AZD0914) belonging to spiropyrimidinetriones was introduced as an antimicrobial compound. The mechanism of its action differs from the mechanisms of all previously and currently used drugs. The ETX0914 pharmacodynamic properties, antimicrobial susceptibility and genetic resistance mechanisms are now extensively studied for the future application as oral monotherapy or in dual combinations with ciprofloxacin, azithromycin, or ceftriaxon (Foerster et al., 2015).

C. trachomatis

Information concerning the occurrence and clinical importance of *C. trachomatis* resistance to antibiotics is scarce and contradictory (Kohlhoff and Hammerschlag, 2015). Cases of multidrug resistance have been reported in *C. trachomatis* (Shkarupeta et al., 2007; Sandoz and Rockey, 2010). For example, failure of treatment with macrolides and doxycycline was reported in patients with chlamydial infection. Clinically isolated strains resistant to doxycycline, azithromycin, josamycin, spiramycin, and ofloxacin were reported, as were multidrug-resistant strains. Although certain molecular markers associated with resistance to macrolides and fluoroquinolones have been described, no functional relationship between the presence of these markers and the efficacy of antibiotic therapy for *Chlamydia* has been established. No mutations were found in the *gyrA*, *gyrB*, *parC*, and *parE* genes (resistance to fluoroquinolones) and in the 23S rRNA V-domain, which contains macrolide resistance-associated mutations in *C. trachomatis* clinical isolates obtained after ineffective therapy of urogenital chlamydiasis with fluoroquinolones and macrolides (Shkarupeta et al., 2007).

It is typical for chlamydia to acquire so-called heterotypic resistance, a form of phenotypic resistance in which a small proportion of an infecting microbial species is capable of expressing resistance at any one time. Strains isolated from patients after the failure of treatment with antimicrobial drugs are fully sensitive to the same drugs *in vitro*, and only a small fraction of the chlamydia population (<1%) survives in the presence of high concentrations of the drugs (Shkarupeta et al., 2007).

Mycoplasna and Ureaplasma spp.

Because members of the genera *Mycoplasma* and *Ureaplasma* have no cell wall, they are insensitive to all types of β-lactam antibiotics (natural susceptibility). Sulfonamide at physiological concentrations also has no effect on these bacteria due to the absence of the metabolic pathway for the synthesis of folic acid. High rates of resistance to erythromycin and tetracycline in clinical specimens (from 73 to 97%) were reported for *Ureaplasma* species and *M. hominis*. Speciation indicated that *U. parvum* was the predominant *Ureaplasma* spp. that conferred antimicrobial resistance. Specimens resistant to macrolides were found, and cases of clinical and microbiological treatment failure with moxifloxacin were also reported (Redelinghuys et al., 2014). An increase in fluoroquinolone-resistant *M. genitalium* strains in Japan has been recently reported, and the prevalence of macrolide and fluoroquinolone resistance-associated mutations in DNA specimens from men with non-gonococcal urethritis has been determined (Kikuchi et al., 2014).

The resistance of *Mycoplasma* and *Ureaplasma* to antibiotics is primarily associated with mutations in the 23S rRNA (macrolides), *gyrA*, *gyrB*, *parC*, or *parE* gene (fluoroquinolones) (**Table 1**). The mutations responsible for macrolide, lincosamide, streptogramin, or ketolide group resistance occur in 23S rRNA at positions 2610, 2611, 2057, 2059, and 2062 in *M. hominis* (*Escherichia coli* numbering) and positions 2058 and 2059 in *M. genitalium*. Deletions and insertions in the L4 ribosomal proteins and mutations in the 23S rRNA at positions 2056, 2057, and 2058 are associated with macrolide resistance in *Ureaplasma* spp. (Couldwell et al., 2013; Salado-Rasmussen and Jensen, 2014; Waites and Xiao, 2015). The efflux genes and *erm* gene that contribute to the resistance of *Ureaplasma* to macrolides have been detected in only one work (Lu et al., 2010) and have not been confirmed by other investigators.

Susceptibility of the *M. hominis* and *Ureaplasma* spp. to tetracyclines was studied in South Africa (Redelinghuys et al., 2014). The high-level resistance to tetracyclines in *M. hominis* and *Ureaplasma* spp. is explained by the presence of the *tet*(M) determinant that provides ribosome protection and represents the sole tetracycline resistance mechanism acquired by clinical isolates of human mycoplasmas (Dégrange et al., 2008). For *M. genitalium*, treatment failures with tetracycline were reported but no genes responsible for the resistance were identified (Waites and Xiao, 2015).

TABLE 1 | Molecular determinants of drug resistance and phenotypic susceptibility in Mycoplasmas and Ureaplasmas.

Antimicrobial drug	Determinants of drug resistance	Range of minimal inhibitory concentrations for resistant isolates (mg/L)
M. genitalium		
Macrolides, lincosamides, streptogramins, ketolides	Mutations in the 23S rRNA gene at positions 2058 and 2059* Mutations in L4 ribosomal protein	16–64 for erythromycin
Tetracyclines	No determinants have been detected for isolates obtained in cases of treatment failures	No data available
Fluoroquinolones	Mutations in the *gyrA, gyrB, parC,* or *parE* genes	No data available
M. hominis		
Macrolides, lincosamides, streptogramins, ketolides	Mutations in the 23S rRNA gene at positions 2610, 2611, 2057, 2059, and 2062*	16–64 for clindamycin
Tetracyclines	*tet*(M) determinant (ribosomal protection)	8–64 for tetracyclines
Fluoroquinolones	Mutations in the *gyrA, gyrB, parC,* or *parE* genes	2–32 for levofloxacin 4–8 for ciprofloxacin
U. urealyticum and U. parvum		
Macrolides, lincosamides, streptogramins, ketolides	Deletions or insertions in L4 ribosomal proteins and/or mutations in the 23S rRNA gene at position 2056, 2057, and 2058 Ribosomal methylation mediated by the *ermB* gene mrsA/mrsB/mrsD efflux pumps	64–128 for erythromycin
Tetracyclines	*tet*(M) determinant (ribosomal protection)	2–32 for tetracyclines
Fluoroquinolones	Mutations in the *gyrA, gyrB, parC,* or *parE* genes	2–16 for levofloxacin

**Escherichia coli numbering system.*

DRUG RESISTANCE OF BV ASSOCIATED BACTERIA

G. vaginalis

G. vaginalis is treated with metronidazole and clindamycin but only limited data are available with respect to its resistance (Nagaraja, 2008; Tomusiak et al., 2011). The putative mechanism for tetracycline resistance is the presence of the *tetM* gene, which is found in tetracycline-resistant strains of *G. vaginalis* (Harwich et al., 2010). Resistance to metronidazole has been found in some *G. vaginalis* strains. The proposed mechanisms of resistance include (Löfmark et al., 2010):

- A suppressed rate of activation of the drug inside the cell through its reduction;
- Increased activity of DNA repair systems;
- Increased activity of enzymes that consume oxygen (i.e., catalase, peroxidase, and superoxide reductase);
- Accelerated clearance of the drug from the cell by active efflux.

The most well-characterized mechanism of resistance to metronidazole is the inactivation or deletion of genes with nitroreductase activity (Dhand and Snydman, 2009). Some isolates have nitroreductase genes; however, the correlation between these genes and metronidazole resistance has not been studied.

Recent whole-genome sequencing studies have revealed that *G. vaginalis* has a population structure that consists of four clades: clades 1 and 3 are associated with bacterial vaginosis and clades 2 and 4 are not. Metronidazole susceptibility is associated with the population structure, with clade 3 and 4 isolates showing 100% resistance to this drug whereas the resistance of clade 1 and 2 are 35 and 7.1%, respectively (Schuyler et al., 2015b).

B. fragilis

Recently, an increasing resistance to different antimicrobial drugs has been reported for *B. fragilis*. Resistant strains were discovered in both European countries and the United States. (Eitel et al., 2013). Multidrug-resistant *B. fragilis* isolates bearing parallel resistance to imipenem, amoxicillin and metronidazole or clindamycin were also found in Russia (Shilnikova and Dmitrieva, 2015). Antibiotic resistance is spread horizontally among the *B. fragilis* group of clinical isolates due to the antibiotic resistance genes carried on conjugative and mobilizable plasmids, conjugative transposons and integrated genetic elements (Eitel et al., 2013).

The most important mechanism of resistance of *B. fragilis* to β-lactam antibiotics is the production of β-lactamases (Edwards, 1997). The *cepA* gene encodes β-lactamase, which is able to destroy penicillins and most cephalosporins (except cefoxitin). Resistance to cefoxitin-resistant strains was explained by the presence of the *cfxA* gene located on the MTn4555 transposon. Resistance to carbapenems was explained by the presence of the *cfiA* gene in the bacterial chromosome. Because the *cfiA* gene may be expressed differently or even be silenced, different levels of carbapenem resistance may be detected. As recently shown (Eitel et al., 2013), the *cfxA* gene is not a major factor in determining cefoxitin resistance, *cfxA* was found with a higher prevalence in non-fragilis *Bacteroides* strains than in *B. fragilis*.

Metronidazole remains the drug of choice for the treatment of infections caused by *B. fragilis,* although metronidazole-resistant strains have been described in the literature (Brook, 2004). The resistance is due to the presence of the nitroimidazole resistance genes *nimA-nimG* on plasmids or on chromosomes (Carlier et al., 1997).

B. fragilis resistance to tetracycline originates from the presence of the *tetQ* gene (ribosome protection mechanism) and the *tetX* and *tetX1* genes encoding FAD-dependent monooxygenases that are able to destroy tetracycline.

B. fragilis resistance to clindamycin occurs via two mechanisms. First, the *ermB*, *ermF,* and *ermG* genes encoding various N^6-methyltransferases modify the 23S RNA. Several transferable plasmids can cause resistance [pBF4, pBFTM10 (pCP1), and pB1136]. The *ermF* resistance gene was found on transposons Tn4351 (pBF4), Tn4400 (pBFTM10), and Tn4551 (pB1136). Among the possible clindamycin resistance genes, *ermF* was the most common and had the largest effect on clindamycin resistance after the *linA* gene. The second mechanism is the action of the efflux pumps encoded by the *msrSA* and *mefA* genes. The *msrSA* gene was first described for *Staphylococcus aureus* and was later also found in *Bacteroides.* The presence of the *ermG-mefA-msrSA* combination was confirmed for clindamycin-resistant *B. fragilis* strains (Eitel et al., 2013).

Members of the *Bacteroides* genus were originally resistant to first and second generation fluoroquinolones. Resistance to the next generation fluoroquinolones appeared in the last few years; however, fluoroquinolones of the third and fourth generations are still effective against *B. fragilis.* The BexA efflux pump encoded by the *bexA* gene may be responsible for the resistance of *B. fragilis* to fluoroquinolones and the elevated moxifloxacin MIC values. The BexA pump belongs to the MATE class. It was first described for *Bacteroides thetaiotaomicron*; disruption of BexA in *B. thetaiotaomicron* made the bacteria more susceptible to norfloxacin, ciprofloxacin, and ethidium bromide. The BexA protein sequence is homologous to the protein sequence of NorM, which is a multidrug efflux transporter of *Vibrio parahaemolyticus* (Miyamae et al., 2001).

A. vaginae

Some studies demonstrated that *A. vaginae* could exhibit a high level of resistance to metronidazole (Geißdörfer et al., 2003). For example, several isolates of *A. vaginae* described in De Backer et al. (2006) were found to be highly resistant to metronidazole and susceptible to clindamycin, which are the two preferred antibiotics for the treatment of bacterial vaginosis; however, a large amount of variability in the susceptibility to metronidazole was reported (ranging from 2 to more than 256 mg/L). The authors concluded that metronidazole resistance was not an intrinsic feature of *A. vaginae.* Further research is required to clarify whether this metronidazole resistance might be acquired by the presence and activation of *nim*-genes encoding an alternative reductase that can convert nitroimidazole to a nontoxic derivative, thereby circumventing the toxic effect that causes breakage of the DNA (Löfmark et al., 2010).

A draft genome sequence of a metronidazole-susceptible (MIC 16 mg/L) vaginal isolate of *A. vaginae* (strain 44061) was recently published (Schuyler et al., 2015a). This information will be useful for comparative studies of the mechanism and the molecular basis of metronidazole resistance in *A. vaginae.*

M. mulieris

In different studies, the resistance of *M. mulieris* to metronidazole varied from 50 to 81%. The MIC_{90} of metronidazole was 128 mg/L. Reports have suggested that 4% of *Mobiluncus* species are clindamycin-resistant (Spiegel, 1987; Bahar et al., 2005). A high prevalence of metronidazole-resistant *Mobiluncus* species (81%) was found among Turkish women with gynecological infections including bacterial vaginosis (Bahar et al., 2005). Notably, the *tetQ* gene that was associated with resistance to tetracycline was found in *Mobiluncus.*

CONCLUSION

The emergence of resistance to antimicrobials is a natural consequence of the evolutionary process under increasing pressure from chemotherapy. As a result, resistance of STD pathogens appears to not only natural β-lactam antibiotics, but also to fully synthetic drugs such as fluoroquinolones. In the ongoing war between the disease and its effective treatment, a detailed understanding of the mechanisms of action of antibiotics and the emergence of resistance is necessary to modify existing drugs and to develop new ones directed against new targets. An ever-increasing range of reproductive tract bacterial infections calls for developing rapid, sensitive, and reliable methods that are able to determine resistance to available antimicrobials in individual patients as early as possible. At the same time, the recommended therapeutic regimen should take into account the regional occurrence of resistance to specific drugs obtained by constant monitoring. Moreover, for adequate therapy of diseases of the urogenital tract, in particular, for targeted selection of drugs, it is very important to take into account the possible polymicrobial character of a disease and to be able to simultaneously identify several STD pathogens and BV associated bacteria in individual clinical samples. These strategies will allow the use of existing drugs for a longer time with better efficiency and suppress the occurrence of multidrug-resistant bacterial microflora generated by repetitive failures of treatment with already inefficient antibiotics.

AUTHOR CONTRIBUTIONS

BS and ED were the primary authors, conceived the study, and drafted the manuscript for publication. AR participated in writing Chapter Brief Description of the Most Common Bacterial Infection of the Human Reproductive System and the Drugs Used to Treat Them. AL wrote Section *T. pallidum*. DV, XP, and AK participated in writing Section *N. gonorrhoeae* of Chapter Drug Resistance of Std Pathogens. DD participated in writing Sections *C. trachomatis* and Mycoplasna and Ureaplasma spp. of Chapter Drug Resistance of Std Pathogens. DG wrote Chapter Drug Resistance of BV Associated Bacteria, and reviewed the initial and revised versions of the manuscript. All authors read and approved the final manuscript.

ACKNOWLEDGMENTS

We are grateful to Dr. Danila Zimenkov for his useful remarks. We are especially grateful to Dr. Alexander Kolchinsky (Champaign, IL, USA) for his assistance in the preparation of this manuscript.

REFERENCES

Africa, C. W., Nel, J., and Stemmet, M. (2014). Anaerobes and bacterial vaginosis in pregnancy: virulence factors contributing to vaginal colonisation. *Int. J. Environ. Res. Public Health* 11, 6979–7000. doi: 10.3390/ijerph110706979

Alvarez-Ortega, C., Olivares, J., and Martinez, J. L. (2013). RND multidrug efflux pumps: what are they good for? *Front. Microbiol.* 4:7. doi: 10.3389/fmicb.2013.00007

Bahar, H., Torun, M. M., Öçer, F., and Kocazeybek, B. (2005). *Mobiluncus* species in gynaecological and obstetric infections: antimicrobial resistance and prevalence in a Turkish population. *Int. J. Antimicrob. Agents* 25, 268–271. doi: 10.1016/j.ijantimicag.2004.09.019

Bai, Z.-G., Yang, K.-H., Liu, Y.-L., Tian, J.-H., Ma, B., Mi, D.-H., et al. (2008). Azithromycin vs benzathine penicillin G for early syphilis: a meta-analysis of randomized clinical trials. *Int. J. STD AIDS* 19, 217–221. doi: 10.1258/ijsa.2007.007245

Brook, I. (2004). Urinary tract and genito-urinary suppurative infections due to anaerobic bacteria. *Int. J. Urol.* 11, 133–141. doi: 10.1111/j.1442-2042.2003.00756.x

Carlier, J. P., Sellier, N., Rager, M. N., and Reysset, G. (1997). Metabolism of a 5-nitroimidazole in susceptible and resistant isogenic strains of *Bacteroides fragilis Antimicrob. Agents Chemother.* 41, 1495–1499.

CDC (2015). *Sexually Transmitted Disease Surveillance 2014. Atlanta: U.S. Department of Health and Human Services.*

Couldwell, D. L., Tagg, K. A., Jeoffreys, N. J., and Gilbert, G. L. (2013). Failure of moxifloxacin treatment in *Mycoplasma genitalium* infections due to macrolide and fluoroquinolone resistance. *Int. J. STD AIDS* 24, 822–828. doi: 10.1177/0956462413502008

Cruz, A. R., Pillay, A., Ramirez, L. G., Chi, H., Valencia, C., Alexander, N., et al. (2013). Molecular typing and detection of macrolide resistance mutations in *T.pallidum* strains from Cali, Colombia. *Sex. Transm. Infect.* 89, A234. doi: 10.1136/sextrans-2013-051184.0729

De Backer, E., Verhelst, R., Verstraelen, H., Claeys, G., Verschraegen, G., Temmerman, M., et al. (2006). Antibiotic susceptibility of *Atopobium vaginae*. *BMC Infect. Dis.* 6:51. doi: 10.1186/1471-2334-6-51

Dégrange, S., Renaudin, H., Charron, A., Bébéar, C., and Bébéar, C. M. (2008). Tetracycline resistance in *Ureaplasma* spp. and *Mycoplasma hominis*: prevalence in Bordeaux, France, from 1999 to 2002 and description of two *tet*(M)-positive isolates of *M. hominis* susceptible to tetracyclines. *Antimicrob. Agents Chemother.* 52, 742–744. doi: 10.1128/aac.00960-07

Dhand, A., and Snydman, D. (2009). "Mechanism of resistance in metronidazole," in *Antimicrobial Drug Resistance. Infectious Disease.* ed D. Mayers (New York, NY: Humana Press), 223–227.

Edwards, J. L., and Butler, E. K. (2011). The Pathobiology of *Neisseria gonorrhoeae* lower female genital tract infection. *Front. Microbiol.* 2:102. doi: 10.3389/fmicb.2011.00102

Edwards, R. (1997). Resistance to beta-lactam antibiotics in *Bacteroides* spp. *J. Med. Microbiol.* 46, 979–986. doi: 10.1099/00222615-46-12-979

Eitel, Z., Sóki, J., Urbán, E., and Nagy, E. (2013). The prevalence of antibiotic resistance genes in *Bacteroides fragilis* group strains isolated in different European countries. *Anaerobe* 21, 43–49. doi: 10.1016/j.anaerobe.2013.03.001

Endimiani, A., Guilarte, Y., Tinguely, R., Hirzberger, L., Selvini, S., Lupo, A., et al. (2014). Characterization of *Neisseria gonorrhoeae* isolates detected in Switzerland (1998-2012): emergence of multidrug-resistant clones less susceptible to cephalosporins. *BMC Infect. Dis.* 14:106. doi: 10.1186/1471-2334-14-106

Foerster, S., Golparian, D., Jacobsson, S., Hathaway, L. J., Low, N., Shafer, W. M., et al. (2015). Genetic resistance determinants, *in vitro* time-kill curve analysis and pharmacodynamic functions for the novel topoisomerase ii inhibitor ETX0914 (AZD0914) in *Neisseria gonorrhoeae*. *Front. Microbiol.* 6:1377. doi: 10.3389/fmicb.2015.01377

Galimand, M., Gerbaud, G., and Courvalin, P. (2000). Spectinomycin resistance in *Neisseria* spp. due to mutations in 16S rRNA. *Antimicrob. Agents Chemother.* 44, 1365–1366. doi: 10.1128/aac.44.5.1365-1366.2000

Geißdörfer, W., Böhmer, C., Pelz, K., Schoerner, C., Frobenius, W., and Bogdan, C. (2003). Tuboovarian abscess caused by *Atopobium vaginae* following transvaginal oocyte recovery. *J. Clin. Microbiol.* 41, 2788–2790. doi: 10.1128/jcm.41.6.2788-2790.2003

Golparian, D., Shafer, W. M., Ohnishi, M., and Unemo, M. (2014). Importance of multidrug efflux pumps in the antimicrobial resistance property of clinical multidrug-resistant isolates of *Neisseria gonorrhoeae*. *Antimicrob. Agents Chemother.* 58, 3556–3559. doi: 10.1128/aac.00038-14

Harwich, M., Alves, J., Buck, G., Strauss, J., Patterson, J., Oki, A., et al. (2010). Drawing the line between commensal and pathogenic *Gardnerella vaginalis* through genome analysis and virulence studies. *BMC Genomics* 11:375. doi: 10.1186/1471-2164-11-375

Helm, R. A., Barnhart, M. M., and Seifert, H. S. (2007). *piQ* missense mutations have diverse effects on PilQ multimer formation, piliation, and pilus function in *Neisseria gonorrhoeae*. *J. Bacteriol.* 189, 3198–3207. doi: 10.1128/jb.01833-06

Hu, M., Nandi, S., Davies, C., and Nicholas, R. A. (2005). High-Level chromosomally mediated tetracycline resistance in *Neisseria gonorrhoeae* results from a point mutation in the *rpsJ* gene encoding ribosomal protein S10 in combination with the *mtrR* and *penB* resistance determinants. *Antimicrob. Agents Chemother.* 49, 4327–4334. doi: 10.1128/aac.49.10.4327-4334.2005

Ilina, E., Malakhova, M., Bodoev, I., Filimonova, A., Oparina, N., and Govorun, V. (2013). Mutation in ribosomal protein S5 leads to spectinomycin resistance in *Neisseria gonorrhoeae*. *Front. Microbiol.* 4:186. doi: 10.3389/fmicb.2013.00186

Ilina, E. N., Vereshchagin, V. A., Borovskaya, A. D., Malakhova, M. V., Sidorenko, S. V., Al-Khafaji, N. C., et al. (2008). Relation between genetic markers of drug resistance and susceptibility profile of clinical *Neisseria gonorrhoeae* strains. *Antimicrob. Agents Chemother.* 52, 2175–2182. doi: 10.1128/aac.01420-07

Jeverica, S., Golparian, D., Matičič M., Potočnik, M., Mlakar, B., and Unemo, M. (2014). Phenotypic and molecular characterization of *Neisseria gonorrhoeae* isolates from Slovenia, 2006–12: rise and fall of the multidrug-resistant NG-MAST genogroup 1407 clone? *J. Antimicrob. Chemother.* 69, 1517–1525. doi: 10.1093/jac/dku026

Josey, W. E., and Schwebke, J. R. (2008). The polymicrobial hypothesis of bacterial vaginosis causation: a reassessment. *Int. J. STD AIDS* 19, 152–154. doi: 10.1258/ijsa.2007.007260

Kalra, A., Palcu, C. T., Sobel, J. D., and Akins, R. A. (2007). Bacterial vaginosis: culture-and PCR-based characterizations of a complex polymicrobial disease's pathobiology. *Curr. Infect. Dis. Rep.* 9, 485–500. doi: 10.1007/s11908-007-0074-4

Katz, A. R., Komeya, A. Y., Soge, O. O., Kiaha, M. I., Lee, M. V. C., Wasserman, G. M., et al. (2012). *Neisseria gonorrhoeae* with high-level resistance to azithromycin: case report of the first isolate identified in the United States. *Clin. Infect. Dis.* 54, 841–843. doi: 10.1093/cid/cir929

Katz, K. A., and Klausner, J. D. (2008). Azithromycin resistance in *Treponema pallidum*. *Curr. Opin. Infect. Dis.* 21, 83–91. doi: 10.1097/QCO.0b013e3282f44772

Kikuchi, M., Ito, S., Yasuda, M., Tsuchiya, T., Hatazaki, K., Takanashi, M., et al. (2014). Remarkable increase in fluoroquinolone-resistant *Mycoplasma genitalium* in Japan. *J. Antimicrob. Chemother.* 69, 2376–2382. doi: 10.1093/jac/dku164

Kirkcaldy, R. D., Kidd, S., Weinstock, H. S., Papp, J. R., and Bolan, G. A. (2013). Trends in antimicrobial resistance in *Neisseria gonorrhoeae* in the USA: the Gonococcal Isolate Surveillance Project (GISP), January 2006–June 2012. *Sex. Transm. Infect.* 89, iv5–iv10. doi: 10.1136/sextrans-2013-051162

Klausner, J. D., and Kerndt, P. (2013). Cephalosporin resistance in *Neisseria gonorrhoeae* infections. *JAMA* 309, 1989. doi: 10.1001/jama.2013.4078

Knapp, J. S., Fox, K. K., Trees, D. L., and Whittington, W. L. (1997). Fluoroquinolone resistance in *Neisseria gonorrhoeae*. *Emerg. Infect. Dis.* 3, 33–39. doi: 10.3201/eid0301.970104

Kohlhoff, S. A., and Hammerschlag, M. R. (2015). Treatment of chlamydial infections: 2014 update. *Expert Opin. Pharmacother.* 16, 205–212. doi: 10.1517/14656566.2015.999041

Kubanova, A. A., Kubanov, A. A., Frigo, N. V., Volkov, I. A., Rotanov, S. V., and Suvorova, A. A. (2013). First experience of molecular typing and determining the antibiotic resistance of syphilis pathogen *Treponema pallidum* in the Russian Federation. *Vestn. Dermatol. Venerol.* 3, 34–36. Available online at: http://www.vestnikdv.ru/archive_eng.php?target=13_03_04; http://www.vestnikdv.ru/archive/13_03_04.pdf

Kubanova, A. A., Kubanov, A. A., Kozhushnaia, O. S., Vorob'ev, D. V., Solomka, V. S., and Frigo, N. V. (2014). The role of some individual amino acid substitutions in penicillin-binding protein (PBP2) of *Neisseria gonorrhoeae* in the emergence of resistance to ceftriaxone. *Mol. Biol. (Mosk).* 48, 977–982. doi: 10.1134/S0026893314060119

Kubanova, A., Frigo, N., Kubanov, A., Sidorenko, S., Lesnaya, I., Polevshikova, S., et al. (2010). The Russian gonococcal antimicrobial susceptibility programme (RU-GASP)–national resistance prevalence in 2007 and 2008, and trends during 2005-2008. *Euro. Surveill.* 15, 19533. Available online at: http://www.eurosurveillance.org/ViewArticle.aspx?ArticleId=19533; http://www.eurosurveillance.org/images/dynamic/EE/V15N14/art19533.pdf

Kubanova, A., Kubanov, A., Frigo, N., Solomka, V., Semina, V., Vorobyev, D., et al. (2014). Russian gonococcal antimicrobial susceptibility programme (RU-GASP) – resistance in *Neisseria gonorrhoeae* during 2009-2012 and NG-MAST genotypes in 2011 and 2012. *BMC Infect. Dis.* 14:342. doi: 10.1186/1471-2334-14-342

Larsen, B., and Hwang, J. (2010). *Mycoplasma, Ureaplasma*, and adverse pregnancy outcomes: a fresh look. *Infect. Dis. Obstet. Gynecol.* 2010:521921. doi: 10.1155/2010/521921. Available online at: http://www.hindawi.com/journals/idog/2010/521921/cta/

Lewis, D. A., Sriruttan, C., Müller, E. E., Golparian, D., Gumede, L., Fick, D., et al. (2013). Phenotypic and genetic characterization of the first two cases of extended-spectrum-cephalosporin-resistant *Neisseria gonorrhoeae* infection in South Africa and association with cefixime treatment failure. *J. Antimicrob. Chemother.* 68, 1267–1270. doi: 10.1093/jac/dkt034

Li, X.-Z., Plésiat, P., and Nikaido, H. (2015). The challenge of efflux-mediated antibiotic resistance in gram-negative bacteria. *Clin. Microbiol. Rev.* 28, 337–418. doi: 10.1128/cmr.00117-14

Lindberg, R., Fredlund, H., Nicholas, R., and Unemo, M. (2007). *Neisseria gonorrhoeae* isolates with reduced susceptibility to cefixime and ceftriaxone: association with genetic polymorphisms in *penA, mtrR, porB1b, and ponA*. *Antimicrob. Agents Chemother.* 51, 2117–2122. doi: 10.1128/aac.01604-06

Löfmark, S., Edlund, C., and Nord, C. E. (2010). Metronidazole is still the drug of choice for treatment of anaerobic infections. *Clin. Infect. Dis.* 50, S16–S23. doi: 10.1086/647939

Lu, C., Ye, T., Zhu, G., Feng, P., Ma, H., Lu, R., et al. (2010). Phenotypic and genetic characteristics of macrolide and lincosamide resistant *Ureaplasma urealyticum* isolated in Guangzhou, China. *Curr. Microbiol.* 61, 44–49. doi: 10.1007/s00284-009-9574-9

Luna, V. A., Cousin, S., Whittington, W. L. H., and Roberts, M. C. (2000). Identification of the conjugative mef gene in clinical *Acinetobacter junii* and *Neisseria gonorrhoeae* isolates. *Antimicrob. Agents Chemother.* 44, 2503–2506. doi: 10.1128/aac.44.9.2503-2506.2000

Margolis, E., and Fredricks, D. N. (2015). "Bacterial vaginosis-associated vacteria," in *Molecular Medical Microbiology, 2nd Edn*, ed Y.-W. Schwartzman (Boston, MA: Academic Press), 1487–1496.

Martin, D. H. (2012). The microbiota of the vagina and its influence on women's health and disease. *Am. J. Med. Sci.* 343, 2–9. doi: 10.1097/MAJ.0b013e31823ea228

Matějková, P., Flasarová M., Zákoucká H., Bořek, M.,Křemenová S., Arenberger, P., et al. (2009). Macrolide treatment failure in a case of secondary syphilis: a novel A2059G mutation in the *23S rRNA* gene of *Treponema pallidum* subsp. *pallidum*. *J. Med. Microbiol.* 58, 832–836. doi: 10.1099/jmm.0.007542-0

Menard, J. P. (2011). Antibacterial treatment of bacterial vaginosis: current and emerging therapies. *Int. J. Womens Health* 3, 295–305. doi: 10.2147/IJWH.S23814

Miyamae, S., Ueda, O., Yoshimura, F., Hwang, J., Tanaka, Y., and Nikaido, H. (2001). A MATE family multidrug efflux transporter pumps out fluoroquinolones in *Bacteroides thetaiotaomicron*. *Antimicrob. Agents Chemother.* 45, 3341–3346. doi: 10.1128/AAC.45.12.3341-3346.2001

Morita-Ishihara, T., Unemo, M., Furubayashi, K., Kawahata, T., Shimuta, K., Nakayama, S., et al. (2014). Treatment failure with 2 g of azithromycin (extended-release formulation) in gonorrhoea in Japan caused by the international multidrug-resistant ST1407 strain of *Neisseria gonorrhoeae*. *J. Antimicrob. Chemother.* 69, 2086–2090. doi: 10.1093/jac/dku118

Nagaraja, P. (2008). Antibiotic resistance of *Gardnerella vaginalis* in recurrent bacterial vaginosis. *Indian J. Med. Microbiol.* 26, 155–157. doi: 10.4103/0255-0857.40531

Ng, L.-K., Martin, I., Liu, G., and Bryden, L. (2002). Mutation in 23s rRNA associated with macrolide resistance in *Neisseria gonorrhoeae*. *Antimicrob. Agents Chemother.* 46, 3020–3025. doi: 10.1128/aac.46.9.3020-3025.2002

Nguyen, F., Starosta, A. L., Arenz, S., Sohmen, D., Dönhöfer, A., and Wilson Daniel, N. (2014). Tetracycline antibiotics and resistance mechanisms. *Biol. Chem.* 395, 559–575. doi: 10.1515/hsz-2013-0292

Ohnishi, M., Golparian, D., Shimuta, K., Saika, T., Hoshina, S., Iwasaku, K., et al. (2011). Is *Neisseria gonorrhoeae* initiating a future era of untreatable gonorrhea?: detailed characterization of the first strain with high-level resistance to ceftriaxone. *Antimicrob. Agents Chemother.* 55, 3538–3545. doi: 10.1128/aac.00325-11

Olesky, M., Zhao, S., Rosenberg, R. L., and Nicholas, R. A. (2006). Porin-mediated antibiotic resistance in *Neisseria gonorrhoeae*: ion, solute, and antibiotic permeation through PIB proteins with *penB* mutations. *J. Bacteriol.* 188, 2300–2308. doi: 10.1128/jb.188.7.2300-2308.2006

Patel, A., Chaudhry, U., Sachdev, D., Sachdeva, P., Bala, M., and Saluja, D. (2011). An insight into the drug resistance profile & mechanism of drug resistance in *Neisseria gonorrhoeae*. *Indian J. Med. Res.* 134, 419–431. Available online at: http://icmr.nic.in/ijmr/2011/october/1003.pdf

Pottumarthy, S., Fritsche, T. R., and Jones, R. N. (2006). Activity of gemifloxacin tested against *Neisseria gonorrhoeae* isolates including antimicrobialresistant phenotypes. *Diagn. Microbiol. Infect. Dis.* 54, 127–134. doi: 10.1016/j.diagmicrobio.2005.08.013

Redelinghuys, M. J., Ehlers, M. M., Dreyer, A. W., Lombaard, H. A., and Kock, M. M. (2014). Antimicrobial susceptibility patterns of *Ureaplasma* species and *Mycoplasma hominis* in pregnant women. *BMC Infect. Dis.* 14:171. doi: 10.1186/1471-2334-14-171

Rossolini, G. M., Arena, F., Pecile, P., and Pollini, S. (2014). Update on the antibiotic resistance crisis. *Curr. Opin. Pharmacol.* 18, 56–60. doi: 10.1016/j.coph.2014.09.006

Rouquette-Loughlin, C., Dunham, S. A., Kuhn, M., Balthazar, J. T., and Shafer, W. M. (2003). The NorM efflux pump of *Neisseria gonorrhoeae* and *Neisseria meningitidis* recognizes antimicrobial cationic compounds. *J. Bacteriol.* 185, 1101–1106. doi: 10.1128/jb.185.3.1101-1106.2003

Rouquette-Loughlin, C. E., Balthazar, J. T., and Shafer, W. M. (2005). Characterization of the MacA-MacB efflux system in *Neisseria gonorrhoeae*. *J. Antimicrob. Chemother.* 56, 856–860. doi: 10.1093/jac/dki333

Salado-Rasmussen, K., and Jensen, J. S. (2014). *Mycoplasma genitalium* testing pattern and macrolide resistance: a Danish nationwide retrospective survey. *Clin. Infect. Dis.* 59, 24–30. doi: 10.1093/cid/ciu217

Sandoz, K. M., and Rockey, D. D. (2010). Antibiotic resistance in *Chlamydiae*. *Future Microbiol.* 5, 1427–1442. doi: 10.2217/fmb.10.96

Schuyler, J. A., Mordechai, E., Adelson, M. E., Gygax, S. E., and Hilbert, D. W. (2015a). Draft genome sequence of a metronidazole-susceptible *Atopobium vaginae* isolate. *Genome Announc.* 3:e0991-15. doi: 10.1128/genomeA.00991-15

Schuyler, J. A., Mordechai, E., Adelson, M. E., Sobel, J. D., Gygax, S. E., and Hilbert, D. W. (2015b). Identification of intrinsically metronidazole-resistant clades of *Gardnerella vaginalis*. *Diagn. Microbiol. Infect. Dis.* 84, 1–3. doi: 10.1016/j.diagmicrobio.2015.10.006. Available online at: http://www.dmidjournal.com/article/S0732-8893%2815%2900360-0/abstract

Shafer, W., and Folster, J. (2006). Towards an understanding of chromosomally mediated penicillin resistance in *Neisseria gonorrhoeae*: evidence for a porin-efflux pump collaboration. *J. Bacteriol.* 188, 2297–2299. doi: 10.1128/JB.188.7.2297-2299.2006

Sharkey, L. K. R., Edwards, T. A., and O'Neill, A. J. (2016). ABC-F Proteins mediate antibiotic resistance through ribosomal protection. *MBio* 7:e01975-15. doi: 10.1128/mBio.01975-15. Available online at: http://mbio.asm.org/content/7/2/e01975-15.abstract

Shilnikova, I. I., and Dmitrieva, N. V. (2015). Evaluation of antibiotic susceptibility of *Bacteroides*, *Prevotella* and *Fusobacterium* species isolated from patients of the N. *N. Blokhin Cancer Research Center, Moscow, Russia*. *Anaerobe* 31, 15–18. doi: 10.1016/j.anaerobe.2014.08.003

Shkarupeta, M. M., Lazarev, V. N., Akopian, T. A., Afrikanova, T. S., and Govorun, V. M. (2007). Analysis of antibiotic resistance markers in *Chlamydia trachomatis* clinical isolates obtained after ineffective antibiotic therapy. *Bull. Exp. Biol. Med.* 143, 713–717. doi: 10.1007/s10517-007-0221-9

Spiegel, C. A. (1987). Susceptibility of *Mobiluncus* species to 23 antimicrobial agents and 15 other compounds. *Antimicrob. Agents Chemother.* 31, 249–252. doi: 10.1128/aac.31.2.249

Spratt, B. G. (1988). Hybrid penicillin-binding proteins in penicillin-resistant strains of *Neisseria gonorrhoeae*. *Nature* 332, 173–176. doi:10.1038/332173a0

Stamm, L. (2012). "Antibiotic resistance in *Treponema pallidum* subsp. pallidum, the syphilis agent," in *The Pathogenic Spirochetes: strategies for evasion of host immunity and persistence*, ed M. E. Embers (New York, NY: Springer), 213–228.

Stamm, L. V. (2010). Global challenge of antibiotic-resistant *Treponema pallidum*. *Antimicrob. Agents Chemother.* 54, 583–589. doi: 10.1128/aac.01095-09

Stamm, L. V., and Bergen, H. L. (2000). A point mutation associated with bacterial macrolide resistance is present in both 23S rRNA genes of an erythromycin-resistant *Treponema pallidum* clinical isolate. *Antimicrob. Agents Chemother.* 44, 806–807. doi: 10.1128/aac.44.3.806-807.2000

Sun, J., Deng, Z., and Yan, A. (2014). Bacterial multidrug efflux pumps: mechanisms, physiology and pharmacological exploitations. *Biochem. Biophys. Res. Commun.* 453, 254–267. doi: 10.1016/j.bbrc.2014.05.090

Thakur, S. D., Starnino, S., Horsman, G. B., Levett, P. N., and Dillon, J. R. (2014). Unique combined *penA/mtrR/porB* mutations and NG-MAST strain types associated with ceftriaxone and cefixime MIC increases in a 'susceptible' *Neisseria gonorrhoeae* population. *J. Antimicrob. Chemother.* 69, 1510–1516. doi: 10.1093/jac/dkt543

Tipple, C., McClure, M. O., and Taylor, G. P. (2011). High prevalence of macrolide resistant *Treponema pallidum* strains in a London centre. *Sex. Transm. Infect.* 87, 486–488. doi: 10.1136/sextrans-2011-050082

Tomberg, J., Unemo, M., Davies, C., and Nicholas, R. A. (2010). Molecular and structural analysis of mosaic variants of penicillin-binding protein 2 conferring decreased susceptibility to expanded-spectrum cephalosporins in *Neisseria gonorrhoeae*: role of epistatic mutations. *Biochemistry* 49, 8062–8070. doi: 10.1021/bi101167x

Tomberg, J., Unemo, M., Ohnishi, M., Davies, C., and Nicholas, R. A. (2013). Identification of amino acids conferring high-level resistance to expanded-spectrum cephalosporins in the *penA* gene from *Neisseria gonorrhoeae* strain H041. *Antimicrob. Agents Chemother.* 57, 3029–3036. doi: 10.1128/aac.00093-13

Tomusiak, A., Strus, M., and Heczko, P. (2011). Antibiotic resistance of *Gardnerella vaginalis* isolated from cases of bacterial vaginosis. *Ginekol. Pol.* 82, 900–904. Available online at: https://journals.viamedica.pl/ginekologia_polska/article/view/46253/33042

Tucker, J. D., and Cohen, M. S. (2011). China's syphilis epidemic: epidemiology, proximate determinants of spread, and control responses. *Curr. Opin. Infect. Dis.* 24, 50–55. doi: 10.1097/QCO.0b013e32834204bf

Turovskiy, Y., Cheryian, T., Algburi, A., Wirawan, R. E., Takhistov, P., Sinko, P. J., et al. (2012). Susceptibility of *Gardnerella vaginalis* biofilms to natural antimicrobials subtilosin, ϵ-poly-L-lysine, and lauramide arginine ethyl ester. *Infect. Dis. Obstet. Gynecol.* 2012:284762. doi: 10.1155/2012/284762. Available online at: http://www.hindawi.com/journals/idog/2012/284762/cta/

Unemo, M. (2015). Current and future antimicrobial treatment of gonorrhoea - the rapidly evolving *Neisseria gonorrhoeae* continues to challenge. *BMC Infect. Dis.* 15:364. doi: 10.1186/s12879-015-1029-2

Unemo, M., Golparian, D., and Hellmark, B. (2014). First three *Neisseria gonorrhoeae* isolates with high-level resistance to azithromycin in Sweden: a threat to currently available dual-antimicrobial regimens for treatment of gonorrhea? *Antimicrob. Agents Chemother.* 58, 624–625. doi: 10.1128/aac.02093-13

Unemo, M., Golparian, D., Nicholas, R., Ohnishi, M., Gallay, A., and Sednaoui, P. (2012). High-level cefixime- and ceftriaxone-resistant *Neisseria gonorrhoeae* in France: novel *penA* mosaic allele in a successful international clone causes treatment failure. *Antimicrob. Agents Chemother.* 56, 1273–1280. doi: 10.1128/aac.05760-11

Unemo, M., Golparian, D., Skogen, V., Olsen, A. O., Moi, H., Syversen, G., et al. (2013). *Neisseria gonorrhoeae* strain with high-level resistance to spectinomycin due to a novel resistance mechanism (mutated ribosomal protein S5) verified in Norway. *Antimicrob. Agents Chemother.* 57, 1057–1061. doi: 10.1128/aac.01775-12

Unemo, M., and Nicholas, R. A. (2012). Emergence of multidrug-resistant, extensively drug-resistant and untreatable gonorrhea. *Future Microbiol.* 7, 1401–1422. doi: 10.2217/fmb.12.117

Unemo, M., and Shafer, W. M. (2014). Antimicrobial resistance in *Neisseria gonorrhoeae* in the 21st century: past, evolution, and future. *Clin. Microbiol. Rev.* 27, 587–613. doi: 10.1128/cmr.00010-14

Vasilevsky, S., Greub, G., Nardelli-Haefliger, D., and Baud, D. (2014). Genital *Chlamydia trachomatis*: understanding the roles of innate and adaptive immunity in vaccine research. *Clin. Microbiol. Rev.* 27, 346–370. doi: 10.1128/CMR.00105-13

Veal, W. L., Nicholas, R. A., and Shafer, W. M. (2002). Overexpression of the MtrC-MtrD-MtrE efflux pump due to an mtrr mutation is required for chromosomally mediated penicillin resistance in *Neisseria gonorrhoeae*. *J. Bacteriol.* 184, 5619–5624. doi: 10.1128/jb.184.20.5619-5624.2002

Vereshchagin, V. A., Ilina, E. N., Malakhova, M. V., Zubkov, M. M., Sidorenko, S. V., Kubanova, A. A., et al. (2004). Fluoroquinolone-resistant *Neisseria gonorrhoeae* isolates from Russia: molecular mechanisms implicated. *J. Antimicrob. Chemother.* 53, 653–656. doi: 10.1093/jac/dkh145

Verhelst, R., Verstraelen, H., Claeys, G., Verschraegen, G., Delanghe, J., Van Simaey, L., et al. (2004). Cloning of 16S rRNA genes amplified from normal and disturbed vaginal microflora suggests a strong association between *Atopobium vaginae*, *Gardnerella vaginalis* and bacterial vaginosis. *BMC Microbiol.* 4:16. doi: 10.1186/1471-2180-4-16

Verstraelen, H., and Verhelst, R. (2009). Bacterial vaginosis: an update on diagnosis and treatment. *Expert Rev. Anti Infect. Ther.* 7, 1109–1124. doi: 10.1586/eri.09.87

Waites, K. B., and Xiao, L. (2015). "Chapter 89 - Mycoplasmas and ureaplasmas of humans," in *Molecular Medical Microbiology, 2nd Edn*, ed Y.-W. Schwartzman (Boston, MA: Academic Press), 1587–1609.

WHO (2013). *Baseline Report on Global Sexually Transmitted Infection Surveillance 2012.* Geneva: WHO Press.

WHO (2014a). *Report on Global Sexually Transmitted Infection Surveillance 2013.* Geneva: WHO Press.

WHO (2014b). *Antimicrobial Resistance: Global Report on Surveillance.* Geneva: WHO Press.

Workowski, K. A., and Bolan, G. A. (2015). Sexually transmitted diseases treatment guidelines, 2015. *MMWR Recomm. Rep.* 64, 1–137. Available online at: http://www.cdc.gov/mmwr/preview/mmwrhtml/rr6403a1.htm; http://www.cdc.gov/mmwr/pdf/rr/rr6403.pdf

Zarantonelli, L., Borthagaray, G., Lee, E.-H., and Shafer, W. M. (1999). Decreased azithromycin susceptibility of *Neisseria gonorrhoeae* due to *mtrR* mutations. *Antimicrob. Agents Chemother.* 43, 2468–2472.

Zeth, K., Kozjak-Pavlovic, V., Faulstich, M., Fraunholz, M., Hurwitz, R., Kepp, O., et al. (2013). Structure and function of the PorB porin from disseminating *Neisseria gonorrhoeae. Biochem. J.* 449, 631–642. doi: 10.1042/BJ20121025

Zhao, S., Tobiason, D. M., Hu, M., Seifert, H. S., and Nicholas, R. A. (2005). The penC mutation conferring antibiotic resistance in *Neisseria gonorrhoeae* arises from a mutation in the PilQ secretin that interferes with multimer stability. *Mol. Microbiol.* 57, 1238–1251. doi: 10.1111/j.1365-2958.2005.04752.x

7

IncF Plasmid Diversity in Multi-Drug Resistant *Escherichia coli* Strains from Animals in China

Qiu-E. Yang [1‡], *Jian Sun* [1‡], *Liang Li* [1], *Hui Deng* [1], *Bao-Tao Liu* [1†], *Liang-Xing Fang* [1], *Xiao-Ping Liao* [1] *and Ya-Hong Liu* [1,2*]

[1] Laboratory of Veterinary Pharmacology, College of Veterinary Medicine, South China Agricultural University, Guangzhou, China, [2] Jiangsu Co-Innovation Centre for Prevention and Control of Important Animal Infectious Diseases and Zoonoses, Yangzhou, China

***Correspondence:**
Ya-Hong Liu,
Laboratory of Veterinary Pharmacology, College of Veterinary Medicine, South China Agricultural University, 483 Wushan Street, Tianhe District, Guangzhou 510642, China
gale@scau.edu.cn

[†] Present Address:
Bao-Tao Liu,
College of Animal Science and Technology, Qingdao Agricultural University, Qingdao, China

[‡] These authors have contributed equally to this work.

The purpose of this study was to characterize a collection of 103 multidrug resistance IncF plasmids recovered from *Escherichia coli* of food producing and companion animals between 2003 and 2012. A total of 103 incF plasmids were characterized using an established PCR-based IncF replicon sequence typing (RST) system to identify FII, FIA, and FIB (FAB) groups. Plasmids were also analyzed using-restriction fragment length polymorphism (RFLP). Antibiotic Resistance determinants $bla_{\text{CTX-M}}$, plasmid-mediated quinolone resistance (PMQR) genes and *rmtB* and plasmid addiction systems (PAS) were identified by PCR screening. A total of 20 different RSTs from 103 IncF plasmids were identified. The groups F2 and F33 with the RST formulae A-: B- were the most frequently encountered types (63.1%). The antibiotic resistance genes (ARGs) $bla_{\text{CTX-M}}$, *rmtB,* and *oqxB* were carried by 82, 37, and 34 IncF plasmids, respectively. Most of these plasmids carried more than one resistance gene (59.2%, 61/103). The IncF plasmids also had a high frequency of addiction systems (mean 2.54) and two antisense RNA-regulated systems (*hok–sok* and *srnBC*) and a protein antitoxin-regulated system (*pemKI*) were the most prevalent. Not surprisingly, RFLP profiles among the IncF plasmids were diverse even though some shared identical IncF-RSTs. This is the first extensive study of IncF plasmid-positive *E. coli* isolates from animals in China. Our results demonstrate that IncF is the most prevalent plasmid family in *E. coli* plasmids and they commonly carry multiple resistance determinants that render them resistant to different antibiotic classes simultaneously. IncF plasmids also harbor addiction systems, promoting their stability and maintenance in the bacterial host, under changing environmental conditions.

Keywords: *Escherichia coli*, IncF plasmid, multi-resistance, addiction systems, RFLP

Introduction

Increasing antibiotic resistance in bacteria has potentially disastrous consequences for human and animal health around the world. Recent studies have demonstrated that plasmids act as efficient vehicles for the spread of antibiotic resistance genes (ARGs) more frequently than previously believed (Taylor et al., 2004; García-Fernández et al., 2009; Dolejska et al., 2011; Accogli et al., 2013; Carattoli, 2013; Dahmen et al., 2013b). Thus far, 27 different plasmid incompatibility (Inc.) groups are recognized in the Enterobacteriaceae

(Couturier et al., 1988; Carattoli et al., 2005; Villa et al., 2010). A smaller number of particular plasmid families play a major role in the diffusion of specific resistance genes among Enterobacteriaceae and are the most frequently encountered. The IncF plasmids represent one of the most prevalent incompatibility types, and have been identified worldwide in Enterobacteriaceae from different origins and sources (Carattoli, 2009; Mathers et al., 2015). Currently, a total of 924 plasmids have been deposited at the plasmid multilocus sequence typing (pMLST) database (http://pubmlst.org/plasmid/, 30 January, 2015). Of these, 214 plasmids belong to IncF group and 158 of them (73.8%) recovered from *Escherichiacoli* could be classified in 90 different subgroups on the basis of their FII, FIA and FIB (FAB) alleles.

IncF plasmids have systems which guarantee their autonomous replication but also encode addiction systems frequently based on toxin-antitoxin factors. These systems contribute to control their copy number and ensurethe instable inheritance during cell division (Cohen, 1976; Kado, 1998; Hayes, 2003). In our previous studies, we found that IncF plasmids could integrate a wide range of genes conferring resistance to all major classes of antimicrobials including β-lactams, aminoglycosides, tetracyclines, chloramphenicol, and quinolones (Liao et al., 2013; Liu et al., 2013). The extended-spectrum β-lactamases (ESBLs), especially those of the CTX-M type, are often associated with plasmid-mediated quinolone resistance (PMQR) and aminoglycoside resistance genes. Plasmids belonging to the IncF group have been the primary hosts for these traits (Boyd et al., 2004; Yao et al., 2011; Matsumura et al., 2013; Ogbolu et al., 2013).

The spread of such multidrug resistance plasmids among Enterobacteriaceae strains could also affect clinical treatments. For instance, IncF-$bla_{\text{CTX-M}}$ association was observed from both human and animal *E. coli* isolates such as the IncF-like plasmid R100 involved in the dissemination of $bla_{\text{CTX-M-14}}$ in Hong Kong, United Kingdom and France (Woodford et al., 2009; Ho et al., 2012; Dahmen et al., 2013a). The genes *rmtB*, *qepA*, *qnr*, *fosA3*, and *oqxAB* have been recently identified on IncF plasmids in *E. coli* from China, Korea and Spain (Tamang et al., 2008; Li et al., 2012; Ruiz et al., 2012; Ho et al., 2013). All together, the IncF-related family has the potential to be a major contributor worldwide to the diffusion of different resistance genes.

In general, the IncF plasmids are not a homogeneous group and vary in size (50–200 kb) and replicon type (Garcillán-Barcia et al., 2009; de Been et al., 2014; Lanza et al., 2014). Most importantly, plasmids encoding virulence-associated traits fall almost exclusively within IncF group (Johnson and Nolan, 2009). Therefore, knowledge of the prevalence and IncF plasmid subtypes in resistant populations could be a useful aid in exploring novel plasmid-targeting strategiesto treat resistant bacteria (Osborn et al., 2000; DeNap and Hergenrother, 2005; Baquero et al., 2011). We investigated variations in IncF plasmids and the phylogenetic relationship among IncF plasmids from different sources using RST and RFLP analyses. This study characterized IncF plasmids according to resistance genes, genetic relatedness and addiction systems in 103 *E. coli* isolates from pigs, poultry and companion animals.

Materials and Methods

Transconjugants and Antibiotic Susceptibility Testing

A total of non-duplicate 795 *E. coli* were isolated from animals between 2002 and 2012, according to the data published in our previous study (Liao et al., 2013; Liu et al., 2013, 2014). Among them, 696 *E. coli* were isolated from liver, heart or faces samples of diseased food-producing animals including 318 from avian (177 from ducks, 110 from chicken and 31 from geese) and 378 from pigs. The food-producing animals originated from more than 80 farms all over Guangdong province. The remaining 99 isolates were from rectal swab samples of pets including 71 dogs and 28 cats in five animal hospitals in Guangdong province. Further information about these animals, the underlying disease and possible antimicrobial pretreatment were unfortunately not available. One suspected colony with typical *E. coli* morphology and size was selected from all agar plates of each sample and was identified by Matrix Assisted Laser Desorption/lionization Time-of-Flight mass spectrometry (MALDI-TOF VITEK MS RUO System) using the Saramis™ database (bioMérieux, France). The genetic relatedness among partial *E. coli* isolates randomly selected were determined by pulsed-field gel electrophoresis (PFGE) with *XbaI* according to a protocol described previously (Gautom, 1997). Isolates encoding $bla_{\text{CTX-M}}$, *rmtB* and/or PMQR gene (535/795), were selected for conjugation experiments by the broth-mating method using streptomycin-resistance *E. coli* C600 as the recipient. Transconjugants were selected on MacConkey agar plates containing streptomycin (1000 mg/L) and cefotaxime (2 mg/L)/amikacin (32 mg/L)/olaquindox (64 mg/L), respectively. The transconjugants harboring $bla_{\text{CTX-M}}$, *rmtB*, and/or PMQR gene mentioned above were confirmed by PCR as previously.

One hundred and three transconjugants, each carrying one single IncF plasmid, were selected from a collection of clonally unrelated *E. coli* strains (15 pets, 43 avian, and 45 pigs) in our study. Table S1 contains detailed information for this population. Within this group 28 IncF plasmids had been previously characterized (Liao et al., 2013; Liu et al., 2013, 2014). Antimicrobial susceptibility tests were determined by agar dilution method on Mueller-Hinton agar plates. The antimicrobial drugs studied included quinolones (nalidixicacid), fluoroquinolones (ciprofloxacin, enrofloxacin, and levofloxacin), ampicillin, third-generation cephalosporins (ceftiofur, cefotaxime and ceftazidime), aminoglycoside (streptomycin, amikacin, kanamycin, and gentamycin) and other antimicrobials (olaquindox, chloramphenicol, florfenicol, and tetracyclines). The susceptibility tests were carried out and evaluated according to the guidelines of the Clinical and Laboratory Standards Institute (CLSI). The breakpoints for each antimicrobial were those recommended by the CLSI (M100-S19), CLSI (Vet01-A4/Vet01-S2), and DANMAP 98 (olaquindox) (Clinical and Laboratory Standards Institute, 2008, 2013). *E. coli* ATCC 25922 was used for quality control purposes.

TABLE 1 | The distribution of addiction systems and resistance genes according to FAB type identified in the 103 multi-resistance plasmids.

FAB	No. (size: kb)	Addiction systems (No.)							Mean	*Resistance genes (No.)											
		hok-sok	*pemKI*	*snrBC*	*vagCD*	*ccdAB*	*pndAC*	Total		M55	M14	M27	M65	M15	M3	M24	*rmtB*	*oqxB*	*qnrB*	*qnrS*	*qepA*
F2:A-:B-	35(70∼194)	28	18	0	3	14	3	66	1.9	5	8	14	2	0	1	1	16	11	3	5	6
F2:A1:B-	3(120∼145)	3	0	3	3	0	0	9	3	1	2	0	0	0	0	0	0	0	0	1	0
F2:A1:B1	2(145∼194)	2	1	2	2	2	0	9	4.5	0	0	0	0	0	0	0	2	1	0	1	0
F2:A-:B10	1(∼120)	1	0	1	1	0	0	3	3	0	1	0	0	0	0	0	0	0	0	0	0
F14:A-:B-	1(ND)	0	1	0	1	0	0	2	2	0	1	0	0	0	0	0	0	1	0	0	0
F16:A-:B-	3(∼97)	3	1	1	0	0	0	5	1.7	0	0	0	0	0	0	0	0	3	0	2	0
F16:A-:B1	1(∼60)	1	1	0	0	1	0	3	3	1	0	0	0	0	0	0	0	0	0	0	0
F18:A-:B-	3(135∼145)	3	3	3	0	0	0	9	3	1	1	0	1	0	0	0	0	1	0	0	0
F18:A-:B1	1(145∼194)	8	8	9	1	2	1	29	2.9	5	0	0	0	0	0	0	1	6	0	0	0
F18:A-:B8	1(∼194)	1	0	1	0	1	0	3	3	0	0	0	0	0	0	0	0	1	0	0	0
F31:A4:B1	3(∼194)	1	3	3	2	3	0	12	4	0	0	0	0	3	0	0	0	0	0	0	0
F33:A-:B-	30(60∼194)	26	25	29	1	1	2	84	2.8	16	0	0	9	0	0	0	17	8	0	0	0
F33:A1:B-	1(ND)	1	0	0	1	1	0	3	3	0	1	0	0	0	0	0	0	0	0	0	0
F33:A-:B1	1(ND)	1	1	1	0	0	0	3	3	0	0	0	0	0	0	0	1	1	0	0	0
F35:A-:B-	3(∼97)	3	0	3	2	1	0	9	3	0	3	0	0	0	0	0	0	0	0	0	0
F36:A1:B1	1(∼160)	1	1	1	0	1	0	4	4	0	1	0	0	0	0	0	0	0	0	0	0
F43:A-:B-	1(∼110)	1	0	0	0	1	0	2	2	0	1	0	0	0	0	0	0	0	0	0	0
F43:A3:B-	1(∼145)	1	1	1	1	1	0	5	5	1	0	0	0	0	0	0	0	0	0	1	0
F46:A-:B24	1(∼130)	1	0	1	0	0	0	2	2	0	0	0	0	0	0	0	0	1	0	1	0
F58:A-:B-	1(∼145)	0	0	0	0	0	0	0	0	0	1	0	1	0	0	0	0	0	0	0	0
Total No.	103	86	64	59	18	29	6	262	2.54	30	20	14	13	3	1	1	37	34	3	11	6

**M55/14/27/65/15/3/24 is resistance genes abbreviations for $bla_{CTX-M-55/14/27/65/15/3/24}$, respectively.*

ND, not determined.

Detection of Antimicrobial Resistance Genes

The total DNA of transconjugants harvested from LB broth were extracted by TIANPrep Plasmid Mini Kit (TIANGEN Biotech, Beijing, China), according to the manufacturer's instructions. The bla_{CTX-M}, *rmtB*, and PMQR genes were screened by PCR using primers as described previously (Cano et al., 2009; Wang et al., 2012). The bla_{CTX-M}, *rmtB*, and *oqxB*-positive transconjugants were also evaluated for the presence of other PMQR genes (*qnrA*, *qnrB*, *qnrC*, *qnrD*, *qnrS*, and *qepA*). PCR products were sequenced and compared with the reported sequences from GenBank (www.ncbi.nlm.nih.gov/genbank/).

IncF Plasmid Analysis

Plasmid DNA was extracted by QIAGENPrep Plasmid Midi Kit (QIAGEN, Hilden, Germany), according to the manufacturer's instructions. PCR-base replicon typing (PBRT) was performed on all transconjugants carrying a single plasmid, as previously described (Carattoli et al., 2005). To better characterize IncF, replicon sequencing typing (RST) was performed according to protocols described previously (Villa et al., 2010), and alleles were assigned by comparing the amplicon sequence to the plasmid MLST database (http://pubmlst.org/plasmid/).

Plasmid sizes in the transconjugants were determined by pulsed-field gel electrophoresis using nuclease S1 (TaKaRa Biotechnology, Dalian, China) digestion of plasmid DNA prepared in agarose blocks (S1-PFGE). DNA fragments were separated by PFGE on a CHEF-DR III apparatus (Bio-Rad, Hercules, CA, USA) for 15 h at 6 V/cm at 14°C with an initial pulse time of 1 s and a final pulse time of 12 s. Southern hybridization was performed following S1-PFGE using bla_{CTX-M}, *rmtB*, and *oqxB*-specific digoxigen in (DIG)-labeled probes. Hybridization was detected using the DIG Nucleic Acid Detection Kit (Roche Diagnostics). All plasmids were also analyzed by restriction fragment length polymorphism (RFLP) as following: Plasmid DNA was digested with *EcoRI* and electrophoresed in 1.0% agarose at 5 V/cm for 2 h. DNA was visualized by EtBr staining. Cluster analysis of digestion patterns generated dendrograms and plasmid similarity was measured using BioNumerics software (Applied Maths, Sint-Martens-Latem, Belgium) using the Dice Similarity Index (DSI) (tolerance 1.5% and optimization 1.5%. Plasmids with a DSI ≥80% were assigned to the same cluster (designated with numbers 1, 2, 3, and 4). Letters were used to discriminate RFLP patterns assigned to the same clusterthat differed by one or two restriction bands (i.e., 1a, 1b, 1c etc.).

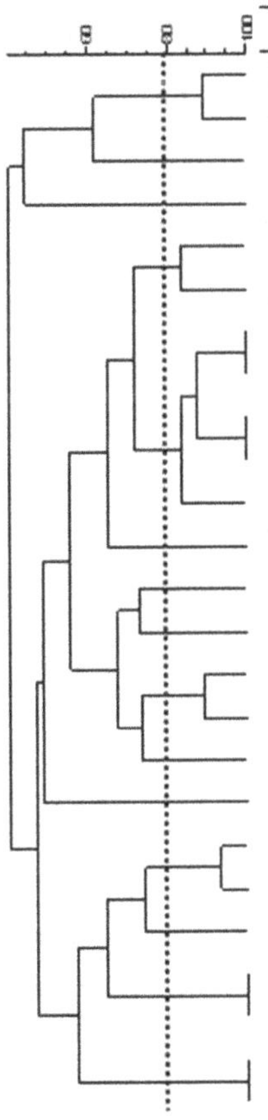

Strains	Year	source	Resistance Phenotype[a]	Size (kb)	Resistance Genes	RFLP[b]
FS006	2011	pig	C-S-A-H-F-G-R-CT-O	90	$bla_{CTX-M-14}$	F2-1a
43	2008	pig	C-S-A	97	$bla_{CTX-M-55}$	F2-1b
S74	2012	pig	C-S-A-G-A-K-R-CT	194	$bla_{CTX-M-14}$, *oqx*B	F2-2
7zu	2010	pig	C-S-A-G-M-R-CT-O	80	*oqx*B, *qep*A	F2-3
FS11Z2C	2012	pig	C-S-A-G-M-R-CT	97	$bla_{CTX-M-27}$, *rmt*B	F2-4a
A6	2007	avian	C-S-A-T-R-CT	70	$bla_{CTX-M-65}$, *oqx*B, *qnr*S, *qep*A	F2-4b
FS11Z1F	2012	pig	C-S-A	97	$bla_{CTX-M-14}$	F2-5a
FS11Z1S	2012	pig	C-A-CT	97	$bla_{CTX-M-14}$	F2-5a
1162	2010	pig	CTZ-A-H-F-R	135	$bla_{CTX-M-14}$	F2-5b
FS11Z1	2012	pig	C-S-A-G-A-K-D-R-CT	195	$bla_{CTX-M-14}$, *rmt*B	F2-5b
A5	2010	pet	C-A-G-K-R-CT	145	$bla_{CTX-M-14}$	F2-5c
S87	2008	pig	C-S-A-T-R-CT	97	$bla_{CTX-M-27}$	F2-6
70ZU	2010	pig	C-S-A-H-F.G-R-CT-O	70	*bla*ctx-m-24, *oqx*B	F2-7
FS044	2011	pig	C-S-A-H-G-K-CT-F	190	$bla_{CTX-M-27}$, *rmt*B	F2-8
A62	2007	avian	C-S-A-T-G-M-K-R-CT	97	$bla_{CTX-M-27}$, *rmt*B	F2-9a
FSD160	2009	avian	C-S-A-G-M-K-R-CT	194	$bla_{CTX-M-55}$	F2-9b
A83	2007	avian	C-S-A-F-T-G-M-K-D-R-CT	97	$bla_{CTX-M-27}$, *rmt*B	F2-10
5wei	2010	pig	N-C-S-A-H-F-O-M-G-K-CT	100	$bla_{CTX-M-65}$, *oqx*B,	F2-11
A84	2007	avian	C-S-A-G-K-R-CT	ND	*oqx*B, *qnr*S	F2-12a
A90	2005	avian	C-S-R-CT-O	ND	$bla_{CTX-M-27}$, *oqx*B, *qep*A, *rmt*B	F2-12b
A61	2007	avian	C-S-A-G-M-K-R-CT-O	97	$bla_{CTX-M-27}$, *rmt*B, *qnr*S, *oqx*B, *qep*A	F2-13
A72	2007	avian	C-S-A-F-G-M-K-R-CT-O	97	$bla_{CTX-M-27}$, *rmt*B	F2-14a
S22	2004	pig	C-S-A-T-G-M-K-R-CT	97	$bla_{CTX-M-27}$, *rmt*B	F2-14a
FS9Y2C	2012	avian	P-S-A-F-T-M-O	194	$bla_{CTX-M-55}$	F2-15a
S116	2007	pig	C-S-A-H-F-T-R-O-CT	80	$bla_{CTX-M-27}$	F2-15a

FIGURE 1 | RFLP patterns and characterization of multi-resistance 25 F2: A-: B- plasmids.

Identification of Plasmid Addiction Systems

Plasmid-mediated addiction systems were identified using primers and amplification conditions were previously described (Mnif et al., 2010). We screened for 8 major addiction systems: *ccdA-ccdB* (involved in cell division), *pemK-pemI* (for plasmid emergency maintenance), *relB-relE* (relaxed control of stable RNA), *parD-parE* (DNA replication), *vagC-vagD* (virulence-associated protein), *hok-hok* (host-killing), *snrB-snrC* (RNA stability), and *pndA-pndC* (promotion of nucleic acid).

Statistical Analysis

Statistical significance for the comparison of prevalence data and proportions was determined by the x^2-test. p-values less than 0.05 were deemed to be statistically significant.

Results

Antibiotic Resistance Phenotypes

A total of 103 transconjugants were examined in this study and 96% exhibited multi-drug resistance phenotypes with to ampicillin and streptomycin. More than half of the isolates also showed resistance tocefotaxime, ceftriaxone, gentamicin, kanamycin and ceftiofur (Table S1). The antimicrobial resistance rates to other antibiotics tested as follows: amikacin (43.7%), olaquindox (42.7%), tetracycline (40.8%), chloramphenicol (34.0%), and florfenicol (26.2%). Most of these isolates were still susceptible to levofloxacin, enrofloxacin and ciprofloxacin.

Detection of Resistance Genes

Results of screening for resistance genes among 103 transconjugants are shown in Table S1. The predominant resistance genes identified were bla_{CTX-M}, *rmtB*, and *oqxB* found in 82, 37, and 34 IncF-type plasmids, respectively. Interestingly, there was a range of bla_{CTX-M} genotypes including M55 (n = 30), M14 (n = 20), M27 (n = 14), M65 (n = 13), M15 (n = 3) and M24 and M3 (1 each). A smaller subset also harbored *qnrS*, *qepA*, and *qnrB* genes (11, 6, and 3, respectively). Sixty-one plasmids carried more than one resistance gene, and the most prevalent combinations were bla_{CTX-M}-*rmtB* (n = 28) and bla_{CTX-M}-*oqxAB* (n = 15). The *qnrA*, *qnrC*, and *qnrD* loci were not found in any of the plasmids tested.

Characterization of IncF Plasmids

S1-PFGE and Southern blot hybridization analysis showed that all the 103 multi-drug resistant strains contained plasmids ranging in size from 60 to 194 kb (**Table 1**). This group contained very diverse IncF-RST patterns. A total of 20 IncF-RSTs were found that had replicon FII alone or in combination with FIA or FIB. Various alleles were observed for each of FII (F2, F14, F16, F18, F31, F33, F35, F36, F43, F46, and F58), FIA (A-, A1, A3, and A4) and FIB (B-, B1, B8, B10, and B24) replicons. Meanwhile, we found identical combinations were detected in a number of different plasmids; F2: A-: B- (n = 35) and F33: A-: B- (n = 30) were the most common. Curiously, more than half of F2: A-: B- positive *E. coli* strains (54.8%, 19/35) were recovered from pigs, while F33: A-: B- (46.7%, 14/30) and F18: A-: B- (50.0%, 5/10) were mainly found in *E. coli* strains recovered from avians.

Further analysis of IncF plasmids bearing multi-resistance genes was performed to see whether a particular resistance gene was associated with a specific plasmid backbone defined by replicon type and addiction system content. Notably, there was higher prevalence of resistance genes located on F2: A- B- and F33: A-: B- plasmids than on the remaining replicon types (**Table 1**). For instance, $bla_{CTX-M-27}$, *qepA*, and *qnrS* were preferentially associated with the F2: A-: B-. The $bla_{CTX-M-55}$, which was the most common identified β-lactamase in our study, combined with F33: A-: B-; while *rmtB* and *oqxB* were mainly found in F2: A-: B- and F33: A-: B-.

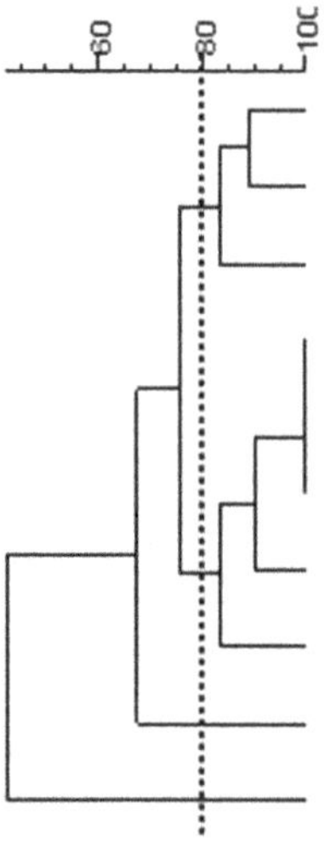

Strains	Year	Source	Resistance Phenotype[a]	Size (kb)	Resistance Genes	RFLP[b]
FS3Z3C	2012	pig	C-S-A-K-R-G-F	145	$bla_{CTX-M-55}$, *oqxB*, *rmtB*	F18-1a
FSD155	2009	avian	C-S-A-H-R-G	ND	$bla_{CTX-M-55}$	F18-1b
33	2010	pet	C-S-A-K-R-G	145	$bla_{CTX-M-55}$, *oqxB*,	F18-1c
A26	2003	avian	C-S-A-H-F-T-A-D-R	145	*oqxB*	F18-2a
A58	2004	avian	S-A-H-T-G-K-D-O	145	*oqxB*	F18-2a
Z1	2004	pig	S-A-H-T-K-D-O	145	*oqxB*	F18-2a
S106	2007	avian	S-A-H-F-G-O	ND	*oqxB*	F18-2b
FS12Y1C	2012	avian	N-S-A-H-T-M-D-O	145	$bla_{CTX-M-55}$	F18-2c
32	2008	pet	C-S-A-G	194	$bla_{CTX-M-14}$	F18-3
LJC8	2010	pig	C-S-A-R	ND	$bla_{CTX-M-55}$	F18-4

FIGURE 2 | RFLP patterns and characterization of multi-resistance 10 F18: A-: B1 plasmids.

In order to assess relationships among the different replicon types of 103 IncF plasmids encoding variable resistance determinants, RFLP analysis was conducted which allowed visualization of variable clustering. However, our RFLP results showed diverse plasmid profiles even among identical IncF-RST groups. For instance, among 27/30 F33: A-: B- and 25/35 F2: A-: B- plasmids, 12 and 15 RFLP patterns were identified, respectively. In addition, antimicrobial susceptibility, plasmid size and antimicrobial resistance genes varied (**Figures 1–3**).

Addiction Systems

Of the eight addiction systems, the most frequently represented systems were *hok-sok* ($n = 86$), followed by *pemKI* ($n = 64$), *snrBC* ($n = 59$), *ccdAB* ($n = 29$), *vagCD* ($n = 18$), and *pndAC* ($n = 6$). None of the IncF-type plasmids harbored *parDE* and *relBE*. The average mean of addiction system was 2.54 with a range of 0–5 per plasmid. Interestingly, when the replicon FII was associated with FIA and FIB, the isolate also carried more addiction systems than in the absence of this association (**Table 1**). For instance, between the groups F2: A1: B1 and F2: A-: B-, there was a mean of 4.5 vs. 1.9, and the combination of F16: A-: B1 and F16: A-: B- with the mean of 3.0 vs. 1.7.

The number of different types of addiction systems also varied between the most prevalence replicon types in this study, F2: A-: B- and F33: A-: B-. The number of *snrBC* loci on F33: A-: B- was significantly higher than on F2: A-: B- ($P < 0.01$). In contrast, this number was reversed in the case of the *ccdAB* system (**Table 1**).

Discussion

In the present study, the prevalence of the resistance determinants bla_{CTX-M}, PMQR genes and *rmtB* in IncF plasmids from farm animals and pets in China was investigated and the

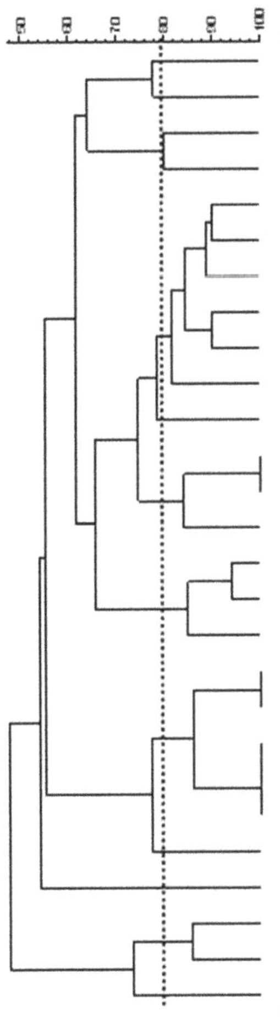

Strains	Year	source	Resistance Phenotype[a]	Size(kb)	Resistance Genes	RFLP[b]
85chang	2010	avian	C-S-A-F-G-M-K-R-CT-O	170	*oqx*B	F33-1
P161	2008	pet	C-S-A-R-CT	120	$bla_{CTX-M-65}$, *rmt*B	F33-2
FS5E1D	2012	avian	C-S-A-H-F-M-G-K-CT-R	100	$bla_{CTX-M-55}$, *oqx*B,	F33-3a
FS6J1W	2012	avian	C-S-A-CT-G	ND	*oqx*B	F33-3b
FS8J4C	2012	avian	C-S-A-R-CT	97	$bla_{CTX-M-65}$	F33-4a
S55-2	2012	pig	C-S-A-T-G-M-K-R-CT-O	ND	*rmt*B	F33-4b
38	2010	pet	C-S-A-G-M-K-R-CT	100	$bla_{CTX-M-65}$, *rmt*B	F33-4c
FS1Z1X	2012	pig	C-S-A-G-M-R-CT	90	$bla_{CTX-M-55}$, *rmt*B	F33-4d
FS6Y1G	2012	avian	C-A-H-F-R	97	$bla_{CTX-M-55}$, *rmt*B	F33-4e
FS11Z5F	2012	pig	C-S-A-M-G-CT-K	90	$bla_{CTX-M-55}$, *rmt*B	F33-4f
FS13Z2C	2012	pig	C-S-R-CT	ND	$bla_{CTX-M-55}$	F33-5
FS2Y3G	2012	avian	C-S-A-R-CT	60	$bla_{CTX-M-55}$	F33-6a
NND6	2010	avian	C-S-A-R	90	$bla_{CTX-M-55}$	F33-6a
FS4Y2C	2012	avian	N-S-A-T-G-M-O	145	$bla_{CTX-M-14}$, *rmt*B	F33-6b
2YC2	2011	avian	C-S-A-H-F-M-G-K-CT-R	ND	$bla_{CTX-M-55}$, *rmt*B	F33-7a
FS13Z3C	2012	pig	N-C-S-M-F-A-T-G-K-R-CT	120	$bla_{CTX-M-55}$, *rmt*B	F33-7b
FS11Y2G	2012	avian	C-S-A-F-M-G-K-CT	120	$bla_{CTX-M-55}$, *rmt*B	F33-7c
50-2	2010	pet	C-S-A-G-M-K-R-CT-O	97	$bla_{CTX-M-65}$, *rmt*B	F33-8a
FS2Y1X	2012	avian	S-A-H-T-M-D-O-	100	$bla_{CTX-M-55}$, *oqx*B,	F33-8b
3-3-2	2008	pig	C-S-A-K-R-CT	60	$bla_{CTX-M-55}$	F33-8c
B7	2010	pet	C-S-A-G-M-K	90	*oqx*B, *rmt*B	F33-8c
S104	2012	pig	C-S-A-H-G-M-K-R-CT	97	$bla_{CTX-M-65}$	F33-8c
FS5Z6D	2012	pig	C-S-A-M-G-R-CT	97	$bla_{CTX-M-55}$, *rmt*B	F33-9
S68	2010	pig	S-A-H-F-G-O	ND	$bla_{CTX-M-65}$, *oqx*B,	F33-10
42-2	2010	avian	C-S-A-H-F-T-K-R	100	$bla_{CTX-M-55}$, *oqx*B,	F33-11a
1-5-1	2008	pig	C-S-A-G-M-K-R-CT	97	$bla_{CTX-M-65}$, *rmt*B	F33-11b
FS6Y4C	2012	avian	S-A-H-T-M-D-O-	90	$bla_{CTX-M-55}$, *rmt*B	F33-12

FIGURE 3 | RFLP patterns and characterization of multi-resistance 27 F33: A-: B- plasmids. The scale on the top left of the figure indicates the percentage of similarity for the *EcoR*I restriction profiles of the IncF plasmids. [a]Antimicrobial for which the plasmids MICs fell within the resistant range; Antimicrobial abbreviations: A, ampicillin; S, streptomycin; M, amikacin; K, kanamycin; G, gentamycin; R, ceftriaxone; C, cefotaxime; CT, ceftiofur; N, nalidixic acid; P, ciprofloxacin; E, enrofloxacin; L, levoflox-acin; O, olaquindox; T, tetracycline; H, chloramphenicol and F, florfenicol. [b]Plasmids with a DSI ≥80% were assigned to the same cluster (designated with numbers 1, 2, 3, 4 etc.). Letters were used to discriminate RFLP patterns assigned to the same cluster, but differing by one or two restriction bands (i.e., 1a, 1b, 1c etc.). ND, not determined.

characteristics of IncF plasmids were elucidated. One-hundred and three IncF plasmids were recovered, the majority from pigs and avians (85.4%, 88/103), and the remaining obtained from pets (14.6%, 15/103), demonstrating that IncF plasmids are prevalent among multi-drug resistant *E. coli* strains from animals in China. The IncF plasmids identified in our study were associated with multidrug resistance profiles that conferred resistance to different classes of antimicrobials simultaneously. Most of IncF plasmids harbored $bla_{\text{CTX-M}}$ and, frequently carried other resistance genes including *qnr*, *qepA*, *oqxB*, and *rmtB*. These results are in agreement with previous findings that the *rmtB* and PMQR genes are often linked with $bla_{\text{CTX-M}}$- located on the same plasmid (Dhanji et al., 2011; Li et al., 2012; Matsumura et al., 2013; Chen et al., 2014). Together, these data suggest that the spread of multiple ARGs on the same plasmid has been an important dissemination mechanism of multidrug resistance (Liebert et al., 1999).

The most impressive finding in this study was the diversity of IncF plasmids. The result is similar to previous reports that showed IncF plasmids are not a homogeneous group (Osborn et al., 2000; Coque et al., 2008; Villa et al., 2010; Shin et al., 2012). Moreover, heterogeneous RFLP patterns among identical IncF-RST groups indicate that the cargos such as resistance genes are also likely associated with the diversity of IncF plasmids. Interestingly, we identified some particular resistance genes were associated with the specific plasmid backbone defined by replicon type. For instance, $bla_{\text{CTX-M-3}}$ was located on F2: A-: B-, whereas it has been previously on detected IncL/M plasmids (Golebiewski et al., 2007). As for $bla_{\text{CTX-M-14}}$, which was primarily found on F2: A-: B- in our study, but in Spain and France, this gene was presented on the IncK plasmids (Diestra et al., 2009; Valverde et al., 2009). Although the movements of these resistance genes were attributed to transposable elements, it is certain that the epidemic plasmids may accelerate their widespread dissemination.

Interestingly, although RFLP patterns were diverse among the plasmids, some with the same IncF-RST grouping did show similar RFLP patterns with minor variations. These data agree with previous studies reporting that IncF plasmids form a very heterogeneous group (Dahmen et al., 2013b). Thus, the extensive diversity of RFLP patterns among IncF plasmids from the collection of *E. coli* used in this study may be due to frequent recombination and acquisition resistance genes between the plasmids (Partridge et al., 2011; Wiedenbeck and Cohan, 2011; Cain and Hall, 2012).

In contrast to RFLP patterns, the content of addiction systems seemed to differ by replicon type. For instance, the *snrBC* system was widely represented in F33: A-: B- but absent in F2: A-: B-, while *ccdAB* was associated with F2: A-: B-. This finding indicates a linkage between addiction systems and specific plasmid backbones, but this must be investigated further. As previously reported, plasmid addiction systems (PAS) contribute to the stability and maintenance of plasmids and they have been shown to facilitate plasmid dissemination even in the absence of antibiotic selection (Hayes, 2003; Moritz and Hergenrother, 2007). Together, these data suggest a hypothesis that the diversity of IncF plasmids can be driven by a combination of acquired multiple resistance genes and addiction modules. In this way, host maintenance would be facilitated by their spread in the *E. coli* population.

In conclusion, we identified extensive diversity of RSTs, plasmid sizes, addiction systems and RFLP patterns among IncF plasmids, carrying $bla_{\text{CTX-M}}$ or PMQR or aminoglycoside resistance genes. Considering the fact that the IncF plasmids have been common reservoirs for diffusion of resistance genes, its wide dissemination among Enterobacteriaceae especially among *E. coli* could pose a serious threat to public health.

Acknowledgments

This work was supported by the Program for Changjiang Scholars and Innovative Research Team in University of Ministry of Education of China (Grant No. IRT13063), the National Natural Science Foundation and Natural Science Foundation of Guangdong Province, China (Grant No. U1201214), the Natural Science Foundation of Guangdong Province (Grant No. S2012030006590) and the National Natural ScienceFunds of China (Grant No. 31402247).

References

Accogli, M., Fortini, D., Giufrè, M., Graziani, C., Dolejska, M., Carattoli, A., et al. (2013). IncI1 plasmids associated with the spread of CMY-2, CTX-M-1 and SHV-12 in *Escherichia coli* of animal and human origin. *Clin. Microbiol. Infect.* 19, E238–E240. doi: 10.1111/1469-0691.12128

Baquero, F., Coque, T. M., and de la Cruz, F. (2011). Ecology and evolution as targets: the need for novel eco-evo drugs and strategies to fight antibiotic resistance. *Antimicrob. Agents Chemother.* 55, 3649–3660. doi: 10.1128/AAC.00013-11

Boyd, D. A., Tyler, S., Christianson, S., McGeer, A., Muller, M. P., Willey, B. M., et al. (2004). Complete nucleotide sequence of a 92-kilobase plasmid harboring the CTX-M-15 extended-spectrum beta-lactamase involved in an outbreak in long-term-care facilities in Toronto, Canada. *Antimicrob. Agents Chemother.* 48, 3758–3764. doi: 10.1128/AAC.48.10.3758-3764.2004

Cain, A. K., and Hall, R. M. (2012). Evolution of a multiple antibiotic resistance region in IncHI1 plasmids: reshaping resistance regions *in situ*. *J. Antimicrob. Chemother.* 67, 2848–2853. doi: 10.1093/jac/dks317

Cano, M. E., Rodriguez-Martinez, J. M., Aguero, J., Pascual, A., Calvo, J., Garcia-Lobo, J. M., et al. (2009). Detection of plasmid-mediated quinolone resistance genes in clinical isolates of *Enterobacter* spp. in Spain. *J. Clin. Microbiol.* 47, 2033–2039. doi: 10.1128/JCM.02229-08

Carattoli, A. (2009). Resistance plasmid families in Enterobacteriaceae. *Antimicrob. Agents Chemother.* 53, 2227–2238. doi: 10.1128/AAC.01707-08

Carattoli, A. (2013). Plasmids and the spread of resistance. *Int. J. Med. Microbiol.* 303, 298–304. doi: 10.1016/j.ijmm.2013.02.001

Carattoli, A., Bertini, A., Villa, L., Falbo, V., Hopkins, K. L., and Threlfall, E. J. (2005). Identification of plasmids by PCR-based replicon typing. *J. Microbiol. Methods* 63, 219–228. doi: 10.1016/j.mimet.2005.03.018

Chen, X., He, L., Li, Y., Zeng, Z., Deng, Y., Liu, Y., et al. (2014). Complete sequence of a F2:A-:B- plasmid pHN3A11 carrying *rmtB* and *qepA*, and its dissemination in China. *Vet Microbiol.* 174, 267–271. doi: 10.1016/j.vetmic.2014.08.023

Clinical and Laboratory Standards Institute. (2008). *Performance Standards for Antimi-crobial Susceptibility Testing; Eighteenth Informational Supplement.* Document M100-S18. Wayne, PA: CLSI.

Clinical and Laboratory Standards Institute. (2013). *Performance Standards for Antimi-crobial Disk and Dilution Susceptibility Tests for Bacteria Isolated from Animals; Approved Standard-fourth Edition and Supplement.* Documents VET01-A4E and VET01-S2E. Wayne, PA: CLSI.

Cohen, S. N. (1976). Transposable genetic elements and plasmid evolution. *Nature* 263, 731–738. doi: 10.1038/263731a0

Coque, T. M., Novais, A., Carattoli, A., Poirel, L., Pitout, J., Peixe, L., et al. (2008). Dissemination of clonally related *Escherichia coli* strains expressing extended-spectrum beta-lactamase CTX-M-15. *Emerg. Infect. Dis.* 14, 195–200. doi: 10.3201/eid1402.070350

Couturier, M., Bex, F., Bergquist, P. L., and Maas, W. K. (1988). Identification and classification of bacterial plasmids. *Microbiol. Rev.* 52, 375–395.

Dahmen, S., Madec, J. Y., and Haenni, M. (2013a). F2: A-: B- plasmid carrying the extended-spectrum beta-lactamase $bla_{(CTX-M-55/57)}$ gene in Proteus mirabilis isolated from a primate. *Int. J. Antimicrob. Agents* 41, 594–595. doi: 10.1016/j.ijantimicag.2013.02.004

Dahmen, S., Métayer, V., Gay, E., Madec, J. Y., and Haenni, M. (2013b). Characterization of extended-spectrum beta-lactamase (ESBL)-carrying plasmids and clones of Enterobacteriaceae causing cattle mastitis in France. *Vet Microbiol.* 162, 793–799. doi: 10.1016/j.vetmic.2012.10.015

de Been, M., Lanza, V. F., de Toro, M., Scharringa, J., Dohmen, W., Du, Y., et al. (2014). Dissemination of cephalosporin resistance genes between *Escherichia coli* strains from farm animals and humans by specific plasmid lineages. *PLoS Genet.* 10:e1004776. doi: 10.1371/journal.pgen.1004776

DeNap, J. C., and Hergenrother, P. J. (2005). Bacterial death comes full circle: targeting plasmid replication in drug-resistant bacteria. *Org. Biomol. Chem.* 3, 959–966. doi: 10.1039/b500182j

Dhanji, H., Murphy, N. M., Akhigbe, C., Doumith, M., Hope, R., Livermore, D. M., et al. (2011). Isolation of fluoroquinolone-resistant O25b:H4-ST131 *Escherichia coli* with CTX-M-14 extended-spectrum beta-lactamase from UK river water. *J. Antimicrob. Chemother.* 66, 512–516. doi: 10.1093/jac/dkq472

Diestra, K., Juan, C., Curiao, T., Moyá, B., Mirá, E., Oteo, J., et al. (2009). Characterization of plasmids encoding *bla*ESBL and surrounding genes in Spanish clinical isolates of *Escherichia coli* and *Klebsiella pneumoniae.* *J. Antimicrob. Chemother.* 63, 60–66. doi: 10.1093/jac/dkn453

Dolejska, M., Duskova, E., Rybarikova, J., Janoszowska, D., Roubalova, E., Dibdakova, K., et al. (2011). Plasmids carrying $bla_{CTX-M-1}$ and *qnr* genes in *Escherichia coli* isolates from an equine clinic and a horseback riding centre. *J. Antimicrob. Chemother.* 66, 757–764. doi: 10.1093/jac/dkq500

García-Fernández, A., Fortini, D., Veldman, K., Mevius, D., and Carattoli, A. (2009). Characterization of plasmids harbouring *qnrS1*, *qnrB2* and *qnrB19* genes in *Salmonella.* *J. Antimicrob. Chemother.* 63, 274–281. doi: 10.1093/jac/dkn470

Garcillán-Barcia, M. P., Francia, M. V., and de la Cruz, F. (2009). The diversity of conjugative relaxases and its application in plasmid classification. *FEMS Microbiol. Rev.* 33, 657–687. doi: 10.1111/j.1574-6976.2009.00168.x

Gautom, R. K. (1997). Rapid pulsed-field gel electrophoresis protocol for typing of *Escherichia coli* O157:H7 and other gram-negative organisms in 1 day. *J. Clin. Microbiol.* 35, 2977–2980.

Golebiewski, M., Kern-Zdanowicz, I., Zienkiewicz, M., Adamczyk, M., Zylinska, J., Baraniak, A., et al. (2007). Complete nucleotide sequence of the pCTX-M-3 plasmid and its involvement in spread of the extended-spectrum beta-lactamase gene $bla_{CTX-M-3}$. *Antimicrob. Agents Chemother.* 51, 3789–3795. doi: 10.1128/AAC.00457-07

Hayes, F. (2003). Toxins-antitoxins: plasmid maintenance, programmed cell death, and cell cycle arrest. *Science* 301, 1496–1499. doi: 10.1126/science.1088157

Ho, P. L., Chan, J., Lo, W. U., Law, P. Y., and Chow, K. H. (2013). Plasmid-mediated fosfomycin resistance in *Escherichia coli* isolated from pig. *Vet. Microbiol.* 162, 964–967. doi: 10.1016/j.vetmic.2012.09.023

Ho, P. L., Lo, W. U., Yeung, M. K., Li, Z., Chan, J., Chow, K. H., et al. (2012). Dissemination of pHK01-like incompatibility group IncFII plasmids encoding CTX-M-14 in *Escherichia coli* from human and animal sources. *Vet Microbiol.* 158, 172–179. doi: 10.1016/j.vetmic.2012.02.004

Johnson, T. J., and Nolan, L. K. (2009). Pathogenomics of the virulence plasmids of *Escherichia coli.* *Microbiol. Mol. Biol. Rev.* 73, 750–774. doi: 10.1128/MMBR.00015-09

Kado, C. I. (1998). Origin and evolution of plasmids. *Antonie Van Leeuwenhoek* 73, 117–126. doi: 10.1023/A:1000652513822

Lanza, V. F., de Toro, M., Garcillán-Barcia, M. P., Mora, A., Blanco, J., Coque, T. M., et al. (2014). Plasmid flux in *Escherichia coli* ST131 sublineages, analyzed by plasmid constellation network (PLACNET), a new method for plasmid reconstruction from whole genome sequences. *PLoS Genet.* 10:e1004766. doi: 10.1371/journal.pgen.1004766

Li, D. X., Zhang, S. M., Hu, G. Z., Wang, Y., Liu, H. B., Wu, C. M., et al. (2012). Tn3-associated *rmtB* together with *qnrS1*, *aac(6′)-Ib-cr* and $bla_{CTX-M-15}$ are co-located on an F49:A-:B- plasmid in an *Escherichia coli* ST10 strain in China. *J. Antimicrob. Chemother.* 67, 236–238. doi: 10.1093/jac/dkr428

Liao, X. P., Liu, B. T., Yang, Q. E., Sun, J., Li, L., Fang, L. X., et al. (2013). Comparison of plasmids coharboring 16s rrna methylase and extended-spectrum beta-lactamase genes among *Escherichia coli* isolates from pets and poultry. *J. Food Prot.* 76, 2018–2023. doi: 10.4315/0362-028X.JFP-13-200

Liebert, C. A., Hall, R. M., and Summers, A. O. (1999). Transposon Tn21, flagship of the floating genome. *Microbiol. Mol. Biol. Rev.* 63, 507–522.

Liu, B. T., Li, L., Fang, L. X., Sun, J., Liao, X. P., Yang, Q. E., et al. (2014). Characterization of plasmids carrying *oqxAB* in *bla*-negative *Escherichia coli* isolates from food-producing animals. *Microb. Drug Resist.* 20, 641–650. doi: 10.1089/mdr.2014.0022

Liu, B. T., Yang, Q. E., Li, L., Sun, J., Liao, X. P., Fang, L. X., et al. (2013). Dissemination and characterization of plasmids carrying *oqxAB*-bla_{CTX-M} genes in *Escherichia coli* isolates from food-producing animals. *PLoS ONE* 8:e73947. doi: 10.1371/journal.pone.0073947

Mathers, A. J., Peirano, G., and Pitout, J. D. (2015). The role of epidemic resistance plasimds and international high-risk clones in the spread of multidrug-resistant in Enterobacteriaceae. *Clin. Microbiol. Rev.* 28, 565–591. doi: 10.1128/CMR.00116-14

Matsumura, Y., Yamamoto, M., Nagao, M., Ito, Y., Takakura, S., Ichiyama, S., et al. (2013). Association of fluoroquinolone resistance, virulence genes, and IncF plasmids with extended-spectrum-beta-lactamase-producing *Escherichia coli* sequence type 131 (ST131) and ST405 clonal groups. *Antimicrob. Agents Chemother.* 57, 4736–4742. doi: 10.1128/AAC.00641-13

Mnif, B., Vimont, S., Boyd, A., Bourit, E., Picard, B., Branger, C., et al. (2010). Molecular characterization of addiction systems of plasmids encoding extended-spectrum beta-lactamases in *Escherichia coli.* *J. Antimicrob. Chemother.* 65, 1599–1603. doi: 10.1093/jac/dkq181

Moritz, E. M., and Hergenrother, P. J. (2007). Toxin-antitoxin systems are ubiquitous and plasmid-encoded in vancomycin-resistant *enterococci.* *Proc. Natl. Acad. Sci. U.S.A.* 104, 311–316. doi: 10.1073/pnas.06011 68104

Ogbolu, D. O., Daini, O. A., Ogunledun, A., Terry Alli, O. A., and Webber, M. A. (2013). Dissemination of IncF plasmids carrying beta-lactamase genes in Gram-negative bacteria from Nigerian hospitals. *J. Infect. Dev. Ctries.* 7, 382–390. doi: 10.3855/jidc.2613

Osborn, A. M., da Silva Tatley, F. M., Steyn, L. M., Pickup, R. W., and Saunders, J. R. (2000). Mosaic plasmids and mosaic replicons: evolutionary lessons from the analysis of genetic diversity in IncFII-related replicons. *Microbiology* 146, 2267–2275. doi: 10.1099/00221287-146-9-2267

Partridge, S. R., Zong, Z., and Iredell, J. R. (2011). Recombination in IS26 and Tn2 in the evolution of multi-resistance regions carrying blaCTX-M-15 on conjugative IncF pla-smids from *Escherichia coli.* *Antimicrob. Agents Chemother.* 55, 4971–4978. doi: 10.1128/AAC.00025-11

Ruiz, E., Sáenz, Y., Zarazaga, M., Rocha-Gracia, R., Martínez-Martinez, L., Arlet, G., et al. (2012). *qnr*, *aac(6′)-Ib-cr* and *qepA* genes in *Escherichia coli* and *Klebsiella* spp.: genetic environments and plasmid and chromosomal location. *J. Antimicrob. Chemother.* 67, 886–897. doi: 10.1093/jac/dkr548

Shin, J., Choi, M. J., and Ko, K. S. (2012). Replicon sequence typing of IncF plasmids and the genetic environments of $bla_{CTX-M-15}$ indicate multiple acquisitions of $bla_{CTX-M-15}$ in *Escherichia coli* and *Klebsiella pneumoniae* isolates from South Korea. *J. Antimicrob. Chemother.* 67, 1853–1857. doi: 10.1093/jac/dks143

Tamang, M. D., Seol, S. Y., Oh, J. Y., Kang, H. Y., Lee, J. C., Lee, Y. C., et al. (2008). Plasmid-mediated quinolone resistance determinants *qnrA*, *qnrB*, and *qnrS* among clinical isolates of Enterobacteriaceae in a Korean hospital. *Antimicrob. Agents Chemother.* 52, 4159–4162. doi: 10.1128/AAC.01633-07

Taylor, D. E., Gibreel, A., Lawley, T. D., and Tracz, D. M. (2004). "Antibiotic resistance plasmids," in *Plasmid Biology*, eds B. Funnell and G. Phillips (Washington, DC: ASM Press), 473–491.

Valverde, A., Cantón, R., Garcillán-Barcia, M. P., Novais, A., Galán, J. C., Alvarado, A., et al. (2009). Spread of *bla*(CTX-M-14) is driven mainly by IncK plasmids disseminated among *Escherichia coli* phylogroups A, B1, and D in Spain. *Antimicrob. Agents Chemother.* 53, 5204–5212. doi: 10.1128/AAC.01706-08

Villa, L., García-Fernández, A., Fortini, D., and Carattoli, A. (2010). Replicon sequence typing of IncF plasmids carrying virulence and resistance determinants. *J. Antimicrob. Chemother.* 65, 2518–2529. doi: 10.1093/jac/dkq347

Wang, Y., He, T., Han, J., Wang, J., Foley, S. L., Yang, G., et al. (2012). Prevalence of ESBLs and PMQR genes in fecal *Escherichia coli* isolated from the non-human primates in six zoos in China. *Vet Microbiol.* 159, 53–59. doi: 10.1016/j.vetmic.2012.03.009

Wiedenbeck, J., and Cohan, F. M. (2011). Origins of bacterial diversity through horizontal genetic transfer and adaptation to new ecological niches. *FEMS Microbiol. Rev.* 35, 957–976. doi: 10.1111/j.1574-6976.2011.00292.x

Woodford, N., Carattoli, A., Karisik, E., Underwood, A., Ellington, M. J., and Livermore, D. M. (2009). Complete nucleotide sequences of plasmids pEK204, pEK499, and pEK516, encoding CTX-M enzymes in three major *Escherichia coli* lineages from the United Kingdom, all belonging to the international O25:H4-ST131 clone. *Antimicrob. Agents Chemother.* 53, 4472–4482. doi: 10.1128/AAC.00688-09

Yao, Q., Zeng, Z., Hou, J., Deng, Y., He, L., Tian, W., et al. (2011). Dissemination of the *rmtB* gene carried on IncF and IncN plasmids among Enterobacteriaceae in a pig farm and its environment. *J. Antimicrob. Chemother.* 66, 2475–2479. doi: 10.1093/jac/dkr328

8

Antibiotic Resistance and *mecA* Characterization of Coagulase-Negative Staphylococci Isolated from three Hotels in London, UK

Zhen Xu, Hermine V. Mkrtchyan and Ronald R. Cutler**

School of Biological and Chemical Sciences, Queen Mary University of London, London, UK

Correspondence:
Hermine V. Mkrtchyan and Ronald R. Cutler, School of Biological and Chemical Sciences, Queen Mary University of London, Mile End Road, London E1 4NS, UK
h.mkrtchyan@qmul.ac.uk; r.cutler@qmul.ac.uk

Antibiotic resistance in bacteria isolated from non-healthcare environments, is a potential problem to public health. In our survey a total of 71 coagulase negative staphylococci (CNS) belonging to 11 different species were isolated from three large hotels in London, UK. The most prevalent species was *Staphylococcus haemolyticus*, with *S. hominis*, *S. warneri*, *S. cohnii*, and *Staphylococcus epidermidis* commonly detected. Antimicrobial susceptibilities and carriage of the *mecA* gene were determined for all of these isolates. Most (85.9%) staphylococci were resistant to multiple antibiotics with all displaying increased susceptibility toward penicillin, fusidic acid, erythromycin, and cefepime. Twenty-one (29.5%) of the isolates were *mecA* positive, however MIC values to oxacillin, normally associated with the carriage of *mecA*, varied widely in this group (from 0.06 to 256 mg/L). Fifteen of the twenty-one *mecA* positive isolates carried SCC*mec* of these seven were type V, one type I, one type II, and one type IV. Additionally, five of these 15 isolates carried a previously unreported type, 1A, which involves an association between class A *mec* complex and *ccr* type 1. The remaining six of the 21 isolates were non-typeable and carried a combination of class A *mec* complex and *ccrC*. In addition to this, we also report on new MLST types which were assigned for five *S. epidermidis* isolates. Four out of these five isolates had MICs between 0.06 and 256 mg/L to oxacillin and would be regarded as clinically susceptible but one isolate had a high oxacillin MIC of 256 mg/L. We demonstrated widespread multiple drug resistance among different staphylococcal species isolated from non-healthcare environments highlighting the potential for these species to act as a reservoir for methicillin and other forms of drug resistance.

Keywords: antibiotic resistance, coagulase-negative staphylococci, *mecA* gene, SCC*mec* typing, MLST

Introduction

Coagulase-negative staphylococci (CNS) are opportunistic pathogens that have emerged as a major cause of nosocomial infections often associated with healthcare settings (Bouchami et al., 2011a; Zong et al., 2011). *S. epidermidis, S. haemolyticus,* and *S. hominis* are amongst the CNS which can be responsible for a wide range of illnesses from minor skin infections to life threatening diseases (Huebner and Goldmann, 1999; Basaglia et al., 2003). In addition to this, the treatment of CNS infections has become more difficult, as many isolates in hospitals carry multiple drug resistance (Bouchami et al., 2011b) due to an increase of ineffectiveness of a wide range of antibiotics (John and Harvin, 2007). Methicillin resistance is commonly associated with the carriage of the *mecA* gene that encodes for penicillin binding protein PBP2a and has a low affinity for β-lactam antibiotics (Tulinski et al., 2012). The *mecA* gene is located on a mobile genetic element called the staphylococcal cassette chromosome *mec* (SCC*mec*) (Milheiriço et al., 2007). There are 11 SCC*mec* types currently reported and typing is based on different combinations of *mec* types (A, B, C1, C2, and D) and *ccr* types (*ccrAB1, ccrAB2, ccrAB3, ccrAB4, and ccrC*) (IWG-SCC, 2009; Shore et al., 2011).

The spread of methicillin resistant *S. aureus* (MRSA) outside of hospital settings, has been reported by several authors and their studies demonstrated that non-healthcare settings, including fire stations, student housing sites/common areas, public buses can be reservoir for MRSA (Roberts et al., 2011a,b; Simões et al., 2011). We have previously reported on the isolation of methicillin resistant coagulase negative staphylococci (MRCNS) from non-hospital restrooms (Mkrtchyan et al., 2013). In this current study we report on the wide variety of antibiotic resistance patterns and the molecular characterization of *mecA* positive determinants that we have isolated from non-healthcare environments.

Materials and Methods

Screening of Staphylococcal Isolates

With the permission of the hotel management/owners, we sampled three hotels in London, UK. The results from each hotel were reported to each manager/owner for their information. The sampling was of inanimate objects only. Eighty-eight randomly selected sites in 32 different hotel rooms were sampled using COPAN dry swabs (Copan Diagnostics Inc., USA).

In addition to these samples, 12 air samples were also collected from 12 randomly selected rooms using a high volume air sampler (Cherwell SAS Super 100, Cherwell Laboratories, UK). The airflow of sample collection was between 200 and 1000 l per min.

All specimens were inoculated onto Nutrient Agar (Nutrient Agar, Oxoid, Basingstoke, UK) and Mannitol Salt Agar plates (Oxoid Basingstoke, UK). These cultures were incubated aerobically at 37°C for 24–72 h.

Identification of Environment Staphylococci

All isolates were initially screened using conventional methods including microscopy (Gram film), catalase and coagulase testing. Prolex™ staph latex kits (ProLab Diagnostics, Neston, UK) were used to identify CNS and *S. aureus.* All potential staphylococcal isolates were then fully identified using a Matrix-assisted laser desorption ionization time flight mass-spectroscopy (MALDI-TOF-MS, Microflex LT, Bruker Daltonics, Coventry, UK) in a positive linear mode (2000–20,000 m/z range). Samples were prepared as described previously (Mkrtchyan et al., 2013). In brief, 3–5 colonies of fresh cultures were added into 300 μl distilled water and mixed with 900 μl absolute ethanol. The suspension was centrifuged for 2 min at 13,000 × g and the pellets were re-suspended in 25 μl of 70% formic acid and then mixed with 25 μl pure acetonitrile. The mixture was centrifuge for 2 min at 13,000 × g. One microliter aliquots of the obtained supernatant were spotted on the MALDI target plate and overlaid with 1 μl of α-Cyano-4-hydroxycinnamic acid (HCCA) matrix (Bruker Daltonics, Coventry, UK). The resulting spectra for each isolate was analyzed by MALDI-Biotyper 3.0 software (Bruker Daltonics, Coventry, UK). *Escherichia coli* DH5α (Bruker Daltonics, Coventry, UK) was used as a standard for calibration and quality control.

Antimicrobial Susceptibility Testing for All Staphylococci

The susceptibility of 12 antibiotics was tested using standard disk diffusion method as previously described (Andrews and Howe, 2011). This included amoxicillin (10 μg); cefepime (30 μg); chloramphenicol (30 μg); erythromycin (5 μg); fusidic acid (10 μg); gentamicin (10 μg); mupirocin (20 μg); oxacillin (1 μg); penicillin (1 unit); streptomycin (10 μg); tetracycline (10 μg); vancomycin (5 μg). The categories susceptible, intermediate resistant or resistant were assigned on the basis of the Guidelines for Susceptibility Testing (Andrews and Howe, 2011). The Minimum Inhibitory Concentrations (MIC) for oxacillin were additionally evaluated using "M.I.C. evaluators" (Oxoid Ltd., Basingstoke, UK).

Detection of *mecA* Gene and Staphylococci Cassette Chromosome *mec* (SCC*mec*) Typing

The detection of *mecA* gene was carried out using primers and methods as described previously (Hanssen et al., 2004). SCC*mec* typing was performed to *mecA* positive isolates using PCR as described previously, and the isolates were investigated using primers for *mec* and *ccr* complexes (Kondo et al., 2007).

MLST Typing of *Staphylococcus epidermidis*

S. epidermidis isolates were further analyzed by Multi Locus Sequence Typing (MLST) for seven housekeeping genes, as has been described previously (Thomas et al., 2007). Sequence types were determined by comparing the alleles to those in the *S. epidermidis* database (www.mlst.net).

Amplicons were sequenced by Eurofins MWG GmBH (Ebersberg, Germany) using ABI 3730XL DNA analyser. Sequence similarity searches were carried out using BLAST tool (http://www.ncbi.nlm.nih.gov/BLAST).

Southern Blotting of *mecA* Positive Isolates with Low Oxacillin MIC

S. hominis which had the lowest MIC to oxacillin was selected for southern blotting. *S. aureus* NCTC6571 was used as a negative control. *ClaI*-digested genomic DNA were transferred to a nitrocellulose membrane (Roche Diagnostics Ltd., West Sussex, UK) as recommended by the manufacturers (GE health care UK Ltd., Buckinghamshire, UK). Hybridization was carried out with a DNA probe for *mecA* at 68°C, and using the DIG luminescence detection kit according to the manufacturer's instructions (Roche Diagnostics Limited, Charles Avenue, Burgess Hill, West Sussex, UK).

Results

Sample Collection

A total of 71 staphylococcal isolates were recovered in this study, this included 62 from hotel surfaces and nine collected from hotel air samples.

Identification of Environmental Staphylococci

We identified 71 staphylococcal isolates as belonging to 11 different staphylococcal species. These included *S. haemolyticus* ($n = 34$), *S. hominis* ($n = 12$), *S. warneri* ($n = 5$), *S. cohnii* ($n = 5$), *S. epidermidis* ($n = 5$), *S. lugdunensis* ($n = 3$), *S. pettenkoferi* ($n = 2$), *S. capitis* ($n = 2$), *S. sciuri* ($n = 1$), *S. pasteuri* ($n = 1$), and *S. equorum* ($n = 1$).

Antibiotic Susceptibilities for All Staphylococci

All isolates were tested for their susceptibility to 12 commonly used antibiotics. We found that all isolates showed resistance to at least one antibiotic. In addition to this, 61 (86%) out of 71 staphylococcal isolates were resistant to two or more of the 12 antibiotics evaluated (**Tables 1**, **2**). Fifty-two (73%) staphylococcal isolates were resistant to penicillin and 50 (70%) were resistance to fusidic acid, 35 (49%) to erythromycin, 24 (34%) to amoxycillin, 23 (32%) to tetracycline, 20 (28%) to cefepime, 20 (28%) to vancomycin, 18 (25%) to mupirocin, 14 (20%) to oxacillin, 13 (18%) to chloramphenicol, 8 (11%) to gentamicin, and 7 (10%) to streptomycin. Among all staphylococci species *S. haemolyticus* was predominantly resistant to erythromycin (59%), followed by *S. epidermidis* to amoxicillin 60% and tetracycline 60% respectively and *S. cohnii* to erythromycin (80%), whereas *S. haemolyticus* (ID 54) and *S. pasteuri* (ID 68) were susceptible to almost all antibiotics tested except for streptomycin (**Tables 1**, **2**).

Determination of MICs to Oxacillin and SCC*mec* Typing

Twenty-one of the *mecA* positive isolates were multiple drug resistant however we found that susceptibility to oxacillin was

TABLE 1 | Molecular characterisation of antibiotic resistant and *mecA* gene positive coagulase negative staphylococci isolated from hotel and air samples.

ID	Species	Source	AM	CEF	CHL	ERY	FC	GEN	MUP	PG	STR	TET	VAN	*mecA*	*mec*	*ccr*	SCC*mec*	MIC/Ox (mg/L)
1	*S. cohnii*	HAS	S	R	S	S	R	S	R	R	I	S	S	+	Class C	C	V	2
2	*S. cohnii*	HAS	S	R	R	R	R	S	S	R	R	R	R	+	Class A	C	NT	1
3	*S. epidermidis*	DSH	R	R	S	R	R	R	R	R	I	R	S	+	Class B	2	IV	256
4	*S. epidermidis*	DSH	R	S	S	I	S	S	S	R	S	R	S	+	Class A	1	1A	0.12
5	*S. haemolyticus*	HAS	S	R	S	R	R	S	S	R	R	R	S	+	Class A	C	NT	256
6	*S. haemolyticus*	DSH	S	R	R	R	R	S	R	R	I	S	R	+	Class C	C	V	256
7	*S. haemolyticus*	DSH	R	R	R	S	R	R	S	R	R	R	R	+	Class A	2	II	256
8	*S. haemolyticus*	DSH	R	R	S	R	R	R	S	R	R	S	S	+	Class C	C	V	8
9	*S. haemolyticus*	DSH	R	R	S	R	R	S	S	R	I	S	S	+	Class C	C	V	8
10	*S. haemolyticus*	DSH	S	R	R	S	R	S	R	R	I	R	R	+	Class A	1	1A	1
11	*S. haemolyticus*	HAS	S	S	R	R	R	S	R	R	R	R	R	+	Class C	C	V	0.5
12	*S. haemolyticus*	DSH	R	S	S	S	R	S	S	R	I	S	R	+	Class C	C	V	0.25
13	*S. haemolyticus*	DSH	R	S	S	S	S	S	S	R	I	R	S	+	Class B	1	I	0.12
14	*S. hominis*	DSH	S	S	R	S	R	S	S	R	S	S	R	+	Class A	1	1A	8
15	*S. hominis*	DSH	R	S	S	R	R	S	R	R	S	R	R	+	Class A	1	1A	0.12
16	*S. hominis*	DSH	R	R	S	R	R	S	R	R	I	S	S	+	Class A	1	1A	0.06
17	*S. lugdunensis*	DSH	S	S	S	R	S	S	S	R	I	S	S	+	Class A	C	NT	0.5
18	*S. pettenkoferi*	DSH	R	R	R	R	R	R	S	R	R	R	R	+	Class A	C	NT	8
19	*S. sciuri*	DSH	S	R	R	S	R	S	S	R	I	S	R	+	Class A	C	NT	16
20	*S. warneri*	DSH	S	S	S	R	S	S	S	R	I	S	S	+	Class A	C	NT	0.25
21	*S. warneri*	DSH	S	S	S	S	R	S	S	R	I	S	R	+	Class C	C	V	0.25

DSH, different sites from hotels; HAS, hotel air samples; AM, amoxicillin (10 µg); CEP, cefepime (30 µg); CHL, chloramphenicol (30 µg); ERY, erythromycin (5 µg); FC, fusidic acid (10 µg); GEN, gentamicin (10 µg); MUP, mupirocin (20 µg); PG, penicillin (1 unit); STR, streptomycin (10 µg); TET, tetracycline (10 µg); VAN, vancomycin (5 µg); R, resistance; S, sensitive; I, intermediate; MIC/Ox, minimum inhibitory concentration Oxacillin; NT, not typeable.

TABLE 2 | Molecular characterisation of antibiotic resistant but *mecA* gene negative, coagulase negative staphylococci isolated from hotel and air samples.

ID	Species	Source	AMO	CEF	CHL	ERY	FC	GEN	MUP	PG	STR	TET	VAN	OX
22	*S. capitis*	DSH	S	S	S	S	S	S	R	R	S	S	S	S
23	*S. capitis*	DSH	S	S	S	S	R	S	S	R	I	S	S	S
24	*S. cohnii*	DSH	R	S	S	R	R	S	S	R	S	S	R	S
25	*S. cohnii*	DSH	R	S	S	R	S	S	R	R	S	S	S	S
26	*S. cohnii*	DSH	S	S	R	R	R	S	S	R	S	S	S	S
27	*S. epidermidis*	DSH	S	S	S	S	R	S	S	R	I	S	R	S
28	*S. epidermidis*	DSH	R	S	R	R	R	S	S	R	I	R	S	S
29	*S. epidermidis*	DSH	S	R	R	S	R	S	R	R	I	S	R	S
30	*S. equorum*	DSH	S	S	S	S	S	S	S	R	I	S	S	S
31	*S. haemolyticus*	DSH	R	S	S	R	S	R	S	S	I	R	S	S
32	*S. haemolyticus*	DSH	R	R	S	R	R	S	S	R	S	S	S	S
33	*S. haemolyticus*	DSH	S	S	S	R	R	R	R	R	I	S	R	S
34	*S. haemolyticus*	DSH	S	S	S	R	S	S	S	S	I	S	S	S
35	*S. haemolyticus*	DSH	S	S	S	R	R	S	R	R	S	S	S	S
36	*S. haemolyticus*	DSH	S	S	S	R	R	S	R	R	I	S	S	S
37	*S. haemolyticus*	DSH	R	S	S	R	R	S	S	R	I	S	S	S
38	*S. haemolyticus*	DSH	S	R	S	R	R	S	S	S	S	S	R	S
39	*S. haemolyticus*	DSH	S	S	S	R	R	S	S	S	I	S	S	S
40	*S. haemolyticus*	DSH	S	R	S	R	S	S	S	S	I	R	S	S
41	*S. haemolyticus*	DSH	S	S	S	S	R	S	S	R	I	S	R	S
42	*S. haemolyticus*	DSH	S	S	S	S	R	S	S	R	I	S	S	S
43	*S. haemolyticus*	DSH	S	R	R	R	S	S	S	S	I	R	S	S
44	*S. haemolyticus*	DSH	S	S	S	R	S	S	S	S	I	R	R	S
45	*S. haemolyticus*	DSH	R	R	S	S	R	S	S	R	I	R	S	S
46	*S. haemolyticus*	DSH	R	S	S	R	S	S	S	R	I	S	S	S
47	*S. haemolyticus*	DSH	R	S	S	R	R	S	S	R	I	S	R	S
48	*S. haemolyticus*	DSH	S	S	S	S	S	S	S	S	I	R	S	S
49	*S. haemolyticus*	DSH	S	S	S	R	S	S	S	S	I	R	S	S
50	*S. haemolyticus*	DSH	S	S	S	S	R	S	S	R	I	R	S	S
51	*S. haemolyticus*	DSH	S	S	S	S	R	S	R	S	S	S	S	S
52	*S. haemolyticus*	HAS	S	S	S	S	R	R	S	S	I	R	S	S
53	*S. haemolyticus*	HAS	S	R	S	S	R	S	S	S	I	S	S	S
54	*S. haemolyticus*	HAS	S	S	S	S	S	S	S	S	I	S	S	S
55	*S. haemolyticus*	HAS	R	R	R	S	R	S	R	R	R	R	S	S
56	*S. hominis*	DSH	S	S	S	R	R	S	S	S	S	S	S	S
57	*S. hominis*	DSH	S	S	S	R	R	S	R	R	S	S	S	S
58	*S. hominis*	DSH	R	S	S	S	R	S	S	R	I	S	S	S
59	*S. hominis*	DSH	R	S	S	S	S	S	S	R	S	S	S	S
60	*S. hominis*	DSH	S	S	S	S	S	S	S	R	S	S	S	S
61	*S. hominis*	DSH	S	S	S	R	S	S	S	S	S	S	S	S
62	*S. hominis*	DSH	S	S	S	S	R	S	S	R	I	R	S	S
63	*S. hominis*	DSH	S	S	S	I	R	S	S	S	S	S	S	S
64	*S. hominis*	DSH	S	S	S	S	R	S	S	S	S	S	S	S
65	*S. lugdunensis*	DSH	S	S	S	S	R	S	R	R	I	S	S	S
66	*S. lugdunensis*	HAS	S	S	S	S	R	S	S	R	I	S	S	S
67	*S. pettenkoferi*	DSH	S	S	S	S	S	S	S	R	I	S	S	S
68	*S. pasteuri*	DSH	S	S	S	S	S	S	S	S	I	S	S	S
69	*S. warneri*	DSH	R	S	S	S	R	R	R	S	I	S	S	S
70	*S. warneri*	DSH	R	S	S	R	R	S	S	R	I	R	S	S
71	*S. warneri*	DSH	S	S	S	S	R	S	S	R	I	S	R	S

DSH, different sites from hotels; HAS, hotel air samples; AMO, amoxicillin (10 μg); CEP, cefepime (30 μg); CHL, chloramphenicol (30 μg); ERY, erythromycin (5 μg); FC, fusidic acid (10 μg); GEN, gentamicin (10 μg); MUP, mupirocin (20 μg); OX, Oxacillin (1 μg); PEN, penicillin (1 unit); STR, streptomycin (10 μg); TET, tetracycline (10 μg); VAN, vancomycin (5 μg); R, resistant; S, sensitive; I, intermediate.

highly variable with MICs ranging from 0.06 to 256 mg/L. Carriage of *mecA* did not always result in isolates demonstrating significant levels of resistance to oxacillin. Seven of the 21 isolates which were *mecA* positive were found to have MICs below 0.5 mg/L to oxacillin (**Table 1**).

SCC*mec* types were assigned in 15 out of the 21 *mecA* positive isolates. Seven isolates harbored SCC*mec* type V ($n = 7$), and one isolate each harbored SCC*mec* type I ($n = 1$), type II ($n = 1$), and type IV ($n = 1$). Five isolates harbored a new SCC*mec* type 1A, which carried combination of class A *mec* complex and *ccr* type 1. The six isolates that were non-typeable, carried a combination of class A *mec* complex and *ccrC* (**Table 1**).

MLST Typing of *Staphylococcus epidermidis*

MLST typing revealed that all five *S. epidermidis* isolates contained novel MLST types. These types were assigned as ST515, ST516, ST517, ST518, and ST519.

Southern Blotting of *mecA* Positive Isolates with Low Oxacillin MIC

There were also seven isolates that were *mecA* positive but had low MICs to oxacillin. In order to fully confirm that these isolates were indeed *mecA* positive, we selected the isolate from this group with the lowest oxacillin MIC (*S. hominis*, isolate 16, oxacillin MIC 0.06 mg/L, **Table 1**) and confirmed that it was indeed *mecA* positive using Southern blotting.

Discussion

The potential threat of antibiotic resistance in environmental/non-healthcare associated bacteria is a concern for public health. Most of the studies on methicillin resistance in staphylococci focus on MRSA and CNS strains isolated from hospital patients (Zong et al., 2011; Brennan et al., 2012; Kinnevey et al., 2013). We have previously reported on the high levels of antibiotic resistance that can be found in bacteria isolated from non-healthcare restrooms (Mkrtchyan et al., 2013). The aim of this current study was to evaluate the levels antibiotic resistance, the carriage of *mecA*, and the diversity of SCC*mec* elements in other staphylococci isolated from high-throughput, non-healthcare environments, in this case hotels.

Bacterial Isolates

A total of 71 staphylococcal isolates belonging to 11 different species recovered from hotel rooms. Within this group, we found that 61 out of 71 isolates (85.9%) were resistant to two or more antibiotics, including one isolate was resistant to 10 antibiotics; 1–9 antibiotics, four isolates were resistant to eight antibiotics; 4–7 antibiotics; 5–6 antibiotics; 7–5 antibiotics; 13–4 antibiotics; 14–3 antibiotics and 12–2 antibiotics (**Tables 1, 2**). In addition to this the MICs to oxacillin varied widely from 0.06 to 256 mg/L, and although *mecA* genes were detected in 21 isolates, seven of these demonstrated only low levels of methicillin resistance. This is the NCCLS standard level for determining resistance in CNS which are *mecA* positive (Hussain et al., 2000).

SCC*mec* Typing

SCC*mec* types were assigned for the 21 isolates mentioned above. Type V was the most common (7 isolates). This is consistent with some previously published works carried out with clinical isolates (Zong et al., 2011). We did however also identify types I, II, and IV in our isolates, whereas types III, VI, VII, VIII, IX, X, and XI were not detected. It has been reported by others that the distribution of SCC*mec* types in MRCNS varies and may depend on the human host and geographical locations of the isolates were obtained from (Oliveira et al., 2006; IWG-SCC, 2009; Zhang et al., 2009; Zong et al., 2011). In addition to this, in previous papers, SCC*mec* types I, II, III, and V were found to be the most common in environmental isolates, such isolates were taken from areas such as public beaches (Soge et al., 2009).

The structural diversity of SCC*mec* has been reported in hospital environments (Ruppé et al., 2009; Barbier et al., 2011; Zong et al., 2011) with high throughputs of patients. It also possible that the SCC*mec* variations we observed were similarly related to the high throughput of people in the hotels tested (Barbier et al., 2011). In addition to this, we found associations between SCC*mec* carriage and certain species, for example SCC*mec* type V was preferentially associated with *S. haemolyticus*, *S. hominis*, *S. warneri*, *S. epidermidis*, and *S. sciuri*. Previously, with clinical isolates, type V SCC*mec* was reported to be associated mainly with *S. haemolyticus* (Zong et al., 2011).

Apart from the variations in the classified SCC*mec* types isolated, we also reported on 11 unclassified SCC*mec* types. Six of these had a combination of class A *mec* complex and *ccrC* and five had a combination of class A *mec* complex and *ccr* type 1. The latter has been reported by other workers to be a new type 1A (Bouchami et al., 2011b).

MLST Types

Finally to emphasis the wide range of genetic variability that exists among these isolates, we also report new MLST types were assigned for five *S. epidermidis* isolates. Interestingly, four of these were determined to be clinically susceptible to oxacillin, whereas one was highly resistant to oxacillin (MIC of 256 mg/L) (Hussain et al., 2000). To date, studies on *S. epidermidis* have been focused on clinical isolates (Li et al., 2009), we believe that this is the first report to include the molecular characterisation of *S. epidermidis* isolated from non-healthcare sources.

In conclusion, public environments are potential reservoirs of multidrug resistant staphylococci. The characterization of an *S. epidermidis* isolate type with an MIC to oxacillin of 256 mg/L is of particular interest and requires further investigation with regard to its classification within the existing SCC*mec* typing system. We also aim in the future to look into the genetics of these isolates for other 11 antibiotics used in this study. Moreover, we have several other studies on-going which are looking at the bacterial populations in non-healthcare environments that will allow us to compare these samples with those from the current as well as previous studies. The dissemination of multidrug resistance in non-healthcare environments is evidence that infection control measures in the hospitals and in public places are ineffective in limiting the spread of such clones and that these environments are a source of antibiotic resistant pathogens.

References

Andrews, J. M., and Howe, R. A. (2011). BSAC standardized disc susceptibility testing method (version 10). *J. Antimicrob. Chemother.* 66, 2726–2757. doi: 10.1093/jac/dkr359

Barbier, F., Lebeaux, D., Hernandez, D., Delannoy, A. S., Caro, V., François, P., et al. (2011). High prevalence of the arginine catabolic mobile element in carriage isolates of methicillin-resistant *Staphylococcus epidermidis*. *J. Antimicrob. Chemother.* 66, 29–36. doi: 10.1093/jac/dkq410

Basaglia, G., Moras, L., Bearz, A., Scalone, S., and Paoli, P. D. (2003). *Staphylococcus cohnii* septicaemia in a patient with colon cancer. *J. Med. Microbiol.* 52, 101–102. doi: 10.1099/jmm.0.05002-0

Bouchami, O., Achour, W., Mekni, M. A., Rolo, J., and Ben Hassen, A. (2011a). Antibiotic resistance and molecular characterization of clinical isolates of methicillin-resistant coagulase-negative staphylococci isolated from bacteremic patients in oncohematology. *Folia Microbiol. (Praha)* 56, 122–130. doi: 10.1007/s12223-011-0017-1

Bouchami, O., Ben Hassen, A., de Lencastre, H., and Miragaia, M. (2011b). Molecular epidemiology of methicillin-resistant *Staphylococcus hominis* (MRSHo): low clonality and reservoirs of SCC*mec* structural elements. *PLoS ONE* 6:e21940. doi: 10.1371/journal.pone.0021940

Brennan, G. I., Shore, A. C., Corcoran, S., Tecklenborg, S., Coleman, D. C., and O'Connell, B. (2012). Emergence of hospital- and community-associated panton-valentine leukocidin-positive methicillin-resistant *Staphylococcus aureus* genotype ST772-MRSA-V in Ireland and detailed investigation of an ST772-MRSA-V cluster in a neonatal intensive care unit. *J. Clin. Microbiol.* 50, 841–847. doi: 10.1128/JCM.06354-11

Hanssen, A. M., Kjeldsen, G., and Sollid, J. U. (2004). Local variants of Staphylococcal cassette chromosome *mec* in sporadic methicillin-resistant *Staphylococcus aureus* and methicillin-resistant coagulase-negative Staphylococci: evidence of horizontal gene transfer? *Antimicrob. Agents Chemother.* 48, 285–296. doi: 10.1128/AAC.48.1.285-296.2004

Huebner, J., and Goldmann, D. A. (1999). Coagulase-negative staphylococci: role as pathogens. *Annu. Rev. Med.* 50, 223–236. doi: 10.1146/annurev.med.50.1.223

Hussain, Z., Stoakes, L., Massey, V., Diagre, D., Fitzgerald, V., El Sayed, S., et al. (2000). Correlation of oxacillin MIC with *mecA* gene carriage in coagulase-negative staphylococci. *J. Clin. Microbiol.* 38, 752–754.

IWG-SCC. (2009). Classification of staphylococcal cassette chromosome *mec* (SCC*mec*): guidelines for reporting novel SCC*mec* elements. *Antimicrob. Agents Chemother.* 53, 4961–4967. doi: 10.1128/AAC.00579-09

John, J. F., and Harvin, A. M. (2007). History and evolution of antibiotic resistance in coagulase-negative staphylococci: susceptibility profiles of new anti-staphylococci agents. *Ther. Clin. Risk Manag.* 3, 1143–1152.

Kinnevey, P. M., Shore, A. C., Brennan, G. I., Sullivan, D. J., Ehricht, R., Monecke, S., et al. (2013). Emergence of sequence type 779 methicillin-resistant *Staphylococcus aureus* harboring a novel pseudo staphylococcal cassette chromosome *mec* (SCC*mec*)-SCC-SCCCRISPR composite element in Irish hospitals. *Antimicrob. Agents Chemother.* 57, 524–531. doi: 10.1128/AAC.01689-12

Kondo, Y., Ito, T., Ma, X. X., Watanabe, S., Kreiswirth, B. N., Etienne, J., et al. (2007). Combination of multiplex PCRs for staphylococcal cassette chromosome *mec* type assignment: rapid identification system for *mec*, *ccr*, and major differences in junkyard regions. *Antimicrob. Agents Chemother.* 51, 264–274. doi: 10.1128/AAC.00165-06

Li, M., Wang, X., Gao, Q., and Lu, Y. (2009). Molecular characterization of *Staphylococcus epidermidis* strains isolated from a teaching hospital in Shanghai, China. *J. Med. Microbiol.* 58, 456–461. doi: 10.1099/jmm.0.007567-0

Milheiriço, C., Oliveira, D. C., and de Lencastre, H. (2007). Update to the multiplex PCR strategy for assignment of *mec* element types in *Staphylococcus aureus*. *Antimicrob. Agents Chemother.* 51, 3374–3377. doi: 10.1128/AAC.00275-07

Mkrtchyan, H. V., Russell, C. A., Wang, N., and Cutler, R. R. (2013). Could public restrooms be an environment for bacterial resistomes? *PLoS ONE* 8:e54223. doi: 10.1371/journal.pone.0054223

Oliveira, D. C., Milheiriço, C., and de Lencastre, H. (2006). Redefining a structural variant of staphylococcal cassette chromosome *mec*, SCC*mec* type VI. *Antimicrob. Agents Chemother.* 50, 3457–3459. doi: 10.1128/AAC.00629-06

Roberts, M. C., Soge, O. O., No, D., Beck, N. K., and Meschke, J. S. (2011a). Isolation and characterization of methicillin-resistant *Staphylococcus aureus* from fire stations in two northwest fire districts. *Am. J. Infect. Control.* 39, 382–389. doi: 10.1016/j.ajic.2010.09.008

Roberts, M. C., Soge, O. O., No, D., Helgeson, S. E., and Meschke, J. S. (2011b). Characterization of Methicillin-resistant *Staphylococcus aureus* isolated from public surfaces on a university campus, student homes and local community. *J. Appl. Microbiol.* 110, 1531–1537. doi: 10.1111/j.1365-2672.2011.05017.x

Ruppé, E., Barbier, F., Mesli, Y., Maiga, A., Cojocaru, R., Benkhalfat, M., et al. (2009). Diversity of staphylococcal cassette chromosome *mec* structures in methicillin-resistant *Staphylococcus epidermidis* and *Staphylococcus haemolyticus* strains among outpatients from four countries. *Antimicrob. Agents Chemother.* 53, 442–449. doi: 10.1128/AAC.00724-08

Shore, A. C., Deasy, E. C., Slickers, P., Brennan, G., O'Connell, B., Monecke, S., et al. (2011). Detection of staphylococcal cassette chromosome *mec* type XI carrying highly divergent *mecA*, *mecI*, *mecR1*, blaZ, and *ccr* genes in human clinical isolates of clonal complex 130 methicillin-resistant *Staphylococcus aureus*. *Antimicrob. Agents Chemother.* 55, 3765–3773. doi: 10.1128/AAC.00187-11

Simões, R. R., Aires-de-Sousa, M., Conceição, T., Antunes, F., da Costa, P. M., and de Lencastre, H. (2011). High prevalence of EMRSA-15 in Portuguese public buses: a worrisome finding. *PLoS ONE* 6:e17630. doi: 10.1371/journal.pone.0017630

Soge, O. O., Meschke, J. S., No, D. B., and Roberts, M. C. (2009). Characterization of methicillin-resistant *Staphylococcus aureus* and methicillin-resistant coagulase-negative *Staphylococcus* spp. isolated from US West Coast public marine beaches. *J. Antimicrob. Chemother.* 64, 1148–1155. doi: 10.1093/jac/dkp368

Thomas, J. C., Vargas, M. R., Miragaia, M., Peacock, S. J., Archer, G. L., and Enright, M. C. (2007). Improved multilocus sequence typing scheme for *Staphylococcus epidermidis*. *J. Clin. Microbiol.* 45, 616–619. doi: 10.1128/JCM.01934-06

Tulinski, P., Fluit, A. C., Wagenaar, J. A., Mevius, D., van de Vijver, L., and Duim, B. (2012). Methicillin-resistant coagulase-negative staphylococci on pig farms as a reservoir of heterogeneous staphylococcal cassette chromosome *mec* elements. *Appl. Environ. Microbiol.* 78, 299–304. doi: 10.1128/AEM.05594-11

Zhang, K., McClure, J. A., Elsayed, S., and Conly, J. M. (2009). Novel staphylococcal cassette chromosome *mec* type, tentatively designated type VIII, harboring class A *mec* and type 4 *ccr* gene complexes in a Canadian epidemic strain of methicillin-resistant *Staphylococcus aureus*. *Antimicrob. Agents Chemother.* 53, 531–540. doi: 10.1128/AAC.01118-08

Zong, Z., Peng, C., and Lü, X. (2011). Diversity of SCC*mec* elements in methicillin-resistant coagulase-negative staphylococci clinical isolates. *PLoS ONE* 6:e20191. doi: 10.1371/journal.pone.0020191

9

Genomic Microbial Epidemiology is Needed to Comprehend the Global Problem of Antibiotic Resistance and to Improve Pathogen Diagnosis

*Ethan R. Wyrsch[1], Piklu Roy Chowdhury[1,2], Toni A. Chapman[2], Ian G. Charles[3], Jeffrey M. Hammond[2] and Steven P. Djordjevic[1]**

[1] The ithree Institute, University of Technology Sydney, Sydney, NSW, Australia, [2] NSW Department of Primary Industries, Elizabeth Macarthur Agricultural Institute, Sydney, NSW, Australia, [3] Institute of Food Research, Norwich Research Park, Norwich, UK

***Correspondence:**
Steven P. Djordjevic
steven.djordjevic@uts.edu.au

Contamination of waste effluent from hospitals and intensive food animal production with antimicrobial residues is an immense global problem. Antimicrobial residues exert selection pressures that influence the acquisition of antimicrobial resistance and virulence genes in diverse microbial populations. Despite these concerns there is only a limited understanding of how antimicrobial residues contribute to the global problem of antimicrobial resistance. Furthermore, rapid detection of emerging bacterial pathogens and strains with resistance to more than one antibiotic class remains a challenge. A comprehensive, sequence-based genomic epidemiological surveillance model that captures essential microbial metadata is needed, both to improve surveillance for antimicrobial resistance and to monitor pathogen evolution. *Escherichia coli* is an important pathogen causing both intestinal [intestinal pathogenic *E. coli* (IPEC)] and extraintestinal [extraintestinal pathogenic *E. coli* (ExPEC)] disease in humans and food animals. ExPEC are the most frequently isolated Gram negative pathogen affecting human health, linked to food production practices and are often resistant to multiple antibiotics. Cattle are a known reservoir of IPEC but they are not recognized as a source of ExPEC that impact human or animal health. In contrast, poultry are a recognized source of multiple antibiotic resistant ExPEC, while swine have received comparatively less attention in this regard. Here, we review what is known about ExPEC in swine and how pig production contributes to the problem of antibiotic resistance.

Keywords: multiple antibiotic resistance, animal production, environmental pollutants, genomic epidemiology, agriculture, *Escherichia coli*

ANTIMICROBIAL RESISTANCE IN AGRICULTURAL AND CLINICAL SETTINGS

Meat production farming practices have increased in scale over the past 30 years (Landers et al., 2012) and are predicted to continue to increase in line with rising incomes in low- and middle-income countries (Van Boeckel et al., 2015). This rationalization of farming has led to intensification of animal production and greater reliance on antimicrobials to control infectious disease, improve feed conversion efficiency, and promote animal growth (Levy, 1992; Sarmah et al., 2006; FAO, 2009; Krishnasamy et al., 2015; Van Boeckel et al., 2015). Modeling studies estimate that global antimicrobial consumption will increase by 67% from an estimated 63,151 tons in 2010 to 105,596 tons in 2030 (Van Boeckel et al., 2015). Much of this rise in consumption is expected to come from China, India, Russia, South Africa, and Brazil; countries where meat consumption is growing due to rising incomes (Van Boeckel et al., 2015). Large scale animal production facilities generate huge volumes of animal waste that is contaminated with veterinary antibiotics. While estimates vary, it is thought that in the USA, 11–14 million kilograms of antibiotics are used annually in the production of animals for food (i.e., livestock; Institute of Medicine; National Research Council; Panel on Animal Health, 1999; Landers et al., 2012). Almost half of these are used for non-therapeutic purposes, which is significantly more than the estimated 1.4 million kilograms of antibiotics used in human medicine (Institute of Medicine; National Research Council; Panel on Animal Health, 1999). Many classes of antibiotics are used in animal production including β-lactams, sulfonamides, tetracyclines, streptogramins, macrolides, lincosamides, polyethers, quinoxalines, elfamycins, glycolipids, arsenicals, and polypeptides (Sarmah et al., 2006). How these compounds are modified within the animal, how they persist in soils and waterways after they are excreted, and their fate when animal slurries are used to fertilize pastures are complex and poorly understood (Sarmah et al., 2006; Zhu et al., 2013). Antimicrobial residues that contaminate groundwater tables, aquatic environments, and land used for crop production exert selection pressure on microbial populations that may promote the lateral transfer of resistance and virulence genes between populations, and contributes to the emergence of novel pathogenic profiles (Venturini et al., 2010, 2013; Baquero and Tobes, 2013; Baquero et al., 2013; Roy Chowdhury et al., 2015). It is perhaps unsurprising that commensal gastrointestinal bacterial populations are commonly resistant to more than one antimicrobial (Bettelheim et al., 2003; Diarrassouba et al., 2007; Bailey et al., 2010) and consequently the frequency of community-acquired infections with resistance to multiple antimicrobials are also increasing (Onken et al., 2015; Paniagua-Contreras et al., 2015; Yahiaoui et al., 2015). Furthermore, surveys have shown the presence of antibiotic resistance genes in the gastrointestinal tracts of humans and animals that have never received antibiotic interventions, specifically in: human feces from remote communities (Bartoloni et al., 2009; Ruppe et al., 2009; Eisenberg et al., 2012), migratory bird populations (Foti et al., 2011; Carroll et al., 2015; Jamborova et al., 2015; Stedt et al., 2015) and various wildlife species (Allen et al., 2010; Baez et al., 2015; Jobbins and Alexander, 2015; Katakweba et al., 2015). This demonstrates that resistance genes in host bacteria can readily spread to naïve microbial populations via waterways, air currents, road incursions into remote areas, animal and bird migration, and land clearance (Tsubokura et al., 1995; Middleton and Ambrose, 2005; Ewers et al., 2009). The application of manure onto pasture from ruminants that have not received recent antibiotic therapy is known to stimulate the expansion of resident flora encoding resistance to β-lactam antibiotics (Udikovic-Kolic et al., 2014). These observations demonstrate our limited understanding of the impact of the application animal waste to agriculture. The mechanisms by which mobile elements flux through microbial populations are not fully understood, but it is clear that efforts must be made to reduce environmental contamination sourced from human and animal effluent.

Antimicrobial resistance is largely an ecological problem (Summers, 2002, 2006; Stokes and Gillings, 2011; Landers et al., 2012; Berendonk et al., 2015; Gillings et al., 2015). In general, studies have focused on the emergence and carriage of resistance genes in certain key microbial populations, without an appreciation for the wider complexity of the problem, or its origins. Hence, there are numerous under-reported microbial sources of resistance genes. Antibiotic resistance genes often traffic in association with transposons that carry mercury resistance operons; these play an important role in transforming mercury to less biologically toxic forms, thereby regulating the availability of toxic mercury compounds in the environment. Mercury-resistance gene operons have evolved as key components of Tn3-family transposons and these transposons are globally disseminated. Mercury has been released into the environment via geological processes over millions of years and, although anthropogenic activity over the past two centuries has contributed significantly to the release of mercury into waterways and the atmosphere, it is likely that mercury levels were higher prior to the industrial revolution than they are now as a result of extensive volcanic activity (Osborn et al., 1997; Barkay et al., 2003). Despite this, large scale surveillance studies of antimicrobial resistance fail to screen microbial populations for the presence of mercury-resistance genes (Djordjevic et al., 2013). Resistance genes can also accumulate in microbial populations in soils that have been fertilized with animal waste and treated effluent (Heuer and Smalla, 2007; Chee-Sanford et al., 2009; Heuer et al., 2011a,b; Kristiansson et al., 2011; Baquero et al., 2013; Berendonk et al., 2015). Meat, seafood, and vegetables are also important and under-recognized sources of antimicrobial resistance genes in bacteria (Johnson et al., 2005a; Agerso et al., 2014; Kim and Woo, 2014; Ahmed and Shimamoto, 2015a,b; Ben Said et al., 2015; Le et al., 2015; van Hoek et al., 2015; Zhang et al., 2015; Zurfluh et al., 2015).

Anthropogenic industrial processes generate heavy metals including cadmium, lead, arsenic, copper, silver, and a wide range of synthetic organic compounds that pollute natural ecosystems. As such, heavy metal contamination represents yet another selective pressure for the development of antimicrobial resistance (Baker-Austin et al., 2006; Castillo et al., 2008; Li et al., 2010; Zhu et al., 2013). Genes coding for resistance to silver, copper, arsenic and antimony are associated with complex resistance gene loci in bacteria resistant to more than one antimicrobial and have great significance to human, livestock, and plant health (Berg et al., 2005; Seiler and Berendonk, 2012; Hobman and Crossman, 2015; Bondarczuk et al., 2016). The widespread occurrence of genes coding for resistance to heavy metals has, in part, been demonstrated in studies using information mined from publicly available genome sequences highlighting the value of genomic surveillance studies (Hobman and Crossman, 2015).

Genome-wide studies of genes coding for resistance to antibiotics, biocides and heavy metals have shed light on how these genes co-assemble on mobile genetic elements. In an analysis of 2522 fully sequenced bacterial genomes and 4582 plasmid sequences, Pal et al. (2015) were able to identify examples where antimicrobial resistance genes co-occurred. The authors found that the most likely co-selection scenario occurred in bacterial strains that carried plasmid-borne antibiotic resistance genes and biocide/heavy metal resistance genes on the same chromosome. A plasmid localized gene cluster coding for a cadmium/zinc resistance gene (*cadD*) with aminoglycoside and macrolide resistance genes was also identified (Pal et al., 2015). Resistance to these combinations of antimicrobials would benefit bacterial populations found in intensive animal production systems where cadmium and zinc are both used to promote growth and aminoglycosides and macrolides are frequently administered for the treatment of Gram-negative and Gram-positive infections, respectively (Castillo et al., 2008; Li et al., 2010). It is clear that plasmids can carry combinations of genes coding for resistance to more than one microbial agent alongside genes coding for resistance to biocides and heavy metals. Invariably these plasmids are large, conjugative and commonly found in pathogens from hospital and intensive farming environments (Chen et al., 2007; Woodford et al., 2009; Venturini et al., 2010, 2013; Pal et al., 2015). Sub-lethal levels of antibacterial biocides and heavy metals found in mildly polluted aquatic and land-based ecosystems may be sufficient to maintain these mobile elements carrying multiple antibiotic, biocide and heavy metal resistance genes (Stepanauskas et al., 2006; Gullberg et al., 2014).

Although plasmids can vary in size and coding ability, their size is generally positively correlated with the size of the host chromosome (Smillie et al., 2010). Plasmids conferring multiple-drug resistance are usually large, as they code for a suite of resistance genes, alongside associated integrons, transposition factors, and genes for heavy metal resistance, which can be in excess of 20,000 bp or more in size. Small plasmids that acquire resistance to more than one antimicrobial are, however, not without precedent. Labar et al. (2012) described the sequence of a small plasmid (pASL01A; 27,072 bp) that codes for resistance to ampicillin, streptomycin, sulfonamides, trimethoprim, and mercury (Labar et al., 2012). Most of the plasmid (21,904 bp) is comprised of a Tn*21* derivate mercury resistance transposon that carries a class 1 integron with a trimethoprim resistance *dfrA7* gene cassette and Tn*6029C* (Roy Chowdhury et al., 2015). Tn*6029C* comprises a $bla_{\text{TEM}-1}$-IS*26*-*repA/C*-*sul2*-*strA*-*strB* gene cluster flanked by direct copies of IS*26* (Labar et al., 2012; Roy Chowdhury et al., 2015). The plasmid backbone (5,168 bp) and related plasmids are widespread in enterobacterial populations in Africa (Labar et al., 2012).

Antimicrobials, including heavy metals, are used widely in animal production to treat clinical disease, to prevent disease outbreaks during critical or vulnerable periods, and to promote growth (McEwen and Fedorka-Cray, 2002; Landers et al., 2012). The use of antibiotics to promote growth is a phenomenon whereby animals receiving very low doses of antimicrobials appear healthier and grow larger (Roy Chowdhury et al., 2014). Although, the mechanism for this growth promoting effect is still poorly understood, the majority of pigs produced in the USA are exposed to tetracyclines and tylosin to prevent disease and promote growth (Apley et al., 2012). While these approaches have proved effective in controlling disease and aiding farms globally, the uninhibited use of antimicrobials also provides the selection pressure that drives antimicrobial resistance (Pulcini and Gyssens, 2013). As such, concerted efforts to reduce the use of antimicrobials in food production should be a priority.

Given that the persistence and spread of resistance is intrinsically linked with the presence and activity of antimicrobials, it is significant that 30–90% of ingested antibiotics are excreted in an un-metabolized or only partially metabolized form (Sarmah et al., 2006) into waste treatment plants and animal waste-holding facilities. Antibiotic residues are known to persist in secondary effluent despite the treatment process (Sarmah et al., 2006; Watkinson et al., 2007; Martinez, 2008; Le-Minh et al., 2010; Bondarczuk et al., 2016). Furthermore, the pH, temperature, nutrient concentration, and bacterial loads in waste treatment plants are conducive to the evolution and spread of antimicrobial resistance (and virulence) genes (Andersen, 1993; Dolejska et al., 2011). This is in part evidenced by an increase in the presence of the class 1 integrase gene, a reliable proxy for resistance to more than one antimicrobial in bacterial populations sampled in wastewater treatment plants (LaPara et al., 2011; Ma et al., 2013; Gillings et al., 2015), and an increase in the number of resistance genes in wastewater treatment plants and rural domestic wastewater treatment systems (Gao et al., 2012; Chen and Zhang, 2013; Ju et al., 2015; Mao et al., 2015). This indicates that controlling the use of antimicrobials is a prerequisite for slowing the development and spread of pathogens with multiple antimicrobial resistance mechanisms.

ANTIMICROBIAL RESISTANCE IN *Escherichia coli*

Escherichia coli is a widespread and abundant organism capable of causing a wide range of gastrointestinal and extra-intestinal diseases. It can survive and proliferate in a diversity of terrestrial and aquatic environments (van Elsas et al., 2011). As such, its genetic profile is shaped profoundly by horizontal gene transfer, and it is a useful marker species for understanding how antimicrobial resistance and virulence genes accumulate over evolutionary time. Horizontal gene transfer events are known to generate novel combinations of putative and established virulence factors, and generate novel pathotypes of *E. coli* (Wu et al., 2007; Bielaszewska et al., 2014). Although, *E. coli* is a commensal inhabitant of the gastrointestinal tract of warm-blooded animals, pathotypes have evolved that cause intestinal [intestinal pathogenic *E. coli* (IPEC)] and extra-intestinal [extraintestinal pathogenic *E. coli* (ExPEC)] diseases. Different pathotypes of *E. coli* cause diarrheal disease, hemolytic uremic syndrome (HUS), urinary tract infection (UTI), pyelonephritis, septicemia, meningitis, and respiratory disease (pneumonia) in humans and animals. Known IPEC pathotypes include the attaching and effacing *E. coli* (AEEC), Shiga-toxigenic *E. coli* (STEC), enteroaggregative *E. coli* (EAEC), enterotoxigenic *E. coli* (ETEC), enteroinvasive *E. coli* (EIEC), diffuse adhering *E. coli* (DAEC) and the recently described enteroaggregative hemorrhagic *E. coli* (EAHEC; Kaper et al., 2004; Brzuszkiewicz et al., 2011). EHEC are a subgroup of STEC, which colonizes the terminal regions of the gastrointestinal tract of ruminants. It is notable that different serotypes of *E. coli* preferentially colonize different ruminant hosts (Djordjevic et al., 2001, 2004; Hornitzky et al., 2002) and carry different Shiga toxin gene variants (Ramachandran et al., 2001; Brett et al., 2003a,b). These studies underscore the importance of understanding the ecology of disease-causing organisms and how niche adaptation influences lateral gene transfer. Notably, however, ruminants are not a recognized source of ExPEC (Manges and Johnson, 2015).

Many recent molecular surveillance studies on *E. coli* report the frequency of genes that code for extended-spectrum beta lactamase enzymes (ESBL's), which are indicative of resistance to penicillin, cephalosporin, and other clinically important antibiotics, but fail to screen for resistance to the older, first generation antibiotics (Bean et al., 2009; Ewers et al., 2012; Glasner et al., 2013; Roschanski et al., 2015). Genes that code for resistance to first generation antibiotics are often carried in bacteria containing class 1 integrons (Johnson et al., 2005b; Jakobsen et al., 2011; Hansen et al., 2014). From a diagnostic perspective, recent genomic studies on an outbreak of EAHEC and EAEC strain O104:H4, highlighted this issue (Ahmed et al., 2012). EAHEC is a recently emerged *E. coli* pathotype and EAEC strain O104:H4 has acquired the Shiga toxin gene *stx2a*, a diagnostic marker of EHEC. Outbreak strains were found to be resistant to ampicillin, streptomycin, sulfamethoxazole, trimethoprim, and tetracycline but little effort was given to determining how the genes that coded for these antibiotic resistance phenotypes were assembled (Ahmed et al., 2012). We were subsequently able to show that the genes coding for resistance to these antibiotics were assembled in Tn*6029D*, a transposon that abuts a class 1 integron in a Tn*21*/Tn*1721* hybrid backbone (Roy Chowdhury et al., 2015). The resistance region resided in genomic island 3 which also carried the virulence gene *ag43* encoding a self-associating serine protease auto-transporter, important for biofilm formation. This is an example of how antimicrobial resistance genes and virulence genes co-localize on the same mobile genetic element (Roy Chowdhury et al., 2015). Chromosomal islands are increasingly associated with carriage of class 1 integrons encoding resistance to multiple antibiotics of clinical significance (Roy Chowdhury et al., 2016).

Salmonella genomic island 1 (Boyd et al., 2001; Levings et al., 2005), Salmonella genomic island 2 (Levings et al., 2008) and several large plasmids in EHEC strain O26:H (Venturini et al., 2010), and an atypical EPEC, strain O111 (Venturini et al., 2013) are also examples of virulence and resistance genes being carried on the same mobile element. Strains of *E. coli* that carry genes that are markers for more than one *E. coli* pathotype pose a dilemma for diagnostic laboratories. There are numerous reports describing novel *E. coli* strains with combinations of virulence genes that are diagnostic of more than one *E. coli* pathotype; this suggests that newly emerging strains are increasingly likely to have complex resistance loci facilitated by the clustering of mobile element-associated resistance and virulence genes. In a study of 265 cases of *E. coli* causing UTI, 28 carried virulence genes typical of IPEC (Bielaszewska et al., 2014). Several other examples of hybrid *E. coli* strains have been described and their presence demonstrates the need to have genomic surveillance strategies in place to determine how antibiotic resistance and virulence genes assemble in emerging pathogens (Wallace-Gadsden et al., 2007; Abe et al., 2008; Bielaszewska et al., 2014; Mariani-Kurkdjian et al., 2014).

Extraintestinal pathogenic *E. coli* is a phylogenetically diverse group comprised of a broad range of *E. coli* sequence types (STs). ExPEC are fecal *E. coli* that rarely cause intestinal disease but have acquired a wide variety of virulence gene cargo that facilities their ability to cause disease at extraintestinal sites, particularly in the urinary tract. ExPEC are the most frequently isolated Gram negative bacterial pathogen infecting humans incurring significant mortality and morbidity. Notably, ExPEC are a leading cause of sepsis and are increasingly resistant to multiple antibiotics posing a serious health concern (Manges and Johnson, 2015; Poolman and Wacker, 2016). ExPEC have a fecal origin but rarely cause gastrointestinal disease. The acquisition of a diverse range of virulence factors by lateral gene transfer has armed ExPEC with an ability to cause life-threatening blood-borne, urinary tract, respiratory, skin and soft tissue infections, and meningitis in humans of all ages (Russo and Johnson, 2003; Poolman and Wacker, 2016). ExPEC vary widely in the combinations of putative virulence genes that they carry. Many genes encode for adhesins, iron acquisition systems and other putative virulence attributes and this genetic redundancy complicates efforts to develop broadly applicable molecular diagnostic tests to detect ExPEC (Johnson et al., 2001; Spurbeck et al., 2012). Importantly, livestock are important reservoirs for ExPEC (Ewers et al., 2007, 2009; Manges et al., 2007; Vincent et al., 2010; Nordstrom et al., 2013; Manges and Johnson, 2015). Virulence genes are often shared among *E. coli* isolates from samples collected from humans, and the meat and feces of intensively reared livestock, particularly poultry (Rodriguez-Siek et al., 2005; Vandekerchove et al., 2005; Jakobsen et al., 2010a,b). Consistent with this view, ExPEC carry genes coding for resistance to antimicrobials frequently used in veterinary medicine. Hospital diagnostics laboratories do not screen for most of the antibiotics used in veterinary medicine and so resistance to these is under-reported. In a Chinese study of 315 ExPEC isolates from various pig tissues, more than 63% exhibited resistance to 10 antibiotics including ampicillin, trimethoprim, sulfadimidine, tetracycline, neomycin, streptomycin, and kanamycin (Tan et al., 2012). The genes $bla_{\text{TEM}-1}$ (ampicillin resistance); *strAB* (streptomycin resistance); *sul1* and, *sul2* (sulfonamide resistance); *aphA1* (kanamycin and neomycin resistance); *tetA*, *tetB*, and *tetG* (tetracycline resistance); as well as various *dfrA* genes (trimethoprim resistance) coded for resistance to these antibiotics.

The class 1 integron is widespread in clinical settings. Bacteria that are resistant to more than one antimicrobial often carry class 1 integrons and their presence is a reliable indicator of multiple antimicrobial resistance (Leverstein-van Hall et al., 2003). The class 1 integron structures identified in most clinical samples are thought to be derived from the capture of a chromosomally located class 1 integron, prevalent within environmentally abundant bacterial species belonging to the broad β-proteobacterium group, by a Tn*402* family transposon (Gillings et al., 2008; Gillings, 2014). Global spread of the class 1 integron is in part a result of the propensity for the Tn*402* family of transposons to target *res* sites found on a wide variety of conjugative and mobile plasmids, including the widespread mercury-resistance transposon, Tn*21*, and the broader Tn*3* family (Liebert et al., 1999; Gillings et al., 2008, 2015). For this and a variety of other reasons described below, resistance genes cluster on mobile elements. Clinical class 1 integrons have subsequently evolved, typically by the loss of most of the Tn*402* *tniB* transposition gene, and partial fusion of the *qacE* gene (coding for an efflux pump for disinfectants, Hall et al., 1994; Partridge et al., 2001) with the sulfonamide resistance gene *sul1*. The most commonly observed structure observed in clinical isolates (**Figure 1A**) is comprised of a 5′ conserved segment (5′-CS), a 3′-conserved segment (3′CS) and a variable region inserted in between them. The 5′-CS contains the *intI1* gene encoding the class 1 integrase; the Tn*402* inverted repeat, the two promoters, one required for the transcription of the integrase and the other for the gene cassettes and the *attI1* recombination site. The variable region contains a diverse array of resistance gene cassettes (Partridge et al., 2009) and the associated *attC* sites. The 3′ conserved segment (3′-CS) most frequently contains *qacE*Δ*1* and *sul1* genes, remnants of the transposition module and a terminal Tn*402* inverted repeat. Most gene cassettes found in clinical class 1 integrons from nosocomial and livestock settings code for resistance to trimethoprim (*dfrA*) and aminoglycosides (*aadA*); despite this over 130 different gene cassettes have been described (Partridge et al., 2009) and, to date, 410 annotated variants are recognized (Tsafnat et al., 2011).

Further variation in the structure of the 3′-CS has also been described (Pan et al., 2006; Cain et al., 2010; Dawes et al., 2010; Saenz et al., 2010; Venturini et al., 2010, 2013; Mattiello et al., 2015). In one instance, the 3′-CS was almost completely lost and had been replaced with the compound transposon, Tn*6026* (Venturini et al., 2013). The Tn*6026* structure contains the beta-lactamase $bla_{\text{TEM}-1}$ gene; the sulfonamide resistance gene, *sul2*; the streptomycin resistance gene *strAB*; the neomycin/kanamycin resistance gene, *aphA1* and it is flanked by direct copies of IS*26* (**Figure 1B**). Tn*6026* is located between *attI*, the insertion point of the gene cassette, and the defective *tni* module of a clinical class 1 integron, replacing all but the first 24 bp of the 3′-CS (Cain et al., 2010; Dawes et al., 2010; Venturini et al., 2010, 2013). A *sul3* variant structure associated with IS*26* has also emerged over the last decade from human- and animal-sourced isolates (**Figure 1C**). The first report of *sul3* was from Swiss pigs and humans in Grape et al. (2003) and Perreten and Boerlin (2003). Since then, *sul3* has been reported in samples from a number of countries (Pan et al., 2006; Saenz et al., 2010; Tang et al., 2011; Mattiello et al., 2015; Wyrsch et al., 2015; Moran et al., 2016). These atypical class 1 integrons (**Figure 1**) are often components of larger complex resistance regions, hosted on plasmids that also carry virulence genes (Venturini et al., 2010, 2013).

Small mobile elements, including insertion sequences (IS*1*, IS*26*, IS*Ecp1c*, and IS*6100* are of note), Insertion Sequence Common Regions (ISCRs) and composite transposons formed from two or more IS elements, play an important role in reshaping the 3′-CS of clinical class 1 integrons (Daly et al., 2005; Dionisi et al., 2009; Venturini et al., 2010). The genes *blaSHV-11*, and *blaSHV-12* (coding for β-lactam resistance; Ford and Avison, 2004; Dionisi et al., 2009); *qnrB19* (coding for quinolone resistance; Dionisi et al., 2009); and *aphA1* (coding for kanamycin/neomycin resistance; Cain et al., 2010) have been shown to be flanked by direct copies of IS*26*. The mechanism of action of IS*26* has been the subject of several recent studies (Harmer et al., 2014; Harmer and Hall, 2015; He et al., 2015). These studies show that resistance loci containing IS*26* can be hotspots for the capture of further resistance genes and other genetic cargo flanked by IS*26* and demonstrates the important role of IS*26* and other mobile elements in the assembly and re-assembly of novel complex resistance loci.

Currently, genomic epidemiological surveillance relies heavily on whole genome and metagenomic sequence information generated using short-read (<400 bp) sequencing platforms. A fall in the cost of high throughput, next generation sequencing with platforms that generate short-read lengths means they have become the leading technology for characterizing microbial evolution and uncultured microbial consortia, and to catalog

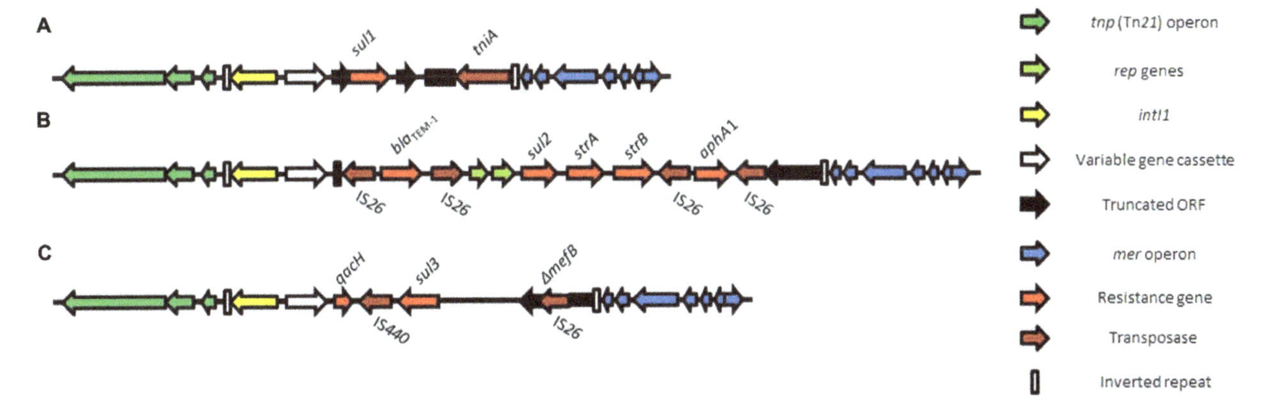

FIGURE 1 | Class 1 integron structures associated with the three sulfonamide resistance gene alleles *sul1* (A), *sul2* (B), and *sul3* (C), shown in a *Tn21* backbone.

antimicrobial resistance and virulence gene carriage. However, short-read sequencing technologies are unable to assemble complex resistance gene loci, or generate complete genome sequences, without which it is difficult to characterize mobile genetic elements rapidly and reliably. These limitations severely restrict efforts to comprehend the role of lateral gene transfer in the evolution of microbial pathogens and antimicrobial resistance, particularly in regards to the microevolutionary events that lead to the generation of novel complex resistance loci. Long-read sequencing technologies have improved significantly over the past 5 years and are beginning to address this shortfall, but are currently either cost prohibitive for large-scale genomic epidemiological surveillance or require further improvements in base call accuracy (Loman and Pallen, 2015).

Genes that code for resistance to older-generation antibiotics are often incorporated within complex resistance regions. In part, this provides a plausible explanation for why these genes persist despite enforced restrictions on prescribing of older-generation antibiotics. In the UK, strict limitations on the prescription of sulfonamide drugs were enforced in Anonymous (1995). However, functional *sul* genes persist in clinically important Gram negative bacteria and their frequency has not declined since the restriction was imposed (Enne et al., 2001; Bean et al., 2005, 2009). A similar scenario unfolded in Finland when trimethoprim was withdrawn from use for the treatment of UTI (Heikkila et al., 1990). In the Enterobacteriaceae, resistance to sulfonamides, trimethoprim, ampicillin, tetracycline, and fluoroquinolones remains high (Enne et al., 2001; Nozarian and Abdollahi, 2015; Paniagua-Contreras et al., 2015; Uzun et al., 2015; Yahiaoui et al., 2015). Carriage rates for *sul1*, *sul2*, or *sul3* genes in *E. coli* isolated from retail meat, livestock, healthy humans, and humans with clinical disease also remains a problem (Enne et al., 2001; Blahna et al., 2006; Frank et al., 2007; Altalhi et al., 2010; Bailey et al., 2010; Saenz et al., 2010; Vogt et al., 2014; Yahiaoui et al., 2015). Carriage of *sul* genes is linked with the presence of both typical and atypical class 1 integrons, including genes that code for resistance to ampicillin, streptomycin, and trimethoprim (Bettelheim et al., 2003; Bean et al., 2009; Bailey et al., 2010; Soufi et al., 2011; Ewers et al., 2014; Yahiaoui et al., 2015). Combinations of genes coding for resistance to first generation antibiotics contribute significantly to the multiple antimicrobial resistance phenotypes observed in commensal *E. coli* (Bettelheim et al., 2003; Vinue et al., 2008, 2010; Bailey et al., 2010). Genetic studies that have examined resistance to a broad spectrum of antibiotics frequently report the presence of $bla_{\text{TEM-1}}$, *sul1*, *sul2*, *strAB*, *tetA*(A), and a range of *aadA* and *dfrA* genes (Soufi et al., 2011; Labar et al., 2012; Ewers et al., 2014; Yamamoto et al., 2014; Yahiaoui et al., 2015). The streptomycin resistance gene, *strAB*, and the *sul2* sulfonamide resistance gene are also spread via small plasmids such as RSF1010 (Yau et al., 2010), and IncQ plasmids that are related to RSF1010 (Tietze et al., 1989). The *strAB* gene and the adjacent inverted repeat IR_R, as seen in RSF1010, probably had their origins in Tn*5393c*, while *sul2* was recruited from a CR2-containing element (Yau et al., 2010). These molecular events describing the evolution of the *sul2-strAB* configuration observed in RSF1010 have been described previously (Yau et al., 2010). The *sul2-strAB* gene cluster and flanking sequences from RSF1010 have been captured onto Tn*21* derivative transposons, on large and small plasmid backbones, and in chromosomal islands; they are often in association with IS*26* and are distributed widely (Daly et al., 2005; Cain et al., 2010; Venturini et al., 2010, 2013; Labar et al., 2012; Reid et al., 2015; Roy Chowdhury et al., 2015).

E. coli IN INTENSIVE PRODUCTION ANIMALS

Porcine Enterotoxigenic *Escherichia coli* (ETEC)

Enterotoxigenic *Escherichia coli* (ETEC) are the causative agents of three distinct diseases in young pigs: neonatal, pre-weaning, and post-weaning diarrhea (Fairbrother et al., 1988; Noamani et al., 2003). These diseases vary in severity and are categorized by the age at which the pig develops symptoms. Diarrhea caused by ETEC strains, generally known as enteric colibacillosis, is a problem in all countries involved in pig production, and various methods have been employed to protect pigs from ETEC infection and any subsequent diarrheal disease. These methods include, but are not limited to, treatment with antibiotics, vaccination, and feed modulation (Fairbrother et al., 2005; Virdi et al., 2013). While these protective steps have helped reduce levels of ETEC infection, particularly in neonatal and pre-weaning colibacillosis, antimicrobial resistance has become a global challenge that is severely limiting antimicrobials as a treatment option.

Pathogenic *E. coli* express a wide variety of functional molecules including toxins, adhesins, autotransporters, and invasins (Nataro and Kaper, 1998; Kaper et al., 2004), which enable the *E. coli* cells to damage host tissues. In porcine ETEC, these molecules, referred to as virulence factors, include heat-stable (ST) and heat-labile (LT) enterotoxins, both of which can cause diarrhea via different molecular pathways within the pig's gastrointestinal tract (Nataro and Kaper, 1998). Various adhesins have evolved in ETEC and are expressed on the bacterial cell surface, allowing adhesion to the host's gastrointestinal tract. In pigs, the K88 (F4), K99 (F5), 987P (F6), F18 and F41 fimbrial adhesins all provide host intestinal cell binding, with K88, K99 and F18 fimbriae being particularly prevalent (Nataro and Kaper, 1998; Nagy and Fekete, 1999; Koh et al., 2008). Interestingly, the K88 and F18 fimbrial adhesins are often associated with pre- and post-weaning diarrhea, whilst the K99 fimbria has been associated with neonatal diarrhea in pigs (DebRoy and Maddox, 2001). These binding effects are thought to be supplemented by other common adhesins coded by genes such as *fimH* (Bouckaert et al., 2006) and *eaeH* (Sheikh et al., 2014), which are known to provide additional post-attachment binding. Chapman et al. (2006) employed multiplex PCR assays targeting 58 virulence genes to screen 52 clinical *E. coli* isolates from episodes of porcine neonatal and post-weaning diarrhea, and 23 commensal *E. coli* isolates from healthy pigs. Of the 58 genes, 17 were useful in distinguishing commensal from clinical *E. coli*, nine of which (*iha*, *hlyA*, *aidA*, *east1*, *aah*, *fimH*, $iroN_{E.coli}$, *traT*, and *saa*) were identified for the first time in clinical porcine isolates in Australia (Chapman et al., 2006).

In an attempt to combat *E. coli* expressing these and other virulence genes, antimicrobials have been employed as both curative and prophylactic medicines on farms worldwide. This has placed a selection pressure on both targeted and surrounding microbial populations, and as such resistance to these antimicrobials has become extremely prevalent. For pathogenic *E. coli* in general, the definition and interpretation of virulence has been tempered based on results from large-scale microbial genome sequencing projects (Falkow, 1988; Pallen and Wren, 2007). ExPEC reside in the gut of their host, often in a commensal state, but have the genetic repertoire of virulence genes that enables them to cause life-threatening extraintestinal infections. Due to the degree of redundancy inherent in many ExPEC virulence genes, it remains a challenge to define virulence in ExPEC. These ExPEC-associated virulence genes have also been found in isolates sourced from humans, poultry and swine but rarely in cattle and other ruminants (Johnson et al., 2001; Tan et al., 2012; Manges and Johnson, 2015). Poultry are a well-recognized reservoir of ExPEC that have the potential to cause human disease but the role of swine in this regard has not been investigated sufficiently.

Current Status of Global Antimicrobial Use and Its Influence on the Porcine *E. coli* Resistome

Rationalization of farming practices has had profound effects on the spread of resistance to antimicrobials, and consequently both human and animal health - and the problem continues to grow (FAO, 2009). An estimated 210 million kilograms of antibiotics are produced annually in China, making it the largest producer and consumer of antibiotics globally. Approximately half of the antibiotics produced are used in livestock production (Hvistendahl, 2012; Zhu et al., 2013). China is also the largest producer and consumer of pork; 690 million pigs were produced in 2011 and 38.1 kg of pork are consumed per person per year (Krishnasamy et al., 2015), now reportedly almost double the pork consumption of the USA population. China is said to contain half the world's pig population, with five times the production rate of the USA (the former largest production center) and a higher per capita meat consumption than any developing nation other than Brazil and Latin America (FAO, 2009). Trends are similar for poultry production in China (Krishnasamy et al., 2015). An estimated 34 million kilograms of antibiotics, particularly tetracyclines, sulfonamides, macrolides, and penicillins were used in Chinese pig production during 2012 (Krishnasamy et al., 2015). Combination therapies of chlortetracycline with sulfathiazole and penicillin, and chlortetracycline with sulfamethazine and penicillin, are used widely. Other individual antibiotics that are used less extensively include tylosin, chlortetracycline, oxytetracycline, bacitracin, and bambermycin amongst others (Krishnasamy et al., 2015). Furthermore, pig production in China is responsible for the production of approximately 618 billion kilograms of manure per annum (Wang et al., 2006), much of which is contaminated with antibiotic residues and heavy metals, particularly tetracyclines, sulfonamides and copper; some residues are present at levels in the order of 100s of milligrams per kilogram (Pan et al., 2011; Qiao et al., 2012; Zhu et al., 2013). Elevated levels of zinc and arsenic have also been detected in these studies. Of 149 unique antimicrobial resistance genes 63 were detected significantly more frequently in microbes from manure at different stages of processing on three large pig production farms in China, compared with microbes in manure from control animals that received no antimicrobials; this included genes coding for resistance to antibiotics used to treat humans (Zhu et al., 2013). Samples of pig manure from China were also rich in microbes carrying transposase genes, notably those belonging to the IS*6*-family, predominantly IS*26* transposase (Zhu et al., 2013).

In the USA, estimates suggest that the usage of tetracyclines is as high as in China, both in the combinations described above, and as stand-alone treatments. Additionally, bacitracin, carbadox, lincomycin, neomycin, penicillin, tiamulin, tilmicosin, tylosin, and viginiamycin have all been used in the USA pig production industry (Apley et al., 2012). The USA and China combined produce the majority of the world's pigs through intensive farming practices (FAO, 2009), with China producing up to five times more than the USA (Krishnasamy et al., 2015). However, other countries also have pig production systems that rely heavily on antibiotic usage. In Alberta, Canada, the same suite of antibiotics is used as in the USA, with the addition of dimetridazole (Rajic et al., 2006). A similar pattern of use has also emerged in an Australian survey of pig production, with the use of apramycin and neomycin, penicillins, macrolides, sulfonamides, tetracyclines, lincomycin and spectinomycin, tiamulin, olaquindox, ceftiofur, and dimetridazole reported (Jordan et al., 2009). A number of these antibiotics, including lincomycin, spectinomycin, and dimetridazole are also used in the treatment of infectious human diseases. In an Australia-wide study of 114 porcine-derived *E. coli*, resistance to numerous antibiotics was common: tetracycline (88.6%), ampicillin (71.05%), trimethoprim/sulfamethoxazole (67.5%), streptomycin (69.3%), chloramphenicol (44.74%), neomycin (35.96%), apramycin (34.21%), gentamicin (28.95%), florphenicol (26.32), cefalotin (24.56%), and spectinomycin (21.93%). Resistance to imipenem and amikacin was not detected (Abraham et al., 2015). Of the 114 isolates evaluated 79% were classified as resistant to antibiotics from three or more different classes. Resistance to extended-spectrum cephalosporins (3%) and fluoroquinolones (1%) was detected in isolates belonging to some *E. coli* lineages (ST117, ST744, ST10, and ST1) albeit infrequently (Abraham et al., 2015).

Colistin is a polymyxin antimicrobial used to treat extensively drug-resistant Gram negative infections. It was first used in the 1950s but its use in humans has declined due to concerns about nephrotoxicity and neurotoxicity (Nation and Li, 2009). China, India, and Europe still use colistin extensively for agricultural purposes. In Europe, colistin is used to treat enterobacterial infections in pigs (neonatal diarrhea), poultry (colibacillosis), cattle (neonatal diarrhea in veal calves), sheep, and goats (Timmerman et al., 2006; Pardon et al., 2012); in 2010 it was the fifth most commonly sold antimicrobial after tetracycline,

TABLE 1 | Molecular characterisation of published antimicrobial resistant, porcine-derived *Escherichia coli* isolates.

Country	Resistance genes detected			Phenotypic resistances tested?	Molecular typing	Prominent Achtman MLSTs	Plasmid typing	Virulence gene detection?	Reference
	Integron associated	Resistance	Beta-lactamases						
Argentina	*intI2*			Yes	Serogrouping			Yes	Moredo et al., 2007, 2015; Pantozzi et al., 2010
Australia	*intI1, intI2, aadA, dfrA, cmlA, cat1, cat2, ereA, aacC4*	*sul1, sul2, sul3, strA, strB, aphA1, tetA, tetB, tetC*	*bla_{TEM}, bla_{CTX-M}, bla_{CMY}*	Yes	RAPD Serogrouping Phylotyping	ST100 ST29 ST90 ST746	Replicon	Yes	Chapman et al., 2006; Wu et al., 2007; Smith et al., 2010; Abraham et al., 2012, 2014, 2015
Austria			*bla_{CTX-M}, bla_{TEM}, bla_{SHV}*	Yes			Replicon		Mayrhofer et al., 2004, 2006; Petternel et al., 2014
Brazil				Yes	ERIC-PCR Serogrouping			Yes	Carvalho et al., 1991; da Costa et al., 2008; Borges et al., 2012; Morales et al., 2012
Canada	*aadA, dfrA, aadB, aacC4, cmlA*	*sul1, sul2, sul3, strA, strB, catA1, aphA, floR, tetA, tetB, tetC*	*bla_{TEM}, bla_{OXA}, bla_{CMY}*	Yes	ERIC-PCR BOX-PCR Serogrouping				Maynard et al., 2003; Lu et al., 2005; Travis et al., 2006; Duriez and Topp, 2007; Kozak et al., 2009a,b; Rosengren et al., 2009; Deckert et al., 2010; Sheikh et al., 2012
China	*intI1, aadA, dfrA*	*sul1, sul2, oqxAB, aac(6)-Ib-cr, qnrA, qnrB, qnrS, qepA, fosA, floR*	*bla_{CTX-M}, bla_{TEM}, bla_{SHV}, bla_{CMY}*	Yes	Serogrouping XbaI PFGE ERIC-PCR Phylogrouping	ST10 ST206	Replicon	Yes	Yang et al., 2004, 2014; Yue et al., 2008; Ho et al., 2009, 2013; Ma et al., 2009; Huang et al., 2012; Tian et al., 2012; Liu et al., 2013; Meng et al., 2014; Xu et al., 2014; Gao et al., 2015; Liao et al., 2015
Denmark	*intI1, aacC4*	*sul1, sul2, sul3*	*bla_{CTX-M}, bla_{TEM}, bla_{CMY}, bla_{SHV}*	Yes	XbaI PFGE Phylogrouping Serogrouping	ST10 ST23	Replicon	Yes	Olesen et al., 2004; Hammerum et al., 2006, 2014; Jensen et al., 2006; Cavaco et al., 2008; Trobos et al., 2009; Jakobsen et al., 2010a,b; Wu et al., 2010; Agerso et al., 2012; Agerso and Aarestrup, 2013; Hansen et al., 2013; Herrero-Fresno et al., 2015
Germany	*intI1, intI2, aadA, dfrA, aadB*	*sul1, sul2, sul3, strA, strB, tetA, tetB, tetM*	*bla_{TEM}, bla_{CTX-M}, bla_{OXA}*	Yes	XbaI PFGE Phylogrouping Serotyping	ST10 ST58 ST167 ST410	Replicon pMLST	Yes	Kadlec and Schwarz, 2008; Schwaiger et al., 2010; Bednorz et al., 2013; Schierack et al., 2013; Fischer et al., 2014; Dahms et al., 2015; Garcia-Cobos et al., 2015

(Continued)

TABLE 1 | Continued

Country	Resistance genes detected			Phenotypic resistances tested?	Molecular typing	Prominent Achtman MLSTs	Plasmid typing	Virulence gene detection?	Reference
	Integron associated	Resistance	Beta-lactamases						
India			*bla*$_{CTX-M}$, *bla*$_{SHV}$, *bla*$_{TEM}$	Yes	Serogrouping			Yes	Murugan et al., 2012; Rajkhowa and Sarma, 2014; Samanta et al., 2015
Italy			*bla*$_{CTX-M}$, *bla*$_{TEM}$	Yes					Stefani et al., 2014; Luppi et al., 2015
Japan	*intI1, aadA, dfrA, cmlA, aacA4*	*cat1, tetA, tetB, tetC*		Yes	PFGE Phylogrouping			Yes	Kijima-Tanaka et al., 2003, 2005; Asai et al., 2005; Harada et al., 2005, 2006; Kumai et al., 2005; Katsunuma et al., 2008; Kojima et al., 2009; Makita et al., 2016
Korea	*intI1, aadA, dfrA, aadB, cmlA*	*aphA, qnrB, qnrS, aac(6)-Ib-cr, tetA*	*bla*$_{TEM}$, *bla*$_{SHV}$, *bla*$_{CTX-M}$	Yes	PFGE HFERP Phylogrouping Serogrouping			Yes	Choi et al., 2002; Han et al., 2002; Kang et al., 2005; Lim et al., 2007, 2009; Rayamajhi et al., 2008; Unno et al., 2010, 2011; Tamang et al., 2012; Lee et al., 2014
Lithuania	*intI1, intI2, aadA, dfrA, estX, sat2*			Yes					Povilonis et al., 2010; Seputiene et al., 2010
Nigeria		*qnrS*	*bla*$_{TEM}$	Yes	ERIC-PCR PFGE Serogrouping		pMLST	Yes	Ojo et al., 2010; Fortini et al., 2011; Adenipekun et al., 2015
Norway	*intI1, intI2, aadA, dfrA, catB, sat1*	*sul1, sul2, strA, strB, tetA, tetB, tetC*	*bla*$_{TEM}$, *bla*$_{OXA}$	Yes	PFGE	ST10 ST168			Sunde et al., 1998; Sunde and Sorum, 1999; Brun et al., 2002; Sunde, 2005; Sunde and Norstrom, 2006; Trobos et al., 2009
Portugal	*intI1, intI2, dfrA, aadA, estX, sat2, catB*	*strA, strB, qnrB, tetA*	*bla*$_{TEM}$, *bla*$_{CTX-M}$, *bla*$_{SHV}$	Yes	XbaI PFGE	ST10	Replicon pMLST RFLP		Machado et al., 2008; Goncalves et al., 2010; Jones-Dias et al., 2013; Ramos et al., 2013; Rodrigues et al., 2013
Spain	*intI1, intI2, aadA, dfrA, cmlA, sat2, linF*	*sul1, sul3, pmrA, pmrB*	*bla*$_{CTX-M}$, *bla*$_{TEM}$, *bla*$_{SHV}$, *bla*$_{OXA}$	Yes	Phylogrouping REP-PCR ERIC-PCR				Brinas et al., 2002; Sabate et al., 2008; Escudero et al., 2010; Marchant and Moreno, 2013; Marchant et al., 2013; Ojer-Usoz et al., 2013; Quesada et al., 2015

(Continued)

TABLE 1 | Continued

Country	Resistance genes detected			Phenotypic resistances tested?	Molecular typing	Prominent Achtman MLSTs	Plasmid typing	Virulence gene detection?	Reference
	Integron associated	Resistance	Beta-lactamases						
Switzerland	*intI1*, *aadA*	*sul1*, *sul2*, *sul3*, *strA*, *strB*, *tetA*, *tetB*, *tetC*	bla_{CTX-M}	Yes	PFGE Serogrouping	ST3 ST529		Yes	Stephan and Schumacher, 2001; Lanz et al., 2003; Perreten and Boerlin, 2003; Zweifel et al., 2006; Stannarius et al., 2009; Endimiani et al., 2012
Taiwan	*intI1*, *aadA*, *dfrA*	*sul1*, *fosA*	bla_{TEM}, bla_{CTX-M}, bla_{CMY}	Yes	XbaI PFGE	ST744 ST2310			Hsu et al., 2006; Tseng et al., 2015
Thailand	*intI1*, *aadA*, *dfrA*, *linF*, *sat1*	*sul1*	bla_{CTX-M}, bla_{TEM}	Yes	Phylogrouping			Yes	Hanson et al., 2002; Phongpaichit et al., 2007; Mathew et al., 2009; Lay et al., 2012; Changkaew et al., 2015
UK	*aadA*	*sul2*, *floR*	bla_{CTX-M}, bla_{SHV}	Yes			pMLST		Jackson, 1981; Enne et al., 2008; Taylor et al., 2008; Freire Martin et al., 2014; Randall et al., 2014; Cheney et al., 2015
USA	*intI1*, *aadA*, *dfrA*, *cmlA*, *sat1*	*cat2*, *flo*, *tetA*, *tetB*, *tetC*, *tetM*		Yes	Serogrouping XbaI PFGE Phylogrouping		Replicon	Yes	Bischoff et al., 2002; Schroeder et al., 2002; Bryan et al., 2004; Singh et al., 2005; Lindsey et al., 2011; Xia et al., 2011; Ju et al., 2012; Tadesse et al., 2012; Roug et al., 2013

penicillins, sulfonamides, and macrolides (European Medicines Agency [EMA], 2013). Colistin is also used in aquaculture (Xu et al., 2012). The recent emergence of colistin resistance in commensal porcine *E. coli* isolates in China via the acquisition of plasmid-mediated *mcr-1* gene has serious implications for the treatment of pan-drug-resistant Gram-negative bacteria, particularly isolates of the extremely drug resistant *Acinetobacter baumannii* and carbapenemase-resistant *Klebsiella pneumoniae* (Liu et al., 2015). The seriousness of this finding is clear due to: (i) high *in vitro* transfer rates among *E. coli* by conjugation and the ability of the *mcr-1* plasmid to transfer and be maintained in globally dispersed pathogenic clones such as *E. coli* ST131, *K. pneumoniae* ST11, and *Pseudomonas aeruginosa*; (ii) the high frequency of carriage of *mcr-1* in *E. coli* from livestock and in retail meats sourced from southern China; (iii) detection of *mcr-1*-like genes in Malaysia (Liu et al., 2016). The apparent high rates of carriage of *mcr-1* in isolates of *E. coli* from animals and the apparent low incidence in human-derived *E. coli* populations has led to speculation that the heavy use of colistin in agriculture in China has been the main driver for the emergence of plasmid-mediated colistin resistance (European Medicines Agency [EMA], 2013; Liu et al., 2016).

Genes conferring antimicrobial resistance have been identified in *E. coli* from diverse pig-related sources (**Table 1**). The genes bla_{TEM}, *sul1/2/3*, *aadA*, *dfrA*, and *tetA/B/C* feature prominently. In order, these genes confer resistance to penicillin, sulfonamides (such as sulphamethoxazole), streptomycin and spectinomycin, trimethoprim, and tetracyclines; all of these are used in the treatment of animals. Additional clinically important cases of resistance are also identified sporadically in the literature, specifically to chloramphenicol (*cmlA*, *cat*), streptothricin (*estX/sat*), florfenicol (*flo*), quinolones (*qnr*), streptomycin (*strAB*), and fosfomycin (*fosA*). There are also a number of known resistance mutations in the *gyr* and *pmr* genes that confer elevated resistance to quinolones and colistin respectively. Already the presence of these genes together in the same isolate and from disparate countries indicates they are both genetically linked in antimicrobial resistance-encoding loci, and globally disseminated. Detection of the genes bla_{OXA}, bla_{SHV}, and bla_{CTX-M} coding for the extended-spectrum beta-lactamases, which are relevant to human medicine, is also of concern (Randall et al., 2014). Of note, these data were collected from a variety of publications for each country, and show some selection bias concerning the genes detected. Whole genome sequencing has become a tool to rectify this bias, and will continue to feature in the detection and characterisation of antimicrobial resistance, its evolution and dissemination (Salipante et al., 2015).

Much needs to be done to reduce the reliance on antimicrobials in food production. There is a growing body

TABLE 2 | Published complete porcine *E. coli* genome and plasmid sequences.

Name	Country	Type	Size (bp)	Achtman MLST/Plasmid Inc.	Disease association/source	GenBank accession	Reference
pND11_107	USA	Plasmid	107,138	I	Neonatal diarrhea	HQ114281	Johnson et al., 2011
pPWD4_103	USA	Plasmid	103,297	I	Post-weaning diarrhea	HQ114284	
pUMNF18_69	USA	Plasmid	69,065	I		CP002891	
pND12_96	USA	Plasmid	92,290	I	Neonatal diarrhea	HQ114282	
UMNK88	USA	Chromosome	5,186,416	ST165 cplx	Post-weaning diarrhea	CP002729	Shepard et al., 2012
pUMNK88_Hly	USA	Plasmid	65,549			CP002733	
pUMNK88_Ent	USA	Plasmid	81,475			CP002732	
pUMNK88_K88	USA	Plasmid	81,883			CP002730	
pUMNK88_91	USA	Plasmid	90,868	I		CP002731	
pUMNK88	USA	Plasmid	160,573	A/C		HQ023862	
pTC1	Hungary	Plasmid	91,019		Weaning diarrhea	CP000913	Fekete et al., 2012
pHK23a	China	Plasmid	73,607	FII	Multi-drug resistant isolate	JQ432559	Ho et al., 2013
pSCEC2	China	Plasmid	135,615	A/C	Maxillary lymph node	KF152885	Zhang et al., 2014
pIFM3804	UK	Plasmid	104,399	I		KF787110	Freire Martin et al., 2014
PCN033	China	Chromosome	4,987,957	ST5147	Extraintestinal infection (brain)	CP006632	Liu et al., 2015
PCN033p1	China	Plasmid	3,319			CP006633	
PCN033p2	China	Plasmid	4,086			CP006634	
PCN033p3	China	Plasmid	161,511			CP006635	
PCN061	China	Chromosome	4,603,777	ST46	Extraintestinal infection (lung)	CP006636	
PCN061p1	China	Plasmid	2,014			CP006637	
PCN061p2	China	Plasmid	5,754			CP006638	
PCN061p3	China	Plasmid	6,222	Q1/FIB/FIC/FII		CP006639	
PCN061p4	China	Plasmid	34,692			CP006640	
PCN061p5	China	Plasmid	103,644	I		CP006641	
PCN061p6	China	Plasmid	145,722	N/FIB/X1		CP006642	
pFSEC-01	China	Plasmid	33,885			KR779901	Zhang et al., 2015
pSD11	China	Plasmid	37,672	X4		KM212169	Sun et al., 2015

of evidence suggesting that food production may be a key driver in the evolution of multiple drug resistance in a number of bacterial species of clinical significance to human health. Livestock represent a reservoir of *E. coli* pathotypes with resistance to more than one antimicrobial. While pigs and poultry are significant sources of ExPEC, cattle are the major reservoirs for Shiga toxin producing *E. coli* (EHEC; Manges and Johnson, 2015) and atypical EPEC (Hornitzky et al., 2005; Dawes et al., 2010). The consequences for the environment of large-scale intensive animal production and a growing human population, estimated to be 9 billion by 2050 (United Nations, 2015) are not fully understood. Much remains to be done to determine how antimicrobial resistance genes are assembled on mobile genetic elements and to identify their unique genetic features. Diagnostics tests that target unique features will be useful in tracking the movement of mobile elements that are carrying complex resistance loci and to identify hotspots where they reside. Metagenomic approaches will have a major role to play in understanding the scale of the antimicrobial resistance problem, detecting and tracking emerging pathogens, and the role of gut flora in human and animal health. Studies on microbial populations from the gastrointestinal tracts of intensively reared livestock are needed to identify and characterize novel pathotypes that will undoubtedly emerge in response to the selection pressures that are commonplace in large-scale animal production facilities. Genomic surveillance studies will have an important role to play in identifying complex resistance loci, particularly how they move through different production systems and natural ecosystems (aquatic and terrestrial), and the impact they have on the carriage of multiple antimicrobial resistance genes in bacteria that colonize and infect humans and animals. Currently, there are just three complete porcine-derived *E. coli* chromosomal sequences published, as well as a variety of complete plasmid sequences, the majority of which have been derived from the study of isolates with closed genome sequences (**Table 2**). This is at odds with the significant role that intensive pig production plays in the release of antibiotic residues into the environment, and we expect more focus to be placed on the sequencing of pig-associated *E. coli* isolates in the near future.

AUTHOR CONTRIBUTIONS

EW drafted an early version of the manuscript and produced the figure and tables. PR and IC contributed to several sections in the manuscript. TC and JH edited drafts of the manuscript. SD wrote most the manuscript.

ACKNOWLEDGMENT

We wish to acknowledge J. K. Pell Consulting for copyediting the manuscript.

REFERENCES

Abe, C. M., Salvador, F. A., Falsetti, I. N., Vieira, M. A., Blanco, J., Blanco, J. E., et al. (2008). Uropathogenic *Escherichia coli* (UPEC) strains may carry virulence properties of diarrhoeagenic *E. coli*. *FEMS Immunol. Med. Microbiol.* 52, 397–406. doi: 10.1111/j.1574-695X.2008.00388.x

Abraham, S., Chin, J., Brouwers, H. J., Zhang, R., and Chapman, T. A. (2012). Molecular serogrouping of porcine enterotoxigenic *Escherichia coli* from Australia. *J. Microbiol. Methods* 88, 73–76. doi: 10.1016/j.mimet.2011.10.016

Abraham, S., Jordan, D., Wong, H. S., Johnson, J. R., Toleman, M. A., Wakeham, D. L., et al. (2015). First detection of extended-spectrum cephalosporin- and fluoroquinolone-resistant *Escherichia coli* in Australian food-producing animals. *J. Glob. Antimicrob. Resist.* 3, 273–277. doi: 10.1016/j.jgar.2015.08.002

Abraham, S., Trott, D. J., Jordan, D., Gordon, D. M., Groves, M. D., Fairbrother, J. M., et al. (2014). Phylogenetic and molecular insights into the evolution of multidrug-resistant porcine enterotoxigenic *Escherichia coli* in Australia. *Int. J. Antimicrob. Agents* 44, 105–111. doi: 10.1016/j.ijantimicag.2014.04.011

Adenipekun, E. O., Jackson, C. R., Oluwadun, A., Iwalokun, B. A., Frye, J. G., Barrett, J. B., et al. (2015). Prevalence and antimicrobial resistance in *Escherichia coli* from food animals in Lagos, Nigeria. *Microb. Drug Resist.* 21, 358–365. doi: 10.1089/mdr.2014.0222

Agerso, Y., and Aarestrup, F. M. (2013). Voluntary ban on cephalosporin use in Danish pig production has effectively reduced extended-spectrum cephalosporinase-producing *Escherichia coli* in slaughter pigs. *J. Antimicrob. Chemother.* 68, 569–572. doi: 10.1093/jac/dks427

Agerso, Y., Aarestrup, F. M., Pedersen, K., Seyfarth, A. M., Struve, T., and Hasman, H. (2012). Prevalence of extended-spectrum cephalosporinase (ESC)-producing *Escherichia coli* in Danish slaughter pigs and retail meat identified by selective enrichment and association with cephalosporin usage. *J. Antimicrob. Chemother.* 67, 582–588. doi: 10.1093/jac/dkr507

Agerso, Y., Jensen, J. D., Hasman, H., and Pedersen, K. (2014). Spread of extended spectrum cephalosporinase-producing *Escherichia coli* clones and plasmids from parent animals to broilers and to broiler meat in a production without use of cephalosporins. *Foodborne Pathog. Dis.* 11, 740–746. doi: 10.1089/fpd.2014.1742

Ahmed, A. M., and Shimamoto, T. (2015a). Molecular analysis of multidrug resistance in Shiga toxin-producing *Escherichia coli* O157:H7 isolated from meat and dairy products. *Int. J. Food Microbiol.* 193, 68–73. doi: 10.1016/j.ijfoodmicro.2014.10.014

Ahmed, A. M., and Shimamoto, T. (2015b). Molecular characterization of multidrug-resistant *Shigella* spp. of food origin. *Int. J. Food Microbiol.* 194, 78–82. doi: 10.1016/j.ijfoodmicro.2014.11.013

Ahmed, S. A., Awosika, J., Baldwin, C., Bishop-Lilly, K. A., Biswas, B., Broomall, S., et al. (2012). Genomic comparison of *Escherichia coli* O104:H4 isolates from 2009 and 2011 reveals plasmid, and prophage heterogeneity, including shiga toxin encoding phage stx2. *PLoS ONE* 7:e48228. doi: 10.1371/journal.pone.0048228

Allen, H. K., Donato, J., Wang, H. H., Cloud-Hansen, K. A., Davies, J., and Handelsman, J. (2010). Call of the wild: antibiotic resistance genes in natural environments. *Nat. Rev. Microbiol.* 8, 251–259. doi: 10.1038/nrmicro2312

Altalhi, A. D., Gherbawy, Y. A., and Hassan, S. A. (2010). Antibiotic resistance in *Escherichia coli* isolated from retail raw chicken meat in Taif, Saudi Arabia. *Foodborne Pathog. Dis.* 7, 281–285. doi: 10.1089/fpd.2009.0365

Andersen, S. R. (1993). Effects of waste water treatment on the species composition and antibiotic resistance of coliform bacteria. *Curr. Microbiol.* 26, 97–103. doi: 10.1007/bf01577343

Anonymous. (1995). Co-trimoxazole use restricted. *Drug Ther. Bull.* 33, 92–93. doi: 10.1136/dtb.1995.331292

Apley, M. D., Bush, E. J., Morrison, R. B., Singer, R. S., and Snelson, H. (2012). Use estimates of in-feed antimicrobials in swine production in the United States. *Foodborne Pathog. Dis.* 9, 272–279. doi: 10.1089/fpd.2011.0983

Asai, T., Kojima, A., Harada, K., Ishihara, K., Takahashi, T., and Tamura, Y. (2005). Correlation between the usage volume of veterinary therapeutic antimicrobials and resistance in *Escherichia coli* isolated from the feces of food-producing animals in Japan. *Jpn. J. Infect. Dis.* 58, 369–372.

Baez, J., Hernandez-Garcia, M., Guamparito, C., Diaz, S., Olave, A., Guerrero, K., et al. (2015). Molecular characterization and genetic diversity of ESBL-producing *Escherichia coli* colonizing the migratory Franklin's gulls (*Leucophaeus pipixcan*) in Antofagasta, North of Chile. *Microb. Drug Resist.* 21, 111–116. doi: 10.1089/mdr.2014.0158

Bailey, J. K., Pinyon, J. L., Anantham, S., and Hall, R. M. (2010). Commensal *Escherichia coli* of healthy humans: a reservoir for antibiotic-resistance determinants. *J. Med. Microbiol.* 59, 1331–1339. doi: 10.1099/jmm.0.022475-0

Baker-Austin, C., Wright, M. S., Stepanauskas, R., and McArthur, J. V. (2006). Co-selection of antibiotic and metal resistance. *Trends Microbiol.* 14, 176–182. doi: 10.1016/j.tim.2006.02.006

Baquero, F., Tedim, A. P., and Coque, T. M. (2013). Antibiotic resistance shaping multi-level population biology of bacteria. *Front. Microbiol.* 4:15. doi: 10.3389/fmicb.2013.00015

Baquero, F., and Tobes, R. (2013). Bloody coli: a gene cocktail in *Escherichia coli* O104:H4. *MBio* 4:e00066-13. doi: 10.1128/mBio.00066-13

Barkay, T., Miller, S. M., and Summers, A. O. (2003). Bacterial mercury resistance from atoms to ecosystems. *FEMS Microbiol. Rev.* 27, 355–384. doi: 10.1016/S0168-6445(03)00046-9

Bartoloni, A., Pallecchi, L., Rodriguez, H., Fernandez, C., Mantella, A., Bartalesi, F., et al. (2009). Antibiotic resistance in a very remote Amazonas community. *Int. J. Antimicrob. Agents* 33, 125–129. doi: 10.1016/j.ijantimicag.2008.07.029

Bean, D. C., Livermore, D. M., and Hall, L. M. (2009). Plasmids imparting sulfonamide resistance in *Escherichia coli*: implications for persistence. *Antimicrob. Agents Chemother.* 53, 1088–1093. doi: 10.1128/AAC.00800-08

Bean, D. C., Livermore, D. M., Papa, I., and Hall, L. M. (2005). Resistance among *Escherichia coli* to sulphonamides and other antimicrobials now little used in man. *J. Antimicrob. Chemother.* 56, 962–964. doi: 10.1093/jac/dki332

Bednorz, C., Guenther, S., Oelgeschlager, K., Kinnemann, B., Pieper, R., Hartmann, S., et al. (2013). Feeding the probiotic *Enterococcus faecium* strain NCIMB 10415 to piglets specifically reduces the number of *Escherichia coli* pathotypes that adhere to the gut mucosa. *Appl. Environ. Microbiol.* 79, 7896–7904. doi: 10.1128/AEM.03138-13

Ben Said, L., Jouini, A., Klibi, N., Dziri, R., Alonso, C. A., Boudabous, A., et al. (2015). Detection of extended-spectrum beta-lactamase (ESBL)-producing *Enterobacteriaceae* in vegetables, soil and water of the farm environment in Tunisia. *Int. J. Food Microbiol.* 203, 86–92. doi: 10.1016/j.ijfoodmicro.2015.02.023

Berendonk, T. U., Manaia, C. M., Merlin, C., Fatta-Kassinos, D., Cytryn, E., Walsh, F., et al. (2015). Tackling antibiotic resistance: the environmental framework. *Nat. Rev. Microbiol.* 13, 310–317. doi: 10.1038/nrmicro3439

Berg, J., Tom-Petersen, A., and Nybroe, O. (2005). Copper amendment of agricultural soil selects for bacterial antibiotic resistance in the field. *Lett. Appl. Microbiol.* 40, 146–151. doi: 10.1111/j.1472-765X.2004.01650.x

Bettelheim, K. A., Hornitzky, M. A., Djordjevic, S. P., and Kuzevski, A. (2003). Antibiotic resistance among verocytotoxigenic *Escherichia coli* (VTEC) and non-VTEC isolated from domestic animals and humans. *J. Med. Microbiol.* 52, 155–162. doi: 10.1099/jmm.0.04903-0

Bielaszewska, M., Schiller, R., Lammers, L., Bauwens, A., Fruth, A., Middendorf, B., et al. (2014). Heteropathogenic virulence and phylogeny reveal phased pathogenic metamorphosis in *Escherichia coli* O2:H6. *EMBO Mol. Med.* 6, 347–357. doi: 10.1002/emmm.201303133

Bischoff, K. M., White, D. G., McDermott, P. F., Zhao, S., Gaines, S., Maurer, J. J., et al. (2002). Characterization of chloramphenicol resistance in beta-hemolytic *Escherichia coli* associated with diarrhea in neonatal swine. *J. Clin. Microbiol.* 40, 389–394. doi: 10.1128/JCM.40.2.389-394.2002

Blahna, M. T., Zalewski, C. A., Reuer, J., Kahlmeter, G., Foxman, B., and Marrs, C. F. (2006). The role of horizontal gene transfer in the spread oftrimethoprim-sulfamethoxazole resistance among uropathogenic *Escherichia coli* in Europe and Canada. *J. Antimicrob. Chemother.* 57, 666–672. doi: 10.1093/jac/dkl020

Bondarczuk, K., Markowicz, A., and Piotrowska-Seget, Z. (2016). The urgent need for risk assessment on the antibiotic resistance spread via sewage sludge land application. *Environ. Int.* 87, 49–55. doi: 10.1016/j.envint.2015.11.011

Borges, C. A., Beraldo, L. G., Maluta, R. P., Cardozo, M. V., Guth, B. E., Rigobelo, E. C., et al. (2012). Shiga toxigenic and atypical enteropathogenic *Escherichia coli* in the feces and carcasses of slaughtered pigs. *Foodborne Pathog. Dis.* 9, 1119–1125. doi: 10.1089/fpd.2012.1206

Bouckaert, J., Mackenzie, J., de Paz, J. L., Chipwaza, B., Choudhury, D., Zavialov, A., et al. (2006). The affinity of the FimH fimbrial adhesin is receptor-driven and quasi-independent of *Escherichia coli* pathotypes. *Mol. Microbiol.* 61, 1556–1568. doi: 10.1111/j.1365-2958.2006.05352.x

Boyd, D., Peters, G. A., Cloeckaert, A., Boumedine, K. S., Chaslus-Dancla, E., Imberechts, H., et al. (2001). Complete nucleotide sequence of a 43-kilobase genomic island associated with the multidrug resistance region of *Salmonella enterica* serovar Typhimurium DT104 and its identification in phage type DT120 and serovar Agona. *J. Bacteriol.* 183, 5725–5732. doi: 10.1128/jb.183.19.5725-5732.2001

Brett, K. N., Hornitzky, M. A., Bettelheim, K. A., Walker, M. J., and Djordjevic, S. P. (2003a). Bovine non-O157 Shiga toxin 2-containing *Escherichia coli* isolates commonly possess stx2-EDL933 and/or stx2vhb Subtypes. *J. Clin. Microbiol.* 41, 2716–2722. doi: 10.1128/jcm.41.6.2716-2722.2003

Brett, K. N., Ramachandran, V., Hornitzky, M. A., Bettelheim, K. A., Walker, M. J., and Djordjevic, S. P. (2003b). stx1c Is the most common Shiga toxin 1 subtype among Shiga toxin-producing *Escherichia coli* isolates from sheep but not among isolates from cattle. *J. Clin. Microbiol.* 41, 926–936. doi: 10.1128/JCM.41.3.926-936.2003

Brinas, L., Zarazaga, M., Saenz, Y., Ruiz-Larrea, F., and Torres, C. (2002). Beta-lactamases in ampicillin-resistant *Escherichia coli* isolates from foods, humans, and healthy animals. *Antimicrob. Agents Chemother.* 46, 3156–3163. doi: 10.1128/AAC.46.10.3156-3163.2002

Brun, E., Holstad, G., Kruse, H., and Jarp, J. (2002). Within-sample and between-sample variation of antimicrobial resistance in fecal *Escherichia coli* isolates from pigs. *Microb. Drug Resist.* 8, 385–391. doi: 10.1089/10766290260469660

Bryan, A., Shapir, N., and Sadowsky, M. J. (2004). Frequency and distribution of tetracycline resistance genes in genetically diverse, nonselected, and nonclinical *Escherichia coli* strains isolated from diverse human and animal sources. *Appl. Environ. Microbiol.* 70, 2503–2507. doi: 10.1128/AEM.70.4.2503-2507.2004

Brzuszkiewicz, E., Thurmer, A., Schuldes, J., Leimbach, A., Liesegang, H., Meyer, F. D., et al. (2011). Genome sequence analyses of two isolates from the recent *Escherichia coli* outbreak in Germany reveal the emergence of a new pathotype: entero-aggregative-haemorrhagic *Escherichia coli* (EAHEC). *Arch. Microbiol.* 193, 883–891. doi: 10.1007/s00203-011-0725-6

Cain, A. K., Liu, X., Djordjevic, S. P., and Hall, R. M. (2010). Transposons related to Tn1696 in IncHI2 plasmids in multiply antibiotic resistant *Salmonella enterica* serovar Typhimurium from Australian animals. *Microb. Drug Resist.* 16, 197–202. doi: 10.1089/mdr.2010.0042

Carroll, D., Wang, J., Fanning, S., and McMahon, B. J. (2015). Antimicrobial resistance in wildlife: implications for public health. *Zoonoses Public Health* 62, 534–542. doi: 10.1111/zph.12182

Carvalho, A. C., Avila, F. A., Schocken-Iturrino, R. P., Quintana, J. L., and Albertini, P. E. (1991). Virulence factors in *Escherichia coli* strains isolated from pigs in the Ribeirao Preto region, State of Sao Paulo, Brazil. *Rev. Elev. Med. Vet. Pays Trop.* 44, 49–52.

Castillo, M., Martin-Orue, S. M., Taylor-Pickard, J. A., Perez, J. F., and Gasa, J. (2008). Use of mannanoligosaccharides and zinc chelate as growth promoters and diarrhea preventative in weaning pigs: effects on microbiota and gut function. *J. Anim. Sci.* 86, 94–101. doi: 10.2527/jas.2005-686

Cavaco, L. M., Frimodt-Moller, N., Hasman, H., Guardabassi, L., Nielsen, L., and Aarestrup, F. M. (2008). Prevalence of quinolone resistance mechanisms and associations to minimum inhibitory concentrations in quinolone-resistant *Escherichia coli* isolated from humans and swine in Denmark. *Microb. Drug Resist.* 14, 163–169. doi: 10.1089/mdr.2008.0821

Changkaew, K., Intarapuk, A., Utrarachkij, F., Nakajima, C., Suthienkul, O., and Suzuki, Y. (2015). Antimicrobial resistance, extended-spectrum beta-lactamase productivity, and class 1 integrons in *Escherichia coli* from healthy swine. *J. Food Prot.* 78, 1442–1450. doi: 10.4315/0362-028X.JFP-14-445

Chapman, T. A., Wu, X. Y., Barchia, I., Bettelheim, K. A., Driesen, S., Trott, D., et al. (2006). Comparison of virulence gene profiles of *Escherichia coli* strains isolated from healthy and diarrheic swine. *Appl. Environ. Microbiol.* 72, 4782–4795. doi: 10.1128/AEM.02885-05

Chee-Sanford, J. C., Mackie, R. I., Koike, S., Krapac, I. G., Lin, Y. F., Yannarell, A. C., et al. (2009). Fate and transport of antibiotic residues and antibiotic resistance genes following land application of manure waste. *J. Environ. Qual.* 38, 1086–1108. doi: 10.2134/jeq2008.0128

Chen, H., and Zhang, M. (2013). Occurrence and removal of antibiotic resistance genes in municipal wastewater and rural domestic sewage treatment systems in eastern China. *Environ. Int.* 55, 9–14. doi: 10.1016/j.envint.2013.01.019

Chen, Y. T., Lauderdale, T. L., Liao, T. L., Shiau, Y. R., Shu, H. Y., Wu, K. M., et al. (2007). Sequencing and comparative genomic analysis of pK29, a 269-kilobase conjugative plasmid encoding CMY-8 and CTX-M-3 beta-lactamases in *Klebsiella pneumoniae. Antimicrob. Agents Chemother.* 51, 3004–3007. doi: 10.1128/AAC.00167-07

Cheney, T. E., Smith, R. P., Hutchinson, J. P., Brunton, L. A., Pritchard, G., and Teale, C. J. (2015). Cross-sectional survey of antibiotic resistance in *Escherichia coli* isolated from diseased farm livestock in England and Wales. *Epidemiol. Infect.* 143, 2653–2659. doi: 10.1017/s0950268814003963

Choi, C., Ham, H. J., Kwon, D., Kim, J., Cheon, D. S., Min, K., et al. (2002). Antimicrobial susceptibility of pathogenic *Escherichia coli* isolated from pigs in Korea. *J. Vet. Med. Sci.* 64, 71–73. doi: 10.1292/jvms.64.71

da Costa, M. M., Drescher, G., Maboni, F., Weber, S., de Avila Botton, S., Vainstein, M. H., et al. (2008). Virulence factors and antimicrobial resistance of *Escherichia coli* isolated from urinary tract of swine in southern of Brazil. *Braz. J. Microbiol.* 39, 741–743. doi: 10.1590/s1517-838220080004000027

Dahms, C., Hubner, N. O., Kossow, A., Mellmann, A., Dittmann, K., and Kramer, A. (2015). Occurrence of ESBL-producing *Escherichia coli* in livestock and farm workers in mecklenburg-western pomerania, Germany. *PLoS ONE* 10:e0143326. doi: 10.1371/journal.pone.0143326

Daly, M., Villa, L., Pezzella, C., Fanning, S., and Carattoli, A. (2005). Comparison of multidrug resistance gene regions between two geographically unrelated *Salmonella* serotypes. *J. Antimicrob. Chemother.* 55, 558–561. doi: 10.1093/jac/dki015

Dawes, F. E., Kuzevski, A., Bettelheim, K. A., Hornitzky, M. A., Djordjevic, S. P., and Walker, M. J. (2010). Distribution of class 1 integrons with IS26-mediated deletions in their 3'-conserved segments in *Escherichia coli* of human and animal origin. *PLoS ONE* 5:e12754. doi: 10.1371/journal.pone.0012754

DebRoy, C., and Maddox, C. W. (2001). Identification of virulence attributes of gastrointestinal *Escherichia coli* isolates of veterinary significance. *Anim. Health Res. Rev.* 2, 129–140.

Deckert, A., Gow, S., Rosengren, L., Leger, D., Avery, B., Daignault, D., et al. (2010). Canadian integrated program for antimicrobial resistance surveillance (CIPARS) farm program: results from finisher pig surveillance. *Zoonoses Public Health* 57(Suppl. 1), 71–84. doi: 10.1111/j.1863-2378.2010.01356.x

Diarrassouba, F., Diarra, M. S., Bach, S., Delaquis, P., Pritchard, J., Topp, E., et al. (2007). Antibiotic resistance and virulence genes in commensal *Escherichia coli* and *Salmonella* isolates from commercial broiler chicken farms. *J. Food Prot.* 70, 1316–1327.

Dionisi, A. M., Lucarelli, C., Owczarek, S., Luzzi, I., and Villa, L. (2009). Characterization of the plasmid-borne quinolone resistance gene qnrB19 in *Salmonella enterica* serovar Typhimurium. *Antimicrob. Agents Chemother.* 53, 4019–4021. doi: 10.1128/AAC.00294-09

Djordjevic, S. P., Hornitzky, M. A., Bailey, G., Gill, P., Vanselow, B., Walker, K., et al. (2001). Virulence properties and serotypes of Shiga toxin-producing *Escherichia coli* from healthy Australian slaughter-age sheep. *J. Clin. Microbiol.* 39, 2017–2021. doi: 10.1128/JCM.39.5.2017-2021.2001

Djordjevic, S. P., Ramachandran, V., Bettelheim, K. A., Vanselow, B. A., Holst, P., Bailey, G., et al. (2004). Serotypes and virulence gene profiles of shiga toxin-producing *Escherichia coli* strains isolated from feces of pasture-fed and lot-fed sheep. *Appl. Environ. Microbiol.* 70, 3910–3917. doi: 10.1128/AEM.70.7.3910-3917.2004

Djordjevic, S. P., Stokes, H. W., and Roy Chowdhury, P. (2013). Mobile elements, zoonotic pathogens and commensal bacteria: conduits for the delivery of resistance genes into humans, production animals and soil microbiota. *Front. Microbiol.* 4:86. doi: 10.3389/fmicb.2013.00086

Dolejska, M., Frolkova, P., Florek, M., Jamborova, I., Purgertova, M., Kutilova, I., et al. (2011). CTX-M-15-producing *Escherichia coli* clone B2-O25b-ST131 and *Klebsiella* spp. isolates in municipal wastewater treatment plant effluents. *J. Antimicrob. Chemother.* 66, 2784–2790. doi: 10.1093/jac/dkr363

Duriez, P., and Topp, E. (2007). Temporal dynamics and impact of manure storage on antibiotic resistance patterns and population structure of *Escherichia coli* isolates from a commercial swine farm. *Appl. Environ. Microbiol.* 73, 5486–5493. doi: 10.1128/AEM.00218-07

Eisenberg, J. N., Goldstick, J., Cevallos, W., Trueba, G., Levy, K., Scott, J., et al. (2012). In-roads to the spread of antibiotic resistance: regional patterns of microbial transmission in northern coastal Ecuador. *J. R. Soc. Interface* 9, 1029–1039. doi: 10.1098/rsif.2011.0499

Endimiani, A., Rossano, A., Kunz, D., Overesch, G., and Perreten, V. (2012). First countrywide survey of third-generation cephalosporin-resistant *Escherichia coli* from broilers, swine, and cattle in Switzerland. *Diagn. Microbiol. Infect. Dis.* 73, 31–38. doi: 10.1016/j.diagmicrobio.2012.01.004

Enne, V. I., Cassar, C., Sprigings, K., Woodward, M. J., and Bennett, P. M. (2008). A high prevalence of antimicrobial resistant *Escherichia coli* isolated from pigs and a low prevalence of antimicrobial resistant *E. coli* from cattle and sheep in Great Britain at slaughter. *FEMS Microbiol. Lett.* 278, 193–199. doi: 10.1111/j.1574-6968.2007.00991.x

Enne, V. I., Livermore, D. M., Stephens, P., and Hall, L. M. (2001). Persistence of sulphonamide resistance in *Escherichia coli* in the UK despite national prescribing restriction. *Lancet* 357, 1325–1328. doi: 10.1016/S0140-6736(00)04519-0

Escudero, E., Vinue, L., Teshager, T., Torres, C., and Moreno, M. A. (2010). Resistance mechanisms and farm-level distribution of fecal *Escherichia coli* isolates resistant to extended-spectrum cephalosporins in pigs in Spain. *Res. Vet. Sci.* 88, 83–87. doi: 10.1016/j.rvsc.2009.05.021

European Medicines Agency [EMA] (2013). *Use of Colistin Products in Animals within the European Union: Development of Resistance and Possible Impact on Human and Animal Health.* London: European Medicines Agency.

Ewers, C., Bethe, A., Semmler, T., Guenther, S., and Wieler, L. H. (2012). Extended-spectrum beta-lactamase-producing and AmpC-producing *Escherichia coli* from livestock and companion animals, and their putative impact on public health: a global perspective. *Clin. Microbiol. Infect.* 18, 646–655. doi: 10.1111/j.1469-0691.2012.03850.x

Ewers, C., Bethe, A., Stamm, I., Grobbel, M., Kopp, P. A., Guerra, B., et al. (2014). CTX-M-15-D-ST648 *Escherichia coli* from companion animals and horses: another pandemic clone combining multiresistance and extraintestinal virulence? *J. Antimicrob. Chemother.* 69, 1224–1230. doi: 10.1093/jac/dkt516

Ewers, C., Guenther, S., Wieler, L. H., and Schierack, P. (2009). Mallard ducks - a waterfowl species with high risk of distributing *Escherichia coli* pathogenic for humans. *Environ. Microbiol. Rep.* 1, 510–517. doi: 10.1111/j.1758-2229.2009.00058.x

Ewers, C., Li, G., Wilking, H., Kiessling, S., Alt, K., Antao, E. M., et al. (2007). Avian pathogenic, uropathogenic, and newborn meningitis-causing *Escherichia coli*: how closely related are they? *Int. J. Med. Microbiol.* 297, 163–176. doi: 10.1016/j.ijmm.2007.01.003

Fairbrother, J. M., Lariviere, S., and Johnson, W. M. (1988). Prevalence of fimbrial antigens and enterotoxins in nonclassical serogroups of *Escherichia coli* isolated from newborn pigs with diarrhea. *Am. J. Vet. Res.* 49, 1325–1328.

Fairbrother, J. M., Nadeau, E., and Gyles, C. L. (2005). *Escherichia coli* in postweaning diarrhea in pigs: an update on bacterial types, pathogenesis, and prevention strategies. *Anim. Health Res. Rev.* 6, 17–39. doi: 10.1079/AHR2005105

Falkow, S. (1988). Molecular Koch's postulates applied to microbial pathogenicity. *Rev. Infect. Dis.* 10(Suppl. 2), S274–S276. doi: 10.1093/cid/10.Supplement_2.S274

FAO (2009). *The State of Food and Agriculture - Livestock in the Balance.* Rome: FAO.

Fekete, P. Z., Brzuszkiewicz, E., Blum-Oehler, G., Olasz, F., Szabo, M., Gottschalk, G., et al. (2012). DNA sequence analysis of the composite plasmid pTC conferring virulence and antimicrobial resistance for porcine enterotoxigenic *Escherichia coli. Int. J. Med. Microbiol.* 302, 4–9. doi: 10.1016/j.ijmm.2011.07.003

Fischer, J., Rodriguez, I., Baumann, B., Guiral, E., Beutin, L., Schroeter, A., et al. (2014). blaCTX-M-(1)(5)-carrying *Escherichia coli* and *Salmonella* isolates from livestock and food in Germany. *J. Antimicrob. Chemother.* 69, 2951–2958. doi: 10.1093/jac/dku270

Ford, P. J., and Avison, M. B. (2004). Evolutionary mapping of the SHV beta-lactamase and evidence for two separate IS26-dependent blaSHV mobilization events from the *Klebsiella pneumoniae* chromosome. *J. Antimicrob. Chemother.* 54, 69–75. doi: 10.1093/jac/dkh251

Fortini, D., Fashae, K., Garcia-Fernandez, A., Villa, L., and Carattoli, A. (2011). Plasmid-mediated quinolone resistance and beta-lactamases in *Escherichia coli* from healthy animals from Nigeria. *J. Antimicrob. Chemother.* 66, 1269–1272. doi: 10.1093/jac/dkr085

Foti, M., Rinaldo, D., Guercio, A., Giacopello, C., Aleo, A., De Leo, F., et al. (2011). Pathogenic microorganisms carried by migratory birds passing through the territory of the island of Ustica, Sicily (Italy). *Avian. Pathol.* 40, 405–409. doi: 10.1080/03079457.2011.588940

Frank, T., Gautier, V., Talarmin, A., Bercion, R., and Arlet, G. (2007). Characterization of sulphonamide resistance genes and class 1 integron gene cassettes in *Enterobacteriaceae*, Central African Republic (CAR). *J. Antimicrob. Chemother.* 59, 742–745. doi: 10.1093/jac/dkl538

Freire Martin, I., AbuOun, M., Reichel, R., La Ragione, R. M., and Woodward, M. J. (2014). Sequence analysis of a CTX-M-1 IncI1 plasmid found in *Salmonella* 4,5,12:i:-, *Escherichia coli* and *Klebsiella pneumoniae* on a UK pig farm. *J. Antimicrob. Chemother.* 69, 2098–2101. doi: 10.1093/jac/dku098

Gao, L., Hu, J., Zhang, X., Wei, L., Li, S., Miao, Z., et al. (2015). Application of swine manure on agricultural fields contributes to extended-spectrum beta-lactamase-producing *Escherichia coli* spread in Tai'an, China. *Front. Microbiol.* 6:313. doi: 10.3389/fmicb.2015.00313

Gao, P., Munir, M., and Xagoraraki, I. (2012). Correlation of tetracycline and sulfonamide antibiotics with corresponding resistance genes and resistant bacteria in a conventional municipal wastewater treatment plant. *Sci. Total Environ.* 42, 173–183. doi: 10.1016/j.scitotenv.2012.01.061

Garcia-Cobos, S., Kock, R., Mellmann, A., Frenzel, J., Friedrich, A. W., and Rossen, J. W. (2015). Molecular typing of *Enterobacteriaceae* from pig holdings in North-Western Germany reveals extended-spectrum and AmpC beta-lactamases producing but no carbapenem resistant ones. *PLoS ONE* 10:e0134533. doi: 10.1371/journal.pone.0134533

Gillings, M. R. (2014). Integrons: past, present, and future. *Microbiol. Mol. Biol. Rev.* 78, 257–277. doi: 10.1128/MMBR.00056-13

Gillings, M. R., Boucher, Y., Labbate, M., Holmes, A., Krishnan, S., Holley, M., et al. (2008). The evolution of class 1 integrons and the rise of antibiotic resistance. *J. Bacteriol.* 190, 5095–5100. doi: 10.1128/JB.00152-08

Gillings, M. R., Gaze, W. H., Pruden, A., Smalla, K., Tiedje, J. M., and Zhu, Y. G. (2015). Using the class 1 integron-integrase gene as a proxy for anthropogenic pollution. *ISME J.* 9, 1269–1279. doi: 10.1038/ismej.2014.226

Glasner, C., Albiger, B., Buist, G., Tambic Andrasevic, A., Canton, R., Carmeli, Y., et al. (2013). Carbapenemase-producing *Enterobacteriaceae* in europe: a survey among national experts from 39 countries, February 2013. *Euro. Surveill.* 18:3. doi: 10.2807/1560-7917.ES2013.18.28.20525

Goncalves, A., Torres, C., Silva, N., Carneiro, C., Radhouani, H., Coelho, C., et al. (2010). Genetic characterization of extended-spectrum beta-lactamases in *Escherichia coli* isolates of pigs from a Portuguese intensive swine farm. *Foodborne Pathog. Dis.* 7, 1569–1573. doi: 10.1089/fpd.2010.0598

Grape, M., Sundstrom, L., and Kronvall, G. (2003). Sulphonamide resistance gene sul3 found in *Escherichia coli* isolates from human sources. *J. Antimicrob. Chemother.* 52, 1022–1024. doi: 10.1093/jac/dkg473

Gullberg, E., Albrecht, L. M., Karlsson, C., Sandegren, L., and Andersson, D. I. (2014). Selection of a multidrug resistance plasmid by sublethal levels of antibiotics and heavy metals. *MBio* 5:e01918-14. doi: 10.1128/mBio.01918-14

Hall, R. M., Brown, H. J., Brookes, D. E., and Stokes, H. W. (1994). Integrons found in different locations have identical 5' ends but variable 3' ends. *J. Bacteriol.* 176, 6286–6294.

Hammerum, A. M., Larsen, J., Andersen, V. D., Lester, C. H., Skovgaard Skytte, T. S., Hansen, F., et al. (2014). Characterization of extended-spectrum beta-lactamase (ESBL)-producing *Escherichia coli* obtained from Danish pigs, pig farmers and their families from farms with high or no consumption of third- or fourth-generation cephalosporins. *J. Antimicrob. Chemother.* 69, 2650–2657. doi: 10.1093/jac/dku180

Hammerum, A. M., Sandvang, D., Andersen, S. R., Seyfarth, A. M., Porsbo, L. J., Frimodt-Moller, N., et al. (2006). Detection of sul1, sul2 and sul3 in sulphonamide resistant *Escherichia coli* isolates obtained from healthy humans, pork and pigs in Denmark. *Int. J. Food Microbiol.* 106, 235–237. doi: 10.1016/j.ijfoodmicro.2005.06.023

Han, D. U., Choi, C., Kim, J., Cho, W. S., Chung, H. K., Ha, S. K., et al. (2002). Anti-microbial susceptibility for east1 + *Escherichia coli* isolated from diarrheic pigs in Korea. *J. Vet. Med. B Infect. Dis. Vet. Public Health* 49, 346–348. doi: 10.1046/j.1439-0450.2002.00577.x

Hansen, F., Olsen, S. S., Heltberg, O., Justesen, U. S., Fuglsang-Damgaard, D., Knudsen, J. D., et al. (2014). Characterization of third-generation cephalosporin-resistant *Escherichia coli* from bloodstream infections in Denmark. *Microb. Drug Resist.* 20, 316–324. doi: 10.1089/mdr.2013.0157

Hansen, K. H., Damborg, P., Andreasen, M., Nielsen, S. S., and Guardabassi, L. (2013). Carriage and fecal counts of cefotaxime M-producing *Escherichia coli* in pigs: a longitudinal study. *Appl. Environ. Microbiol.* 79, 794–798. doi: 10.1128/AEM.02399-12

Hanson, R., Kaneene, J. B., Padungtod, P., Hirokawa, K., and Zeno, C. (2002). Prevalence of *Salmonella* and E. *coli*, and their resistance to antimicrobial agents, in farming communities in northern Thailand. *S. Asian J. Trop. Med. Public Health* 33(Suppl. 3), 120–126.

Harada, K., Asai, T., Kojima, A., Ishihara, K., and Takahashi, T. (2006). Role of coresistance in the development of resistance to chloramphenicol in *Escherichia coli* isolated from sick cattle and pigs. *Am. J. Vet. Res.* 67, 230–235. doi: 10.2460/ajvr.67.2.230

Harada, K., Asai, T., Kojima, A., Oda, C., Ishihara, K., and Takahashi, T. (2005). Antimicrobial susceptibility of pathogenic *Escherichia coli* isolated from sick cattle and pigs in Japan. *J. Vet. Med. Sci.* 67, 999–1003. doi: 10.1292/jvms.67.999

Harmer, C. J., and Hall, R. M. (2015). IS26-mediated precise excision of the IS26-aphA1a translocatable unit. *MBio* 6, e1866–e1815. doi: 10.1128/mBio.01866-15

Harmer, C. J., Moran, R. A., and Hall, R. M. (2014). Movement of IS26-associated antibiotic resistance genes occurs via a translocatable unit that includes a single IS26 and preferentially inserts adjacent to another IS26. *mBio* 5:e01801-14. doi: 10.1128/mBio.01801-14

He, S., Hickman, A. B., Varani, A. M., Siguier, P., Chandler, M., Dekker, J. P., et al. (2015). Insertion Sequence IS26 Reorganises Plasmids in Clinically Isolated Multidrug-Resistant Bacteria by Replicative Transposition. *mBio* 6:e00762. doi: 10.1128/mBio.00762-15

Heikkila, E., Sundstrom, L., and Huovinen, P. (1990). Trimethoprim resistance in *Escherichia coli* isolates from a geriatric unit. *Antimicrob. Agents Chemother.* 34, 2013–2015. doi: 10.1128/AAC.34.10.2013

Herrero-Fresno, A., Larsen, I., and Olsen, J. E. (2015). Genetic relatedness of commensal *Escherichia coli* from nursery pigs in intensive pig production in Denmark and molecular characterization of genetically different strains. *J. Appl. Microbiol.* 119, 342–353. doi: 10.1111/jam.12840

Heuer, H., Schmitt, H., and Smalla, K. (2011a). Antibiotic resistance gene spread due to manure application on agricultural fields. *Curr. Opin. Microbiol.* 14, 236–243. doi: 10.1016/j.mib.2011.04.009

Heuer, H., Solehati, Q., Zimmerling, U., Kleineidam, K., Schloter, M., Muller, T., et al. (2011b). Accumulation of sulfonamide resistance genes in arable soils due to repeated application of manure containing sulfadiazine. *Appl. Environ. Microbiol.* 77, 2527–2530. doi: 10.1128/AEM.02577-10

Heuer, H., and Smalla, K. (2007). Manure and sulfadiazine synergistically increased bacterial antibiotic resistance in soil over at least two months. *Environ. Microbiol.* 9, 657–666. doi: 10.1111/j.1462-2920.2006.01185.x

Ho, P. L., Chan, J., Lo, W. U., Law, P. Y., and Chow, K. H. (2013). Plasmid-mediated fosfomycin resistance in *Escherichia coli* isolated from pig. *Vet. Microbiol.* 162, 964–967. doi: 10.1016/j.vetmic.2012.09.023

Ho, P. L., Wong, R. C., Chow, K. H., and Que, T. L. (2009). Distribution of integron-associated trimethoprim-sulfamethoxazole resistance determinants among *Escherichia coli* from humans and food-producing animals. *Lett. Appl. Microbiol.* 49, 627–634. doi: 10.1111/j.1472-765X.2009.02717.x

Hobman, J. L., and Crossman, L. C. (2015). Bacterial antimicrobial metal ion resistance. *J. Med. Microbiol.* 64, 471–497. doi: 10.1099/jmm.0.023036-0

Hornitzky, M. A., Mercieca, K., Bettelheim, K. A., and Djordjevic, S. P. (2005). Bovine feces from animals with gastrointestinal infections are a source of serologically diverse atypical enteropathogenic *Escherichia coli* and Shiga toxin-producing *E. coli* strains that commonly possess intimin. *Appl. Environ. Microbiol.* 71, 3405-3412. doi: 10.1128/aem.71.7.3405-3412.2005

Hornitzky, M. A., Vanselow, B. A., Walker, K., Bettelheim, K. A., Corney, B., Gill, P., et al. (2002). Virulence properties and serotypes of Shiga toxin-producing *Escherichia coli* from healthy Australian cattle. *Appl. Environ. Microbiol.* 68, 6439-6445. doi: 10.1128/aem.68.12.6439-6445.2002

Hsu, S. C., Chiu, T. H., Pang, J. C., Hsuan-Yuan, C. H., Chang, G. N., and Tsen, H. Y. (2006). Characterisation of antimicrobial resistance patterns and class 1 integrons among *Escherichia coli* and *Salmonella enterica* serovar *Choleraesuis* strains isolated from humans and swine in Taiwan. *Int. J. Antimicrob. Agents* 27, 383-391. doi: 10.1016/j.ijantimicag.2005.11.020

Huang, S. Y., Zhu, X. Q., Wang, Y., Liu, H. B., Dai, L., He, J. K., et al. (2012). Co-carriage of qnrS1, floR, and bla(CTX-M-14) on a multidrug-resistant plasmid in *Escherichia coli* isolated from pigs. *Foodborne Pathog. Dis.* 9, 896-901. doi: 10.1089/fpd.2012.1131

Hvistendahl, M. (2012). Public health. China takes aim at rampant antibiotic resistance. *Science* 336:795. doi: 10.1126/science.336.6083.795

Institute of Medicine; National Research Council; Panel on Animal Health (1999). *The Use of Drugs in Food Animals: Benefits and Risks.* Washington, DC: National Academy Press.

Jackson, G. (1981). A survey of antibiotic resistance of *Escherichia coli* isolated from farm animals in Great Britain from 1971 to 1977. *Vet. Rec.* 108, 325-328. doi: 10.1136/vr.108.15.325

Jakobsen, L., Garneau, P., Kurbasic, A., Bruant, G., Stegger, M., Harel, J., et al. (2011). Microarray-based detection of extended virulence and antimicrobial resistance gene profiles in phylogroup B2 *Escherichia coli* of human, meat and animal origin. *J. Med. Microbiol.* 60, 1502-1511. doi: 10.1099/jmm.0.033993-0

Jakobsen, L., Kurbasic, A., Skjot-Rasmussen, L., Ejrnaes, K., Porsbo, L. J., Pedersen, K., et al. (2010a). *Escherichia coli* isolates from broiler chicken meat, broiler chickens, pork, and pigs share phylogroups and antimicrobial resistance with community-dwelling humans and patients with urinary tract infection. *Foodborne Pathog. Dis.* 7, 537-547. doi: 10.1089/fpd.2009.0409

Jakobsen, L., Spangholm, D. J., Pedersen, K., Jensen, L. B., Emborg, H. D., Agerso, Y., et al. (2010b). Broiler chickens, broiler chicken meat, pigs and pork as sources of ExPEC related virulence genes and resistance in *Escherichia coli* isolates from community-dwelling humans and UTI patients. *Int. J. Food Microbiol.* 142, 264-272. doi: 10.1016/j.ijfoodmicro.2010.06.025

Jamborova, I., Dolejska, M., Vojtech, J., Guenther, S., Uricariu, R., Drozdowska, J., et al. (2015). Plasmid-mediated resistance to cephalosporins and fluoroquinolones in various *Escherichia coli* sequence types isolated from rooks wintering in Europe. *Appl. Environ. Microbiol.* 81, 648-657. doi: 10.1128/AEM.02459-14

Jensen, V. F., Jakobsen, L., Emborg, H. D., Seyfarth, A. M., and Hammerum, A. M. (2006). Correlation between apramycin and gentamicin use in pigs and an increasing reservoir of gentamicin-resistant *Escherichia coli*. *J. Antimicrob. Chemother.* 58, 101-107. doi: 10.1093/jac/dkl201

Jobbins, S. E., and Alexander, K. A. (2015). From whence they came - antibiotic-resistant *Escherischia coli* in African wildlife. *J. Wildl. Dis.* 51, 811-820. doi: 10.7589/2014-11-257

Johnson, J. R., Delavari, P., Kuskowski, M., and Stell, A. L. (2001). Phylogenetic distribution of extraintestinal virulence-associated traits in *Escherichia coli*. *J. Infect. Dis.* 183, 78-88. doi: 10.1086/317656

Johnson, J. R., Kuskowski, M. A., Smith, K., O'Bryan, T. T., and Tatini, S. (2005a). Antimicrobial-resistant and extraintestinal pathogenic *Escherichia coli* in retail foods. *J. Infect. Dis.* 191, 1040-1049. doi: 10.1086/428451

Johnson, J. R., Murray, A. C., Kuskowski, M. A., Schubert, S., Prere, M. F., Picard, B., et al. (2005b). Distribution and characteristics of *Escherichia coli* clonal group A. *Emerg. Infect. Dis.* 11, 141-145. doi: 10.3201/eid1101.040418

Johnson, T. J., Shepard, S. M., Rivet, B., Danzeisen, J. L., and Carattoli, A. (2011). Comparative genomics and phylogeny of the IncI1 plasmids: a common plasmid type among porcine enterotoxigenic *Escherichia coli*. *Plasmid* 66, 144-151. doi: 10.1016/j.plasmid.2011.07.003

Jones-Dias, D., Manageiro, V., Francisco, A. P., Martins, A. P., Domingues, G., Louro, D., et al. (2013). Assessing the molecular basis of transferable quinolone resistance in *Escherichia coli* and *Salmonella* spp. from food-producing animals and food products. *Vet. Microbiol.* 167, 523-531. doi: 10.1016/j.vetmic.2013.08.010

Jordan, D., Chin, J. J., Fahy, V. A., Barton, M. D., Smith, M. G., and Trott, D. J. (2009). Antimicrobial use in the Australian pig industry: results of a national survey. *Aust. Vet. J.* 87, 222-229. doi: 10.1111/j.1751-0813.2009.00430.x

Ju, F., Li, B., Ma, L., Wang, Y., Huang, D., and Zhang, T. (2015). Antibiotic resistance genes and human bacterial pathogens: co-occurrence, removal, and enrichment in municipal sewage sludge digesters. *Water Res.* 91, 1-10. doi: 10.1016/j.watres.2015.11.071

Ju, W., Shen, J., Li, Y., Toro, M. A., Zhao, S., Ayers, S., et al. (2012). Non-O157 Shiga toxin-producing *Escherichia coli* in retail ground beef and pork in the Washington D.C. *area*. *Food Microbiol.* 32, 371-377. doi: 10.1016/j.fm.2012.07.017

Kadlec, K., and Schwarz, S. (2008). Analysis and distribution of class 1 and class 2 integrons and associated gene cassettes among *Escherichia coli* isolates from swine, horses, cats and dogs collected in the BfT-GermVet monitoring study. *J. Antimicrob. Chemother.* 62, 469-473. doi: 10.1093/jac/dkn233

Kang, S. G., Lee, D. Y., Shin, S. J., Ahn, J. M., and Yoo, H. S. (2005). Changes in patterns of antimicrobial susceptibility and class 1 integron carriage among *Escherichia coli* isolates. *J. Vet. Sci.* 6, 201-205.

Kaper, J. B., Nataro, J. P., and Mobley, H. L. (2004). Pathogenic *Escherichia coli*. *Nat. Rev. Microbiol.* 2, 123-140. doi: 10.1038/nrmicro818

Katakweba, A. A., Moller, K. S., Muumba, J., Muhairwa, A. P., Damborg, P., Rosenkrantz, J. T., et al. (2015). Antimicrobial resistance in faecal samples from buffalo, wildebeest and zebra grazing together with and without cattle in Tanzania. *J. Appl. Microbiol.* 118, 966-975. doi: 10.1111/jam.12738

Katsunuma, Y., Hanazumi, M., Fujisaki, H., Minato, H., Kataoka, Y., Sawada, T., et al. (2008). Comparison of pulsed-field gel electrophoresis patterns of antimicrobial-resistant *Escherichia coli* and enterococci isolates from the feces of livestock and livestock farmers in Japan. *J. Gen. Appl. Microbiol.* 54, 39-50. doi: 10.2323/jgam.54.39

Kijima-Tanaka, M., Ishihara, K., Kojima, A., Morioka, A., Nagata, R., Kawanishi, M., et al. (2005). A national surveillance of Shiga toxin-producing *Escherichia coli* in food-producing animals in Japan. *J. Vet. Med. B Infect. Dis. Vet. Public Health* 52, 230-237. doi: 10.1111/j.1439-0450.2005.00852.x

Kijima-Tanaka, M., Ishihara, K., Morioka, A., Kojima, A., Ohzono, T., Ogikubo, K., et al. (2003). A national surveillance of antimicrobial resistance in *Escherichia coli* isolated from food-producing animals in Japan. *J. Antimicrob. Chemother.* 51, 447-451. doi: 10.1093/jac/dkg014

Kim, S., and Woo, G. J. (2014). Prevalence and characterization of antimicrobial-resistant *Escherichia coli* isolated from conventional and organic vegetables. *Foodborne Pathog. Dis.* 11, 815-821. doi: 10.1089/fpd.2014.1771

Koh, S. Y., George, S., Brozel, V., Moxley, R., Francis, D., and Kaushik, R. S. (2008). Porcine intestinal epithelial cell lines as a new in vitro model for studying adherence and pathogenesis of enterotoxigenic *Escherichia coli*. *Vet. Microbiol.* 130, 191-197. doi: 10.1016/j.vetmic.2007.12.018

Kojima, A., Asai, T., Ishihara, K., Morioka, A., Akimoto, K., Sugimoto, Y., et al. (2009). National monitoring for antimicrobial resistance among indicator bacteria isolated from food-producing animals in Japan. *J. Vet. Med. Sci.* 71, 1301-1308. doi: 10.1292/jvms.001301

Kozak, G. K., Boerlin, P., Janecko, N., Reid-Smith, R. J., and Jardine, C. (2009a). Antimicrobial resistance in *Escherichia coli* isolates from swine and wild small mammals in the proximity of swine farms and in natural environments in Ontario, Canada. *Appl. Environ. Microbiol.* 75, 559-566. doi: 10.1128/AEM.01821-08

Kozak, G. K., Pearl, D. L., Parkman, J., Reid-Smith, R. J., Deckert, A., and Boerlin, P. (2009b). Distribution of sulfonamide resistance genes in *Escherichia coli* and *Salmonella* isolates from swine and chickens at abattoirs in Ontario and Quebec, Canada. *Appl. Environ. Microbiol.* 75, 5999-6001. doi: 10.1128/AEM.02844-08

Krishnasamy, V., Otte, J., and Silbergeld, E. (2015). Antimicrobial use in Chinese swine and broiler poultry production. *Antimicrob. Resist. Infect. Control* 4:17. doi: 10.1186/s13756-015-0050-y

Kristiansson, E., Fick, J., Janzon, A., Grabic, R., Rutgersson, C., Weijdegard, B., et al. (2011). Pyrosequencing of antibiotic-contaminated river sediments reveals high levels of resistance and gene transfer elements. *PLoS ONE* 6:e17038. doi: 10.1371/journal.pone.0017038

Kumai, Y., Suzuki, Y., Tanaka, Y., Shima, K., Bhadra, R. K., Yamasaki, S., et al. (2005). Characterization of multidrug-resistance phenotypes and genotypes of *Escherichia coli* strains isolated from swine from an abattoir in Osaka, Japan. *Epidemiol. Infect.* 133, 59-70. doi: 10.1017/S0950268804003280

Labar, A. S., Millman, J. S., Ruebush, E., Opintan, J. A., Bishar, R. A., Aboderin, A. O., et al. (2012). Regional dissemination of a trimethoprim-resistance gene cassette via a successful transposable element. *PLoS ONE* 7:e38142. doi: 10.1371/journal.pone.0038142

Landers, T. F., Cohen, B., Wittum, T. E., and Larson, E. L. (2012). A review of antibiotic use in food animals: perspective, policy, and potential. *Public Health Rep.* 127, 4–22.

Lanz, R., Kuhnert, P., and Boerlin, P. (2003). Antimicrobial resistance and resistance gene determinants in clinical *Escherichia coli* from different animal species in Switzerland. *Vet. Microbiol.* 91, 73–84. doi: 10.1016/S0378-1135(02)00263-8

LaPara, T. M., Burch, T. R., McNamara, P. J., Tan, D. T., Yan, M., and Eichmiller, J. J. (2011). Tertiary-treated municipal wastewater is a significant point source of antibiotic resistance genes into Duluth-Superior Harbor. *Environ. Sci. Technol.* 45, 9543–9549. doi: 10.1021/es202775r

Lay, K. K., Koowattananukul, C., Chansong, N., and Chuanchuen, R. (2012). Antimicrobial resistance, virulence, and phylogenetic characteristics of *Escherichia coli* isolates from clinically healthy swine. *Foodborne Pathog. Dis.* 9, 992–1001. doi: 10.1089/fpd.2012.1175

Le, Q. P., Ueda, S., Nguyen, T. N., Dao, T. V., Van Hoang, T. A., Tran, T. T., et al. (2015). Characteristics of extended-spectrum beta-lactamase-producing *Escherichia coli* in retail meats and shrimp at a local market in Vietnam. *Foodborne Pathog. Dis.* 12, 719–725. doi: 10.1089/fpd.2015.1954

Lee, M., Shin, E., and Lee, Y. (2014). Antimicrobial resistance and integron profiles in multidrug-resistant *Escherichia coli* isolates from pigs. *Foodborne Pathog. Dis.* 11, 988–997. doi: 10.1089/fpd.2014.1795

Le-Minh, N., Khan, S. J., Drewes, J. E., and Stuetz, R. M. (2010). Fate of antibiotics during municipal water recycling treatment processes. *Water Res.* 44, 4295–4323. doi: 10.1016/j.watres.2010.06.020

Leverstein-van Hall, M. A., He, M. B., Ar, T. D., Paauw, A., Fluit, A. C., and Verhoef, J. (2003). Multidrug resistance among *Enterobacteriaceae* is strongly associated with the presence of integrons and is independent of species or isolate origin. *J. Infect. Dis.* 187, 251–259. doi: 10.1086/345880

Levings, R. S., Djordjevic, S. P., and Hall, R. M. (2008). SGI2, a relative of *Salmonella* genomic island SGI1 with an independent origin. *Antimicrob. Agents Chemother.* 52, 2529–2537. doi: 10.1128/AAC.00189-08

Levings, R. S., Lightfoot, D., Partridge, S. R., Hall, R. M., and Djordjevic, S. P. (2005). The genomic island SGI1, containing the multiple antibiotic resistance region of *Salmonella enterica* serovar Typhimurium DT104 or variants of it, is widely distributed in other *S. enterica* serovars. *J. Bacteriol.* 187, 4401–4409. doi: 10.1128/jb.187.13.4401-4409.2005

Levy, S. B. (1992). *The Antibiotic Paradox: How Miracle Drugs Are Destroying the Miracle.* New York, NY: Plenum.

Li, Y. X., Xiong, X., Lin, C. Y., Zhang, F. S., Wei, L., and Wei, H. (2010). Cadmium in animal production and its potential hazard on Beijing and Fuxin farmlands. *J. Hazard. Mater.* 177, 475–480. doi: 10.1016/j.jhazmat.2009.12.057

Liao, X. P., Xia, J., Yang, L., Li, L., Sun, J., Liu, Y. H., et al. (2015). Characterization of CTX-M-14-producing *Escherichia coli* from food-producing animals. *Front. Microbiol.* 6:1136. doi: 10.3389/fmicb.2015.01136

Liebert, C. A., Hall, R. M., and Summers, A. O. (1999). Transposon Tn21, flagship of the floating genome. *Microbiol. Mol. Biol. Rev.* 63, 507–522.

Lim, S. K., Lee, H. S., Nam, H. M., Cho, Y. S., Kim, J. M., Song, S. W., et al. (2007). Antimicrobial resistance observed in *Escherichia coli* strains isolated from fecal samples of cattle and pigs in Korea during 2003-2004. *Int. J. Food Microbiol.* 116, 283–286. doi: 10.1016/j.ijfoodmicro.2006.12.014

Lim, S. K., Lee, H. S., Nam, H. M., Jung, S. C., and Bae, Y. C. (2009). CTX-M-type beta-lactamase in *Escherichia coli* isolated from sick animals in Korea. *Microb. Drug Resist.* 15, 139–142. doi: 10.1089/mdr.2009.0901

Lindsey, R. L., Frye, J. G., Thitaram, S. N., Meinersmann, R. J., Fedorka-Cray, P. J., and Englen, M. D. (2011). Characterization of multidrug-resistant *Escherichia coli* by antimicrobial resistance profiles, plasmid replicon typing, and pulsed-field gel electrophoresis. *Microb. Drug Resist.* 17, 157–163. doi: 10.1089/mdr.2010.0148

Liu, B. T., Yang, Q. E., Li, L., Sun, J., Liao, X. P., Fang, L. X., et al. (2013). Dissemination and characterization of plasmids carrying oqxAB-bla CTX-M genes in *Escherichia coli* isolates from food-producing animals. *PLoS ONE* 8:e73947. doi: 10.1371/journal.pone.0073947

Liu, C., Zheng, H., Yang, M., Xu, Z., Wang, X., Wei, L., et al. (2015). Genome analysis and in vivo virulence of porcine extraintestinal pathogenic *Escherichia coli* strain PCN033. *BMC Genomics* 16:717. doi: 10.1186/s12864-015-1890-9

Liu, Y.-Y., Wang, Y., Walsh, T. R., Yi, L.-X., Zhang, R., Spencer, J., et al. (2016). Emergence of plasmid-mediated colistin resistance mechanism MCR-1 in animals and human beings in China: a microbiological and molecular biological study. *Lancet Infect. Dis.* 16, 161–168. doi: 10.1016/S1473-3099(15)00424-7

Loman, N. J., and Pallen, M. J. (2015). Twenty years of bacterial genome sequencing. *Nat. Rev. Microbiol.* 13, 787–794. doi: 10.1038/nrmicro3565

Lu, Z., Lapen, D., Scott, A., Dang, A., and Topp, E. (2005). Identifying host sources of fecal pollution: diversity of *Escherichia coli* in confined dairy and swine production systems. *Appl. Environ. Microbiol.* 71, 5992–5998. doi: 10.1128/aem.71.10.5992-5998.2005

Luppi, A., Bonilauri, P., Dottori, M., Gherpelli, Y., Biasi, G., Merialdi, G., et al. (2015). Antimicrobial resistance of F4+ *Escherichia coli* isolated from Swine in Italy. *Transbound. Emerg. Dis.* 62, 67–71. doi: 10.1111/tbed.12081

Ma, J., Zeng, Z., Chen, Z., Xu, X., Wang, X., Deng, Y., et al. (2009). High prevalence of plasmid-mediated quinolone resistance determinants qnr, aac(6')-Ib-cr, and qepA among ceftiofur-resistant *Enterobacteriaceae* isolates from companion and food-producing animals. *Antimicrob. Agents Chemother.* 53, 519–524. doi: 10.1128/AAC.00886-08

Ma, L., Zhang, X. X., Zhao, F., Wu, B., Cheng, S., and Yang, L. (2013). Sewage treatment plant serves as a hot-spot reservoir of integrons and gene cassettes. *J. Environ. Biol.* 34, 391–399.

Machado, E., Coque, T. M., Canton, R., Sousa, J. C., and Peixe, L. (2008). Antibiotic resistance integrons and extended-spectrum {beta}-lactamases among *Enterobacteriaceae* isolates recovered from chickens and swine in Portugal. *J. Antimicrob. Chemother.* 62, 296–302. doi: 10.1093/jac/dkn179

Makita, K., Goto, M., Ozawa, M., Kawanishi, M., Koike, R., Asai, T., et al. (2016). Multivariable analysis of the association between antimicrobial use and antimicrobial resistance in *Escherichia coli* isolated from apparently healthy pigs in Japan. *Microb. Drug Resist.* 22, 28–39. doi: 10.1089/mdr.2014.0311

Manges, A. R., and Johnson, J. R. (2015). Reservoirs of extraintestinal pathogenic *Escherichia coli*. *Microbiol. Spectr.* 3. doi: 10.1128/microbiolspec.UTI-0006-2012

Manges, A. R., Smith, S. P., Lau, B. J., Nuval, C. J., Eisenberg, J. N., Dietrich, P. S., et al. (2007). Retail meat consumption and the acquisition of antimicrobial resistant *Escherichia coli* causing urinary tract infections: a case-control study. *Foodborne Pathog. Dis.* 4, 419–431. doi: 10.1089/fpd.2007.0026

Mao, D., Yu, S., Rysz, M., Luo, Y., Yang, F., Li, F., et al. (2015). Prevalence and proliferation of antibiotic resistance genes in two municipal wastewater treatment plants. *Water Res.* 85, 458–466. doi: 10.1016/j.watres.2015.09.010

Marchant, M., and Moreno, M. A. (2013). Dynamics and diversity of *Escherichia coli* in animals and system management of the manure on a commercial farrow-to-finish pig farm. *Appl. Environ. Microbiol.* 79, 853–859. doi: 10.1128/AEM.02866-12

Marchant, M., Vinue, L., Torres, C., and Moreno, M. A. (2013). Change of integrons over time in *Escherichia coli* isolates recovered from healthy pigs and chickens. *Vet. Microbiol.* 163, 124–132. doi: 10.1016/j.vetmic.2012.12.011

Mariani-Kurkdjian, P., Lemaitre, C., Bidet, P., Perez, D., Boggini, L., Kwon, T., et al. (2014). Haemolytic-uraemic syndrome with bacteraemia caused by a new hybrid *Escherichia coli* pathotype. *New Microbes New Infect* 2, 127–131. doi: 10.1002/nmi2.49

Martinez, J. L. (2008). Antibiotics and antibiotic resistance genes in natural environments. *Science* 321, 365–367. doi: 10.1126/science.1159483

Mathew, A. G., Liamthong, S., Lin, J., and Hong, Y. (2009). Evidence of class 1 integron transfer between *Escherichia coli* and *Salmonella* spp. on livestock farms. *Foodborne Pathog. Dis.* 6, 959–964. doi: 10.1089/fpd.2009.0263

Mattiello, S. P., Drescher, G., Barth, V. C. Jr., Ferreira, C. A., and Oliveira, S. D. (2015). Characterization of antimicrobial resistance in *Salmonella enterica* strains isolated from Brazilian poultry production. *Antonie Van Leeuwenhoek* 108, 1227–1238. doi: 10.1007/s10482-015-0577-1

Maynard, C., Fairbrother, J. M., Bekal, S., Sanschagrin, F., Levesque, R. C., Brousseau, R., et al. (2003). Antimicrobial resistance genes in enterotoxigenic *Escherichia coli* O149:K91 isolates obtained over a 23-year period from pigs. *Antimicrob. Agents Chemother.* 47, 3214–3221. doi: 10.1128/AAC.47.10.3214-3221.2003

Mayrhofer, S., Paulsen, P., Smulders, F. J., and Hilbert, F. (2004). Antimicrobial resistance profile of five major food-borne pathogens isolated from beef, pork and poultry. *Int. J. Food Microbiol.* 97, 23–29. doi: 10.1016/j.ijfoodmicro.2004.04.006

Mayrhofer, S., Paulsen, P., Smulders, F. J., and Hilbert, F. (2006). Antimicrobial resistance in commensal *Escherichia coli* isolated from muscle foods as related to the veterinary use of antimicrobial agents in food-producing animals in Austria. *Microb. Drug Resist.* 12, 278–283. doi: 10.1089/mdr.2006.12.278

McEwen, S. A., and Fedorka-Cray, P. J. (2002). Antimicrobial use and resistance in animals. *Clin. Infect. Dis.* 34(Suppl. 3), S93–S106. doi: 10.1086/340246

Meng, Q., Bai, X., Zhao, A., Lan, R., Du, H., Wang, T., et al. (2014). Characterization of Shiga toxin-producing *Escherichia coli* isolated from healthy pigs in China. *BMC Microbiol.* 14:5. doi: 10.1186/1471-2180-14-5

Middleton, J. H., and Ambrose, A. (2005). Enumeration and antibiotic resistance patterns of fecal indicator organisms isolated from migratory Canada geese (*Branta canadensis*). *J. Wildl. Dis.* 41, 334–341. doi: 10.7589/0090-3558-41.2.334

Morales, A. S., Fragoso de Araujo, J., de Moura Gomes, V. T., Reis Costa, A. T., dos Prazeres Rodrigues, D., Porfida Ferreira, T. S., et al. (2012). Colistin resistance in *Escherichia coli* and *Salmonella enterica* strains isolated from swine in Brazil. *Sci. World J.* 2012:109795. doi: 10.1100/2012/109795

Moran, R. A., Holt, K. E., and Hall, R. M. (2016). pCERC3 from a commensal ST95 *Escherichia coli*: a ColV virulence-multiresistance plasmid carrying a sul3-associated class 1 integron. *Plasmid* 84–84, 11–19. doi: 10.1016/j.plasmid.2016.02.002

Moredo, F. A., Pineyro, P. E., Marquez, G. C., Sanz, M., Colello, R., Etcheverria, A., et al. (2015). Enterotoxigenic *Escherichia coli* subclinical infection in pigs: bacteriological and genotypic characterization and antimicrobial resistance profiles. *Foodborne Pathog. Dis.* 12, 704–711. doi: 10.1089/fpd.2015.1959

Moredo, F. A., Vigo, G. B., Cappuccio, J. A., Pineyro, P., Perfumo, C. J., and Giacoboni, G. I. (2007). Antimicrobial resistance of *Escherichia coli* isolated from pigs in Argentina. *Rev. Argent Microbiol.* 39, 227–229.

Murugan, K., Prabhakaran, P., Al-Sohaibani, S., and Sekar, K. (2012). Identification of source of faecal pollution of Tirumanimuttar River, Tamilnadu, India using microbial source tracking. *Environ. Monit. Assess.* 184, 6001–6012. doi: 10.1007/s10661-011-2398-7

Nagy, B., and Fekete, P. Z. (1999). Enterotoxigenic *Escherichia coli* (ETEC) in farm animals. *Vet. Res.* 30, 259–284.

Nataro, J. P., and Kaper, J. B. (1998). Diarrheagenic *Escherichia coli*. *Clin. Microbiol. Rev.* 11, 142–201.

Nation, R. L., and Li, J. (2009). Colistin in the 21st century. *Curr. Opin. Infect. Dis.* 22, 535–543. doi: 10.1097/QCO.0b013e328332e672

Noamani, B. N., Fairbrother, J. M., and Gyles, C. L. (2003). Virulence genes of O149 enterotoxigenic *Escherichia coli* from outbreaks of postweaning diarrhea in pigs. *Vet. Microbiol.* 97, 87–101. doi: 10.1016/j.vetmic.2003.08.006

Nordstrom, L., Liu, C. M., and Price, L. B. (2013). Foodborne urinary tract infections: a new paradigm for antimicrobial-resistant foodborne illness. *Front. Microbiol.* 4:29. doi: 10.3389/fmicb.2013.00029

Nozarian, Z., and Abdollahi, A. (2015). Microbial etiology and antimicrobial susceptibility of bacteria implicated in urinary tract infection in Tehran, Iran. *Iran J. Pathol.* 10, 54–60.

Ojer-Usoz, E., Gonzalez, D., Vitas, A. I., Leiva, J., Garcia-Jalon, I., Febles-Casquero, A., et al. (2013). Prevalence of extended-spectrum beta-lactamase-producing *Enterobacteriaceae* in meat products sold in Navarra, Spain. *Meat Sci.* 93, 316–321. doi: 10.1016/j.meatsci.2012.09.009

Ojo, O. E., Ajuwape, A. T., Otesile, E. B., Owoade, A. A., Oyekunle, M. A., and Adetosoye, A. I. (2010). Potentially zoonotic shiga toxin-producing *Escherichia coli* serogroups in the faeces and meat of food-producing animals in Ibadan, Nigeria. *Int. J. Food Microbiol.* 142, 214–221. doi: 10.1016/j.ijfoodmicro.2010.06.030

Olesen, I., Hasman, H., and Aarestrup, F. M. (2004). Prevalence of beta-lactamases among ampicillin-resistant *Escherichia coli* and *Salmonella* isolated from food animals in Denmark. *Microb. Drug Resist.* 10, 334–340. doi: 10.1089/mdr.2004.10.334

Onken, A., Said, A. K., Jorstad, M., Jenum, P. A., and Blomberg, B. (2015). Prevalence and antimicrobial resistance of microbes causing bloodstream infections in Unguja, Zanzibar. *PLoS ONE* 10:e0145632. doi: 10.1371/journal.pone.0145632

Osborn, A. M., Bruce, K. D., Strike, P., and Ritchie, D. A. (1997). Distribution, diversity and evolution of the bacterial mercury resistance (mer) operon. *FEMS Microbiol. Rev.* 19, 239–262. doi: 10.1111/j.1574-6976.1997.tb00300.x

Pal, C., Bengtsson-Palme, J., Kristiansson, E., and Larsson, D. G. (2015). Co-occurrence of resistance genes to antibiotics, biocides and metals reveals novel insights into their co-selection potential. *BMC Genomics* 16:964. doi: 10.1186/s12864-015-2153-5

Pallen, M. J., and Wren, B. W. (2007). Bacterial pathogenomics. *Nature* 449, 835–842. doi: 10.1038/nature06248

Pan, J. C., Ye, R., Meng, D. M., Zhang, W., Wang, H. Q., and Liu, K. Z. (2006). Molecular characteristics of class 1 and class 2 integrons and their relationships to antibiotic resistance in clinical isolates of *Shigella sonnei* and *Shigella flexneri*. *J. Antimicrob. Chemother.* 58, 288–296. doi: 10.1093/jac/dkl228

Pan, X., Qiang, Z., Ben, W., and Chen, M. (2011). Residual veterinary antibiotics in swine manure from concentrated animal feeding operations in Shandong Province, China. *Chemosphere* 84, 695–700. doi: 10.1016/j.chemosphere.2011.03.022

Paniagua-Contreras, G. L., Monroy-Perez, E., Rodriguez-Moctezuma, J. R., Dominguez-Trejo, P., Vaca-Paniagua, F., and Vaca, S. (2015). Virulence factors, antibiotic resistance phenotypes and O-serogroups of *Escherichia coli* strains isolated from community-acquired urinary tract infection patients in Mexico. *J. Microbiol. Immunol. Infect.* doi: 10.1016/j.jmii.2015.08.005 [Epub ahead of print].

Pantozzi, F. L., Moredo, F. A., Vigo, G. B., and Giacoboni, G. I. (2010). Antimicrobial resistance in indicator and zoonotic bacteria isolated from domestic animals in Argentina. *Rev. Argent Microbiol.* 42, 49–52. doi: 10.1590/s0325-75412010000100011

Pardon, B., Catry, B., Dewulf, J., Persoons, D., Hostens, M., De Bleecker, K., et al. (2012). Prospective study on quantitative and qualitative antimicrobial and anti-inflammatory drug use in white veal calves. *J. Antimicrob. Chemother.* 67, 1027–1038. doi: 10.1093/jac/dkr570

Partridge, S. R., Brown, H. J., Stokes, H. W., and Hall, R. M. (2001). Transposons Tn1696 and Tn21 and their integrons In4 and In2 have independent origins. *Antimicrob. Agents Chemother.* 45, 1263–1270. doi: 10.1128/aac.45.4.1263-1270.2001

Partridge, S. R., Tsafnat, G., Coiera, E., and Iredell, J. R. (2009). Gene cassettes and cassette arrays in mobile resistance integrons. *FEMS Microbiol. Rev.* 33, 757–784. doi: 10.1111/j.1574-6976.2009.00175.x

Perreten, V., and Boerlin, P. (2003). A new sulfonamide resistance gene (sul3) in *Escherichia coli* is widespread in the pig population of Switzerland. *Antimicrob. Agents Chemother.* 47, 1169–1172. doi: 10.1128/AAC.47.3.1169-1172.2003

Petternel, C., Galler, H., Zarfel, G., Luxner, J., Haas, D., Grisold, A. J., et al. (2014). Isolation and characterization of multidrug-resistant bacteria from minced meat in Austria. *Food Microbiol.* 44, 41–46. doi: 10.1016/j.fm.2014.04.013

Phongpaichit, S., Liamthong, S., Mathew, A. G., and Chethanond, U. (2007). Prevalence of class 1 integrons in commensal *Escherichia coli* from pigs and pig farmers in Thailand. *J. Food Prot.* 70, 292–299.

Poolman, J. T., and Wacker, M. (2016). Extraintestinal pathogenic *Escherichia coli*, a common human pathogen: challenges for vaccine development and progress in the field. *J. Infect. Dis.* 213, 6–13. doi: 10.1093/infdis/jiv429

Povilonis, J., Seputiene, V., Ruzauskas, M., Siugzdiniene, R., Virgailis, M., Pavilonis, A., et al. (2010). Transferable class 1 and 2 integrons in *Escherichia coli* and *Salmonella enterica* isolates of human and animal origin in Lithuania. *Foodborne Pathog. Dis.* 7, 1185–1192. doi: 10.1089/fpd.2010.0536

Pulcini, C., and Gyssens, I. C. (2013). How to educate prescribers in antimicrobial stewardship practices. *Virulence* 4, 192–202. doi: 10.4161/viru.23706

Qiao, M., Chen, W., Su, J., Zhang, B., and Zhang, C. (2012). Fate of tetracyclines in swine manure of three selected swine farms in China. *J. Environ. Sci. (China)* 24, 1047–1052. doi: 10.1016/S1001-0742(11)60890-5

Quesada, A., Porrero, M. C., Tellez, S., Palomo, G., Garcia, M., and Dominguez, L. (2015). Polymorphism of genes encoding PmrAB in colistin-resistant strains of *Escherichia coli* and *Salmonella enterica* isolated from poultry and swine. *J. Antimicrob. Chemother.* 70, 71–74. doi: 10.1093/jac/dku320

Rajic, A., Reid-Smith, R., Deckert, A. E., Dewey, C. E., and McEwen, S. A. (2006). Reported antibiotic use in 90 swine farms in Alberta. *Can. Vet. J.* 47, 446–452.

Rajkhowa, S., and Sarma, D. K. (2014). Prevalence and antimicrobial resistance of porcine O157 and non-O157 Shiga toxin-producing *Escherichia coli* from

India. *Trop. Anim. Health Prod.* 46, 931–937. doi: 10.1007/s11250-014-0587-4

Ramachandran, V., Hornitzky, M. A., Bettelheim, K. A., Walker, M. J., and Djordjevic, S. P. (2001). The common ovine Shiga toxin 2-containing *Escherichia coli* serotypes and human isolates of the same serotypes possess a Stx2d toxin type. *J. Clin. Microbiol.* 39, 1932–1937. doi: 10.1128/JCM.39.5.1932-1937.2001

Ramos, S., Silva, N., Dias, D., Sousa, M., Capelo-Martinez, J. L., Brito, F., et al. (2013). Clonal diversity of ESBL-producing *Escherichia coli* in pigs at slaughter level in Portugal. *Foodborne Pathog. Dis.* 10, 74–79. doi: 10.1089/fpd.2012.1173

Randall, L. P., Lemma, F., Rogers, J. P., Cheney, T. E., Powell, L. F., and Teale, C. J. (2014). Prevalence of extended-spectrum-beta-lactamase-producing *Escherichia coli* from pigs at slaughter in the UK in 2013. *J. Antimicrob. Chemother.* 69, 2947–2950. doi: 10.1093/jac/dku258

Rayamajhi, N., Kang, S. G., Lee, D. Y., Kang, M. L., Lee, S. I., Park, K. Y., et al. (2008). Characterization of TEM-, SHV- and AmpC-type beta-lactamases from cephalosporin-resistant *Enterobacteriaceae* isolated from swine. *Int. J. Food Microbiol.* 124, 183–187. doi: 10.1016/j.ijfoodmicro.2008.03.009

Reid, C. J., Roy Chowdhury, P., and Djordjevic, S. P. (2015). Tn6026 and Tn6029 are found in complex resistance regions mobilised by diverse plasmids and chromosomal islands in multiple antibiotic resistant *Enterobacteriaceae. Plasmid* 80, 127–137. doi: 10.1016/j.plasmid.2015.04.005

Rodrigues, C., Machado, E., Peixe, L., and Novais, A. (2013). IncI1/ST3 and IncN/ST1 plasmids drive the spread of blaTEM-52 and blaCTX-M-1/-32 in diverse *Escherichia coli* clones from different piggeries. *J. Antimicrob. Chemother.* 68, 2245–2248. doi: 10.1093/jac/dkt187

Rodriguez-Siek, K. E., Giddings, C. W., Doetkott, C., Johnson, T. J., Fakhr, M. K., and Nolan, L. K. (2005). Comparison of *Escherichia coli* isolates implicated in human urinary tract infection and avian colibacillosis. *Microbiology* 151, 2097–2110. doi: 10.1099/mic.0.27499-0

Roschanski, N., Friese, A., von Salviati-Claudius, C., Hering, J., Kaesbohrer, A., Kreienbrock, L., et al. (2015). Prevalence of carbapenemase producing *Enterobacteriaceae* isolated from German pig-fattening farms during the years 2011 2013. *Vet. Microbiol.* doi: 10.1016/j.vetmic.2015.11.030 [Epub ahead of print].

Rosengren, L. B., Waldner, C. L., and Reid-Smith, R. J. (2009). Associations between antimicrobial resistance phenotypes, antimicrobial resistance genes, and virulence genes of fecal *Escherichia coli* isolates from healthy grow-finish pigs. *Appl. Environ. Microbiol.* 75, 1373–1380. doi: 10.1128/AEM.01253-08

Roug, A., Byrne, B. A., Conrad, P. A., and Miller, W. A. (2013). Zoonotic fecal pathogens and antimicrobial resistance in county fair animals. *Comp. Immunol. Microbiol. Infect. Dis.* 36, 303–308. doi: 10.1016/j.cimid.2012.11.006

Roy Chowdhury, P., Charles, I. G., and Djordjevic, S. P. (2015). A role for Tn6029 in the evolution of the complex antibiotic resistance gene loci in genomic island 3 in enteroaggregative hemorrhagic *Escherichia coli* O104:H4. *PLoS ONE* 10:e0115781. doi: 10.1371/journal.pone.0115781

Roy Chowdhury, P., McKinnon, J., Wyrsch, E., Hammond, J. M., Charles, I. G., and Djordjevic, S. P. (2014). Genomic interplay in bacterial communities: implications for growth promoting practices in animal husbandry. *Front. Microbiol.* 5:394. doi: 10.3389/fmicb.2014.00394

Roy Chowdhury, P., Scott, M., Worden, P., Huntington, P., Hudson, B., Karagiannis, T., et al. (2016). Genomic islands 1 and 2 play key roles in the evolution of extensively drug-resistant ST235 isolates of *Pseudomonas aeruginosa. Open Biol.* 6:150175. doi: 10.1098/rsob.150175

Ruppe, E., Woerther, P. L., Diop, A., Sene, A. M., Da Costa, A., Arlet, G., et al. (2009). Carriage of CTX-M-15-producing *Escherichia coli* isolates among children living in a remote village in Senegal. *Antimicrob. Agents Chemother.* 53, 3135–3137. doi: 10.1128/AAC.00139-09

Russo, T. A., and Johnson, J. R. (2003). Medical and economic impact of extraintestinal infections due to *Escherichia coli*: focus on an increasingly important endemic problem. *Microbes Infect.* 5, 449–456. doi: 10.1016/S1286-4579(03)00049-2

Sabate, M., Prats, G., Moreno, E., Balleste, E., Blanch, A. R., and Andreu, A. (2008). Virulence and antimicrobial resistance profiles among *Escherichia coli* strains isolated from human and animal wastewater. *Res Microbiol* 159, 288–293. doi: 10.1016/j.resmic.2008.02.001

Saenz, Y., Vinue, L., Ruiz, E., Somalo, S., Martinez, S., Rojo-Bezares, B., et al. (2010). Class 1 integrons lacking qacEDelta1 and sul1 genes in *Escherichia coli* isolates of food, animal and human origins. *Vet. Microbiol.* 144, 493–497. doi: 10.1016/j.vetmic.2010.01.026

Salipante, S. J., Roach, D. J., Kitzman, J. O., Snyder, M. W., Stackhouse, B., Butler-Wu, S. M., et al. (2015). Large-scale genomic sequencing of extraintestinal pathogenic *Escherichia coli* strains. *Genome Res.* 25, 119–128. doi: 10.1101/gr.180190.114

Samanta, I., Joardar, S. N., Mahanti, A., Bandyopadhyay, S., Sar, T. K., and Dutta, T. K. (2015). Approaches to characterize extended spectrum beta-lactamase/beta-lactamase producing *Escherichia coli* in healthy organized vis-a-vis backyard farmed pigs in India. *Infect. Genet. Evol.* 36, 224–230. doi: 10.1016/j.meegid.2015.09.021

Sarmah, A. K., Meyer, M. T., and Boxall, A. B. (2006). A global perspective on the use, sales, exposure pathways, occurrence, fate and effects of veterinary antibiotics (VAs) in the environment. *Chemosphere* 65, 725–759. doi: 10.1016/j.chemosphere.2006.03.026

Schierack, P., Rodiger, S., Kuhl, C., Hiemann, R., Roggenbuck, D., Li, G., et al. (2013). Porcine E. *coli:* virulence-associated genes, resistance genes and adhesion and probiotic activity tested by a new screening method. *PLoS ONE* 8:e59242. doi: 10.1371/journal.pone.0059242

Schroeder, C. M., Zhao, C., DebRoy, C., Torcolini, J., Zhao, S., White, D. G., et al. (2002). Antimicrobial resistance of *Escherichia coli* O157 isolated from humans, cattle, swine, and food. *Appl. Environ. Microbiol.* 68, 576–581. doi: 10.1128/AEM.68.2.576-581.2002

Schwaiger, K., Holzel, C., and Bauer, J. (2010). Resistance gene patterns of tetracycline resistant *Escherichia coli* of human and porcine origin. *Vet. Microbiol.* 142, 329–336. doi: 10.1016/j.vetmic.2009.09.066

Seiler, C., and Berendonk, T. U. (2012). Heavy metal driven co-selection of antibiotic resistance in soil and water bodies impacted by agriculture and aquaculture. *Front. Microbiol.* 3:399. doi: 10.3389/fmicb.2012.00399

Seputiene, V., Povilonis, J., Ruzauskas, M., Pavilonis, A., and Suziedeliene, E. (2010). Prevalence of trimethoprim resistance genes in *Escherichia coli* isolates of human and animal origin in Lithuania. *J. Med. Microbiol.* 59, 315–322. doi: 10.1099/jmm.0.015008-0

Sheikh, A., Luo, Q., Roy, K., Shabaan, S., Kumar, P., Qadri, F., et al. (2014). Contribution of the highly conserved EaeH surface protein to enterotoxigenic *Escherichia coli* pathogenesis. *Infect. Immun.* 82, 3657–3666. doi: 10.1128/IAI.01890-14

Sheikh, A. A., Checkley, S., Avery, B., Chalmers, G., Bohaychuk, V., Boerlin, P., et al. (2012). Antimicrobial resistance and resistance genes in *Escherichia coli* isolated from retail meat purchased in Alberta, Canada. *Foodborne Pathog. Dis.* 9, 625–631. doi: 10.1089/fpd.2011.1078

Shepard, S. M., Danzeisen, J. L., Isaacson, R. E., Seemann, T., Achtman, M., and Johnson, T. J. (2012). Genome sequences and phylogenetic analysis of K88- and F18-positive porcine enterotoxigenic *Escherichia coli. J. Bacteriol.* 194, 395–405. doi: 10.1128/JB.06225-11

Singh, R., Schroeder, C. M., Meng, J., White, D. G., McDermott, P. F., Wagner, D. D., et al. (2005). Identification of antimicrobial resistance and class 1 integrons in Shiga toxin-producing *Escherichia coli* recovered from humans and food animals. *J. Antimicrob. Chemother.* 56, 216–219. doi: 10.1093/jac/dki161

Smillie, C., Garcillan-Barcia, M. P., Francia, M. V., Rocha, E. P., and de la Cruz, F. (2010). Mobility of plasmids. *Microbiol. Mol. Biol. Rev.* 74, 434–452. doi: 10.1128/MMBR.00020-10

Smith, M. G., Jordan, D., Chapman, T. A., Chin, J. J., Barton, M. D., Do, T. N., et al. (2010). Antimicrobial resistance and virulence gene profiles in multi-drug resistant enterotoxigenic *Escherichia coli* isolated from pigs with post-weaning diarrhoea. *Vet. Microbiol.* 145, 299–307. doi: 10.1016/j.vetmic.2010.04.004

Soufi, L., Saenz, Y., Vinue, L., Abbassi, M. S., Ruiz, E., Zarazaga, M., et al. (2011). *Escherichia coli* of poultry food origin as reservoir of sulphonamide resistance genes and integrons. *Int. J. Food Microbiol.* 144, 497–502. doi: 10.1016/j.ijfoodmicro.2010.11.008

Spurbeck, R. R., Dinh, P. C. Jr., Walk, S. T., Stapleton, A. E., Hooton, T. M., Nolan, L. K., et al. (2012). *Escherichia coli* isolates that carry vat, fyuA, chuA, and yfcV efficiently colonize the urinary tract. *Infect. Immun.* 80, 4115–4122. doi: 10.1128/IAI.00752-12

Stannarius, C., Burgi, E., Regula, G., Zychowska, M. A., Zweifel, C., and Stephan, R. (2009). Antimicrobial resistance in *Escherichia coli* strains isolated from Swiss weaned pigs and sows. *Schweiz Arch Tierheilkd.* 151, 119–125. doi: 10.1024/0036-7281.151.3.119

Stedt, J., Bonnedahl, J., Hernandez, J., Waldenstrom, J., McMahon, B. J., Tolf, C., et al. (2015). Carriage of CTX-M type extended spectrum beta-lactamases (ESBLs) in gulls across Europe. *Acta Vet. Scand.* 57:74. doi: 10.1186/s13028-015-0166-3

Stefani, S., Giovanelli, I., Anacarso, I., Condo, C., Messi, P., de Niederhausern, S., et al. (2014). Prevalence and characterization of extended-spectrum beta-lactamase-producing *Enterobacteriaceae* in food-producing animals in Northern Italy. *New Microbiol.* 37, 551–555.

Stepanauskas, R., Glenn, T. C., Jagoe, C. H., Tuckfield, R. C., Lindell, A. H., King, C. J., et al. (2006). Coselection for microbial resistance to metals and antibiotics in freshwater microcosms. *Environ. Microbiol.* 8, 1510–1514. doi: 10.1111/j.1462-2920.2006.01091.x

Stephan, R., and Schumacher, S. (2001). Resistance patterns of non-O157 Shiga toxin-producing *Escherichia coli* (STEC) strains isolated from animals, food and asymptomatic human carriers in Switzerland. *Lett. Appl. Microbiol.* 32, 114–117. doi: 10.1046/j.1472-765x.2001.00867.x

Stokes, H. W., and Gillings, M. R. (2011). Gene flow, mobile genetic elements and the recruitment of antibiotic resistance genes into Gram-negative pathogens. *FEMS Microbiol. Rev.* 35, 790–819. doi: 10.1111/j.1574-6976.2011.00273.x

Summers, A. O. (2002). Generally overlooked fundamentals of bacterial genetics and ecology. *Clin. Infect. Dis.* 34(Suppl. 3), S85–S92. doi: 10.1086/340245

Summers, A. O. (2006). Genetic linkage and horizontal gene transfer, the roots of the antibiotic multi-resistance problem. *Anim. Biotechnol.* 17, 125–135. doi: 10.1080/10495390600957217

Sun, J., Deng, H., Li, L., Chen, M. Y., Fang, L. X., Yang, Q. E., et al. (2015). Complete nucleotide sequence of cfr-carrying IncX4 plasmid pSD11 from *Escherichia coli*. *Antimicrob. Agents Chemother.* 59, 738–741. doi: 10.1128/AAC.04388-14

Sunde, M. (2005). Prevalence and characterization of class 1 and class 2 integrons in *Escherichia coli* isolated from meat and meat products of Norwegian origin. *J. Antimicrob. Chemother.* 56, 1019–1024. doi: 10.1093/jac/dki377

Sunde, M., Fossum, K., Solberg, A., and Sorum, H. (1998). Antibiotic resistance in *Escherichia coli* of the normal intestinal flora of swine. *Microb. Drug Resist.* 4, 289–299. doi: 10.1089/mdr.1998.4.289

Sunde, M., and Norstrom, M. (2006). The prevalence of, associations between and conjugal transfer of antibiotic resistance genes in *Escherichia coli* isolated from Norwegian meat and meat products. *J. Antimicrob. Chemother.* 58, 741–747. doi: 10.1093/jac/dkl294

Sunde, M., and Sorum, H. (1999). Characterization of integrons in *Escherichia coli* of the normal intestinal flora of swine. *Microb. Drug Resist.* 5, 279–287. doi: 10.1089/mdr.1999.5.279

Tadesse, D. A., Zhao, S., Tong, E., Ayers, S., Singh, A., Bartholomew, M. J., et al. (2012). Antimicrobial drug resistance in *Escherichia coli* from humans and food animals, United States, 1950-2002. *Emerg. Infect. Dis.* 18, 741–749. doi: 10.3201/eid1805.111153

Tamang, M. D., Nam, H. M., Chae, M. H., Kim, S. R., Gurung, M., Jang, G. C., et al. (2012). Prevalence of plasmid-mediated quinolone resistance determinants among *Escherichia coli* isolated from food animals in Korea. *Foodborne Pathog. Dis.* 9, 1057–1063. doi: 10.1089/fpd.2012.1225

Tan, C., Tang, X., Zhang, X., Ding, Y., Zhao, Z., Wu, B., et al. (2012). Serotypes and virulence genes of extraintestinal pathogenic *Escherichia coli* isolates from diseased pigs in China. *Vet. J.* 192, 483–488. doi: 10.1016/j.tvjl.2011.06.038

Tang, X., Tan, C., Zhang, X., Zhao, Z., Xia, X., Wu, B., et al. (2011). Antimicrobial resistances of extraintestinal pathogenic *Escherichia coli* isolates from swine in China. *Microb. Pathog.* 50, 207–212. doi: 10.1016/j.micpath.2011.01.004

Taylor, N. M., Davies, R. H., Ridley, A., Clouting, C., Wales, A. D., and Clifton-Hadley, F. A. (2008). A survey of fluoroquinolone resistance in *Escherichia coli* and thermophilic Campylobacter spp. on poultry and pig farms in Great Britain. *J. Appl. Microbiol.* 105, 1421–1431. doi: 10.1111/j.1365-2672.2008.03877.x

Tian, G. B., Wang, H. N., Zhang, A. Y., Zhang, Y., Fan, W. Q., Xu, C. W., et al. (2012). Detection of clinically important beta-lactamases in commensal *Escherichia coli* of human and swine origin in western China. *J. Med. Microbiol.* 61, 233–238. doi: 10.1099/jmm.0.036806-0

Tietze, E., Tschape, H., and Voigt, W. (1989). Characterization of new resistance plasmids belonging to incompatibility group IncQ. *J. Basic Microbiol.* 29, 695–706. doi: 10.1002/jobm.3620291013

Timmerman, T., Dewulf, J., Catry, B., Feyen, B., Opsomer, G., de Kruif, A., et al. (2006). Quantification and evaluation of antimicrobial drug use in group treatments for fattening pigs in Belgium. *Prev. Vet. Med.* 74, 251–263. doi: 10.1016/j.prevetmed.2005.10.003

Travis, R. M., Gyles, C. L., Reid-Smith, R., Poppe, C., McEwen, S. A., Friendship, R., et al. (2006). Chloramphenicol and kanamycin resistance among porcine *Escherichia coli* in Ontario. *J. Antimicrob. Chemother.* 58, 173–177. doi: 10.1093/jac/dkl207

Trobos, M., Christensen, H., Sunde, M., Nordentoft, S., Agerso, Y., Simonsen, G. S., et al. (2009). Characterization of sulphonamide-resistant *Escherichia coli* using comparison of sul2 gene sequences and multilocus sequence typing. *Microbiology* 155, 831–836. doi: 10.1099/mic.0.024190-0

Tsafnat, G., Copty, J., and Partridge, S. R. (2011). RAC: repository of antibiotic resistance cassettes. *Database (Oxford)* 2011:bar054. doi: 10.1093/database/bar054

Tseng, S. P., Wang, S. F., Kuo, C. Y., Huang, J. W., Hung, W. C., Ke, G. M., et al. (2015). Characterization of fosfomycin resistant extended-spectrum beta-lactamase-producing *Escherichia coli* isolates from human and pig in Taiwan. *PLoS ONE* 10:e0135864. doi: 10.1371/journal.pone.0135864

Tsubokura, M., Matsumoto, A., Otsuki, K., Animas, S. B., and Sanekata, T. (1995). Drug resistance and conjugative R plasmids in *Escherichia coli* strains isolated from migratory waterfowl. *J. Wildl. Dis.* 31, 352–357. doi: 10.7589/0090-3558-31.3.352

United Nations (2015). *World Population Prospects: The 2015 Revision*. New York, NY: United Nations.

Udikovic-Kolic, N., Wichmann, F., Broderick, N. A., and Handelsman, J. (2014). Bloom of resident antibiotic-resistant bacteria in soil following manure fertilisation. *Proc. Natl. Acad. Sci. U.S.A.* 111, 15202–15207. doi: 10.1073/pnas.1409836111

Unno, T., Han, D., Jang, J., Lee, S. N., Kim, J. H., Ko, G., et al. (2010). High diversity and abundance of antibiotic-resistant *Escherichia coli* isolated from humans and farm animal hosts in Jeonnam Province, South Korea. *Sci. Total Environ.* 408, 3499–3506. doi: 10.1016/j.scitotenv.2010.04.046

Unno, T., Han, D., Jang, J., Widmer, K., Ko, G., Sadowsky, M. J., et al. (2011). Genotypic and phenotypic trends in antibiotic resistant pathogenic *Escherichia coli* isolated from humans and farm animals in South Korea. *Microbes Environ.* 26, 198–204. doi: 10.1264/jsme2.ME10194

Uzun, C., Oncul, O., Gumus, D., Alan, S., Dayioglu, N., and Kucuker, M. A. (2015). Virulence genes and antibiotic susceptibilities of uropathogenic *E. coli* strains. *Clin. Lab.* 61, 941–950.

Van Boeckel, T. P., Brower, C., Gilbert, M., Grenfell, B. T., Levin, S. A., Robinson, T. P., et al. (2015). Global trends in antimicbial use in food animals. *Proc. Natl. Acad. Sci. U.S.A.* 112, 5649–5654. doi: 10.1073/pnas.1503141112

van Elsas, J. D., Semenov, A. V., Costa, R., and Trevors, J. T. (2011). Survival of *Escherichia coli* in the environment: fundamental and public health aspects. *ISME J.* 5, 173–183. doi: 10.1038/ismej.2010.80

van Hoek, A. H., Veenman, C., van Overbeek, W. M., Lynch, G., de Roda Husman, A. M., and Blaak, H. (2015). Prevalence and characterization of ESBL- and AmpC-producing *Enterobacteriaceae* on retail vegetables. *Int. J. Food Microbiol.* 204, 1–8. doi: 10.1016/j.ijfoodmicro.2015.03.014

Vandekerchove, D., Vandemaele, F., Adriaensen, C., Zaleska, M., Hernalsteens, J. P., De Baets, L., et al. (2005). Virulence-associated traits in avian *Escherichia coli*: comparison between isolates from colibacillosis-affected and clinically healthy layer flocks. *Vet. Microbiol.* 108, 75–87. doi: 10.1016/j.vetmic.2005.02.009

Venturini, C., Beatson, S. A., Djordjevic, S. P., and Walker, M. J. (2010). Multiple antibiotic resistance gene recruitment onto the enterohemorrhagic *Escherichia coli* virulence plasmid. *FASEB J.* 24, 1160–1166. doi: 10.1096/fj.09-144972

Venturini, C., Hassan, K. A., Roy Chowdhury, P., Paulsen, I. T., Walker, M. J., and Djordjevic, S. P. (2013). Sequences of two related multiple antibiotic resistance virulence plasmids sharing a unique IS26-related molecular signature isolated from different *Escherichia coli* pathotypes from different hosts. *PLoS ONE* 8:e78862. doi: 10.1371/journal.pone.0078862

Vincent, C., Boerlin, P., Daignault, D., Dozois, C. M., Dutil, L., Galanakis, C., et al. (2010). Food reservoir for *Escherichia coli* causing urinary tract infections. *Emerg. Infect. Dis.* 16, 88–95. doi: 10.3201/eid1601.091118

Vinue, L., Saenz, Y., Rojo-Bezares, B., Olarte, I., Undabeitia, E., Somalo, S., et al. (2010). Genetic environment of sul genes and characterisation of integrons in *Escherichia coli* isolates of blood origin in a Spanish hospital. *Int. J. Antimicrob. Agents* 35, 492–496. doi: 10.1016/j.ijantimicag.2010.01.012

Vinue, L., Saenz, Y., Somalo, S., Escudero, E., Moreno, M. A., Ruiz-Larrea, F., et al. (2008). Prevalence and diversity of integrons and associated resistance genes in faecal *Escherichia coli* isolates of healthy humans in Spain. *J. Antimicrob. Chemother.* 62, 934–937. doi: 10.1093/jac/dkn331

Virdi, V., Coddens, A., De Buck, S., Millet, S., Goddeeris, B. M., Cox, E., et al. (2013). Orally fed seeds producing designer IgAs protect weaned piglets against enterotoxigenic *Escherichia coli* infection. *Proc. Natl. Acad. Sci. U.S.A.* 110, 11809–11814. doi: 10.1073/pnas.1301975110

Vogt, D., Overesch, G., Endimiani, A., Collaud, A., Thomann, A., and Perreten, V. (2014). Occurrence and genetic characteristics of third-generation cephalosporin-resistant *Escherichia coli* in Swiss retail meat. *Microb. Drug Resist.* 20, 485–494. doi: 10.1089/mdr.2013.0210

Wallace-Gadsden, F., Johnson, J. R., Wain, J., and Okeke, I. N. (2007). Enteroaggregative *Escherichia coli* related to uropathogenic clonal group A. *Emerg. Infect. Dis* 13, 757–760. doi: 10.3201/eid1305.061057

Wang, F., Ma, W., Dou, Z., Ma, L., Liu, X., Xu, J., et al. (2006). The estimation of the production amount of animal manure and its environmental effect in China. *China Environ. Sci.* 26, 614–617.

Watkinson, A. J., Murby, E. J., and Costanzo, S. D. (2007). Removal of antibiotics in conventional and advanced wastewater treatment: implications for environmental discharge and wastewater recycling. *Water Res.* 41, 4164–4176. doi: 10.1016/j.watres.2007.04.005

Woodford, N., Carattoli, A., Karisik, E., Underwood, A., Ellington, M. J., and Livermore, D. M. (2009). Complete nucleotide sequences of plasmids pEK204, pEK499, and pEK516, encoding CTX-M enzymes in three major *Escherichia coli* lineages from the United Kingdom, all belonging to the international O25:H4-ST131 clone. *Antimicrob. Agents Chemother.* 53, 4472–4482. doi: 10.1128/AAC.00688-09

Wu, S., Dalsgaard, A., Hammerum, A. M., Porsbo, L. J., and Jensen, L. B. (2010). Prevalence and characterization of plasmids carrying sulfonamide resistance genes among *Escherichia coli* from pigs, pig carcasses and human. *Acta Vet. Scand.* 52:47. doi: 10.1186/1751-0147-52-47

Wu, X. Y., Chapman, T., Trott, D. J., Bettelheim, K., Do, T. N., Driesen, S., et al. (2007). Comparative analysis of virulence genes, genetic diversity, and phylogeny of commensal and enterotoxigenic *Escherichia coli* isolates from weaned pigs. *Appl. Environ. Microbiol.* 73, 83–91. doi: 10.1128/AEM.00990-06

Wyrsch, E., Roy Chowdhury, P., Abraham, S., Santos, J., Darling, A. E., Charles, I. G., et al. (2015). Comparative genomic analysis of a multiple antimicrobial resistant enterotoxigenic *E. coli* O157 lineage from Australian pigs. *BMC Genomics* 16:165. doi: 10.1186/s12864-015-1382-y

Xia, X., Meng, J., Zhao, S., Bodeis-Jones, S., Gaines, S. A., Ayers, S. L., et al. (2011). Identification and antimicrobial resistance of extraintestinal pathogenic *Escherichia coli* from retail meats. *J. Food Prot.* 74, 38–44. doi: 10.4315/0362-028X.JFP-10-251

Xu, X., Cui, S., Zhang, F., Luo, Y., Gu, Y., Yang, B., et al. (2014). Prevalence and characterization of cefotaxime and ciprofloxacin co-resistant *Escherichia coli* isolates in retail chicken carcasses and Ground Pork, China. *Microb. Drug Resist.* 20, 73–81. doi: 10.1089/mdr.2012.0224

Xu, Y., Tian, X., Ren, C., Huang, H., Zhang, X., Gong, X., et al. (2012). Analysis of colistin A and B in fishery products by ultra performance liquid chromatography with positive electrospray ionization tandem mass spectrometry. *J. Chromatogr. B Analyt. Technol. Biomed. Life Sci.* 899, 14–20. doi: 10.1016/j.jchromb.2012.04.028

Yahiaoui, M., Robin, F., Bakour, R., Hamidi, M., Bonnet, R., and Messai, Y. (2015). Antibiotic resistance, virulence, and genetic background of community-acquired uropathogenic *Escherichia coli* from Algeria. *Microb. Drug Resist.* 21, 516–526. doi: 10.1089/mdr.2015.0045

Yamamoto, S., Nakano, M., Kitagawa, W., Tanaka, M., Sone, T., Hirai, K., et al. (2014). Characterization of multi-antibiotic-resistant *Escherichia coli* isolated from beef cattle in Japan. *Microbes Environ.* 29, 136–144. doi: 10.1264/jsme2.ME13173

Yang, H., Chen, S., White, D. G., Zhao, S., McDermott, P., Walker, R., et al. (2004). Characterization of multiple-antimicrobial-resistant *Escherichia coli* isolates from diseased chickens and swine in China. *J. Clin. Microbiol.* 42, 3483–3489. doi: 10.1128/jcm.42.8.3483-3489.2004

Yang, T., Zeng, Z., Rao, L., Chen, X., He, D., Lv, L., et al. (2014). The association between occurrence of plasmid-mediated quinolone resistance and ciprofloxacin resistance in *Escherichia coli* isolates of different origins. *Vet. Microbiol.* 170, 89–96. doi: 10.1016/j.vetmic.2014.01.019

Yau, S., Liu, X., Djordjevic, S. P., and Hall, R. M. (2010). RSF1010-like plasmids in Australian *Salmonella enterica* serovar Typhimurium and origin of their sul2-strA-strB antibiotic resistance gene cluster. *Microb. Drug Resist.* 16, 249–252. doi: 10.1089/mdr.2010.0033

Yue, L., Jiang, H. X., Liao, X. P., Liu, J. H., Li, S. J., Chen, X. Y., et al. (2008). Prevalence of plasmid-mediated quinolone resistance qnr genes in poultry and swine clinical isolates of *Escherichia coli*. *Vet. Microbiol.* 132, 414–420. doi: 10.1016/j.vetmic.2008.05.009

Zhang, R., Sun, B., Wang, Y., Lei, L., Schwarz, S., and Wu, C. (2015). Characterization of a cfr-carrying plasmid from porcine *Escherichia coli* that closely resembles plasmid pEA3 from the plant pathogen *Erwinia amylovora*. *Antimicrob Agents Chemother.* 60, 658–661. doi: 10.1128/AAC.02114-15

Zhang, W. J., Xu, X. R., Schwarz, S., Wang, X. M., Dai, L., Zheng, H. J., et al. (2014). Characterization of the IncA/C plasmid pSCEC2 from *Escherichia coli* of swine origin that harbours the multiresistance gene cfr. *J. Antimicrob. Chemother.* 69, 385–389. doi: 10.1093/jac/dkt355

Zhu, Y. G., Johnson, T. A., Su, J. Q., Qiao, M., Guo, G. X., Stedtfeld, R. D., et al. (2013). Diverse and abundant antibiotic resistance genes in Chinese swine farms. *Proc. Natl. Acad. Sci. U.S.A.* 110, 3435–3440. doi: 10.1073/pnas.1222743110

Zurfluh, K., Poirel, L., Nordmann, P., Klumpp, J., and Stephan, R. (2015). First detection of Klebsiella variicola producing OXA-181 carbapenemase in fresh vegetable imported from Asia to Switzerland. *Antimicrob. Resist. Infect. Control* 4:38. doi: 10.1186/s13756-015-0080-5

Zweifel, C., Schumacher, S., Beutin, L., Blanco, J., and Stephan, R. (2006). Virulence profiles of Shiga toxin 2e-producing *Escherichia coli* isolated from healthy pig at slaughter. *Vet. Microbiol.* 117, 328–332. doi: 10.1016/j.vetmic.2006.06.017

10

CTX-M-27 Producing *Salmonella enterica* Serotypes Typhimurium and Indiana are Prevalent among Food-Producing Animals in China

Wen-Hui Zhang†, Xiang-Yan Lin†, Liang Xu, Xi-Xi Gu, Ling Yang, Wan Li, Si-Qi Ren, Ya-Hong Liu, Zhen-Ling Zeng* and Hong-Xia Jiang*

National Risk Assessment Laboratory for Antimicrobial Resistance of Animal Original Bacteria, College of Veterinary Medicine, South China Agricultural University, Guangzhou, China

***Correspondence:**
Zhen-Ling Zeng
zlzeng@scau.edu.cn;
Hong-Xia Jiang
hxjiang@scau.edu.cn

† These authors have contributed equally to this work.

Salmonella spp. is one of the most important food-borne pathogens causing digestive tract and invasive infections in both humans and animals. Extended-spectrum β-lactamases (ESBLs) especially the CTX-M-type ESBLs are increasingly being reported worldwide and in China. These studies seldom focused on *Salmonella* isolates from food-producing animals. The aim of this study was to characterize the antimicrobial resistance profiles, serotypes and ESBLs and in particular, CTX-M producing *Salmonella* isolates from chickens and pigs in China. *Salmonella* isolates were identified by API20E system and polymerase chain reaction (PCR) assay; serotypes were determined using slide agglutination with hyperimmune sera; antimicrobial susceptibility was tested using the ager dilution method; the prevalence of ESBLs and PMQR genes were screened by PCR; CTX-M-producing isolates were further characterized by conjugation along with genetic relatedness and plasmid replicon type. In total, 159 *Salmonella* strains were identified, among which 95 strains were *Salmonella enterica* serovar Typhimurium, 63 strains were *S. enterica* serovar Indiana, and 1 strain was *S. enterica* serovar Enteritidis. All of these isolates presented multi-drug resistant phenotypes. Forty-five isolates carried bla_{CTX-M} genes, the most common subtype was CTX-M-27(34), followed by CTX-M-65(7) and CTX-M-14(4). Most bla_{CTX-M} genes were transmitted by non-typeable or IncN/IncFIB/IncP/IncA/C/IncHI2 plasmids with sizes ranging from 80 to 280 kb. In particular, all the 14 non-typeable plasmids were carrying $bla_{CTX-M-27}$ gene and had a similar size. PFGE profiles indicated that CTX-M-positive isolates were clonally related among the same serotype, whilst the isolates of different serotypes were genetically divergent. This suggested that both clonal spread of resistant strains and horizontal transmission of the resistance plasmids contributed to the dissemination of $bla_{CTX-M-9G}$-positive *Salmonella* isolates. The presence and spread of CTX-M, especially the CTX-M-27 in *S. enterica* serovars Typhimurium and Indiana from food-producing animals poses a potential threat for public health. Control strategies to limit the dissemination of these strains through the food chain are necessary.

Keywords: *Salmonella*, food-producing animals, serotype, antimicrobial resistance, CTX-M

INTRODUCTION

The emergence of antibiotic-resistant bacteria has become a serious challenge in human and veterinary medicine globally and poses a serious public health threat. Non-typhoidal *Salmonella* (NTS) are a leading cause of bacterial diarrhea worldwide and one of the most important foodborne pathogens. The majorities of human infections by NTS are associated with food product consumption of meat, eggs, milk, seafood, and other fresh products derived from animals (Foley and Lynne, 2008). In the animal husbandry industry, antibiotics are used both for therapy and as growth promoters. Additionally, animals are always a large repository of resistant bacteria. Domestic farm animals, especially poultry and pigs have been shown to be major environmental reservoirs of food-borne NTS (Vo et al., 2006).

Serotyping is a useful classification scheme that allows for trends in *Salmonella* surveillance data to be followed over time. These patterns are also related to the ability to cause disease and with the associated antibiotic resistance profile. Over 2,600 serotypes of *Salmonella* have been identified based on the reactivity of antisera to O and H antigens (Stevens et al., 2009), and there are numerous overlaps between animal and human *Salmonella* serotypes (Alcaine et al., 2006). This suggests that *Salmonella* transmission from animals to humans occurs via the food chain. *Salmonella enterica* serovars Enteritidis and Typhimurium are the most common serotypes in Europe (European Centre for Disease Prevention and Control, 2013). However, serotype distribution is varied in different provinces of China and in total the most prevalent serovars were also Typhimurium and Enteritidis with a rising rate of reports of *S. enterica* serovar Indiana in isolates obtained from animals (Xia et al., 2009; Yang et al., 2010; Lu et al., 2014; Zhang et al., 2014).

It is estimated that that between 1994 and 2005 roughly 22% of foodborne diseases in China were caused by *Salmonella* though there was no official surveillance data (Wang et al., 2007). In 2013, unpublished data from the China CDC surveillance system showed that the carriage rate of human salmonellosis was 549 per 100,000 people. This is more than 33 times higher than human infections in the USA in 2012 (16.4 per 100,000; Centers for Disease Control and Prevention, 2013; Sun et al., 2014). There is also an increasing risk of *Salmonella* spread from animals to humans *via* the food chain due to worldwide distribution of animal food products from China. Extended spectrum cephalosporins (ESCs) and fluoroquinolones are the drugs of choice for treatment of invasive *Salmonella* infections in food animals and for people at risk of such infections (Harrois et al., 2014). This is the focus of current concerns on the emergence of resistance to these drugs. ESCs- and fluoroquinolone-resistant *Salmonella* populations have increased dramatically worldwide (Arlet et al., 2006; Hendriksen et al., 2009; Jiang et al., 2014; Lu et al., 2014). Resistance to cephalosporins is mainly due to the acquisition of extended-spectrum β-lactamases (ESBLs) genes especially the CTX-M type that is primarily carried by transferable plasmids and transposons (Liebana et al., 2013). These plasmids and transposons, in many cases, also carry resistance genes for other antimicrobial classes such as the fluoroquinolones which sometimes limits treatment options (Harrois et al., 2014). Plasmid-mediated quinolone resistance (PMQR) has recently been categorized as containing three distinct resistance mechanisms: (1) Qnr proteins that mediate target protection, (2) A variant of an aminoglycoside acetyltransferase designated AAC(6')-Ib-cr that acetylates ciprofloxacin and norfloxacin and (3) Drug efflux mediated by OqxAB and QepA (Strahilevitz et al., 2009). Although these PMQR determinants confer only low-level fluoroquinolone resistance, their presence can provide a selective advantage for bacteria to develop to high-level quinolone resistance. This occurs by chromosomal mutations in the quinolone resistance-determining regions (QRDRs) of genes encoding target enzymes (Strahilevitz et al., 2009). The situation is especially troubling when ESBL genes and PMQR genes are co-transmitted through transferable plasmids.

Indiscriminate use of antibiotics in both human and veterinary medicine make the ESBLs especially the CTX-M-producing bacteria including *Salmonella* increase rapidly accelerating the spread of antibiotic resistance. There have been several reports regarding characteristics of CTX-M-producing *Salmonella* isolated from food-producing animals in China. However, data on distribution of serotypes and antimicrobial susceptibility of *Salmonella* recovered from animals are available in most of these reports (Yan et al., 2010; Yang et al., 2010; Li R. et al., 2013; Li et al., 2014; Lu et al., 2014; Kuang et al., 2015). The aim of the present study was to investigate the prevalence of antibiotic resistance, serotypes and ESBLs among *Salmonella* isolates from chickens and pigs in China. Plasmids that carried $bla_{\text{CTX-M}}$ genes were also further studied to characterize the mechanism of transfer and dissemination of β-lactamases.

MATERIALS AND METHODS

Salmonella Isolation, Identification, and Serotyping

In 2014, a total of 3850 non-repetitive fecal swabs were collected from healthy chickens and pigs in Guangdong, Shandong, Henan, Hubei provinces of China. Of these samples, 2090 samples were from chickens and 1760 samples were from pigs.

Cotton swabs of feces were inoculated into sterile selenite cystine broth for 24 h at 37°C, and then streaked onto chromogenic medium selective for *Salmonella* (CHROMagar Microbiology, France) and incubated for another 24 h at 37°C. One purple colony was selected from each plate and then confirmed using the API20E system (bioMérieux, Marcy l'Étoile, France) and a PCR assay targeting the *invA* gene (Rahn et al., 1992). *Salmonella* isolates were serotyped using slide agglutination with hyperimmune sera (S&A Company, Bangkok, Thailand) and the results were interpreted according to the Kauffmann–White scheme. All identified isolates were stored at −80°C in Luria–Bertani (LB) broth containing 30% glycerol.

Antimicrobial Susceptibility Testing

The minimum inhibitory concentrations (MICs) of *Salmonella* isolates were determined using the agar dilution method following Clinical and Laboratory Standards Institution guidelines. Sixteen antimicrobials were tested: ampicillin (AMP), cefotaxime (CTX), cefoxitin (CXT), ceftiofur (CTF), ceftazidime (CAZ), ceftriaxone (CTR), nalidixic acid (NAL), ciprofloxacin (CIP), enrofloxacin (ENR), kanamycin (KAN), gentamycin (GEN), amikacin (AMK), tetracycline (TET), chloramphenicol (CHL), florfenicol (FFC) and olaquindox (OLA). The results were interpreted according to the standards described by CLSI (M100-S25) (Clinical and Laboratory Standards Institute [CLSI], 2015) (ampicillin, cefotaxime, ceftiofur, ceftriaxone, cefoxitin, ceftazidime, nalidixic acid, ciprofloxacin, kanamycin, amikacin) and VET01-A4/VET01-S2 (Clinical and Laboratory Standards Institute [CLSI], 2013) (gentamicin, enrofloxacin, tetracycline, chloramphenicol, florfenicol) and the DANMAP 98 (olaquindox). *Escherichia coli* ATCC 25922 was used as quality control.

Detection of β-Lactamase Genes and PMQR Genes

The *Salmonella* isolates harvested from Mueller Hinton (MH) agar plates supplied with 2 mg/L cefotaxime were subjected to screening for ESBL-genes using PCR as described previously (Jiang et al., 2012). The DNA sequences and deduced amino acid sequences were compared with the reported sequences from GenBank[1]. The presence of PMQR determinants [*qnrA, qnrB, qnrS, qnrD, qnrC, aac(6')-Ib-cr,qepA*, and *oqxAB*] was also analyzed using PCR primers and conditions described previously (Jiang et al., 2012). Mutations in QRDR of target genes (*gyrA* and *parC*) were further analyzed in both PMQR and CTX-M-positive isolates as described previously (O'Regan et al., 2009).

Molecular Typing

Genetic relatedness of all bla_{CTX-M} -positive isolates was analyzed by pulsed-field gel electrophoresis (PFGE) after *Xba*I-digested genomic DNA using a CHEF-MAPPER System (Bio-Rad Laboratories, Hercules, CA, USA) as described previously (Jiang et al., 2014). The resulting PFGE patterns were compared using the Dice similarity coefficient of BioNumerics software (Applied Maths, Sint-Martens-Latem, Belgium).

Conjugation and Transformation Experiments

Conjugation experiments were conducted in bla_{CTX-M}-positive strains by liquid mating-out assay in LB-medium using a sodium azide-resistant *E. coli* J53 as the recipient. Transconjugants were selected on MacConkey agar containing cefotaxime (2 mg/L) and sodium azide (300 mg/L). For transformation experiments, plasmid DNA from the bla_{CTX-M}-positive strains were extracted using Qiagen Plasmid Midi Kit according to the manufacturer's instructions (Qiagen, Germany). Purified plasmids were transformed into *E. coli* DH5a (TaKaRa Biotechnology, Dalian, China). Selection of transformants was performed on MacConkey agar containing 2 mg/L cefotaxime. MICs and the presence of bla_{CTX-M} gene of transconjugants and transformants were determined as described above.

Plasmid Characterization

PCR-based replicon typing (PBRT) was performed on transconjugants and transformants using primers as described previously (Carattoli et al., 2005). Then PFGE with S1 nuclease (Takara Biotechnology, Dalian, China) digestion of whole genomic DNA was carried out as described previously (Barton et al., 1995). The resulting gels were analyzed by Southern transfer and probing with a DIG-labeled bla_{CTX-M} gene fragment according to the manufacturer's instructions (DIG High Prime DNA Labeling and Detection Starter Kit I, Roche Applied Science, Mannheim, Germany).

RESULTS

Salmonella Isolation, Identification, and Serotyping

A total of 159 *Salmonella* strains were obtained among which 90 (56.6%) were isolated from pigs and 69 (43.4%) were recovered from chickens. In all, three serotypes were identified in the 159 *Salmonella* isolates and this accounted for 95 strains of *S. enterica* serovar Typhimurium, 63 strains of *S. enterica* serovar Indiana, and 1 strain of *S. enterica* serovar Enteritidis.

The *S. enterica* serovar Typhimurium isolates were distributed as follows: 73.7% from pigs and 26.3% from chickens while the Indiana isolates were almost evenly distributed (50.8% from chickens and 49.2% from pigs, relatively).

Antimicrobial Susceptibility Phenotypes

Among the159 *Salmonella* isolates, resistance was most frequently observed to tetracycline (89.9%), ampicillin (84.9%), and gentamicin (81.1%). Resistance rates of the quinolone antibiotics were all above 50% including resistance to nalidixic acid (77.3%), ciprofloxacin (64.8%), and enrofloxacin (62.9%). Cephalosporin resistance rates ranged from 17.6 to 76.7% with high resistance rates to ceftriaxone (76.7%), ceftiofur (52.8%), and cefotaxime (47.2%). Resistance rates to ceftazidime and cefoxitin were 30.8 and 17.6%, respectively. The presence of resistance to olaquindox, a growth promoter used extensively in pigs and recently prohibited for poultry use, was detected in 65.4% of all isolates (**Table 1**).

All the 159 *Salmonella* isolates were multi-drug resistant displaying resistance to three or more classes of antimicrobials. Higher resistance frequencies were found among *S. enterica* serovar Indiana isolates compared with *S. enterica* serovar Typhimurium isolates. For example, cefotaxime resistance in Indiana and Typhimurium isolates were 71.4 and 30.5%, respectively, while the ciprofloxacin resistance rates were 73.0 and 43.2%, respectively (**Table 2**).

ESBL Characterization

Seventy-five isolates displayed non-wild type MICs for cefotaxime and 45 of these carried bla_{CTX-M} genes, three

[1] www.ncbi.nlm.nih.gov/genbank/

TABLE 1 | Antimicrobial resistance of *Salmonella enterica* isolates from food-producing animals in China.

Antimicrobial agents	Number(%) of resistant isolates (n = 159)
β-Lactams	
Ampicillin	135 (84.9)
Cefotaxime	75 (47.2)
Cefoxitin	28 (17.6)
Ceftiofur	84 (52.8)
Ceftazidime	49 (30.8)
Ceftriaxone	122 (76.7)
Quinolones	
Nalidixic acid	123 (77.4)
Ciprofloxacin	103 (64.8)
Enrofloxacin	100 (62.9)
Aminoglycosides	
Kanamycin	124 (78.0)
Gentamicin	129 (81.1)
Amikacin	9 (5.7)
Other Antibiotics	
Tetracycline	143 (89.9)
Chloramphenicol	126 (79.2)
Florfenicol	124 (78.0)
Olaquindox	104 (65.4)

harbored bla_{CMY-2} one of which coexisted with the CTX-M-encoding gene. For other β-lactamase genes, narrow-spectrum β-lactamase bla_{TEM-1} was present in 86 of the 159 isolates, bla_{SHV-1} and bla_{OXA-1} genes were found in 62 and 55 of these isolates, respectively. No other type of ESBLs gene was found.

For the PMQR genes, three classes of resistance mechanisms were represented: *oqxAB* (78.0%, n = 124); *aac(6')-Ib-cr*(69.2%, n = 110) and *qnr*(17.6%, n = 28). For 28 *qnr* genes, 12 were *qnrD*, 7 were *qnrB*, 5 were *qnrS*, and the remaining 4 were *qnrA*. All *qnr*-positive strains also carried *oqxAB* and/or *aac(6')-Ib-cr*. At least one PMQR gene was found in each CTX-M-producing strains, especially the *aac(6')-Ib-cr +oqxAB* and qnr+*aac(6')-Ib-cr +oqxAB* were found in 17 and 4 of all 45 CTX-M-producing strains, respectively. Mutations in the QRDRs of *gyrA* and *parC* were analyzed among the 45 PMQR and CTX-M-positive isolates. A combination of mutations in *gyrA*83 (S83F) and 87 (D87G) and in *parC* 80(S80R) were found in 35 (77.8%) isolates, a signal mutation in *gyrA* 87 (D87N) without mutation in *parC* was detected in the remaining 10 isolates (**Table 3**).

A total of three different CTX-M ESBLs were detected in these isolates and they all belonged to the CTX-M-9 group with the CTX-M-encoding genes distributed as 34 $bla_{CTX-M-27}$, 7 $bla_{CTX-M-65}$, and 4 $bla_{CTX-M-14}$. The distribution of these three CTX-M subtypes showed no specificity between serotypes and animals and were found in both Indiana and Typhimurium isolates from pigs and chickens. Antimicrobial susceptibility testing demonstrated that CTX-M-27-positive isolates had significantly higher resistance levels than the CTX-M-14 or CTX-M-65 -positive isolates.

TABLE 2 | Antibiotic resistance rate of *Salmonella enterica* serotype Typhimurium and Indiana isolates (%).

Serotype / Antibiotics	AMP	CTF	CTX	CXT	CTZ	CTR	GEN	KAN	AMI	CIP	ENR	NAL	TET	CHL	FFC	OQX
Indiana (63)	93.7	76.2	71.4	19.0	33.3	82.5	88.9	84.1	6.3	73.0	77.8	87.3	96.8	90.5	84.1	68.3
Typhimurium (95)	89.5	37.9	30.5	11.6	29.5	73.7	76.8	74.7	5.3	60.0	52.6	70.5	86.3	72.6	74.7	64.2

TABLE 3 | Characteristics of CTX-M-producing *Salmonella enterica* isolates from food-producing animals in China.

Strain	Source	Serotype	ESBL gene	PMQR	Amino acid substitutions		Co-transferred resistant gene	Plasmid replicon type	Plasmid approx. size(kb)
					gyrA	*parC*			
SP5	Pig	Typhimurium	*bla*$_{\text{CTX-M-14}}$	*aac-(6')-Ib-cr,oqxAB*	D87N	–	*bla*$_{SHV-1}$, *aac-(6')-Ib-cr*	FIB	100
SP85	Pig	Indiana	*bla*$_{\text{CTX-M-27}}$	*aac-(6')-Ib-cr oqxAB*	S83F,D87G	S80R	*bla*$_{OXA-1}$,*aac-(6')-Ib-cr*	NT	100
SP96	Pig	Indiana	*bla*$_{\text{CTX-M-27}}$	*oqxAB*	S83F,D87G	S80R	*bla*$_{SHV-1}$, *oqxAB*	P	150
SP99	Pig	Typhimurium	*bla*$_{\text{CTX-M-27}}$	*qnrB, aac-(6')-Ib-cr,oqxAB*	S83F,D87G	S80R	*aac-(6')-Ib-cr oqxAB*	NT	100
SP101	Pig	Typhimurium	*bla*$_{\text{CTX-M-65}}$	*oqxAB*	D87N	–	*oqxAB*	FIB	150
SP108	Pig	Indiana	*bla*$_{\text{CTX-M-27}}$	*aac-(6')-Ib-cr,oqxAB*	S83F,D87G	S80R	*bla*$_{SHV-1}$, *aac-(6')-Ib-cr*	A/C	150
SP110	Pig	Indiana	*bla*$_{\text{CTX-M-65}}$	*oqxAB*	S83F,D87G	S80R	*bla*$_{SHV-1}$	N	100
SP115	Pig	Indiana	*bla*$_{\text{CTX-M-27}}$	*aac-(6')-Ib-cr,oqxAB*	S83F,D87G	S80R	*aac-(6')-Ib-cr*	NT	100
SP123	Pig	Indiana	*bla*$_{\text{CTX-M-27}}$	*oqxAB*	D87N	–	–	FIB	150
SP125	Pig	Indiana	*bla*$_{\text{CTX-M-27}}$	*oqxAB*	D87N	–	–	FIB	150
SP129	Pig	Typhimurium	*bla*$_{\text{CTX-M-27}}$	*aac-(6')-Ib-cr,oqxAB*	S83F,D87G	S80R	*bla*$_{SHV-1}$,*aac-(6')-Ib-cr*	P	80
SP131	Pig	Indiana	*bla*$_{\text{CTX-M-65}}$	*aac-(6')-Ib-cr,oqxAB*	S83F,D87G	S80R	*bla*$_{SHV-1}$, *aac-(6')-Ib-cr*	N	150
SP132	Pig	Indiana	*bla*$_{\text{CTX-M-27}}$	*oqxAB*	S83F,D87G	S80R	*bla*$_{SHV-1}$, *oqxAB*	N	150
SP2019	Pig	Typhimurium	*bla*$_{\text{CTX-M-14}}$	*aac-(6')-Ib-cr,oqxAB*	D87N	–	*bla*$_{OXA-1}$, *oqxAB*	HI2	280
CL108	Chicken	Indiana	*bla*$_{\text{CTX-M-27}}$	*oqxAB*	S83F,D87G	–	–	NT	100
CL129	Chicken	Indiana	*bla*$_{\text{CTX-M-27}}$	*aac-(6')-Ib-cr*	S83F,D87G	S80R	*bla*$_{SHV-1}$,*aac-(6')-Ib-cr*	FIB	150
CL135	Chicken	Indiana	*bla*$_{\text{CTX-M-27}}$	*oqxAB*	S83F,D87G	S80R	–	NT	100
CL140	Chicken	Indiana	*bla*$_{\text{CTX-M-27}}$	*aac-(6')-Ib-cr*	S83F,D87G	S80R	–	NT	100
CL146	Chicken	Indiana	*bla*$_{\text{CTX-M-27}}$	*qnrD,aac-(6')-Ib-cr,oqxAB*	S83F,D87G	S80R	*bla*$_{SHV-1}$,*aac-(6')-Ib-cr*	NT	100
CL189	Chicken	Indiana	*bla*$_{\text{CTX-M-27}}$	*oqxAB*	S83F,D87G	S80R	*oqxAB*	HI2	200
XC48	Chicken	Typhimurium	*bla*$_{\text{CTX-M-27}}$	*aac-(6')-Ib-cr, oqxAB*	S83F,D87G	S80R	*aac-(6')-Ib-cr*	N	150
XC87	Chicken	Typhimurium	*bla*$_{\text{CTX-M-65}}$	*aac-(6')-Ib-cr,oqxAB*	S83F,D87G	S80R	*aac-(6')-Ib-cr oqxAB*	N,	150
XC134	Chicken	Typhimurium	*bla*$_{\text{CTX-M-14}}$	*aac-(6')-Ib-cr,oqxAB*	S83F,D87G	S80R	*oqxAB*	N,A/C	150
XC164	Chicken	Typhimurium	*bla*$_{\text{CTX-M-27}}$	*oqxAB*	S83F,D87G	S80R	*bla*$_{TEM-1b}$,*oqxAB*	HI2	194
HB73	Chicken	Indiana	*bla*$_{\text{CTX-M-27}}$	*oqxAB*	S83F,D87G	S80R	–	A/C	130
HB137	Chicken	Indiana	*bla*$_{\text{CTX-M-27}}$	*aac-(6')-Ib-cr,oqxAB*	S83F,D87G	S80R	*oqxAB*	NT	100
HB154	Chicken	Indiana	*bla*$_{\text{CTX-M-65}}$	*aac-(6')-Ib-cr,oqxAB*	S83F,D87G	S80R	*aac-(6')-Ib-cr oqxAB*	N,	130
SG36	Chicken	Indiana	*bla*$_{\text{CTX-M-27}}$	*oqxAB*	S83F,D87G	S80R	*bla*$_{SHV-1}$	NT	100
SG119	Chicken	Indiana	*bla*$_{\text{CTX-M-27}}$	*aac-(6')-Ib-cr*	S83F,D87G	S80R	–	NT	100
MM62	Chicken	Enteritidis	*bla*$_{\text{CTX-M-27}}$	*aac-(6')-Ib-cr*	D87N	–	*aac-(6')-Ib-cr*	P	80
PY12	Chicken	Indiana	*bla*$_{\text{CTX-M-14}}$	*aac-(6')-Ib-cr,oqxAB*	D87N	–	*bla*$_{SHV-1}$	N,A/C	130
K13	Chicken	Indiana	*bla*$_{\text{CTX-M-27}}$	*aac-(6')-Ib-cr,oqxAB*	S83F,D87G	S80R	–	NT	100
K14	Chicken	Indiana	*bla*$_{\text{CTX-M-27}}$	*oqxAB*	S83F,D87G	S80R	–	NT	100
K17	Chicken	Typhimurium	*bla*$_{\text{CTX-M-27}}$	*aac-(6')-Ib-cr,oqxAB*	S83F,D87G	S80R	*aac-(6')-Ib-cr*	NT	100
K19	Chicken	Indiana	*bla*$_{\text{CTX-M-65}}$	*aac-(6')-Ib-cr,oqxAB*	S83F,D87G	S80R	*aac-(6')-Ib-cr,oqxAB*	N	150
K21	Chicken	Indiana	*bla*$_{\text{CTX-M-27}}$	*aac-(6')-Ib-cr*	D87N	–	*aac-(6')-Ib-cr*	FIB	150
K46	Chicken	Indiana	*bla*$_{\text{CTX-M-27}}$	*aac-(6')-Ib-cr,oqxAB*	S83F,D87G	S80R	*aac-(6')-Ib-cr,oqxAB*	P	100
K47	Chicken	Indiana	*bla*$_{\text{CTX-M-27}}$	*aac-(6')-Ib-cr*	S83F,D87G	S80R	*aac-(6')-Ib-cr*	NT	100

NT, non-typeable incompatibility (Inc) group plasmid. The underline isolates were transconjugants, the others were transformants.

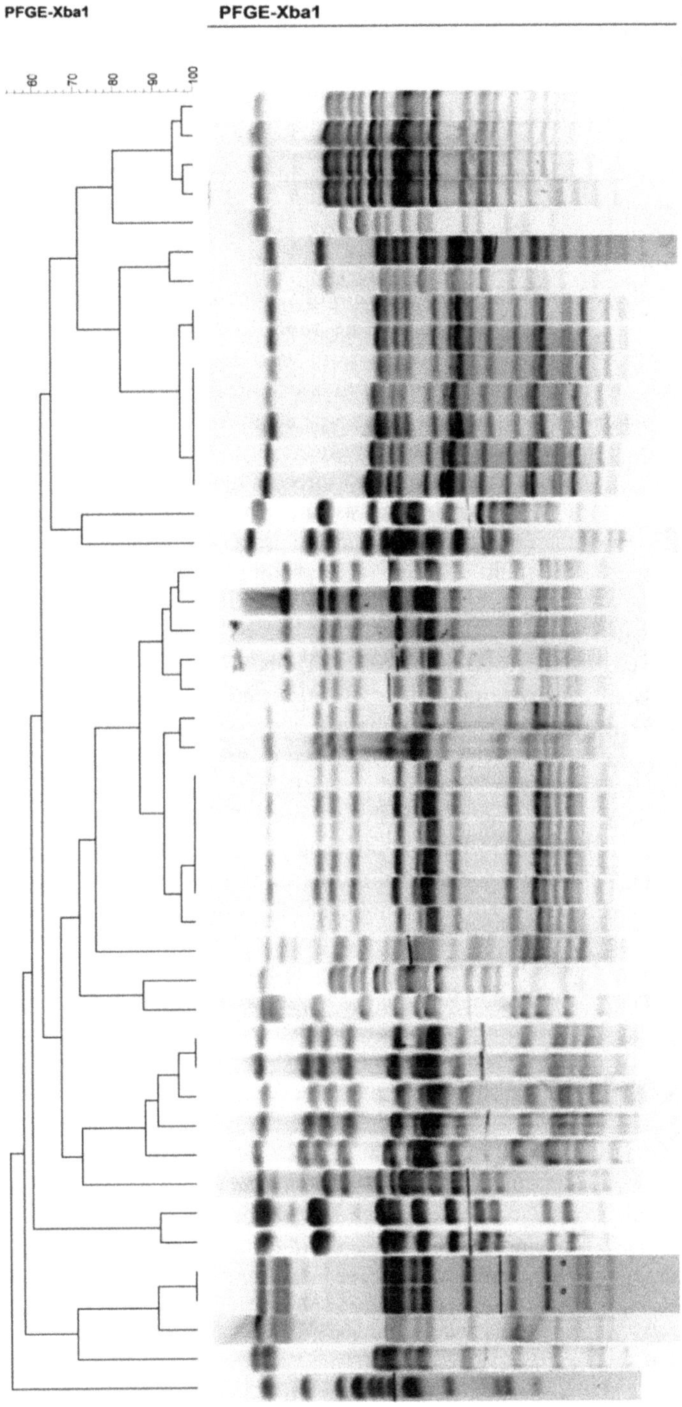

Strain	Serotype	Location	Origin	PFGE
XC48	Typhimurium	XC	C	A
XC87	Typhimurium	XC	C	A
XC134	Typhimurium	XC	C	A
XC164	Typhimurium	XC	C	A
SP129	Typhimurium	MM	P	B
HB73	Indiana	WH	C	C
PY12	Indiana	PY	C	C
CL129	Indiana	CL	C	D
CL189	Indiana	CL	C	D
CL108	Indiana	CL	C	D
CL135	Indiana	CL	C	D
CL140	Indiana	CL	C	D
CL146	Indiana	CL	C	D
JN186	Indiana	JN	C	D
MM62	Enteritidis	MM	C	E
SP131	Indiana	MM	P	F
SP103	Indiana	MM	P	G
SP96	Indiana	MM	P	G
SP85	Indiana	MM	P	G
SP108	Indiana	MM	P	G
SP110	Indiana	MM	P	G
K46	Indiana	YF	C	G
SP91	Indiana	MM	P	G
K13	Indiana	YF	C	G
K14	Indiana	YF	C	G
K17	Indiana	YF	C	G
K21	Indiana	YF	C	G
K47	Indiana	YF	C	G
K19	Indiana	YF	C	G
SP6	Typhimurium	MM	P	H
SP5	Typhimurium	MM	P	I
SP99	Typhimurium	MM	P	I
SP115	Indiana	MM	P	J
SP132	Indiana	MM	P	J
SP123	Indiana	MM	P	J
SP118	Indiana	MM	P	J
SP125	Indiana	MM	P	J
SP101	Typhimurium	MM	P	K
2002	Typhimurium	ZQ	P	L
2019	Typhimurium	ZQ	P	L
HB137	Indiana	WH	C	M
HB154	Indiana	WH	C	M
SG119	Indiana	SG	C	M
SG36	Indiana	SG	C	N
SP95	Indiana	MM	P	O

FIGURE 1 | Pulsed-field gel electrophoresis fingerprinting patterns of *Xba* I-digested total DNA preparations from *Salmonella isolates* harboring CTX-M-encoding genes.

Plasmid Characterization

Six transconjugants and 32 transformants were successfully obtained from 45 bla_{CTX-M}-positive isolates by conjugation/transformation experiments with frequencies of 10^{-8} to 10^{-3} per donor cell. PMQR genes were found to be co-transferred with bla_{CTX-M} genes in 26 (68.4%) transconjugants/transformants and the most common co-transferring pattern was bla_{CTX-M} +*aac(6')-Ib-cr* accounting for 13 of 26 transconjugants/transformants, bla_{CTX-M} +*oqxAB* and bla_{CTX-M} +*aac(6')-Ib-cr* +*oqxAB* accounting for eight and five transconjugants/transformants, respectively. For narrow-spectrum β-lactamases, bla_{SHV-1}, bla_{OXA-1}, and bla_{Tem-1b} were co-transferred with bla_{CTX-M} in 11, 2, and 1 isolates, respectively.

Plasmid replicon typing of transconjugants/transformants revealed that IncN, IncFIB, IncP, IncA/C, and IncHI2 were detected in 9, 6, 4, 4, and 3 transconjugants/transformants, respectively. Two plasmid replicons (IncN in combination with IncA/C) were simultaneously present in 2 CTX-M-14-producing transformants. Surprisingly, the replicon types could not be determined by PBRT in 14 transconjugants/transformants all of which carried the $bla_{CTX-M-27}$ gene (**Table 3**).

Southern blot hybridization suggested that the plasmid sizes of bla_{CTX-M} genes varied between 80 and 280 kb among which the 100 kb ($n = 17$) and 150 kb ($n = 13$) were the most common sizes. Interestingly, the size of all the 14 non-typeable $bla_{CTX-M-27}$ plasmids was ~100 kb.

Pulsed-Field Gel Electrophoresis (PFGE)

A total of 34 different PFGE profiles were obtained from the 45 bla_{CTX-M}-positive isolates (**Figure 1**). These could be grouped into 15 PFGE clusters designated A–O having 85% genetic similarity. Clusters G, D, J, and A accounted for 28.9, 15.6, 11.1, and 8.9% of the isolates, respectively. In addition, all isolates in each cluster had the same serotype and were also isolated from the same province (same or different cities). The exceptions were clusters C and M both of which were comprised of two isolates each from different provinces (Hubei, Henan, or Shan dong provinces).

In the most predominant cluster G, a high similarity of PFGE profiles of the isolates could be found and the isolates were recovered from pigs or chickens in two cities of Guangdong province. Seven isolates in this cluster were recovered from chickens and six were from pigs. In the remaining 14 PFGE clusters, isolates were all recovered from the same origin; either chickens or pigs.

DISCUSSION

In this study, we examined *Salmonella* isolates recovered from food-producing animals to determine their serotypes, antimicrobial susceptibility phenotypes, and genotypes. The results showed that *S. enterica* serovars Typhimurium and Indiana were the prevailing serotypes of *Salmonella* in pigs and chickens. Both serovars were resistant to multiple antimicrobials including ESCs and fluoroquinolones which are often antimicrobials of choice for treating salmonellosis. Resistance to cefotaxime could be explained by the presence of non-typeable and IncN/IncFIB/IncP/IncA/C/IncHI2 plasmids carrying $bla_{CTX-M-9G}$ genes. The high detection rate of PMQR determinants especially *aac(6')-Ib-cr* and *oqxAB* and mutations in QRDR of target genes made an important contribution to the non-wild type MICs of the fluoroquinolones.

Salmonella has various serotypes, and some serotypes may also relate to multidrug-resistant phenotypes (Meunier et al., 2002). The predominant serotypes change over time and differ from one geographical area to another. Additionally, a particular serovar can prevail and emerge within a region for a certain period while being completely absent in other regions. *S. enterica* serovar Indiana is rarely reported worldwide but there have been large-scale food poisoning outbreaks caused by this serotype in both the USA and Europe (Price and Carter, 1967; Campbell and Eckman, 1975). In China, little information about *S. enterica* serovar Indiana was available until this serotype was obtained from a food animal (Yan et al., 2010) and showed resistance to multiple antimicrobial agents. Following this, isolation of *S. enterica* serovar Indiana increased rapidly and it became more and more prevalent in China especially in isolates from veterinary clinics and animal foods. The characteristics of multidrug-resistant Indiana in China were also reported (Xia et al., 2009; Yang et al., 2010; Lu et al., 2014). In the present study, all of the 159 *Salmonella* isolates displayed resistance to three or more classes of antimicrobials, but serovar Indiana isolates showed higher resistance levels than serovar Typhimurium isolates. Our results indicate that the multi-resistant serotype Indiana along with Typhimurium isolates are of high prevalence among food-producing animals in China.

CTX-M type ESBLs have been widely reported globally for many years and there is a strong linkage between their emergence and increasing quinolone resistance in the Enterobacteriaceae (Lavilla et al., 2008). The co-existence or co-transfer of PMQR genes in ESBLs and especially in CTX-M-producing isolates has been also previously described (Liu et al., 2013; Jiang et al., 2014; Li et al., 2014; Yang et al., 2015). These may promote the development of multidrug-resistant isolates under selective pressure of the quinolone and/or cephalosporin (Liu et al., 2013). We found all CTX-M-encoding strains contained at least one PMQR genes especially the *aac(6')-Ib-cr and oqxAB* genes. These two PMQR genes have been shown to accelerate the development of fluoroquinolone resistance in *S. typhimurium* (Wong et al., 2014a) and were frequently co-transferred with bla_{CTX-M} genes. Previous reports showed that *aac(6')-Ib-cr* and *oqxAB* were also prevalent PMQR genes in *E. coli* isolates from humans, animals and the environment (Chen et al., 2012). In general, detection rates of PMQR genes in *Salmonella* were less than those observed in *E. coli*. However, these rates in *Salmonella* increased quickly in China especially *aac(6')-Ib-cr* and *oqxAB*. In the present study, 78.0 and 69.2% harbored *oqxAB* and *aac(6')-Ib-cr*, which is higher than levels previously reported in 2009–2010 (32.3%, 25.8%), 2007–2011(30.8%, 30.8%) and in 2012–2013 (31.7%, 36.5%) in China (Li et al., 2013; Jiang et al., 2014; Li et al., 2014). Our results may indicate that ESBL genes along with PMQR genes are increasing among *Salmonella* strains in China.

The CTX-M type β-lactamases are the most prevalent ESBLs among the Enterobacteriaceae recovered from both animals and humans worldwide (D'Andrea et al., 2013). The spread and characteristics of CTX-M type ESBLs producing pathogenic bacteria had been widely studied previously in China, but works seldom focused on food-borne *Salmonella*. In the present study, 60% of cefotaxime-resistant isolates produced CTX-M type ESBLs and three different CTX-M-9 group variants were detected among which the CTX-M-27 enzyme was the most dominant. Consistent with the results in this study, the CTX-M-27 enzyme was also the main type of ESBL in our previous study with *Salmonella* (Jiang et al., 2014) and we also previously found the CTX-M-27 was the only CTX-M-type ESBLs detected in *Salmonella* isolates of retail pork (unpublished data). However, only two reports were found about CTX-M-27-producing human clinical *Salmonella* strains. One study showed that CTX-M-27-producing isolates of *S. enterica* serotype Livingstone were the cause of a nosocomial outbreak in the neonatal ward, the other study showed $bla_{CTX-M-27}$ along with *oqxAB* on the IncHI2 plasmid which was similar to that of the strain CL189 in our study (Bouallegue-Godet et al., 2005; Wong et al., 2014b). Many reports suggested that CTX-M-14 and CTX-M-55 enzymes were the two most dominant types in *E. coli* obtained from food animals in China (Zheng et al., 2012; Rao et al., 2014). CTX-M-27 in *E. coli* was only sporadically detected in several reports (Liu et al., 2007; Lu et al., 2010; Ho et al., 2011; Ma et al., 2012; Zheng et al., 2012; Rao et al., 2014) among which two studies found its high presence in *E. coli* isolated from duck and environmental samples and aquatic sediment samples (Lu et al., 2010; Ma et al., 2012). Study on isolates from human beings and environmental samples suggested that most CTX-M-27-positive *E. coli* from different hospitals and from rivers and lakes belonged to the O25b-ST131-B2 or B2:ST131 which was strongly associated with potentially severe infections in both humans and animals (Matsumura et al., 2012; Zurfluh et al., 2013; Micenkova et al., 2014). The high prevalence of $bla_{CTX-M-27}$ in *Salmonella* obtained from food animals and in *E. coli* isolates from different sources (human beings, environment, and animals) should be a cause for concern which may be a potential threat to public health.

CTX-M-27 which was first found in a clinical isolate from a French hospital differed from its ancestor-CTX-M-14 only by the substitution D240G, but had significant higher hydrolytic activity against ceftazidime (Bonnet et al., 2003). Previous studies (Rao et al., 2014) suggested that CTX-M-1G-positive isolates had significantly higher resistance rates to cefquinome, ceftazidime, amikacin and fosfomycin when compared to the CTX-M-9G-positive isolates. These authors also compared the activity of different CTX-M variants on cephalosporin resistance and proved that CTX-M-1 group enzymes, especially CTX-M-55, have higher hydrolytic activities against cefquinome than CTX-M-9 group enzymes (except CTX-M-27). All the bla_{CTX-M} genes detected in this study belonged to CTX-M-9 group. When we analyzed the MICs of cephalosporin among different CTX-M-9G variants, we concluded that $bla_{CTX-M-27}$-positive isolates had a higher MIC for cephalosporin in particular to ceftazidime than that in CTX-M-14 and CTX-M-65-producing isolates. There were few differences in the resistance phenotypes of different variants of the CTX-M-9G family of β-lactamases isolates. This may also explain the prevalence of different variants.

In this study, 38 bla_{CTX-M}-positive transconjugants/transformants were obtained, among which 68.4% co-transferred bla_{CTX-M} with *aac(6')-Ib-cr* and/or *oqxAB*, indicating that these fluoroquinolone resistant determinants can be transferred horizontally simultaneous with the transfer of CTX-M-encoding genes. Characterization of bla_{CTX-M} plasmids in the transconjugants/transformants revealed that bla_{CTX-M} genes were located on plasmids of un-typeable and IncN/IncFIB/IncP/IncA/C/IncHI2 replicon types with different plasmid sizes. In particular, we observed that plasmids carrying $bla_{CTX-M-27}$ from epidemiologically unrelated strains (from different geographic regions and sources) had surprisingly similar properties (replicon types and sizes) indicating the presence of epidemic $bla_{CTX-M-27}$ plasmids in China. It's worth noting that the replicon types were untypeable using the current PBRT scheme in half (14/28) of the transconjugants/transformants carrying $bla_{CTX-M-27}$. Previous studies on $bla_{CTX-M-27}$ also found some plasmids could not be determined by PBRT (Ma et al., 2012). Therefore, there may be a new type of plasmid-carrying $bla_{CTX-M-27}$. We have sequenced two $bla_{CTX-M-27}$ plasmids from different sources to further study their characteristics (unpublished data).

Among the five detected plasmid replicons in present study, the IncP type plasmid carrying bla_{CTX-M} in *Salmonella* isolates was reported for the first time. In general, most bla_{CTX-M} genes can be horizontally transferred. Untypeable plasmids and IncN/IncFIB/IncP/IncA/C/IncHI2 plasmids can drive such increased dissemination in *Salmonella* isolates from food animals. To the best of our knowledge, the current study is also the first report about the spread of non-typeable or IncN/IncFIB/IncP/IncA/C/IncHI2 plasmids carrying bla_{CTX-M} genes in *S. enterica* serovars Typhimurium and Indiana isolated from pigs and chickens in China.

PFGE is a gold-standard for *Salmonella* subtyping and has been widely used to determine the relatedness of pathogens to confirm the outbreaks and trace the source of the isolates (White et al., 2007). Fifteen different PFGE clusters (85% genetic similarity) were obtained in this study and these represented a wide variety of genotypes. However, isolates recovered from the same or even different provinces in each identified serovars were highly genetically similar (cluster A, D, G, J and cluster C, M). These may have derived from a specific clone, so the horizontal transmission of the resistance plasmids along with clonal spread of resistant strains were both responsible for dissemination of $bla_{CTX-M-9G}$-positive strains.

All of the 45 $bla_{CTX-M-9G}$-positive *Salmonella* strains were isolated from food animals from different provinces. Therefore, humans can be infected through the consumption of food of animal origin (Thorns, 2000), accelerating the transmission of such *Salmonella* strains. Along with this, food animals trading may be an important source of *Salmonella* colonization as has been previously assumed (Wegener et al., 2003). Though studies proving definitive evidence of ESC-R bacterial transmission from food animals to humans are limited; differences can always be shown when comparing *Salmonella* isolates from humans and the animals. Importantly, previous studies have shown that the same IncN plasmids harboring bla_{CTX-M} are simultaneously present in isolates from pigs and farm workers (Moodley and Guardabassi, 2009). Therefore, further study monitoring and comparing antimicrobial susceptibility, serotypes and ESBL-producing *Salmonella* isolates from both veterinary settings (pets, wild animals, and livestock) and humans (communities and hospitals) in the same geographic region could lead to the discovery of dissemination routes.

CONCLUSION

Multi-drug resistant *S. enterica* serotype Typhimurium and Indiana and especially CTX-M-producing isolates were predominant among food-producing animals in China. Untypeable and IncN/IncFIB/IncP/IncA/C/IncHI2 resistant plasmids harboring bla_{CTX-M} genes and clonal spread of strains were both responsible for dissemination of resistant *Salmonella* isolates. The presence and spread of bla_{CTX-M}, especially the $bla_{CTX-M-27}$ on non-typeable plasmids in *Salmonella* isolates from food-producing animals may pose a potential threat for public health. Proper molecular approaches and hygienic practices are urgently needed to control the dissemination of resistant *Salmonella* strains through food chain. As ceftiofur and cefquinome have been widely used as therapeutic antibiotic in veterinary medicine, the third- and fourth-generation cephalosporins should be used more prudently in animal husbandry in China.

AUTHOR CONTRIBUTIONS

Conceived and designed the experiments: Z-LZ, H-XJ, and Y-HL. Performed the experiments: W-HZ, X-YL, LX, and X-XG. Analyzed the data: W-HZ and X-YL. Contributed reagents/materials/analysis tools: LY, WL, and S-QR. Wrote the paper: W-HZ and H-XJ.

ACKNOWLEDGMENT

This work was supported in-part by the National Natural Science Foundation of China (31272602) and 973 Program (2013CB127203).

REFERENCES

Alcaine, S. D., Soyer, Y., Warnick, L. D., Su, W. L., Sukhnanand, S., Richards, J., et al. (2006). Multilocus sequence typing supports the hypothesis that cow- and human-associated *Salmonella* isolates represent distinct and overlapping populations. *Appl. Environ. Microbiol.* 72, 7575–7585. doi: 10.1128/AEM.01174-06

Arlet, G., Barrett, T. J., Butaye, P., Cloeckaert, A., Mulvey, M. R., and White, D. G. (2006). *Salmonella* resistant to extended-spectrum cephalosporins: prevalence and epidemiology. *Microbes Infect.* 8, 1945–1954. doi: 10.1016/j.micinf.2005.12.029

Barton, B. M., Harding, G. P., and Zuccarelli, A. J. (1995). A general method for detecting and sizing large plasmids. *Anal. Biochem.* 226, 235–240. doi: 10.1006/abio.1995.1220

Bonnet, R., Recule, C., Baraduc, R., Chanal, C., Sirot, D., De Champs, C., et al. (2003). Effect of D240G substitution in a novel ESBL CTX-M-27. *J. Antimicrob. Chemother.* 52, 29–35. doi: 10.1093/jac/dkg256

Bouallegue-Godet, O., Ben, S. Y., Fabre, L., Demartin, M., Grimont, P. A., Mzoughi, R., et al. (2005). Nosocomial outbreak caused by *Salmonella enterica* serotype Livingstone producing CTX-M-27 extended-spectrum beta-lactamase in a neonatal unit in Sousse, Tunisia. *J. Clin. Microbiol.* 43, 1037–1044. doi: 10.1128/JCM.43.3.1037-1044.2005

Campbell, C. W., and Eckman, M. R. (1975). Acute acalculous cholecystitis caused by *Salmonella* Indiana. *JAMA* 233, 815. doi: 10.1001/jama.1975.03260070073030

Carattoli, A., Bertini, A., Villa, L., Falbo, V., Hopkins, K. L., and Threlfall, E. J. (2005). Identification of plasmids by PCR-based replicon typing. *J. Microbiol. Methods* 63, 219–228. doi: 10.1016/j.mimet.2005.03.018

Centers for Disease Control and Prevention (2013). *Trends in Foodborne Illness in the United States 2012.* Available at: http://www.cdc.gov/Features/dsfoodnet 2012/reportcard.html

Chen, X., Zhang, W., Pan, W., Yin, J., Pan, Z., Gao, S., et al. (2012). Prevalence of qnr, aac(6')-Ib-cr, qepA, and oqxAB in *Escherichia coli* isolates from humans, animals, and the environment. *Antimicrob. Agents Chemother.* 56, 3423–3427. doi: 10.1128/AAC.06191-11

Clinical and Laboratory Standards Institute [CLSI] (2013). *Performance Standards for Antimicrobial Disk and Dilution Susceptibility Tests for Bacteria Isolated from Animals; Approved Standard,* 4th Edn and supplement Documents VET 01-A4 and VET01-S2. (Wayne, PA: Clinical, and Laboratory Standards Institute).

Clinical and Laboratory Standards Institute [CLSI] (2015). *Performance Standards for Antimicrobial SusceptibilityTesting,* Twenty-fifth Informational Supplement. CLSI document M100-S25. Wayne, PA: Clinical and Laboratory Standards Institute.

D'Andrea, M. M., Arena, F., Pallecchi, L., and Rossolini, G. M. (2013). CTX-M-type beta-lactamases: a successful story of antibiotic resistance. *Int. J. Med. Microbiol.* 303, 305–317. doi: 10.1016/j.ijmm.2013.02.008

European Centre for Disease Prevention and Control (2013). *Annual epidemiological report Reporting on 2011 Surveillance Data and 2012 Epidemic Intelligence Data.* Stockholm: European Centre for Disease Prevention and Control, 103–108. Available at: http://ecdc.europa.eu/en/publications/_layouts/forms/Publication_DispForm.aspx?List=4f55ad51-4aed-4d32-b960-af70113dbb90&ID=989

Foley, S. L., and Lynne, A. M. (2008). Food animal-associated *Salmonella* challenges: pathogenicity and antimicrobial resistance. *J. Anim. Sci.* 86, E173–E187. doi: 10.2527/jas.2007-0447

Harrois, D., Breurec, S., Seck, A., Delaune, A., Le Hello, S., Pardos, D. L. G. M., et al. (2014). Prevalence and characterization of extended-spectrum beta-lactamase-producing clinical *Salmonella enterica* isolates in Dakar. Senegal, from 1999 to 2009. *Clin. Microbiol. Infect.* 20, O109–O116. doi: 10.1111/1469-0691.12339

Hendriksen, R. S., Mikoleit, M., Kornschober, C., Rickert, R. L., Duyne, S. V., Kjelso, C., et al. (2009). Emergence of multidrug-resistant *salmonella* concord infections in Europe and the United States in children adopted from Ethiopia, 2003–2007. *Pediatr. Infect. Dis. J.* 28, 814–818. doi: 10.1097/INF.0b013e3181a3aeac

Ho, P. L., Chow, K. H., Lai, E. L., Lo, W. U., Yeung, M. K., Chan, J., et al. (2011). Extensive dissemination of CTX-M-producing *Escherichia coli* with multidrug resistance to 'critically important' antibiotics among food animals in Hong Kong, 2008–2010. *J. Antimicrob. Chemother.* 66, 765–768. doi: 10.1093/jac/dkq539

Jiang, H. X., Song, L., Liu, J., Zhang, X. H., Ren, Y. N., Zhang, W. H., et al. (2014). Multiple transmissible genes encoding fluoroquinolone and third-generation cephalosporin resistance co-located in non-typhoidal *Salmonella* isolated from food-producing animals in China. *Int. J. Antimicrob. Agents* 43, 242–247. doi: 10.1016/j.ijantimicag.2013.12.005

Jiang, H. X., Tang, D., Liu, Y. H., Zhang, X. H., Zeng, Z. L., Xu, L., et al. (2012). Prevalence and characteristics of beta-lactamase and plasmid-mediated quinolone resistance genes in *Escherichia coli* isolated from farmed fish in China. *J. Antimicrob. Chemother.* 67, 2350–2353. doi: 10.1093/jac/dks250

Kuang, X., Hao, H., Dai, M., Wang, Y., Ahmad, I., Liu, Z., et al. (2015). Serotypes and antimicrobial susceptibility of *Salmonella* spp. isolated from farm animals in China. *Front. Microbiol.* 6:602. doi: 10.3389/fmicb.2015.00602

Lavilla, S., Gonzalez-Lopez, J. J., Sabate, M., Garcia-Fernandez, A., Larrosa, M. N., Bartolome, R. M., et al. (2008). Prevalence of qnr genes among extended-spectrum beta-lactamase-producing enterobacterial isolates in

Barcelona. *Spain. J. Antimicrob. Chemother.* 61, 291–295. doi: 10.1093/jac/dkm448

Li, L., Liao, X., Yang, Y., Sun, J., Li, L., Liu, B., et al. (2013). Spread of oqxAB in *Salmonella enterica* serotype Typhimurium predominantly by IncHI2 plasmids. *J. Antimicrob. Chemother.* 68, 2263–2268. doi: 10.1093/jac/dkt209

Li, L., Liao, X. P., Liu, Z. Z., Huang, T., Li, X., Sun, J., et al. (2014). Co-spread of oqxAB and blaCTX-M-9G in non-Typhi *Salmonella enterica* isolates mediated by ST2-IncHI2 plasmids. *Int. J. Antimicrob. Agents* 44, 263–268. doi: 10.1016/j.ijantimicag.2014.05.014

Li, R., Lai, J., Wang, Y., Liu, S., Li, Y., Liu, K., et al. (2013). Prevalence and characterization of *Salmonella* species isolated from pigs, ducks and chickens in Sichuan Province. *China. Int. J. Food Microbiol.* 163, 14–18. doi: 10.1016/j.ijfoodmicro.2013.01.020

Liebana, E., Carattoli, A., Coque, T. M., Hasman, H., Magiorakos, A. P., Mevius, D., et al. (2013). Public health risks of enterobacterial isolates producing extended-spectrum beta-lactamases or AmpC beta-lactamases in food and food-producing animals: an EU perspective of epidemiology, analytical methods, risk factors, and control options. *Clin. Infect. Dis.* 56, 1030–1037. doi: 10.1093/cid/cis1043

Liu, B. T., Yang, Q. E., Li, L., Sun, J., Liao, X. P., Fang, L. X., et al. (2013). Dissemination and characterization of plasmids carrying oqxAB-bla CTX-M genes in *Escherichia coli* isolates from food-producing animals. *PLoS ONE* 8:e73947. doi: 10.1371/journal.pone.0073947

Liu, J. H., Wei, S. Y., Ma, J. Y., Zeng, Z. L., Lu, D. H., Yang, G. X., et al. (2007). Detection and characterisation of CTX-M and CMY-2 beta-lactamases among *Escherichia coli* isolates from farm animals in Guangdong Province of China. *Int. J. Antimicrob. Agents* 29, 576–581. doi: 10.1016/j.ijantimicag.2006.12.015

Lu, S. Y., Zhang, Y. L., Geng, S. N., Li, T. Y., Ye, Z. M., Zhang, D. S., et al. (2010). High diversity of extended-spectrum beta-lactamase-producing bacteria in an urban river sediment habitat. *Appl. Environ. Microbiol.* 76, 5972–5976. doi: 10.1128/AEM.00711-10

Lu, Y., Zhao, H., Sun, J., Liu, Y., Zhou, X., Beier, R. C., et al. (2014). Characterization of multidrug-resistant *Salmonella enterica* serovars Indiana and Enteritidis from chickens in Eastern China. *PLoS ONE* 9:e96050. doi: 10.1371/journal.pone.0096050

Ma, J., Liu, J. H., Lv, L., Zong, Z., Sun, Y., Zheng, H., et al. (2012). Characterization of extended-spectrum beta-lactamase genes found among *Escherichia coli* isolates from duck and environmental samples obtained on a duck farm. *Appl. Environ. Microbiol.* 78, 3668–3673. doi: 10.1128/AEM.07507-11

Matsumura, Y., Yamamoto, M., Higuchi, T., Komori, T., Tsuboi, F., Hayashi, A., et al. (2012). Prevalence of plasmid-mediated AmpC beta-lactamase-producing *Escherichia coli* and spread of the ST131 clone among extended-spectrum beta-lactamase-producing E. *coli in Japan. Int. J. Antimicrob. Agents* 40, 158–162. doi: 10.1016/j.ijantimicag.2012.04.013

Meunier, D., Boyd, D., Mulvey, M. R., Baucheron, S., Mammina, C., Nastasi, A., et al. (2002). *Salmonella enterica* serotype Typhimurium DT 104 antibiotic resistance genomic island I in serotype paratyphi B. *Emerg. Infect. Dis.* 8, 430–433. doi: 10.3201/eid0804.010375

Micenkova, L., Siskova, P., Bosak, J., Jamborova, I., Cernohorska, L., and Smajs, D. (2014). Characterization of human uropathogenic ESBL-producing *Escherichia coli* in the Czech Republic: spread of CTX-M-27-producing strains in a university hospital. *Microb. Drug Resist.* 20, 610–617. doi: 10.1089/mdr.2014.0013

Moodley, A., and Guardabassi, L. (2009). Transmission of IncN plasmids carrying blaCTX-M-1 between commensal *Escherichia coli* in pigs and farm workers. *Antimicrob. Agents Chemother.* 53, 1709–1711. doi: 10.1128/AAC.01014-08

O'Regan, E., Quinn, T., Pages, J. M., McCusker, M., Piddock, L., and Fanning, S. (2009). Multiple regulatory pathways associated with high-level ciprofloxacin and multidrug resistance in *Salmonella enterica* serovar enteritidis: involvement of RamA and other global regulators. *Antimicrob. Agents Chemother.* 53, 1080–1087. doi: 10.1128/AAC.01005-08

Price, J. J., and Carter, H. J. (1967). An outbreak of gastroenteritis caused by *Salmonella* indiana. *Public Health Rep.* 82, 551–554. doi: 10.2307/4593068

Rahn, K., De Grandis, S. A., Clarke, R. C., McEwen, S. A., Galan, J. E., Ginocchio, C., et al. (1992). Amplification of an invA gene sequence of *Salmonella typhimurium* by polymerase chain reaction as a specific method of detection of *Salmonella*. *Mol. Cell. Probes* 6, 271–279. doi: 10.1016/0890-8508(92)90002-F

Rao, L., Lv, L., Zeng, Z., Chen, S., He, D., Chen, X., et al. (2014). Increasing prevalence of extended-spectrum cephalosporin-resistant *Escherichia coli* in food animals and the diversity of CTX-M genotypes during 2003-2012. *Vet. Microbiol.* 172, 534–541. doi: 10.1016/j.vetmic.2014.06.013

Stevens, M. P., Humphrey, T. J., and Maskell, D. J. (2009). Molecular insights into farm animal and zoonotic *Salmonella* infections. *Philos. Trans. R. Soc. Lond. B Biol. Sci.* 364, 2709–2723. doi: 10.1098/rstb.2009.0094

Strahilevitz, J., Jacoby, G. A., Hooper, D. C., and Robicsek, A. (2009). Plasmid-mediated quinolone resistance: a multifaceted threat. *Clin. Microbiol. Rev.* 22, 664–689. doi: 10.1128/CMR.00016-09

Sun, J., Ke, B., Huang, Y., He, D., Li, X., Liang, Z., et al. (2014). The molecular epidemiological characteristics and genetic diversity of *Salmonella typhimurium* in Guangdong, China, 2007-2011. *PLoS ONE* 9:e113145. doi: 10.1371/journal.pone.0113145

Thorns, C. J. (2000). Bacterial food-borne zoonoses. *Rev. Sci. Tech.* 19, 226–239.

Vo, A. T., van Duijkeren, E., Fluit, A. C., Heck, M. E., Verbruggen, A., Maas, H. M., et al. (2006). Distribution of *Salmonella enterica* serovars from humans, livestock and meat in Vietnam and the dominance of *Salmonella* Typhimurium phage type 90. *Vet. Microbiol.* 113, 153–158. doi: 10.1016/j.vetmic.2005.10.034

Wang, S., Duan, H., Zhang, W., and Li, J. W. (2007). Analysis of bacterial foodborne disease outbreaks in China between 1994 and 2005. *FEMS Immunol. Med. Microbiol.* 51, 8–13. doi: 10.1111/j.1574-695X.2007.00305.x

Wegener, H. C., Hald, T., Lo, F. W. D., Madsen, M., Korsgaard, H., Bager, F., et al. (2003). *Salmonella* control programs in Denmark. *Emerg. Infect. Dis.* 9, 774–780. doi: 10.3201/eid0907.030024

White, P. L., Naugle, A. L., Jackson, C. R., Fedorka-Cray, P. J., Rose, B. E., Pritchard, K. M., et al. (2007). *Salmonella* Enteritidis in meat, poultry, and pasteurized egg products regulated by the U.S. Food Safety and Inspection Service, 1998 through 2003. *J. Food Prot.* 70, 582–591.

Wong, M. H., Chan, E. W., Liu, L. Z., and Chen, S. (2014a). PMQR genes oqxAB and aac(6')Ib-cr accelerate the development of fluoroquinolone resistance in *Salmonella typhimurium*. *Front. Microbiol.* 5:521. doi: 10.3389/fmicb.2014.00521

Wong, M. H., Yan, M., Chan, E. W., Biao, K., and Chen, S. (2014b). Emergence of clinical *Salmonella enterica* serovar Typhimurium isolates with concurrent resistance to ciprofloxacin, ceftriaxone, and azithromycin. *Antimicrob. Agents Chemother.* 58, 3752–3756. doi: 10.1128/AAC.02770-13

Xia, S., Hendriksen, R. S., Xie, Z., Huang, L., Zhang, J., Guo, W., et al. (2009). Molecular characterization and antimicrobial susceptibility of *Salmonella* isolates from infections in humans in Henan Province, China. *J. Clin. Microbiol* 47, 401–409. doi: 10.1128/JCM.01099-08

Yan, H., Li, L., Alam, M. J., Shinoda, S., Miyoshi, S., and Shi, L. (2010). Prevalence and antimicrobial resistance of *Salmonella* in retail foods in northern China. *Int. J. Food Microbiol.* 143, 230–234. doi: 10.1016/j.ijfoodmicro.2010.07.034

Yang, B., Qu, D., Zhang, X., Shen, J., Cui, S., Shi, Y., et al. (2010). Prevalence and characterization of *Salmonella* serovars in retail meats of marketplace in Shaanxi. *China. Int. J. Food Microbiol.* 141, 63–72. doi: 10.1016/j.ijfoodmicro.2010.04.015

Yang, L., Yang, L., Lu, D. H., Zhang, W. H., Ren, S. Q., Liu, Y. H., et al. (2015). Co-prevalance of PMQR and 16S rRNA methylase genes in clinical *Escherichia coli* isolates with high diversity of CTX-M from diseased farmed pigeons. *Vet. Microbiol.* 178, 238–245. doi: 10.1016/j.vetmic.2015.05.009

Zhang, J., Jin, H., Hu, J., Yuan, Z., Shi, W., Ran, L., et al. (2014). Serovars and antimicrobial resistance of non-typhoidal *Salmonella* from human patients in Shanghai, China, 2006-2010. *Epidemiol. Infect.* 142, 826–832. doi: 10.1017/S0950268813001659

Zheng, H., Zeng, Z., Chen, S., Liu, Y., Yao, Q., Deng, Y., et al. (2012). Prevalence and characterisation of CTX-M beta-lactamases amongst *Escherichia coli* isolates from healthy food animals in China. *Int. J. Antimicrob. Agents* 39, 305–310. doi: 10.1016/j.ijantimicag.2011.12.001

Zurfluh, K., Hachler, H., Nuesch-Inderbinen, M., and Stephan, R. (2013). Characteristics of extended-spectrum beta-lactamase- and carbapenemase-producing *Enterobacteriaceae* Isolates from rivers and lakes in Switzerland. *Appl. Environ. Microbiol.* 79, 3021–3026. doi: 10.1128/AEM.00054-13

11

Serotypes and Antibiotic Susceptibility of *Streptococcus pneumoniae* Isolates from Invasive Pneumococcal Disease and Asymptomatic Carriage in a Pre-vaccination Period, in Algeria

Hanifa Ziane[1], *Vera Manageiro*[2,3]*, *Eugénia Ferreira*[2], *Inês B. Moura*[2], *Soumia Bektache*[1], *Mohamed Tazir*[1] *and Manuela Caniça*[2]

[1] *Service de Microbiologie Médicale, Centre Hospitalo-Universitaire Mustapha Bacha, Faculté de Médecine, Algiers, Algeria,* [2] *National Reference Laboratory of Antibiotic Resistances and Healthcare Associated Infections, Department of Infectious Diseases, National Institute of Health Doutor Ricardo Jorge, Lisbon, Portugal,* [3] *Centre for the Studies of Animal Science, Institute of Agrarian and Agri-Food Sciences and Technologies, University of Oporto, Oporto, Portugal*

***Correspondence:**
Vera Manageiro
vera.manageiro@insa.min-saude.pt

In Algeria, few data is available concerning the distribution of pneumococcal serotypes and respective antibiotic resistance for the current pre-vaccination period, which is a public health concern. We identified the most frequent *Streptococcus pneumoniae* serogroup/types implicated in invasive pneumococcal disease (IPD; $n = 80$) and carriage ($n = 138$) in Algerian children younger than 5 years old. Serogroup/types of 78 IPD isolates were identified by capsular typing using a sequential multiplex PCR. Overall, serotypes 14, 19F, 6B, 23F, 18C, 1, 5, 7F, 19A, and 3 (55% of PCV7 serotypes, 71.3% of PCV10, and 90% of PCV13) were identified. Additionally, 7.5% of the non-vaccine serotypes 6C, 9N/L, 20, 24F, 35B, and 35F, were observed. In the case of *S. pneumoniae* asymptomatic children carriers, the most common serogroup/types were 6B, 14, 19F, 23F, 4, 9V/A, 1, 19A, 6A, and 3 (42.7% of PCV7 serotypes, 44.2% of PCV10, and 58% of PCV13). For 6.1% of the cases co-colonization was detected. Serotypes 14, 1, 5, and 19A were more implicated in IPD ($p < 0.01$), whereas serotype 6A was exclusively isolated from carriers ($p < 0.01$). Deaths associated with IPD were related to serotypes 19A, 14, 18C, and one non-typeable isolate. Among IPD related to vaccine serotypes, the rates of penicillin non-susceptible isolates were higher in no meningitis cases (80%) than in meningitis (66.7%), with serotypes 14, 19A, 19F, and 23F presenting the highest MIC levels ($>2\mu g/ml$). Resistance to cefotaxime was higher in isolates from meningitis (40.5%); however, resistance to erythromycin and co-trimoxazole (>40%) was more pronounced in no-meningeal forms. Overall, our results showed that PCV13 conjugate vaccine would cover up to 90% of the circulating isolates associated with IPD in Algeria, highlighting the importance of monitoring the frequency of *S. pneumoniae* serogroups/types during pre- and post-vaccination periods.

Keywords: pneumococci serotype, antibiotic susceptibility, invasive disease, pneumococcal carriage, children, vaccine, Algeria

INTRODUCTION

Streptococcus pneumoniae remains the leading cause of bacterial infection among children worldwide, being the most common cause of bacterial pneumonia, and an important cause of meningitis and bacteremia. Approximately 800,000 deaths per year occur among children as a result of pneumococcal infection (Johnson et al., 2010). The management of pneumococcal infections has been aggravated by the rapid worldwide increase of resistance to penicillin and other antibiotics, mostly related to the misuse of these drugs in respiratory pathogens (Song et al., 2012; Ginsburg et al., 2013).

Despite the diversity of capsular types, comprising at least 98 distinct serotypes, only some variants are associated with invasive pneumococcal disease (IPD; Caierão et al., 2014; Richter et al., 2014).

Pneumococcal disease is frequently preceded by asymptomatic nasopharyngeal colonization, which can be quite high in early childhood (Bogaert et al., 2004; Miernyk et al., 2011; Satzke et al., 2013). It is generally agreed that most serotypes recovered from IPD are also frequently identified in colonized healthy children (Bogaert et al., 2004; Dias and Caniça, 2007). However, serotype prevalence can change according to age, geography, time, and antibiotic resistance, among other factors (Finland and Barnes, 1977; Hausdorff et al., 2005; Ingels et al., 2012). IPD has also been related to recent respiratory viral infection (Weinberger et al., 2014).

In some countries, the use of effective pneumococcal conjugate vaccines (PCVs) during infancy have contributed to reduce morbidity and mortality associated to IPD, as well as nasopharyngeal colonization by vaccine serotypes (Ghaffar et al., 2004; Millar et al., 2006; Tan, 2012). Despite the availability of these vaccines, pneumococcal infections remain a global problem due to the replacement of vaccine by non-vaccine serotypes, mostly associated with the emergence of multidrug resistant serotypes, such as the serotype 19A (Dias and Caniça, 2007; Dagan et al., 2009; Richter et al., 2014). Thus, due to the widespread phenomena of serotype replacement, PCVs have been substituted by higher valence pneumococcal vaccines (from PCV7 and PCV10 to PCV13) across the world, according with the recommendations of the Centers for Disease Control and Prevention (CDC, 2013).

The monitoring of antibiotic resistance trends and serotype distribution in the pre- and post-vaccination periods is essential to assess the dynamic change of epidemiology. This way, the impact of vaccines and antibiotic use control programmes should be evaluated across countries.

In this study, we analyzed the frequency of serotypes associated to IPD and *S. pneumoniae* asymptomatic carriage among children younger than 5 years old in Algeria, before the introduction of the pneumococcal vaccine, and correlated the isolates antibiotic susceptibility with vaccine serotypes .

MATERIALS AND METHODS

Bacterial Isolates

An overall of 218 *S. pneumoniae* isolates recovered from children <5 years old were collected and studied regarding the serotype. Briefly, 80 IPD isolates [children <1 year old ($n = 44$), 1–2 years old ($n = 20$), and 3–5 years old ($n = 16$)] were collected between the 1st January 2010 and the 31st December 2014. The isolates were recovered from routine microbiological cultures at Laboratory of Clinical Microbiology, at CHU Mustapha Bacha (LCM/CHU), Algiers, Algeria, and at cooperation laboratories in the north ($n = 50$), west ($n = 12$), south ($n = 2$), and northeast ($n = 16$) regions of the country that sent samples and/or isolates to LCM/CHU. Isolates were included if they were obtained from consecutive blood, and cerebrospinal, pleural, peritoneal, ascitic, bone, and joint fluids from patients with symptoms compatible with IPD. Only one isolate per patient was considered .

In addition, all nasopharyngeal cultures ($n = 130$) recovered at LCM/CHU between 2011 and in 2012, from asymptomatic children <5 years old were also included for serotyping evaluation. Each age group of <1 year, 1–2 years, and 3–5 years included 91, 20, and 27 *S. pneumoniae* isolates, respectively. Only one isolate per child was considered, except for eight cultures corresponding to carriers co-colonized with two pneumococcal serogroups/types (in a total of 138 isolates). Authorization for carriage study was approved by "The Direction de la Santé et de la Population de la Wilaya d'Alger," in Algeria.

Culture of sterile body fluids and nasopharyngeal samples at LCM/CHU was carried out by standard protocols. Pneumococcal isolates were identified using classic microbiological tests: colony morphology, optochin susceptibility, and bile solubility (**Figure 1**). Thirty seven *S. pneumoniae* isolates expressing different serogroups/types (1, 3, 4, 5, 6B, 6C, 7F, 7C, 8, 9V, 9N, 10A, 10F, 11A, 12F, 13, 14, 15A, 15B, 16F, 17F, 18C, 19F, 19A, 20, 21, 22F, 23A, 23B, 23F, 24F, 31, 33F, 34, 35A, 35B, and 35F), belonging to the collection of the National Reference Laboratory of Antibiotic Resistances and Healthcare Associated Infections, at National Institute of Health in Portugal, were also used as controls for serotype identification, as previously (Ziane et al., 2015).

DNA Extraction and Multiplex PCRs

To extract DNA from clinical and control *S. pneumoniae* isolates, several colonies were picked from the culture plates. DNA was extracted by the heat lysis method and stored at −20°C until further analysis. The serogroups, and whenever possible the serotypes, of 80 *S. pneumoniae* from IPD and of 138 recovered in asymptomatic carriers were determined by sequential multiplex groups (SMGs), as previously described (Ziane et al., 2015; **Figure 1**).

Quellung Serotyping

In addition to multiplex PCR (Ziane et al., 2015), serogroups/types of all the 80 invasive isolates were determined at LCM/CHU by Quellung reaction with specific type antiserum [Statens-Serum Institute]. Concerning the isolates recovered from carriers, only those determined as serotype 6A/B or as non-typeable by the multiplex PCR method, were characterized by Quellung reaction (**Figure 1**).

PCR Detection of Autolysin (*lytA*) Gene

A primer pair 5′-TCCAGCCTGTAGCCATTTCG-3′ and 5′-GCGGTTGAACTGATTGAAAG-3′ that specifically targeted a

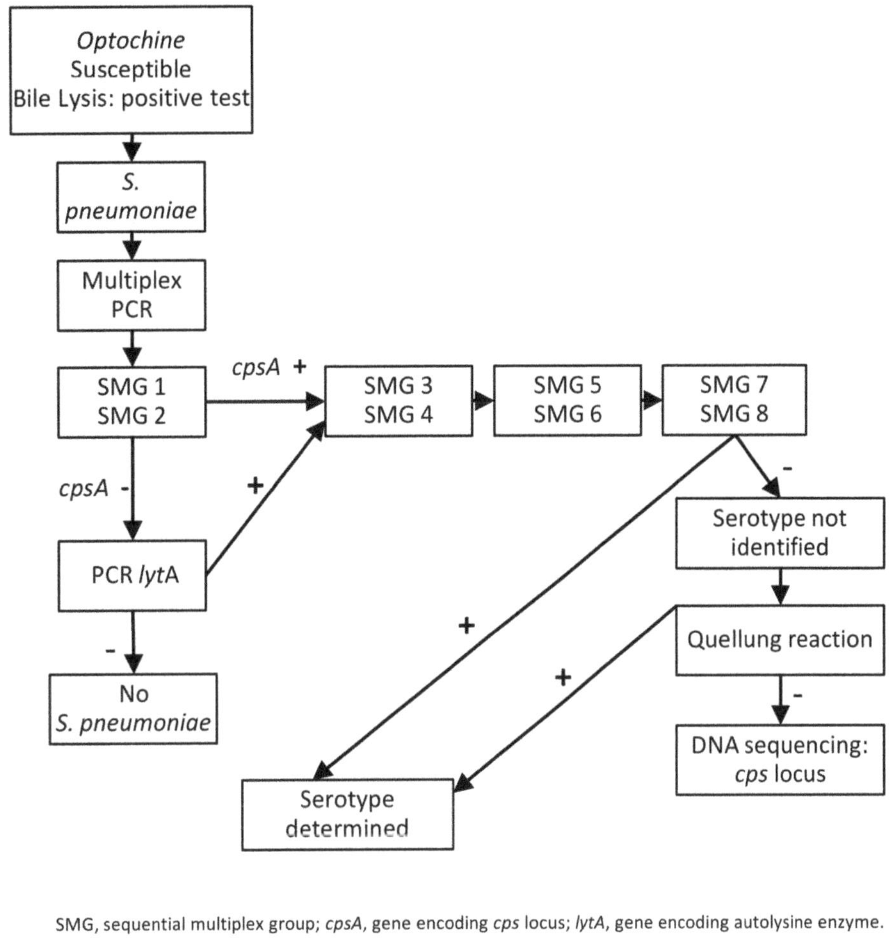

FIGURE 1 | Multiplex PCR scheme used in capsular typing of *S. pneumoniae* isolates from Algeria, and general scheme proposed for usual pneumococcal serotyping.

472 bp internal region of the autolysin (*lytA*) gene was used to the identification of *cps*-negative *S. pneumoniae*. The amplification conditions were: initial denaturation at 94°C for 5 min., followed by 30 cycles of denaturation at 94°C for 30 s, annealing at 56°C for 30 s and extension at 72°C for 30 s, and a final extension at 72°C for 5 min. Positive and negative controls were included in each PCR reaction.

Antibiotic Susceptibility Testing

Susceptibility testing of 72 IPD vaccine serotype isolates and of 8 IPD non-vaccine serotype was carried out by an agar disk diffusion method for four antibiotics (erythromycin, clindamycin, co-trimoxazole, tetracycline), and minimal inhibitory concentration (MIC) was determined using *E*-test method (AB Biodisk) for four β-lactam antibiotics (penicillin, amoxicillin, cefotaxime, and imipenem). Testing conditions and susceptibility interpretation followed the standards proposed by the Clinical and Laboratory Standards Institute (CLSI, 2014). *S. pneumoniae* ATCC 49619 was used as the quality control strain.

Statistical Analysis

OpenEpi software, version 3.03a (Dean et al., 2015), was used for statistical analysis. Fisher exact test was used to assess differences between IPD and carriers groups. One-tail $P \leq 0.05$ were considered to be statistically significant.

RESULTS

IPD Serogroup/Types

Between 2010 and 2014, a total of 207 episodes of IPD were registered at LCM/CHU. Among those, 80 (38.6%) corresponded to children <5 years old and were retained for this study. These 80 IPD cases (**Figure 2**) comprised 56.3% of occurrences in males and 43.7% in females, with 64 cases (80%) being reported to infants (≤2 years old). Overall, the serotypes were identified in 78 isolates, while two were non-typeable (**Table 1**).

Forty-eight (60%) of the total IPD episodes included cases of meningitis [of which 62.5% (30/48) were in infants <1 year old], while 40% (32/80) comprised cases of nonmeningitis [56.3% of

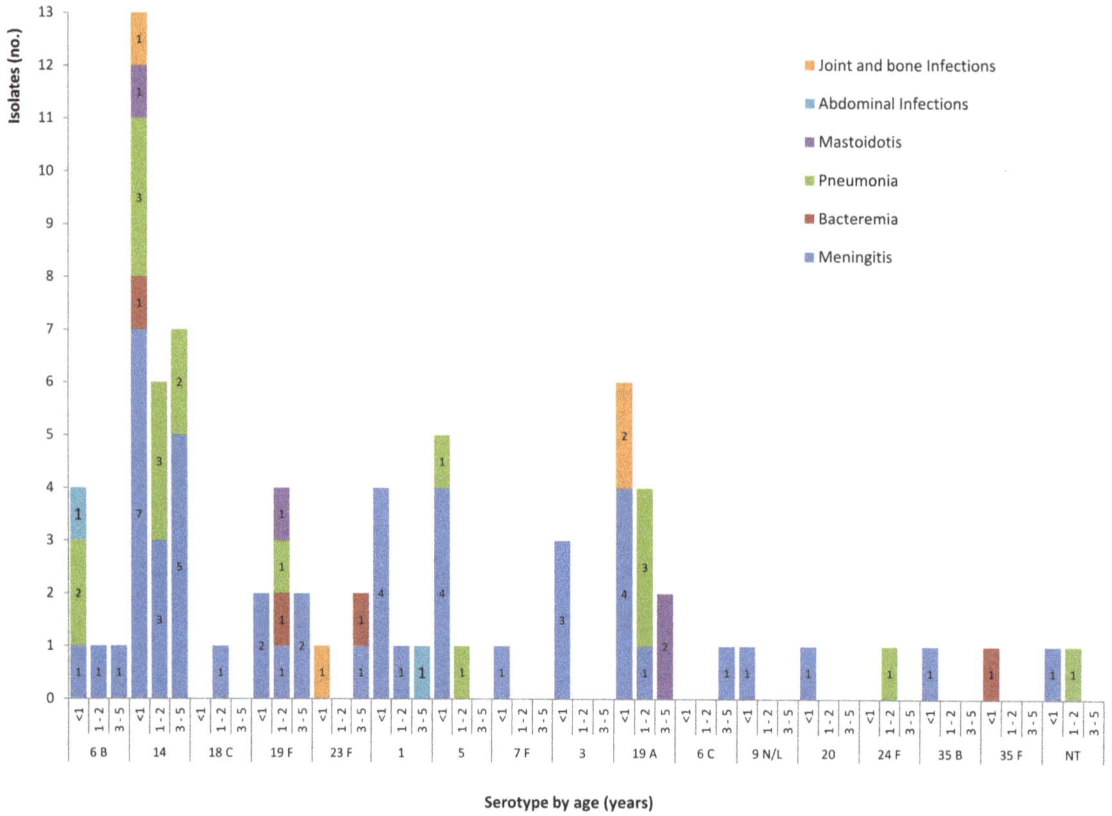

FIGURE 2 | Serogroup/types distribution and age groups in children under 5 years old according to clinical presentations of invasive pneumococcal disease (IPD) episodes. Abdominal infections, *S. pneumoniae* was isolated from ascitic and peritoneal fluids; NT, non-typeable.

which were pleuropneumonia (18/32), including 55.5% (10/18) in infants from 1 to 2 of age; **Figure 2**]. The most frequent serotypes implicated in IPD in this study, which accounted for 87.5% (70/80) of the tested isolates, were in decreasing frequency (**Figure 3**): 14, 19A, 19F, and 1 (from 0 to 5 years old), 5 (from 0 to 2 years old), 6B (from 0 to 5 years old), 3 (from <1 year old), and 23F (from <1 year, and from 3 to 5 years old). Serotypes 14, 1, 19A, 19F, 5, 3, and 6B were the most common in meningitis cases. However, serotypes 14, 19A, 5, and 6B were also implicated in pleuropneumonia, and 19A, 19F, and 14 in bacteremia (**Figure 2**).

Deaths caused by *S. pneumoniae* infection were noticed in 7 IPD cases (7/80, 8.8%) associated with meningitis (6/7, 85.7%), and pneumonia (1/7, 14.3%). Serotypes 19A and 14 were cause of death in 3 (42.8%), and 2 (28.6%) cases, respectively. The two remaining death cases were caused by serotype 18C, and one non-typeable isolate.

A total of 44 pneumococcal isolates expressed the serotypes included in PCV7, which would reflect the coverage of 55% (44/80) (**Figure 4**; **Table 1**). The coverage of PCV10 would be of 71.3% (57/80), because there were 13 isolates expressing serotypes 1 (6/57, 10.5%), 5 (6/57, 10.5%), and 7F (1/57, 1.8%). The coverage of PCV13 would reach up to 90% (72/80) (**Figure 4**, **Table 1**). All PCVs would cover the three age groups included in the study. Non-vaccine serogroup/types were expressed in 7.5% (6/80) with one isolate of each: 6C/D, 9N/L, 20, 24F, 35B, and 35F.

Serogroup/Types Characterization of Nasopharyngeal Isolates

The serogroup/type of 138 isolates, identified in 130 nasopharyngeal cultures from colonized children <5 years old, was determined by multiplex PCR method, using the same scheme as for IPD isolates (**Figure 1**): 117 (83.6%) *S. pneumoniae* were characterized at the serogroup/type level [101 (86.3%) children carried a single serogroup/type, whereas eight children (8/132, 6.1%) were co-colonized with pneumococci belonging to two different serogroup/types]. Furthermore, of the 18 isolates that remained non-typeable by multiplex PCR reactions, 3 were assigned to serogroup/type 15, 19A, and 20 by the Quellung reaction (**Table 1**). Serogroup 6A/B was differentiated by Quellung reaction into serotype 6B ($n = 16$) and serotype 6A ($n = 13$).

The most common serogroup/type was 6 ($n = 31$) [divided in 6A ($n = 13$), 6B ($n = 16$) (both included in PCV13 and PCV7, respectively), and 6C/D ($n = 2$)]; it was followed by serogroup/type 14 ($n = 13$), 19F ($n = 12$), and 23F ($n = 11$; **Figure 4**; **Table 1**). All these four serogroup/types were identified in the three age groups defined: <1 year, 1–2 years, and 3–5 years (**Figure 3**). The remaining conjugate vaccine serotypes identified in asymptomatic children carriers of *S. pneumoniae* included 19A ($n = 5$), 4 ($n = 4$), 9V/A ($n = 3$), 1 ($n = 2$), and 3 ($n = 1$). Non-conjugate vaccine serotypes accounted for

TABLE 1 | *S. pneumoniae* conjugate vaccines PCV7, PCV10, and PCV13 and non conjugate vaccine serotypes implicated in IPD cases and in nasopharyngeal carriage, according to the age groups.

Serotypes/Age(years)	IPD				Nasopharyngeal carriage				Global total	*P*-value[a]
	<1	1–2	3–5	Total	<1	1–2	3–5	Total		
PCV7 SEROTYPES										
4					1	1	2	4	4	0.161
6 B	4	1	1	6	12	2	2	16	22	0.245
9V/A						1	2	3	3	0.256
14	13	6	7	26	4	4	5	13	39	<0.01
18 C		1		1					1	0.364
19 F	2	4	2	8	6	5	1	12	20	0.449
23 F	1		2	3	8	1	2	11	14	0.182
Subtotal	20	12	12	44	31	14	14	59	103	0.045
ADDITIONAL PCV10 SEROTYPES										
1	4	1	1	6	2			2	8	0.028
5	5	1		6					6	<0.01
7 F	1			1					1	0.364
Subtotal	10	2	1	13	2			2	15	<0.01
ADDITIONAL PCV13 SEROTYPES										
3	3			3			1	1	4	0.138
6A					11	1	1	13	13	<0.01
19 A	6	4	2	12	5[b]			5[b]	17	<0.01
Subtotal	9	4	2	15	16	1	2	19	34	0.203
NON CONJUGATE VACCINE SEROTYPES										
6 C			1	1	1		1	2	3	0.700
8							1	1	1	0.636
9 N/L	1			1					1	0.364
10A					1			1	1	0.636
11A/D					3			3	3	0.256
15							1[c]	1[c]	1	0.636
15 A/F					3	1	2	6	6	0.064
15B/C					5			5	5	0.116
16F					1			1	1	0.636
17F					1			1	1	0.636
20	1			1	1[c]			1[c]	2	0.700
23A					1	1		2	2	0.404
23B					3		1	4	4	0.161
24 F		1		1	1		1	2	3	0.700
33F/A/37					1			1	1	0.636
34					4		1	5	5	0.116
35 B	1			1	3		1	4	5	0.401
35 F	1			1					1	0.364
Subtotal	4	1	1	6	29	2	9	40	46	<0.01
Total Typeable	43	19	16	78	78	17	25	120	198	<0.01
Non typeable	1	1		2	13	3	2	18	20[d]	<0.01
Global Total	44	20	16	80	91	20	27	138	218	

[a]*One-tail P ≤ 0.05 were considered to be statistically significant.*
[b]*Four isolates were serotyped by Multiplex PCR and one was serotyped by Quellung reaction.*
[c]*Isolates serotyped only by Quellung reaction.*
[d]*Three Multiplex PCR non-typeable isolates were serotyped only by Quellung reaction (serotypes 19A[b], 15[c], and 20[c]).*

29% (40/138), identified by both PCR ($n = 38$) and Quellung reaction ($n = 2$). These serotypes were mostly identified as 15A/F, 15B/C, 34, 23B, 35B, and 11A/D. Globally, the section of the study that included the carrier patients allowed the identification of 120 isolates at serogroup/type level, and the evaluation of 18 non-typeable isolates.

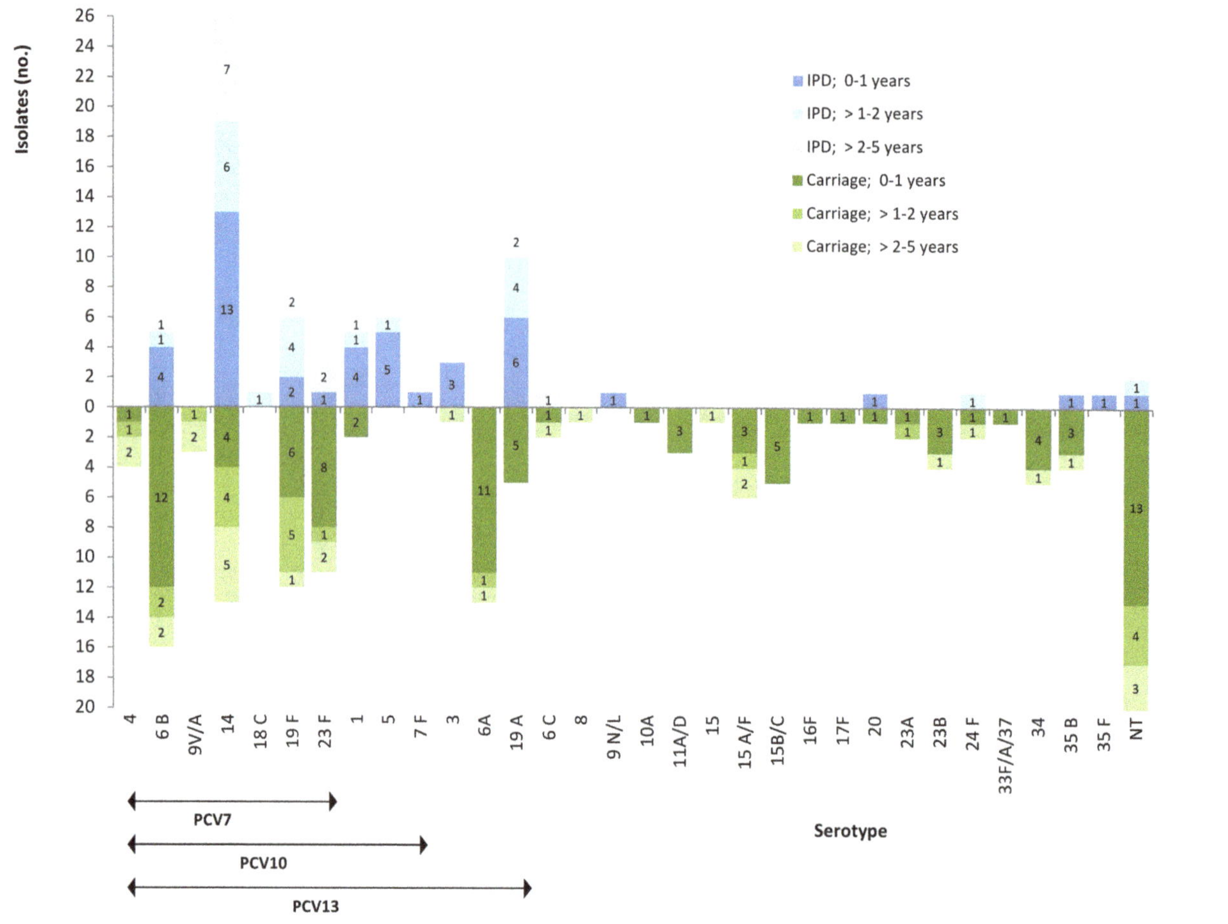

FIGURE 3 | Distribution of serogroup/types and pneumococcal conjugate vaccine (PCV) coverage for invasive pneumococcal disease (IPD) (n = 80) and nasopharyngeal (n = 140) isolates in children aged 5 years and less, shown by age group. NT, non-typeable.

Overall, 4.1% (09/218) of the isolates lacked the *cpsA* gene. However, the presence of the *lytA* gene confirmed the identification of *S. pneumoniae* specie. In addition, the sequential multiplex PCR scheme (**Figure 1**) used in our study demonstrated a specific identification of each serogroup/type in 90.8% (198/218) of the isolates analyzed: among the 80 IPD and the 138 nasopharyngeal *S. pneumoniae* isolates, 97.5% (78/80) and 86.9% (120/138) were positively serotyped by sequential multiplex PCR, respectively ($p < 0.01$; **Table 1**).

Antibiotic Susceptibility and Vaccine Serotype

Among *S. pneumoniae* vaccine serotypes (n = 72) from meningitis (n = 39) we identified 66.7% isolates penicillin non-susceptible (MIC ≥ 0.12 μg/ml) with 25.6% showing high level of resistance (MIC 2–4 μg/ml; **Table 2**). Isolates non-susceptible to cefotaxime and imipenem corresponded to 40.5 and 43.2%, respectively. However, high level of resistance was noticed for imipenem only in 5.4% isolates.

From no meningitis infections (n = 25), 80% of the isolates were penicillin non-susceptible with 12% of high level of resistance (MIC = 4–8 μg/ml). Intermediate resistance to amoxicillin and cefotaxime was 9.1 and 8.3%, respectively. High level of resistance to amoxicillin was observed in 4.5% isolates (MIC 8 μg/ml).

Non-susceptibility to erythromycin, clindamycin, co-trimoxazole, and tetracycline occurred in lower frequencies in isolates from meningitis (42.5, 40, 53.8, and 27.2%, respectively) than in isolates from no meningitis infections (74.1, 66.7, 75, and 46.2%, respectively).

High level of resistance for vaccine serotypes was observed in serotypes 14, 19A, 19F, and 23F. Overall, the vaccine serotypes 14, 19A, 19F, 23F, 6B, and 5 presented higher rates of resistance (90–100%) than the eight non-vaccine serotypes (6C, 9N, 20, 24F, 35B, 35F, non-typable; $p < 0.05$; data not shown).

DISCUSSION

S. pneumoniae remains the leading cause of bacterial infection among children worldwide, including numerous cases of invasive disease associated high morbidity and mortality rates (Harboe et al., 2010; Adegbola et al., 2014). The pneumococcal

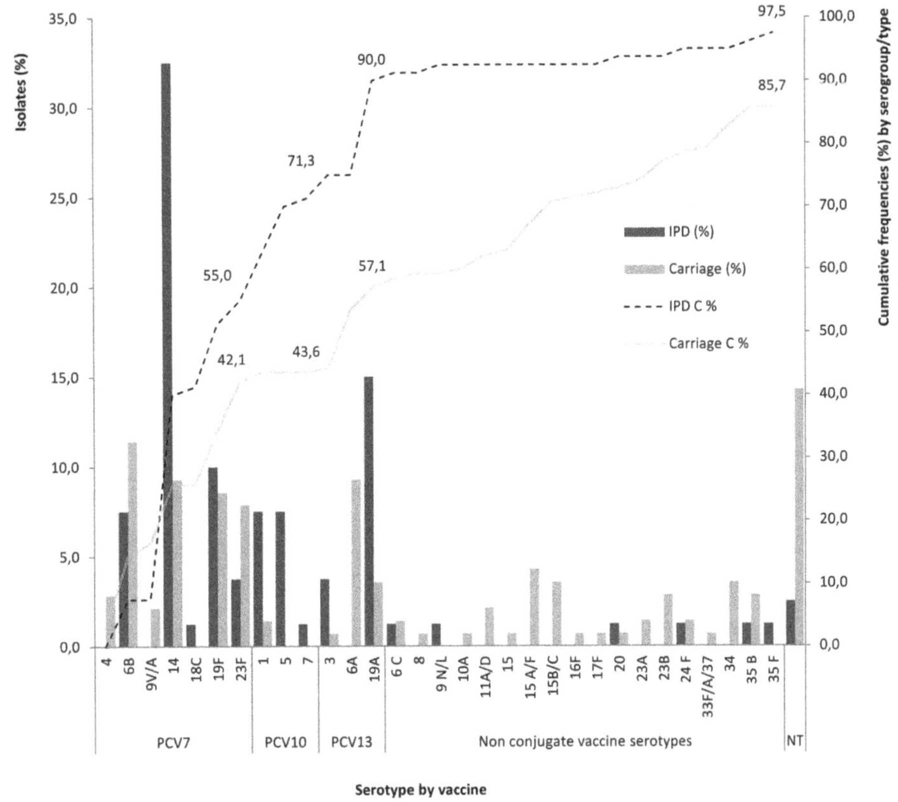

FIGURE 1 | Rate of serogroup/type cumulative coverage (C %) in each conjugate vaccine (PCV7, PCV10, PCV13) for *S. pneumoniae* recovered from invasive pneumococcal disease (IPD) and asymptomatic carriers less than 5 years old, from Algeria. NT, non-typeable.

epidemiology regarding capsular types and antibiotic resistance varies geographically and temporally in terms of origin of the isolates (infections or carriage), clinical presentation, pathogenicity (Hausdorff et al., 2005; Harboe et al., 2010; Ingels et al., 2012; Geno et al., 2015), and the methods used for serotyping (Turner et al., 2011; Song et al., 2012; Geno et al., 2015). Although antibiotic susceptibility and serotype data remains insufficient in many countries such as Algeria, its collection and evaluation is essential for the treatment of pneumococcal infections and for the usage of conjugate vaccines (Ramdani-Bouguessa and Rahal, 2003; Tali-Maamar et al., 2012; Ziane et al., 2012; Ramdani-Bouguessa et al., 2015).

Thus, the main goal of this study was to analyze the frequency of serotypes associated to IPD and *S. pneumoniae* asymptomatic carriage in Algeria, in children <5 years old before the introduction of the pneumococcal vaccine. To accomplish our purpose, we used the more recent IPD samples studied in the country (Ramdani-Bouguessa and Rahal, 2003; Tali-Maamar et al., 2012; Ziane et al., 2012; Ramdani-Bouguessa et al., 2015). It is worth mentioning that a molecular approach was here applied for the first time to isolates recovered in this country in the context of a monitoring survey of *S. pneumoniae* serogroup/types (Ziane et al., 2015).

In this study, meningitis represented 60% of the clinical presentation of IPD, with 79.2% registered in children younger than 2 years old. Pleuropneumonia was reported in 22.5% of the total IPD cases, with the majority being manifested in infants (88.8%, 16/18). Differently from bacteremia, mastoiditis, and abdominal infections, the bone and joint infections were noted exclusively in infants with up to 1 year old. Indeed, IPD occurs mostly in children under the age of 5 years, especially within the subgroup of those under 2 years of age (Tan, 2012). The prevalence of *S. pneumoniae* carriage in healthy children younger than 5 years old can fluctuate between 20 and 93.4% in low income countries, being superior than what is stated for lower-middle income countries (from 6.5 to 69.8%), as reported by Adegbola et al. (2014). In addition, the density of pneumococcal nasopharyngeal carriage seems to decrease in higher age groups, with the children being more competent than adults in the transmission of pneumococci (Roca et al., 2012).

Mortality rate of pneumococcal invasive diseases may range from 10 to 30%, according with the studies of Pebody et al. (2006), and Bravo (2009). Although it has been reported that the highest *S. pneumoniae*-associated morbidity and mortality rates are in Africa and Asia (Johnson et al., 2010; Turner et al., 2011), in our study the case fatality was 8.8%, mainly comprising meningitis related with vaccine serotypes (85.7%).

Overall, we identified serogroups 14, 19, 23, and 6 as the most common among IPD and nasopharyngeal carriers (**Figure 2**).

TABLE 2 | Antibiotic susceptibility of 72 isolates of vaccine serotypes[a], according to site infection.

Antibiotic[b, c] site of infection	Antibiotic susceptibility (%)				Total no. of isolates ($n = 72$)	Breakpoint[b, c] (CLSI, 2014)	
	S	I	R	IR		S≤	R≥
PENICILLIN G							
Meningitis	33.3	–	66.7	66.7	39	0.06	0.12
PARENTERAL PENICILLIN PG							
No meningitis	88.0	8.0	4.0	12.0	25	2	8
ORAL PENICILLIN							
No meningitis	20.0	32.0	48.0	80.0	25	0.06	2
AMOXICILLIN							
No meningitis	86.4	9.1	4.5	13.6	22	2	8
CEFOTAXIME							
Meningitis	59.5	40.5	0.0	40.5	37	0.5	2
No meningitis	91.7	8.3	0.0	8.3	24	1	4
IMIPENEM							
Meningitis	56.8	37.8	5.4	43.2	37	0.12	1
ERYTHROMYCIN							
Meningitis	57.5	0.0	42.5	42.5	40	≥21	≤15
No meningitis	25.9	0.0	74.1	74.1	27	≥21	≤15
CLINDAMYCIN							
Meningitis	60.0	0.0	40.0	40.0	40	≥19	≤15
No meningitis	33.3	0.0	66.7	66.7	27	≥19	≤15
CO-TRIMOXAZOLE							
Meningitis	46.2	2.6	51.2	53.8	39	≥19	≤15
No meningitis	25.0	0.0	75.0	75.0	24	≥19	≤15
TETRACYCLINE							
Meningitis	71.8	2.6	25.6	27.2	39	≥28	≤24
No meningitis	57.7	3.8	42.3	46.2	26	≥28	≤24

[a] *Includes serogroups/types: 1 ($n = 6$), 3 ($n = 3$), 5 ($n = 6$), 6B ($n = 6$), 7 ($n = 1$), 14 ($n = 26$), 18C ($n = 1$), 19A ($n = 12$), 19F ($n = 8$), and 23F ($n = 3$).*
[b] *Susceptibility testing by E-test method (MIC determination), for penicillin, amoxicillin, cefotaxime, and imipenem.*
[c] *Susceptibility testing by agar disk diffusion method, for erythromycin, clindamycin, co-trimoxazole, tetracycline.*
S, Susceptible; I, Intermediate; R, resistant; IR, non-susceptible.

Among IPD isolates, serotypes 14, 19A, 19F, 6B, 1, and 5 were the most frequent, which shows some differences from data described for other periods in Algeria. For instance, the serogroups/types 1 and 5 were the most common for the period of 1996–2000 (Ramdani-Bouguessa and Rahal, 2003), the serogroups/types 14, 19F, 23F, and 6B for the periods of 2001–2010 and 2005–2011 (Tali-Maamar et al., 2012; Hecini-Hannachi et al., 2014), and serogroups/types 14, 19F, 6B, 1, and 19A for the period of 2005–2012 (Ramdani-Bouguessa et al., 2015). In Tunisia, the most prevalent serogroups for IPD in children were nearly the same: 19, 14, 23, and 4 (Charfi et al., 2012). Internationally, among the 98 known pneumococcal serotypes 11 of them account for more than 70% of IPD, in children younger than 5 years old, with serotypes 1, 5, 6A, 6B, 14, 19F, 23F being the most common (Johnson et al., 2010). Indeed, it has been described that a restricted number of serotypes is in the origin of the majority of the IPD cases worldwide. To summarize, since the report of the first studies concerning the distribution of IPD serotypes in Algeria, there was an emergence of serotype 19A, which is one of most common causes of invasive disease in developed countries in children (Geno et al., 2015). Furthermore, the studied isolates expressing serotype 19A were assigned to ST276 (M. Caniça, personal communication), which is one of the most predominant sequence-types within this serotype (Reinert et al., 2010; Ramos et al., 2014).

Some of the *S. pneumoniae* serotypes are more prone to successfully colonize the nasopharynx, being in advantage to cause invasive disease. The carriage of *S. pneumoniae* may play an important role in the pathogenesis of IPD and in the transmission of this bacterium (Roca et al., 2012). Indeed, vaccination often brings a decrease in the reduction of vaccine serotype *S. pneumoniae* isolates, and a raise in carriage of non-vaccine serotype isolates (Dias and Caniça, 2007).

In this study, it is essential not only to emphasize the differences in serotype distribution (in IPD and asymptomatic carriage), but also to consider the presence of non-vaccine types (such as 15, 35B, and 34), particularly in carriage, despite the unavailability of pneumococcal vaccines in Algeria (**Figure 2**). Thus, when comparing serotype rate for IPD and nasopharyngeal carriage, serotypes 14, 1, 5, and 19A were more implicated in IPD than in carriage ($p < 0.01$), whereas serotype 6A was exclusively isolated from carriers ($p < 0.01$; **Table 2**).

Non-typeable isolates by PCR methods should be typed by Quellung reaction in order to monitor and detect the emergence of *S. pneumoniae* serotype variants, and if this test is negative, the isolates should be sequenced for the *cps* locus to characterize variants (Bentley et al., 2006). In fact, the *cpsA* gene is common within most encapsulated *S. pneumoniae*, being a highly conserved region of the *cps* locus in all known pneumococcal *cps* operons (Bentley et al., 2006; Pai et al., 2006; Jin et al., 2009). However, the absence of *cpsA* amplification in the multiplex PCR scheme has been reported among rough strains, and pneumococci with mutated capsular genes, or without the *cps* locus (Pai et al., 2006; Ahn et al., 2012; Richter et al., 2013). Previous studies have also reported absence of *cpsA* gene by PCR-based serotyping of *S. pneumoniae* in 1–3% of the cases, particularly among serotypes 38 and 25F (da Gloria Carvalho et al., 2010; Jourdain et al., 2011). In this study, 4.1% of the isolates lacked the *cpsA* gene.

Among the *cpsA* negative isolates, the detection of the *lytA* gene resolved the *S. pneumoniae* specie (Moreno et al., 2005). Thus, we propose the scheme in **Figure 1** for pneumococcal serotyping that will extend the application of multiplex PCR in laboratories, and concentrate the use of conventional method in reference laboratories only.

Similarly to other countries (Flasche et al., 2011; Ahn et al., 2012; Steens et al., 2013; von Gottberg et al., 2014), we noticed in Algeria an increase of serotypes covered by the different PCVs, particularly among IPD (**Figure 4**). These new data suggests an increase in the frequency of serotypes included in PCV13 in Algeria, in comparison with the 74.2% registered between 2005 and 2011 (Hecini-Hannachi et al., 2014), but similar to what was observed from 2005 to June 2012 (86.8%; Ramdani-Bouguessa et al., 2015).

Concerning the antibiotic resistance of *S. pneumoniae* from vaccine serotypes, the rates obtained were higher in no meningitis infections probably due to the large use of these antibiotics in the treatment of respiratory or urinary tract infections in Algeria. Tetracycline resistance rate might be explained by a lesser use of this antibiotic.

Rates of *S. pneumoniae* non-susceptible to penicillin vary in the country according to the study periods. Therefore, Algerian studies reported 34.6% of penicillin non-susceptible *S. pneumoniae* in 2003 (Ramdani-Bouguessa and Rahal, 2003), 25.2% in 2001–2010, mostly from meningitis, and 4.4% of high level resistance to cefotaxime (Tali-Maamar et al., 2012). A later study, conducted on invasive and non-invasive pneumococcal disease in children, identified 48% of penicillin non-susceptible isolates, mainly in no meningeal infections (Ramdani-Bouguessa et al., 2015). Rates of 48.5% and 45% have been reported in Morocco and Tunisia, respectively (Charfi et al., 2012; Elmdaghri et al., 2012).

In our study, the decreased susceptibility to penicillin is significantly associated with both vaccine serotypes and non-vaccine serotypes ($p < 0.05$; data not shown), but the vaccine serotypes 14, 19A, 19F, and 23F, showed the highest levels of penicillin resistance (MIC Peni G > 2μg/ml). These data is in agreement to earlier reports from Algeria (Ramdani-Bouguessa and Rahal, 2003; Hecini-Hannachi et al., 2014), Tunisia (Charfi et al., 2012), Morocco, (Elmdaghri et al., 2010), and France (Varon, 2012), where the serotypes 14, 19F, 23F, 6B were described as the most resistant. However, in France, after the introduction of PCV13, the serotypes 19A, 19F, 15A, 35B, and 24F emerged as those with higher resistance (Varon et al., 2015).

The fluctuations of *S. pneumoniae* circulating serotypes and its relation with antibiotic resistance and the PCVs coverage, reinforces the importance of *S. pneumoniae* serogroup/type identification and studies of antibiotic susceptibility, in pre- and post-vaccination periods, particularly in countries with few data, such as Algeria. These will help guide the treatment and will motivate the implementation of strategies for prevention of pneumococcal disease.

AUTHOR CONTRIBUTIONS

HZ designed the study, performed experiments, analyzed the data, and wrote the manuscript. VM analyzed the data and reviewed the manuscript. EF performed experiments and reviewed the manuscript. IM performed experiments and reviewed the manuscript. SB performed experiments. MT reviewed the manuscript. MC designed the study, analyzed the data and reviewed the manuscript. All authors read and approved the final manuscript.

ACKNOWLEDGMENTS

The authors thank D. Jones-Dias for her suggestions for the manuscript. Additionally, the authors thank to R. Touati, F. Z. Iles, N. Abdelaziz, S. Benada, N. Haddadi, and A. Mertani, for their technical assistance and support during the study. The authors also thank to all collaborators in the north, western, south and northeast regions of the country who sent isolates to LCM/CHU (S. Bekhoucha, S. Zouagui, Z. Guechi, S. Mahrane, A. Azzam, D. Haouchine, L. Oussadou, D. Touati, S. Azzoug, M. Naim, F. Z. Henniche, N. Aggoune, K. Lassas, S. Azrou, F. Lalaoui, F. Sahli) as well as to the clinical collaborators (T. Annane, N. Bouhafs, A. Laraba, S. Kermani, S. Bouziane, and M. Neggazi).

REFERENCES

Adegbola, R. A., DeAntonio, R., Hill, P. C., Roca, A., Usuf, E., Hoet, B., et al. (2014). Carriage of *Streptococcus pneumoniae* and other respiratory bacterial pathogens in low and lower-middle income countries: a systematic review and meta-analysis. *PLoS ONE* 9:e103293. doi: 10.1371/journal.pone.0103293

Ahn, J. G., Choi, S. Y., Kim, D. S., and Kim, K. H. (2012). Enhanced detection and serotyping of *Streptococcus pneumoniae* using multiplex polymerase chain reaction. *Korean J. Pediatr.* 55, 424–429. doi: 10.3345/kjp.2012.55.11.424

Bentley, S. D., Aanensen, D. M., Mavroidi, A., Saunders, D., Rabbinowitsch, E., Collins, M., et al. (2006). Genetic analysis of the capsular biosynthetic locus from all 90 pneumococcal serotypes. *PLoS Genet.* 2:e31. doi: 10.1371/journal.pgen.0020031

Bogaert, D., De Groot, R., and Hermans, P. W. (2004). *Streptococcus pneumoniae* colonisation: the key to pneumococcal disease. *Lancet Infect. Dis.* 4, 144–154. doi: 10.1016/S1473-3099(04)00938-7

Bravo, L. C. (2009). Overview of the disease burden of invasive pneumococcal disease in Asia. *Vaccine* 27, 7282–7291. doi: 10.1016/j.vaccine.2009.04.046

Caierão, J., Hawkins, P., Sant'anna, F. H., da Cunha, G. R., d'Azevedo, P. A., McGee, L., et al. (2014). Serotypes and genotypes of invasive *Streptococcus pneumoniae* before and after PCV10 implementation in southern Brazil. *PLoS ONE* 9:e111129. doi: 10.1371/journal.pone.0111129

Centers for Disease Control and Prevention (CDC) (2013). Progress in introduction of pneumococcal conjugate vaccine - worldwide, 2000-2012. *Morb Mortal Wkly Rep* 62, 308–311.

Charfi, F., Smaoui, H., and Kechrid, A. (2012). Non-susceptibility trends and serotype coverage by conjugate pneumococcal vaccines in a Tunisian paediatric population: a 10-year study. *Vaccine* 30(Suppl. 6), G18–G24. doi: 10.1016/j.vaccine.2012.07.017

Clinical and Laboratory Standards Institute (CLSI) (2014). *Performance Standards for Antimicrobial Susceptibility Testing. Approved Standard M100-S24.* Wayne, PA: Clinical and Laboratory Standards Institute (CLSI).

Dagan, R., Givon-Lavi, N., Leibovitz, E., Greenberg, D., and Porat, N. (2009). Introduction and proliferation of multidrug-resistant *Streptococcus pneumoniae* serotype 19A clones that cause acute otitis media in an unvaccinated population. *J. Infect. Dis.* 199, 776–785. doi: 10.1086/597044

da Gloria Carvalho, M., Pimenta, F. C., Jackson, D., Roundtree, A., Ahmad, Y., Millar, E. V., et al. (2010). Revisiting pneumococcal carriage by use of broth enrichment and PCR techniques for enhanced detection of carriage and serotypes. *J. Clin. Microbiol.* 48, 1611–1618. doi: 10.1128/JCM.02243-09

Dean, A. G., Sullivan, K. M., and Soe, M. M. (2015). *OpenEpi: Open Source Epidemiologic Statistics for Public Health, Version.* Available online at: www.OpenEpi.com, updated 2015/05/04 (Accessed July 12, 2015).

Dias, R., and Caniça, M. (2007). Invasive pneumococcal disease in Portugal prior to and after the introduction of pneumococcal heptavalent conjugate vaccine. *FEMS Immunol. Med. Microbiol.* 51, 35–42. doi: 10.1111/j.1574-695X.2007.00283.x

Elmdaghri, N., Belabbes, H., Najib, J., Zerouali, K., and Benbachir, M. (2010). Changing epidemiology of *Streptococcus pneumoniae* in Morocco, 2006–2008. *Clin. Microbiol. Infect.* 16, S600–S601. doi: 10.1111/j.1469-0691.2010.03239.x

Elmdaghri, N., Benbachir, M., Belabbes, H., Zaki, B., and Benzaid, H. (2012). Changing epidemiology of pediatric *Streptococcus pneumoniae* isolates before vaccine introduction in Casablanca (Morocco). *Vaccine* 30(Suppl. 6), G46–G50. doi: 10.1016/j.vaccine.2012.10.044

Finland, M., and Barnes, M. W. (1977). Changes in occurrence of capsular serotypes of *Streptococcus pneumoniae* at Boston City Hospital during selected years between 1935 and 1974. *J. Clin. Microbiol.* 5, 154–166.

Flasche, S., Van Hoek, A. J., Sheasby, E., Waight, P., Andrews, N., Sheppard, C., et al. (2011). Effect of pneumococcal conjugate vaccination on serotype-specific carriage and invasive disease in England: a cross-sectional study. *PLoS Med.* 8:e1001017. doi: 10.1371/journal.pmed.1001017

Geno, K. A., Gilbert, G. L., Song, J. Y., Skovsted, I. C., Klugman, K. P., Jones, C., et al. (2015). Pneumococcal capsules and their types: past, present, and future. *Clin. Microbiol. Rev.* 28, 871–899. doi: 10.1128/CMR.00024-15

Ghaffar, F., Barton, T., Lozano, J., Muniz, L. S., Hicks, P., Gan, V., et al. (2004). Effect of the 7-valent pneumococcal conjugate vaccine on nasopharyngeal colonization by *Streptococcus pneumoniae* in the first 2 years of life. *Clin. Infect. Dis.* 39, 930–938. doi: 10.1086/423379

Ginsburg, A. S., Tinkham, L., Riley, K., Kay, N. A., Klugman, K. P., and Gill, C. J. (2013). Antibiotic non-susceptibility among *Streptococcus pneumoniae* and *Haemophilus influenzae* isolates identified in African cohorts: a meta-analysis of three decades of published studies. *Int. J. Antimicrob. Agents* 42, 482–491. doi: 10.1016/j.ijantimicag.2013.08.012

Harboe, Z. B., Benfield, T. L., Valentiner-Branth, P., Hjuler, T., Lambertsen, L., Kaltoft, M., et al. (2010). Temporal trends in invasive pneumococcal disease and pneumococcal serotypes over 7 decades. *Clin. Infect. Dis.* 50, 329–337. doi: 10.1086/649872

Hausdorff, W. P., Feikin, D. R., and Klugman, K. P. (2005). Epidemiological differences among pneumococcal serotypes. *Lancet Infect. Dis.* 5, 83–93. doi: 10.1016/S1473-3099(05)70083-9

Hecini-Hannachi, A., Bentchouala, C., Lezzar, L. A., Belabed, K., Laouar, H., and Smati, F. (2014). Serotypes and antimicrobial resistance of invasive *Streptococcus pneumoniae* isolates from East Algeria (2005-2011). *Afr. J. Microbiol. Res.* 8, 167–177. doi: 10.5897/AJMR2013.5833

Ingels, H., Rasmussen, J., Andersen, P. H., Harboe, Z. B., Glismann, S., Konradsen, H., et al. (2012). Impact of pneumococcal vaccination in Denmark during the first 3 years after PCV introduction in the childhood immunization programme. *Vaccine* 30, 3944–3950. doi: 10.1016/j.vaccine.2012.03.060

Jin, P., Kong, F., Xiao, M., Oftadeh, S., Zhou, F., Liu, C., et al. (2009). First report of putative *Streptococcus pneumoniae* serotype 6D among nasopharyngeal isolates from Fijian children. *J. Infect. Dis.* 200, 1375–1380. doi: 10.1086/606118

Johnson, H. L., Deloria-Knoll, M., Levine, O. S., Stoszek, S. K., Freimanis Hance, L., Reithinger, R., et al. (2010). Systematic evaluation of serotypes causing invasive pneumococcal disease among children under five: the pneumococcal global serotype project. *PLoS Med.* 7:e1000348. doi: 10.1371/journal.pmed.1000348

Jourdain, S., Drèze, P. A., Vandeven, J., Verhaegen, J., Van Melderen, L., and Smeesters, P. R. (2011). Sequential multiplex PCR assay for determining capsular serotypes of colonizing *S. pneumoniae. BMC Infect. Dis.* 11:100. doi: 10.1186/1471-2334-11-100

Miernyk, K., Debyle, C., Harker-Jones, M., Hummel, K. B., Hennessy, T., Wenger, J., et al. (2011). Serotyping of *Streptococcus pneumoniae* isolates from nasopharyngeal samples: use of an algorithm combining microbiologic, serologic, and sequential multiplex PCR techniques. *J. Clin. Microbiol.* 49, 3209–3214. doi: 10.1128/JCM.00610-11

Millar, E. V., O'Brien, K. L., Watt, J. P., Bronsdon, M. A., Dallas, J., Whitney, C. G., et al. (2006). Effect of community-wide conjugate pneumococcal vaccine use in infancy on nasopharyngeal carriage through 3 years of age: a cross-sectional study in a high-risk population. *Clin. Infect. Dis.* 43, 8–15. doi: 10.1086/504802

Moreno, J., Hernández, E., Sanabria, O., and Castañeda, E. (2005). Detection and serotyping of *Streptococcus pneumoniae* from nasopharyngeal samples by PCR-based multiplex assay. *J. Clin. Microbiol.* 43, 6152–6154. doi: 10.1128/JCM.43.12.6152-6154.2005

Pai, R., Gertz, R. E., and Beall, B. (2006). Sequential multiplex PCR approach for determining capsular serotypes of *Streptococcus pneumoniae* isolates. *J. Clin. Microbiol.* 44, 124–131. doi: 10.1128/JCM.44.1.124-131.2006

Pebody, R. G., Hellenbrand, W., D'Ancona, F., Ruutu, P., and European Union funded Pnc−EURO contributing group (2006). Pneumococcal disease surveillance in Europe. *Euro Surveill.* 11, 171–178.

Ramdani-Bouguessa, N., and Rahal, K. (2003). Serotype distribution and antimicrobial resistance of *Streptococcus pneumoniae* isolated in Algiers, Algeria. *Antimicrob. Agents Chemother.* 47, 824–826. doi: 10.1128/AAC.47.2.824-826.2003

Ramdani-Bouguessa, N., Ziane, H., Bekhoucha, S., Guechi, Z., Azzam, A., Touati, D., et al. (2015). Evolution of antimicrobial resistance and serotype distribution of *Streptococcus pneumoniae* isolated from children with invasive and noninvasive pneumococcal diseases in Algeria from 2005 to 2012. *New Microbes New Infect.* 6, 42–48. doi: 10.1016/j.nmni.2015.02.008

Ramos, V., Parra, E. L., Duarte, C., and Moreno, J. (2014). Characterization of *Streptococcus pneumoniae* invasive serotype 19A isolates recovered in Colombia. *Vaccine* 32, 755–758. doi: 10.1016/j.vaccine.2013.12.024

Reinert, R., Jacobs, M. R., and Kaplan, S. L. (2010). Pneumococcal disease caused by serotype 19A: review of the literature and implications for future vaccine development. *Vaccine* 28, 4249–4259. doi: 10.1016/j.vaccine.2010.04.020

Richter, S. S., Diekema, D. J., Heilmann, K. P., Dohrn, C. L., Riahi, F., and Doern, G. V. (2014). Changes in pneumococcal serotypes and antimicrobial resistance after introduction of the 13-valent conjugate vaccine in the United States. *Antimicrob. Agents Chemother.* 58, 6484–6489. doi: 10.1128/AAC.03344-14

Richter, S. S., Heilmann, K. P., Dohrn, C. L., Riahi, F., Diekema, D. J., and Doern, G. V. (2013). Evaluation of pneumococcal serotyping by multiplex PCR and Quellung reactions. *J. Clin. Microbiol.* 51, 4193–4195. doi: 10.1128/JCM.0 1876-13

Roca, A., Bottomley, C., Hill, P. C., Bojang, A., Egere, U., Antonio, M., et al. (2012). Effect of age and vaccination with a pneumococcal conjugate vaccine on the density of pneumococcal nasopharyngeal carriage. *Clin. Infect. Dis.* 55, 816–824. doi: 10.1093/cid/cis554

Satzke, C., Turner, P., Virolainen-Julkunen, A., Adrian, P. V., Antonio, M., Hare, K. M., et al. (2013). Standard method for detecting upper respiratory carriage of *Streptococcus pneumoniae*: updated recommendations from the World Health Organization Pneumococcal Carriage Working Group. *Vaccine* 32, 165–179. doi: 10.1016/j.vaccine.2013.08.062

Song, J. H., Dagan, R., Klugman, K. P., and Fritzell, B. (2012). The relationship between pneumococcal serotypes and antibiotic resistance. *Vaccine* 30, 2728–2737. doi: 10.1016/j.vaccine.2012.01.091

Steens, A., Bergsaker, M. A., Aaberge, I. S., Ronning, K., and Vestrheim, D. F. (2013). Prompt effect of replacing the 7-valent pneumococcal conjugate vaccine with the 13-valent vaccine on the epidemiology of invasive pneumococcal disease in Norway. *Vaccine* 31, 6232–6238. doi: 10.1016/j.vaccine.2013.10.032

Tali-Maamar, H., Laliam, R., Bentchouala, C., Touati, D., Sababou, K., Azrou, S., et al. (2012). Reprint of: serotyping and antibiotic susceptibility of *Streptococcus pneumoniae* strains isolated in Algeria from 2001 to 2010. *Vaccine* 30, G25–G31. doi: 10.1016/j.vaccine.2012.11.019

Tan, T. Q. (2012). Pediatric invasive pneumococcal disease in the United States in the era of pneumococcal conjugate vaccines. *Clin. Microbiol. Rev.* 25, 409–419. doi: 10.1128/CMR.00018-12

Turner, P., Hinds, J., Turner, C., Jankhot, A., Gould, K., Bentley, S. D., et al. (2011). Improved detection of nasopharyngeal cocolonization by multiple pneumococcal serotypes by use of latex agglutination or molecular serotyping by microarray. *J. Clin. Microbiol.* 49, 1784–1789. doi: 10.1128/JCM.00157-11

Varon, E. (2012). Epidemiology of *Streptococcus pneumoniae*. *Med. Mal. Infect.* 42, 361–365. doi: 10.1016/j.medmal.2012.04.002

Varon, E., Cohen, R., Béchet, S., Doi, C., and Levy, C. (2015). Invasive disease potential of pneumococci before and after the 13-valent pneumococcal conjugate vaccine implementation in children. *Vaccine* 33, 6178–6185. doi: 10.1016/j.vaccine.2015.10.015

von Gottberg, A., de Gouveia, L., Tempia, S., Quan, V., Meiring, S., von Mollendorf, C., et al. (2014). Effects of vaccination on invasive pneumococcal disease in South Africa. *N. Engl. J. Med.* 371, 1889–1899. doi: 10.1056/NEJMoa1401914

Weinberger, D. M., Grant, L. R., Steiner, C. A., Weatherholtz, R., Santosham, M., Viboud, C., et al. (2014). Seasonal drivers of pneumococcal disease incidence: impact of bacterial carriage and viral activity. *Clin. Infect. Dis.* 58, 188–194. doi: 10.1093/cid/cit721

Ziane, H., Manageiro, V., Ferreira, E., Bektache, S., Tazir, M., and Caniça, M. (2015). Capsular typing of *Streptococcus pneumoniae* isolated in an Algerian Hospital using a new multiplex PCR-based scheme. *J. Microbiol. Methods* 119, 243–246. doi: 10.1016/j.mimet.2015.11.002

Ziane, H., Ramdani-Bouguess, N., Bektache, S., Bekhoucha, S., Zouagui, S., Haouchine, D., et al. (2012). "Antimicrobial susceptibility and serotype distribution of *Streptococcus pneumoniae* isolates in children in Algeria: 2005 to 2011," in *30th Annual Meeting of the European Society for Paediatric Infectious Diseases* (Greece).

12

Breaking the Spell: Combating Multidrug Resistant 'Superbugs'

*Shahper N. Khan and Asad U. Khan**

Interdisciplinary Biotechnology Unit, Aligarh Muslim University, Aligarh, India

Correspondence:
Asad U. Khan
asad.k@rediffmail.com

Multidrug-resistant (MDR) bacteria have become a severe threat to community wellbeing. Conventional antibiotics are getting progressively more ineffective as a consequence of resistance, making it imperative to realize improved antimicrobial options. In this review we emphasized the microorganisms primarily reported of being resistance, referred as ESKAPE pathogens (*Enterococcus faecium*, *Staphylococcus aureus*, *Klebsiella pneumoniae*, *Acinetobacter baumanii*, *Pseudomonas aeruginosa*, and *Enterobacteriaceae*) accentuating their capacity to "escape" from routine antimicrobial regimes. The upcoming antimicrobial agents showing great potential and can serve as alternative therapeutic options are discussed. We also provided succinct overview of two evolving technologies; specifically network pharmacology and functional genomics profiling. Furthermore, *In vivo* imaging techniques can provide novel targets and a real time tool for potential lead molecule assessment. The employment of such approaches at prelude of a drug development process, will enables more informed decisions on candidate drug selection and will maximize or predict therapeutic potential before clinical testing.

Keywords: multidrug-resistant, drug development, functional genomics, network pharmacology, *in vivo* imaging

INTRODUCTION

A change in the pattern of serious hospital infection after the introduction of antibiotics was noticed early in the antibiotic era. Furthermore with the triumph of the penicillin discovery and the synthesis of antibacterial sulfonamides in the initial half of the 20th century, the modern antimicrobial revolution started. There onward, newer antimicrobial were reported and several semi-synthetic and synthetic antibacterial agents came into existence. Antimicrobial drugs have cured plenty of cases with life-threatening bacterial infections and relieved patients' agony. Unfortunately, unrestrained use of antibacterial past 50 years has wielded selection pressure on susceptible bacteria stains, which attributed to the endurance of drug resistance (Levy and Marshall, 2004; Tacconelli, 2009), among them some are resistant to more than one antibiotic. Presently, the treatment of these infections has once again becomes increasingly complicated as microorganisms are becoming resistance to the available antimicrobial options (Pitout and Laupland, 2008; Nordmann et al., 2011; Khan and Nordmann, 2012a; Labro and Bryskier, 2014). With course of time, sustained selective pressure by various antibiotics has culminated into organisms augmenting ancillary resistance mechanisms that led to multidrug resistance (MDR)—novel penicillin-binding proteins (PBPs), enzyme dependant drug alteration, altered membrane permeability, mutated drug targets and increased efflux pump expression. Further to mention few most challenging MDR organisms presently being encountered includes the so called ESKAPE pathogens like *Pseudomonas aeruginosa*, *Acinetobacter baumannii*, *Escherichia coli*, and *Klebsiella neumoniae* with extended-spectrum β-lactamases (ESBL), vancomycin resistant enterococci (VRE), methicillin-resistant *Staphylococcus aureus* (MRSA), vancomycin-resistant MRSA strains, extensively drug-resistant (XDR) *Mycobacterium tuberculosis* and newly identified transmissible carbapenamase, New Delhi metallo-beta-lactamases (NDM) in Enterobacteriaceae (Alekshun and Levy, 2007; Gootz, 2010; Khan and Nordmann, 2012b). Carbapenems were the only sensitive antibiotics for the treatment of MDR coliforms but the development of carbapenem resistance recently is a matter of great concern. Efforts directed toward identifying newer antibiotics were formerly an exquisite research area and development priority among pharmaceutical giants but poor success rate has dampens the interest. Further studies comprehending resistance illustrates that the evolution and spread of antimicrobial resistance (AMR) is in fact, a very convoluted issue. Hence, a sole target will not ensure eradication of AMR; rather a coordinated multidisciplinary approach is needed to tackle this problem (Smith et al., 2009; Cantas et al., 2013). Mortality rates and length of hospital stay associated with the treatment of drug resistant infections are about twice as big when patients infected with drug sensitive bacteria of the same species, thereby ensuing inflation in healthcare costs.

The aim of this article is to emphasize the ever growing problem of antimicrobial resistance, counting in the present approaches to limit the spread of MDR. We specifically highlighted how the emerging technologies could be a great promise for new antimicrobial discovery.

FAILURE OF PRESENT MEASURES TO COMBAT MDR

Multidrug-resistant is prevalent in nature, and the strategy of eliminating resistance genes makes no sense, as the natural function of most resistance genes is not primarily confirming MDR (Morar and Wright, 2010). Most probably, there is a huge "intrinsic resistome" in bacterial organisms, composed of various genes with diverse phylogeny which contribute to resistance only on interaction with the antibiotic (Fajardo et al., 2008; Girgis et al., 2009; Sommer et al., 2009). Possible strategy to combat with emerging drug resistance is to control the emergence, selection, and spread of MDR strains of bacteria from hospital settings and community (Wright, 2009). The conventional strategies of combating the emergence and spread of MDR atypically relies on the discovery of newer drugs (Wright, 2009; Nordmann et al., 2012), reduction in antibiotic induced bacterial mutation, genetics dependant recombination and horizontal-transfer at lower concentration of drugs (Couce and Blázquez, 2009), suppression of phenotypic traits of resistance (Udekwu et al., 2009), use of combinations therapy (De Cristóbal et al., 2008), including antagonistic drugs (Drew, 2009), early intensive (frontline) therapy, maintaining a low bacterial density (Motter, 2010), and lately, surveillance of hypermutable organisms (Oliver et al., 2000; Carattoli, 2009) and targeting regulating functions necessary for infection (Dandekar and Dandekar, 2010; Greenberg et al., 2010). In essence, these preventive measures are proving increasingly inadequate in the existing global scenario of MDR (Boucher et al., 2009). Averting the spread of resistance can apparently be significant for the person, but exhibits weak impact on the community (Durante-Mangoni and Zarrilli, 2011). Procedures that might work in the initial phase of the development of resistance in hospitals or nations with low rates of MDR, may not be competent enough in regions with prevailing higher resistance frequency (De Gelder et al., 2007). Reports from regions with low levels of MDR such as Sweden, revealed that discontinuance of trimethoprim use for 2 years had no impact on the resistance rate of *Escherichia coli*. That was further linked to the extensive dissemination of trimethoprim resistance genes (*dfr*) along with other resistance determinants, thus encouraging co-selection of *dfr* with other resistance genes as well (Brolund et al., 2010). In a global scenario, eventually, resistance commencing in these heavily contaminated "sources of resistance" will infest areas that are still cleaner (Thaller et al., 2010). Thus, antibiotic resistance keep evolving to attain higher antibiotic resistance exhibiting elevated bacterial genetic evolvability, a phenomenon known as "genetic capitalism", where the rich tends to become richer. It refers to further adaptive potential of an organism to enrich their resistance mechanism either via mutational or gene acquisition events.

POTENTIAL THERAPEUTIC INTERVENTIONS

Molecules Targeting Protein Synthesis

Among the many exploited targets the one, which has been frequently approved by nature and by many successful clinical trial is the ribosome. Many antibiotics targeting protein synthesis are in development or in different phases of clinical trials as a prospective remedy of temperate-to-serious community acquired bacterial infections: solithromycin, cethromycin, omadacycline, CEM-102, GSK1322322, radezolid, and tedizolid. Interestingly, antibiotics targeting the cellular protein synthesis, TP-434, GSK2251052, and plazomicin, are reported to have a range that covers drug resistant gram negative class of bacteria. Among which, TP-434 (**Figure 1**) is a C7, C9 di-substituted broad-spectrum tetracycline based antibiotic was discovered and being developed by Tetraphase Pharmaceuticals, MA, showed effective mechanism-driven impediment of protein synthesis in a coupled transcription/translation assay [half maximal inhibitory concentration (IC_{50}) = 0.29 μg/mL] and a competition assay employing radio labeled tetracycline (Grossman et al., 2012). Furthermore, TP-434 activity is also reported against tetracycline-specific efflux proteins (including *mepA*) genes bearing stains, ribosomal defense mechanisms and for enzymes capable of destructing tetracycline antibiotics (Sutcliffe et al., 2013). Further, TP-434 is insusceptible to $bla_{\text{NDM}-1}$ positive carbapenemase that has recently been reported in enterobacteriaceae. Plazomicin (ACHN-490, **Figure 1**), a "neoglycoside," a semisynthetic drug evolved from sisomicin with considerably enhanced efficacy toward amikacin and gentamicin resistant bacteria (Aggen et al., 2010; Armstrong and Miller, 2010). The minimum inhibitory concentration (MIC) $_{50/90}$ reported for plazomicin ranges in 0.5–1 μg/mL against resistant *K. pneumoniae*, including the serine

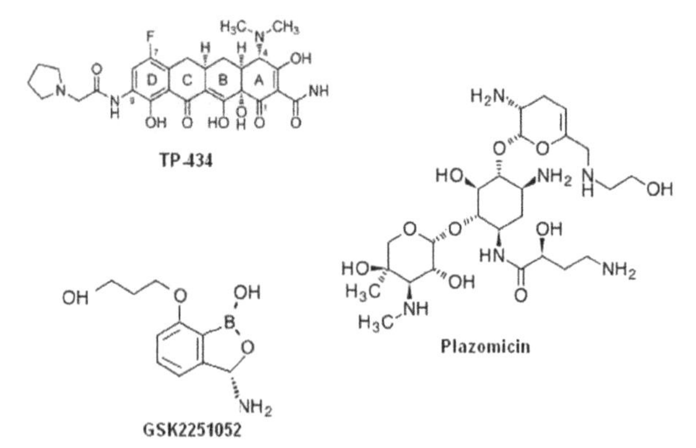

FIGURE 1 | Chemical structure of protein synthesis inhibitors as promising antimicrobial agents.

carbapenemase KPC strains and 1/2 μg/mL against 493 strains of MRSA positive bacteria (Tenover et al., 2011). Whereas, MICs tested against 65 carbapenem resistant enterobacteriaceae was found to be ≤2 μg/mL except for NDM metallo-β-lactamase producers (Livermore et al., 2011). Plazomicin has successfully concluded a level 2 in global multilocation indiscriminate double blind trial evaluating its efficacy relative to levofloxacin, a gold standard for complex urinary tract infection (cUTI) and acute pyelonephritis (AP) and now registered in a level 3 trial stage (ClinicalTrials.gov identifier: NCT01970371). GSK2251052 (**Figure 1**), is a novel boron derivative that interacts with the leucyl-tRNA synthetase at adenosine ribose (A76) termini with an IC_{50} of 0.31 μM, thereby aborting protein synthesis (Goldstein et al., 2013). The compound has shown variable range of $MIC_{50/90}$ for various rampant gram negative aerobic and anaerobic bacteria and anaerobic gram-positive strains (Mendes et al., 2013). Further, in an *in vitro* potency test against bla_{NDM-1} producing enterobacteriaceae isolates, MIC_{90} of the compound was reported to be 1 μg/mL, with a range of 0.5–2 μg/mL. This novel antibiotic has also shown is activity toward category A and B bacterial biothreat infections, with MIC_{90} concentration in the rage of 0.12–2 μg/ml (Heine et al., 2011). When tested on healthy cohort as single IV doses of 200, 400, 900, 2,000, or 3,000 mg (1-hour infusion) and as multiple ascending doses (MADs) of 500, 750, 1,200, or 2,000 mg two times a day for 8 days (500 mg) or 14 days (all other cohorts) was well taken, with no severe implications leading to patients withdrawal but a recent article reports development of some resistance toward it due to specific mutations in the LeuRS editing domain (O'Dwyer et al., 2015). A review by Sutcliffe on antibiotics targeting protein synthesis describes them in detail (Sutcliffe, 2011). Specifically, Dewan et al. (2014) describes in detail the importance aminoacyl-tRNA synthetases as a therapeutic target for novel antibiotic development.

Peptides

Combinational administration of antimicrobial peptides (AMP's) with other antimicrobials has been recommended as an alternative strategy for enhanced therapeutic outcomes. They act by affecting cell membrane integrity, inhibiting protein and cell wall synthesis, altering enzyme activity, and others (Guilhelmelli et al., 2013). Their discrete therapeutic potency and less side effects makes AMP's interesting candidates for concurrent or subsequent use in diverse bacterial infections. AMP's are recently regarded as a viable option for eradicating the multidrug resistant micro-organisms, based on their distinct mechanism of action than that of the presently used antibiotics (Fjell et al., 2011; Nan et al., 2012). Till date, more than 3700 AMP's have already been reported and characterized from flora, faunna, and other sources (Tossi and Sandri, 2002). AMP's can also be produced synthetically and moreover, recombinant AMP's can be yielded by various recombinant cell and/or organisms (Yu et al., 2010). A good number of synthetic AMPs are being tested in clinical trials and in excess of 15 peptides or mimetics are in (or have completed) clinical testing as antimicrobial agents. In a phase 1/2 of clinical testing, the AMP hLF1–11 (1–11 amino acids long amino-terminal of human lactoferrin) was found to be risk free with no after effects when delivered intravenously (Velden et al., 2009). Two peptides, pexignan and omiganan have exhibited efficacy in Phase III clinical trials but waiting for approval. Pexiganan (Lipsky et al., 2008), a derived from magainin, demonstrated similar effectiveness to an oral fluoroquinolone for treating patients with diabetes foot ulcer but was not approved by the US Food and Drug Administration, although there is indication that it might resurface in clinical trials. Omiganan (MBI226), a derivative of indolicidin, proved competent in drastically limiting catheter colonization and microbial tunnel infections during catheterization (ClinicalTrials.gov identifier: NCT00608959). AMP's when tested for treating UTI, the most common infections in hospital settings and well documented in general population, seems to work best due to the optimum environment where peptides naturally, exhibit their potency (Lupetti et al., 2003; Melendez-Alafort et al., 2004). Cudic et al. (2003), illustrated that higher salt concentrations decreases the antimicrobial activity of various AMP's, however, lactoferricins and derivates thereof, are quite active against UTI, regardless of limited antimicrobial activity at higher salt concentration as suggested in *in vitro* settings. Probably, the peptide is effective in eradicating urinary tract infections at remote sites, likely through passive or active transfer of the peptide to the contagion site via renal discharge (Del Olmo et al., 2009; Fornili et al., 2010).

Administration of antimicrobial peptides treated equipment offers potential microbial protection, although the attrition in antimicrobial attributes due to cross linking of the peptide to solid supports must be addressed (Onaizi and Leong, 2011). There are satisfying instances for cationic peptides possessing clinical efficacy (Gordon et al., 2005); polymyxin a cationic lipopeptide is the last resort treatment for multi-drug resistant *Pseudomonas* and *Acinetobacter* infections, the gramicidin S a cyclic cationic peptide is frequently prescribed in topical and eye infections, and the cationic nisin antibiotic is already an approved food supplement in Europe. As per our inference, the increasing accessibility and exploitation of high throughput involved strategies has shown substantial prospects to improve the search for the next generation therapeutic peptides and peptide mimetic as antimicrobials not only specific for bacteria that are resistant to existing antibiotics but also for eliminating other disease causing bugs like protozoa, helminthes, insects and fungi (Bommarius and Kalman, 2009; Tavares et al., 2013).

Vaccines

Rational designing of vaccines have markedly improved with the advancement of recombinant DNA technology against complex human pathologies. In spite of extraordinary performances in pre-clinical and clinical testing, only few recombinant vaccines are deemed safe for humans use till date. Wherein, extensive screening procedures for its production and speculations about their use might be accountable. Recent application of new approaches like systems biology and advanced immunology to better understand mechanism of vaccines is propelling the evolution of vaccinology. Moreover, the outcomes of synthetic biology in vaccine design as evident in the first synthetic bacterium, demonstrates its distinction and rational attributes. Over the last few years there have been several excellent research articles describing strategies of creating the 'optimal' vaccine, as well as highlighting the significant challenges of developing an effective vaccines (Otto, 2010; Wu et al., 2012). Inactivated bacterial strains have shown to be extremely immunogenic against Gram-negative bacteria and exhibit protective immunity against several other bacterial infections. However, its applicability in human is limited due to the presence of lipopolysaccharide induced endotoxin levels. Nevertheless, in a recent report it was suggested that lipopolysaccharide impaired and inactivated *A. baumannii* whole cells can induce protection against *A. baumannii* infections. In which, the endotoxins levels were found to be reduced (<1.0 toxin unit/10^6 cells) relative to the wild type strain, as on inactivation of lipopolysaccharide due to a mutation in the lpxD gene (García-Quintanilla et al., 2014). Vaccines, intended at combat *P. aeruginosa* infections in cystic fibrosis have been developed and are under different clinical phases, though none has been recommended for use (Johansen and Gøtzsche, 2015). Besides the ongoing improvement in whole-cell enterotoxigenic *Escherichia coli* (ETEC) vaccine development the research on subunit or polypeptide vaccines, offers great therapeutic promise. Recent article by Zhang and Sack (2015), has critically summarizes the progress in the development of ETEC vaccine.

Despite the daunting odds of success, there are at least seven active vaccine efforts are ongoing in different stages of clinical development (GlaxoSmithKline/Nabi, Pfizer/Inhibitex, Sanofi Pasteur/Syntiron, Novartis, Novadigm, Integrated Biotherapeutics, and Vaccine Research International). Several studies have been conducted to evaluate the potential of vaccination with microbial surface components illustrating adhesive matrix molecules (MSCRAMMs) whole protein or subunit offers superior protection against staphylococcal infection. Earlier reported, recombinant parts of collagen adhesin (CNA) were shown to provide immunity in a murine model of sepsis (Kuklin et al., 2006). Shkreta et al. (2004) illustrated the protective potential of both clumping factor A (ClfA) and Fibronectin binding protein (FnBP) as an optimal vaccination strategy in bovine mastitis model, eliciting cellular and humoral immune response providing partial protection against *Staphylococcal mastitis*. Recently in an *In silico* analysis, potential multisubunit vaccine targets like ClfA, ron-regulated surface determinant (IsdB) and gamma hemolysin (Hlg) were predicted against *S. aureus* (Delfani et al., 2015). Likewise, several extracellular and surface protein factors in combination with aluminum hydroxide have shown to induce high and broad protection against *S. aureus* (Bagnoli et al., 2015).

Another promising alternative to vaccine prophylaxis against bacterial pathogenesis is the 'DNA-vaccine', wherein DNA sequence encodes the antigen(s) against which an immune response is sought. It will be less labor intensive and may offer a unique method for vaccination (Tang et al., 1992). Though to obtain an improved immunogenic response of DNA vaccines entails detailed familiarity of underlying mechanism through which DNA vaccines provide immunity to the patient and needs the right combination adjuvants as crucial molecules for strengthening the response (Coban et al., 2008). In implant infections caused by *S. aureus*, MSCRAMM is reported to act as an excellent immunogen for an anti-*Staphylococcus* vaccine. A survey comprising multiple studies in where MSCRAMMs of staphylococcal are exploited as the immunogenic entity, which can implemented following the start of infection as presented in a recent review by Arciola et al., where the authors suggests a "Decalogue" for a rational selection of specific target in constructing DNA vaccines to impede infections in implants (Arciola et al., 2009). Another proposed strategy to induce protective immunity against infectious diseases is the application of live attenuated vaccines. Recent studes illustrates that nasopharyngeal colonization with *Streptococcus pneumoniae* induces protective immunity against subsequent invasive infection, suggesting live vaccination through attenuated bacteria could be a treatment of choice in future. However the bacterial attributes influencing the strength of this adaptive immune response are still to be explored (Cohen et al., 2012).

THE SEARCH OF NOVEL ANTIMICROBIALS

Concept of Network Pharmacology

The conception of directed "magic bullets" has long been a therapeutic goal to achieve since Paul Ehrlich (Strebhardt and Ullrich, 2008) and a realistic standard in drug development for past three decades. The central concept of drug development is the notion of developing maximally selective molecules directed to discrete drug targets. Conversely, current therapeutics affects multiple proteins rather than discrete target to execute its effect. Development in the area of systems biology further indicates phenotypic robustness and a network structure implying that specific ligands, compared to multi-target ones, exhibit inferior to expected clinical potency. This revised paradigm about polypharmacology offers improved strategy to rise upon the major pitfalls in new antibiotic development, i.e., efficacy and toxicity. Combining system biology with polypharmacology brings in the opportunity of increasing the existing druggable targets. Nevertheless, the coherent design of polypharmacology needs to fulfill the requirement for new procedures to confirm target associations and augment structure-activity interactions while preserving drug like attributes. Progresses in similar avenues are paying the path toward the next paradigm in novel antibiotic discovery as 'network pharmacology'.

The notion about 'one drug for one target' has affected various facets of drug development approach, like disease categorization, target validation, drug design, and planning of clinical testing. Though, a growing data in post-genomics research is suggesting a more complicated scenario in drug action. An interesting research by Yildirim et al. (2007), illustrates not only the existence of several keys for each lock but also a single key for multiple locks. Employing network analysis of combined profiles and a network distance metric, can differentiate between soothing drugs, which ease symptoms, and drugs affecting directly the concern disease genes. Furthermore, the trends in recent years toward the drugs that target the genes associated with disease were emphasized by the network distance metric. It has been well accepted that many effective drugs in therapeutic areas as varied as oncology, psychiatry and antimicrobials affects multiple rather than single targets (Paolini et al., 2006; Tian and Liu, 2012). Many efficient antibiotics are directed toward multiple proteins concurrently rather than individual protein (Lange et al., 2007). For instance, the antimicrobial property of beta-lactams is reliant on the inhibition of more than one PBPs. Indeed, as multiple PBPs can be eliminated with least effect on phenotype (Denome et al., 1999), the approach of lone target essentiality may not have revealed this significant group of antimicrobial drug targets. Likewise, fluoroquinolone based antibiotics can inhibit more than one target proteins ParC and GyrA (Janoir et al., 1996). D-Cycloserine is reported to inhibit four proteins, dimer of alanine racemases and D-Ala-D-Ala ligases. Similarly, fosfomycin circumvent the excess of UDP *N*-acetylglucosamine enolpyruvyl transferases by restraining them both. Consequently, any effort in the direction of drug designing for combating drug resistance, could consider the development of procedures to identify and evaluate which group of targets can be repressed by one single drug and are indispensible, either alone ('dualessentials') or when taken together ('synthetic lethals').

Network biology is suggested to play imperative role in drug target characterization. Is it feasible to recognize drug targets by tracing their location in a biological network? When the researchers mapped drug targets against human protein interaction data, result suggests that drug targets tend to have more interactions than average proteins but fewer interactions than crucial proteins to a statistically significant degree (Hopkins, 2007, 2008). The findings about the linkage among drug targets that are not exclusively essential, opens up the avenues for statistical analysis to serve as a vital tool for scoring them. Conventionally, medicinal chemists considered the design of ligands with multiple activities with apprehension, skeptical about conjugated ligands with high molecular weights complex and/or their structure-activity relationships (Hopkins et al., 2006; Morphy and Rankovic, 2006). Though, polypharmacology of standard drugs illustrates that a more opportunistic plan exploring multi-target action could be more efficient. Employing chemogenomics along with network biology will bring in a efficient network-pharmacology approach to drug design (Keiser et al., 2007; Morphy and Rankovic, 2007). Developing strategy to assist polypharmacology will further help to predict better efficacy and redundant off-target properties.

Functional Genomics in Drug Designing

The tremendous advancement in the technology for genome screening had a substantial impact on all biological sciences, including antimicrobial research. Since the decoding of the *Haemophilus influenza* genome (Fleischmann et al., 1995), various other bacterial genomes were deduced. Complete genomes of >180 bacteria were sequenced and are now freely accessible, including various imperative disease causing pathogens (e.g., http://www.genomenewsnetwork.org/resources/sequenced_genomes/genome_guide_p1.shtml). Therefore, the drug development industry exploited the sequencing data as the basis for a rational, target-specific novel drug designing approach to complement the conventional strategy. Central to the paradigm shift was the idea of the occurrence of the so-far unexploited targets with the prospective for effective and discerning antibiotics for broad spectrum of bacterial infections (McDevitt et al., 2002; Gwynn et al., 2010; Brunschweiger and Hall, 2012). An array of genomics platforms are employed in the present antiinfectious drug development process to lay more proficient procedure compared to conventional strategy. Herein, we proposed a more robust strategy as an alternative for the discovery of next generation antibiotics (**Figure 2**), which includes all possible coverage for better output. Including knockout analyses and mutation studies in the strategy will enhance the prioritization and validation of prospective novel drug target by questioning its importance for bacterial existence. Applications of genetically manipulated cell, along with holistic profiling strategies like 'OMICS,' i.e., transcriptomic and proteomic are contributory in verifying the mode of action (MOA) while screening lead molecules from target assays. Functional genomics strategies also offers vital clues on the mechanism of lead molecules screened through the empiric approach for novel antibacterial discovery. Furthermore, comparing genomes facilitates the identification of proteins that are conserved across the clinically critical pathogens, assisting functional characterization of new genes and identification of novel targets. Genome wide gene silencing studies facilitate an approximation of the number of genes necessary for survival of various bacterial species. The inference on the role of same gene product essentiality ('ortholog') in different species will augment the feasibility of such targets. While selecting a target diverse criterion, such as screening competence, drug like attributes and metabolical context are of a great significance. Although, data on these features are often not accessible and even some targets are not completely characterized. The number of uncharacterized targets typically increases when focusing on attributes preserved in a selective group of pathogens (narrowed range of bacteria). Growth studies with different supplements, cytological assessment, transcriptome, proteome analyses, and metabolic labeling experiments of conditional mutants may assist in the evaluation of corresponding functional genes. Further interesting strategy to explore novel drug is to evaluate the

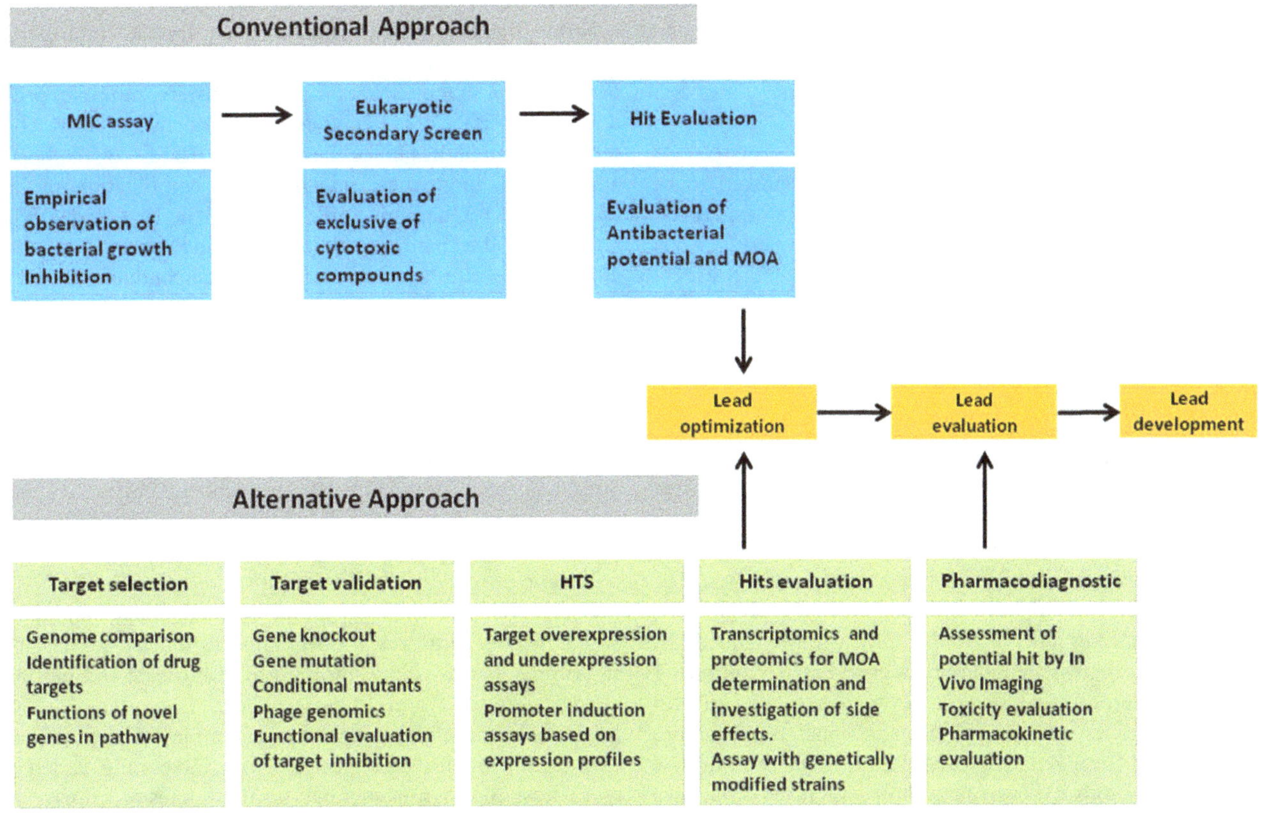

FIGURE 2 | Alternative approach for the discovery of next generation antibiotics.

molecular action of bacteriophages to arrest critical cellular pathways. As done by Liu et al. (2004), on sequencing 26 *S. aureus* phages thirty one (31) novel polypeptide were identified that on expression exhibit cell death in *S. aureus*. Affinity chromatography illustrates the role of DnaI as a target protein, a requisite protein for primosome activity on the initiation of DNA replication. Such screening techniques can be further extended to other species as well and could be instrumental in proving imperative information and as screening tools for novel or unexplored targets. In addition functional genomics applications have proved to be indispensable for expediting the characterization of mechanism of action for novel compounds with antinfectious activity and offers novel mechanism based screening options by generating and characterizing point mutations that confers drug resistance. In general conditional mutants with target gene repression illustrate an increase in sensitivity toward that target specific inhibitor. When analyzed, the relative growth suppression of these mutants to the wild type enables an easy validation confirming the mechanism of novel drugs/hits, as reported by DeVito et al. (2002) and Forsyth et al. (2002).

An approach of global expression profiling can revolutionize the analysis of drug targets holistically as never before. As whole genome profiling offers the static blueprint of cells attributes, as being highly dynamic in nature the transcriptome and proteome are appropriate to obtain snapshots of that cell physiology when challenged by environmental alterations, exposure to stress or antibiotic administration. As application of a DNA microarray provides direct assessment of the mRNA of the gene of interest, the proteomic profiling by 2D gel electrophoresis involves an implicit protein atlas needed initially to confirm the identity of each protein (as determined by mass spectrometry) to its spot location on the 2D gel (Brötz-Oesterhelt et al., 2005). The expression profiles resulted from these techniques illustrates the molecular insight of the adaptive physiology of bacteria like the regulatory mechanism, signal transduction and the underlying metabolism that influence the phenotypic outcomes. Transcriptome as well as proteome profiling were widely used to study the physiology of bacteria in response to various environmental stresses provided particularly useful information about the underlying network of adaptive responses. As a proof-of-concept is the *B. subtilis* mutant down regulating the peptide deformylase, wherein the proteomic profiling of this strain matched adequately well with the wild-type strain exposed to the deformylase inhibitor actinonin (Bandow et al., 2003). Furthermore, bacterial acetyl-CoA carboxylase (ACC) is recently been suggested as the target of moiramide B based on a reference compilation of transcriptome profiles (Freiberg et al., 2004, 2005). In a recent interesting work Murray et al. (2015) has employed expression- and fitness-based genomic strategies to validate role of genetic loci exhibiting drug resistance in human pathogen *P. aeruginosa*. Signifying that gene expression standalone is not a reliable predictor of resistance determinants. Moreover when combine together, whole genome expression and fitness correlation may offer better mechanistic perceptions about multidrug resistance.

In Vivo Imaging Technologies

Recently, *in vivo* imaging techniques are being proved to be a powerful complement to various platforms of antimicrobial resistance and drug discovery (Probst et al., 2012; Roda and Guardigli, 2012). It may not only minimize the use of histopathological examination of autopsies but also be helpful in limiting the animal sacrifice and cost for *in vivo* drug-kinetic studies. Hence, we propose that improvement of intravital dynamic monitoring strategies to probe cellular phenotypes will reflect as wise drug development investment. Real time monitoring enables a faster readout of drug action in the complex model organisms, thus facilitating comprehensive assessment of drug profiling *in vivo*. Moreover, this could enable lead optimization and medicinal chemistry can be directed by instructive functional *in vivo* response data. The clinical reliability of highthroughput screens and *in vivo* monitoring strategies are yet to be fully comprehended. In particular, the progress in bioluminescence based monitoring of disease progression *in vivo* is ever increasing. Further identifies underlying physiology, such as signal transduction, proliferation and cell renewal to be examined in the purview of an intact organism. Two commonly employed strategies for incorporating bioluminescent marker in a model organism are: First is the *lux* operon from *Photorhabdus luminescens* or *Xenorhabdus luminescens,* encodes genes to produce luciferase and its substrate luciferin constitutively, and glow even absence of any exogenous substrate. The *lux* operon gets stably incorporated to other bacterial species but fail to integrate in higher species, though continuous efforts are make to use it as a reporter in mammalian system. The second strategy for bioluminescent probes uses enzyme luciferase from firefly (*Photinus pyralis*) or sea pansy (*Renilla reniliformis*), as firefly and Renilla luciferase require two distinct substrates, which make it possible to link them with two different biological processes in the same research model (Bhaumik and Gambhir, 2002; Ng et al., 2011). However, each reporter differs in the pharmacokinetic of their substrate, as on intraperitoneal administration of luciferin, firefly luciferase bioluminescence attain saturation in about 5–10 min and stays almost constant for 30 min (Paroo et al., 2004), however, renilla luciferase reach to its maxima in 1 min on intravenous coelenterazine administration and declines back in 10 min (Bhaumik and Gambhir, 2002). This technology can be successfully employed to study a variety of infection and their progression in animal models (**Figure 3**). Also manifested by the work of other researchers, that bioluminescence imaging can be used to validate new features in host-pathogen interactions. Furthermore developments in the live cell-fluorescent reporter molecules, brings in the opportunity to adopt *in vivo* monitoring applications in drug development (Carragher et al., 2012).

Past few years, array of nanoparticles have emerged with a promise of superior atttributes for *in vivo* fluorescence imaging technology. Besides providing dynamic size range, these particles offers diverse structural and optical properties with superior signals strength compared to organic fluorophores, providing more sensitive visualization of even sparse biomarkers. Furthermore, nanoparticles can incorporate multiple probes due larger surface area, facilitating multivalent targeting. Above mentioned attributes make these nanocarriers fit for therapeutic applications, biomedical imaging or a combination of both (theranostics). Quantum dots (QDs) are the best characterized and most studied nanocrystals (Mandal and Parvin, 2011; Li et al., 2012). These minute nanomaterials are semiconductive in nature and have an adjustable emission fluorescence that can be adjusted by regulating their synthesis (Bentolila et al., 2009). Furthermore can be visualized in a wide, from the ultraviolet to the near infrared exhibit higher intensity and photoresistant attributes. Recently, QDs treated with coordination complexes were used to specifically visualize a rough *Escherichia coli* mutant facilitating optical detection in murine infection model (Leevy et al., 2008). Various other nanoparticles that have been developed for *in vivo* fluorescence imaging applications are metallic, hybrid, C dots, polymeric or biodegradable in nature (Coto-García et al., 2011). Recent development in capturing detailed images and image based analysis softwares are beginning to impact the design of algorithms that can be customized to fit intricate and pertinent biological models and tissue specimen (Jones et al., 2009). Amendable image analyzing software's can leverage quantitative data from complex biological systems, integrating varied cell types, fresh biopsies, or material from cell lines or primary cells for efficient mimicking of the cellular environment. Therefore, high-resolution *in vivo* imaging should facilitate drug discovery per se and understanding of the drug therapeutic effectiveness (**Table 1**), and will apparently increase the success rate in clinical testing by providing pertinent biological perspective to genomic and proteomic approaches.

CONCLUSION AND FUTURE PERSPECTIVE

The yin and yang of novel antibiotic discovery swings around from a serious need for antibiotics to eradicate drug resistant bacteria to antimicrobial agents. Ever increasing resistance despite the rigorous attempts for control use of antibiotics and sanitize hospitals routinely is the driver for the need of next generation antibiotics. These bacteria "superbugs" have escaped the clinical settings and attain the status of community acquired pathogens. Besides the upcoming promising antiinfective agents as discussed in this article earlier, there is the need to adopt alternative approaches for the discovery of next generation of antibiotics. The strategies discussed in this review are network pharmacology and functional genomics in complement with *in vivo* imaging platforms. The network pharmacology encompasses systems biology, network analysis, connectivity, redundancy, and pleiotropy to improve clinical efficacy and understanding side effects and toxicity. Functional genomics techniques are proved to be indispensible for *in vitro* target authentication and elucidating mechanism of action of novel antibacterial. In addition, the

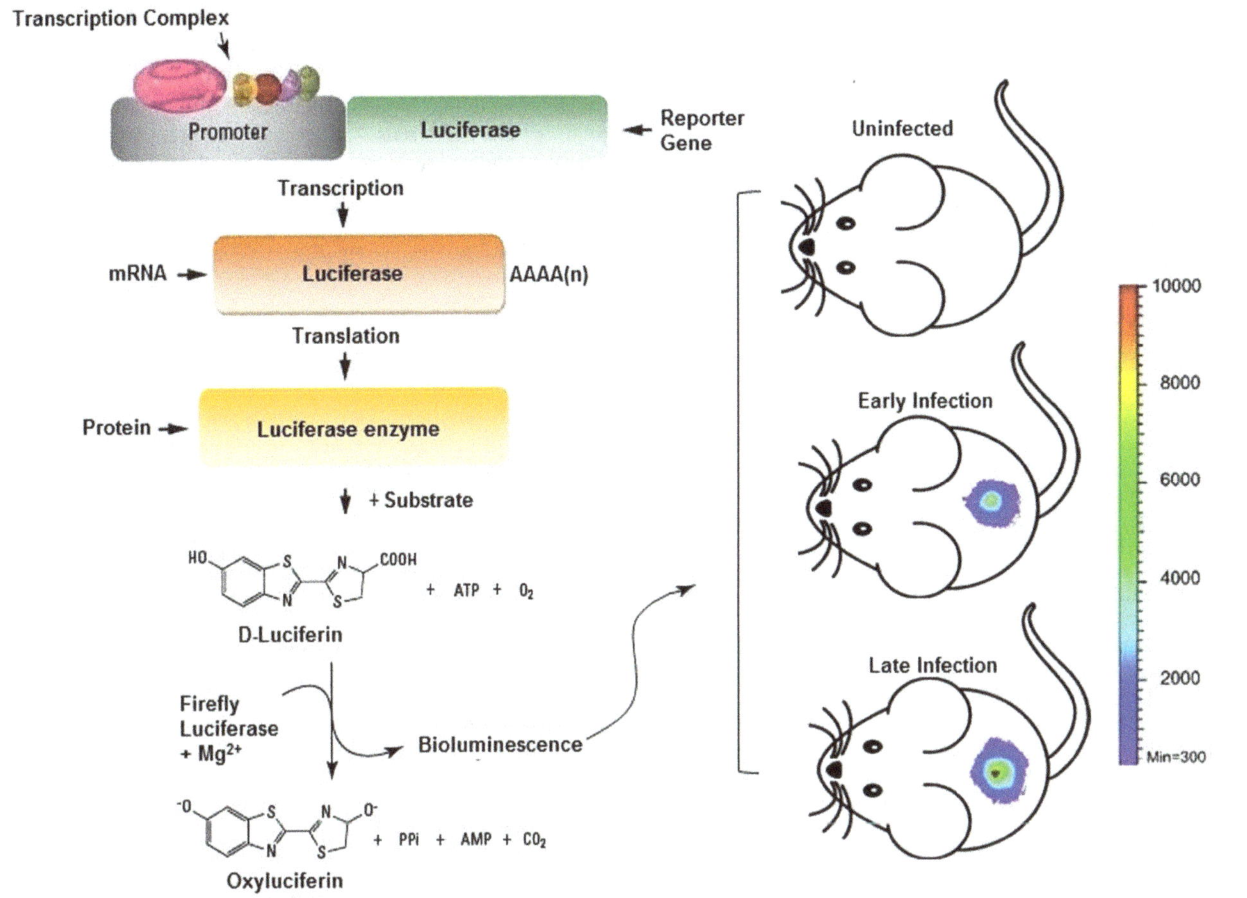

FIGURE 3 | Scheme representing the usage of *in vivo* imaging technique for the assessment of bacterial infection in murine model. The bacterial cells bearing plasmid with reporter genes expressed will provide luminescence signals when injected with appropriate substrate provides real time readout for the extent of infection and/or therapeutic efficacy.

TABLE 1 | Potential applications of *in vivo* imaging in drug discovery.

Assessment of disease model efficiency	Disease model can be assessed for the optimal engraftment or infection from orthotropic cells before treatment regimes
Potential hit screening	Evaluation of MIC values across multiple pathways to determine the response of target activity
Biomarker discovery	Detection of post-translational markers of therapeutic relevance from clinical biopsy or body fluids
Identify drug–target mechanisms	Identification and validation of drug combination strategies and synergism of drugs
Predictive *in vivo* pharmacodynamics	Monitor organ-specific response and correlate with functional drug response
Drug candidate profiling *in vitro*	Establish broad pathway-activity mechanisms
Confirming functional genomics screens and pathways	Characterize impact of knockdown of genes on key pathways

approach of functional genomics not only relies on target-based screening but also supports the traditional screening strategy by predicting novel mechanism for hits and natural products with potential antibacterial activity and unknown targets. Complementary to approach of drug discovery, *in vivo* imaging is an economical, user friendly and radioactive free tool that can extract quick semi-qualitative or quantitative information representing physiological milieu from the cellular to the computable form. Key for best realization of imaging and post-translational pathway modeling approaches into routine antibiotic discovery relies on its early integration with target specific drug development efforts. Validating efficiency and safety profiles of hit molecules in pathological models, before cost intensive medicinal approaches, offer a perfect solution for reducing the unsustainable expense. In summary, there is strong likelihood that the combination of both the traditional and genomics-based approaches, together with the live cell visualization techniques, will led to better strategies for the discovery of newer antibiotics to combat the emergence of bacterial resistance.

AUTHOR CONTRIBUTIONS

SNK wrote review article. AUK guided and gave idea of writing.

ACKNOWLEDGMENTS

Author acknowledges DBT, government of India for the support and internal facilities of the department. This work was supported by internal funds of Interdisciplinary Biotechnology Unit and DBT-BUILDER program, AMU. The authors have no other applicable memberships or financial involvement with any group or entity with a financial interest in or financial conflict with the subject matter or materials conversed in the manuscript. No writing assistance was utilized in the production of this manuscript. We highly appreciate the reviewers for constructive criticism.

REFERENCES

Aggen, J. B., Armstrong, E. S., Goldblum, A. A., Dozzo, P., Linsell, M. S., Gliedt, M. J., et al. (2010). Synthesis and spectrum of the neoglycoside ACHN-490. *Antimicrob. Agents Chemother.* 54, 4636–4642. doi: 10.1128/AAC.00572-10

Alekshun, M. N., and Levy, S. B. (2007). Molecular mechanisms of antibacterial multidrug resistance. *Cell* 128, 1037–1050. doi: 10.1016/j.cell.2007.03.004

Arciola, C. R., Speziale, P., and Montanaro, L. (2009). Perspectives on DNA vaccines. Targeting staphylococcal adhesins to prevent implant infections. *Int. J. Artif. Organs* 32, 635–641.

Armstrong, E. S., and Miller, G. H. (2010). Combating evolution with intelligent design: the neoglycoside ACHN-490. *Curr. Opin. Microbiol.* 13, 565–573. doi: 10.1016/j.mib.2010.09.004

Bagnoli, F., Fontana, M. R., Soldaini, E., Mishra, R. P., Fiaschi, L., Cartocci, E., et al. (2015). Vaccine composition formulated with a novel TLR7-dependent adjuvant induces high and broad protection against *Staphylococcus aureus*. *Proc. Natl. Acad. Sci. U.S.A.* 112, 3680–3685. doi: 10.1073/pnas.1424924112

Bandow, J. E., Becher, D., Büttner, K., Hochgräfe, F., Freiberg, C., Brötz, H., et al. (2003). The role of peptide deformylase in protein biosynthesis: a proteomic study. *Proteomics* 3, 299–306. doi: 10.1002/pmic.200390043

Bentolila, L. A., Ebensteinn, Y., and Weiss, S. (2009). Quantum dots for in vivo small-animal imaging. *J. Nucl. Med.* 50, 493–496. doi: 10.2967/jnumed.108.053561

Bhaumik, S., and Gambhir, S. (2002). Optical imaging of *Renilla* luciferase reporter gene expression in living mice. *Proc. Natl. Acad. Sci. U.S.A.* 99, 377–382. doi: 10.1073/pnas.012611099

Bommarius, B., and Kalman, D. (2009). Antimicrobial and host defense peptides for therapeutic use against multidrug-resistant pathogens: new hope on the horizon. *IDrugs* 12, 376–380.

Boucher, H. W., Talbot, G. H., Bradley, J. S., Edwards, J. E., Gilbert, D., Rice, L. B., et al. (2009). Bad bugs, no drugs: no ESKAPE! An update from the Infectious Diseases Society of America. *Clin. Infect. Dis.* 48, 1–2. doi: 10.1086/595011

Brolund, A., Sundqvist, M., Kahlmeter, G., and Grape, M. (2010). Molecular characterisation of trimethoprim resistance in *Escherichia coli* and *Klebsiella pneumoniae* during a two year intervention on trimethoprim use. *PLoS ONE* 5:e9233. doi: 10.1371/journal.pone.0009233

Brötz-Oesterhelt, H., Bandow, J. E., and Labischinski, H. (2005). Bacterial proteomics and its role in antibacterial drug discovery. *Mass. Spectrom. Rev.* 24, 549–565. doi: 10.1002/mas.20030

Brunschweiger, A., and Hall, J. (2012). A decade of the human genome sequence–how does the medicinal chemist benefit? *Chem. Med. Chem.* 7, 194–203. doi: 10.1002/cmdc.201100498

Cantas, L., Shah, S. Q., Cavaco, L. M., Manaia, C. M., Walsh, F., Popowska, M., et al. (2013). A brief multi-disciplinary review on antimicrobial resistance in medicine and its linkage to the global environmental microbiota. *Front. Microbiol.* 4:96. doi: 10.3389/fmicb.2013.00096

Carattoli, A. (2009). Resistance plasmid families in *Enterobacteriaceae*. *Antimicrob. Agents Chemother.* 53, 2227–2238. doi: 10.1128/AAC.01707-08

Carragher, N. O., Brunton, V. G., and Frame, M. C. (2012). Combining imaging and pathway profiling: an alternative approach to cancer drug discovery. *Drug Discov. Today* 17, 203–214. doi: 10.1016/j.drudis.2012.02.002

Coban, C., Koyama, S., Takeshita, F., Akira, S., and Ishii, K. J. (2008). Molecular and cellular mechanisms of DNA vaccines. *Hum. Vaccin.* 4, 453–456. doi: 10.4161/hv.4.6.6200

Cohen, J. M., Chimalapati, S., and de Vogel, C. (2012). Contributions of capsule, lipoproteins and duration of colonisation towards the protective immunity of prior *Streptococcus pneumoniae* nasopharyngeal colonisation. *Vaccine* 30, 4453–4459. doi: 10.1016/j.vaccine.2012.04.080

Coto-García, A. M., Sotelo-González, E., and Fernández-Argüelles, M. T. (2011). Nanoparticles as fluorescent labels for optical imaging and sensing in genomics and proteomics. *Anal. Bioanal. Chem.* 399, 29–42. doi: 10.1007/s00216-010-4330-3

Couce, A., and Blázquez, J. (2009). Side effects of antibiotics on genetic variability. *FEMS Microbiol. Rev.* 33, 531–538. doi: 10.1111/j.1574-6976.2009.00165.x

Cudic, M., Lockatell, C. V., Johnson, D. E., and Otvos, L. Jr. (2003). In vitro and in vivo activity of an antibacterial peptide analog against uropathogens. *Peptides* 24, 807–820. doi: 10.1016/S0196-9781(03)00172-4

Dandekar, T., and Dandekar, G. (2010). Pharmacogenomic strategies against microbial resistance: from bright to bleak to innovative. *Pharmacogenomics* 11, 1193–1196. doi: 10.2217/pgs.10.18

De Cristóbal, R. E., Vincent, P. A., and Salomón, R. A. (2008). A combination of sbmA and tolC mutations in *Escherichia coli* K-12 Tn10-carrying strains results in hypersusceptibility to tetracycline. *J. Bacteriol.* 190, 1491–1494. doi: 10.1128/JB.01844-07

De Gelder, L., Ponciano, J. M., Joyce, P., and Top, E. M. (2007). Stability of a promiscuous plasmid in different hosts: no guarantee for a long-term relationship. *Microbiology* 153, 452–463. doi: 10.1099/mic.0.2006/001784-0

Del Olmo, A., Morales, P., and Nuñez, M. (2009). Bactericidal activity of lactoferrin and its amidated and pepsin-digested derivatives against *Pseudomonas fluorescens* in ground beef and meat fractions. *J. Food Prot.* 72, 760–765.

Delfani, S., Imani Fooladi, A. A., Mobarez, A. M., Emaneini, M., Amani, J., and Sedighian, H. (2015). In silico analysis for identifying potential vaccine candidates against *Staphylococcus aureus*. *Clin. Exp. Vaccine Res.* 1, 99–106. doi: 10.7774/cevr.2015.4.1.99

Denome, S. A., Elf, P. K., Henderson, T. A., Nelson, D. E., and Young, K. D. (1999). *Escherichia coli* mutants lacking all possible combinations of eight penicillin binding proteins: viability, characteristics, and implications for peptidoglycan synthesis. *J. Bacteriol.* 181, 3981–3993.

DeVito, J. A., Mills, J. A., Liu, V. G., Agarwal, A., Sizemore, C. F., Yao, Z., et al. (2002). An array of targetspecific screening strains for antibacterial discovery. *Nat. Biotechnol.* 20, 478–483. doi: 10.1038/nbt0502-478

Dewan, V., Reader, J., and Forsyth, K. M. (2014). Role of aminoacyl-tRNA synthetases in infectious diseases and targets for therapeutic development. *Top. Curr. Chem.* 344, 293–329. doi: 10.1007/128_2013_425

Drew, R. H. (2009). Antimicrobial stewardship programs: how to start and steer a successful program. *J. Manag. Care Pharm.* 15, S18–S23. doi: 10.1007/128_2013_425

Durante-Mangoni, E., and Zarrilli, R. (2011). Global spread of drug-resistant *Acinetobacter baumannii*: molecular epidemiology and management of antimicrobial resistance. *Future Microbiol.* 6, 407–422. doi: 10.2217/fmb.11.23

Fajardo, A., Martínez-Martín, N., Mercadillo, M., Galán, J. C., Ghysels, B., Matthijs, S., et al. (2008). The neglected intrinsic resistome of bacterial pathogens. *PLoS ONE* 3:e1619. doi: 10.1371/journal.pone.0001619

Fjell, C. D., Hiss, J. A., Hancock, R. E., and Schneider, G. (2011). Designing antimicrobial peptides: form follows function. *Nat. Rev. Drug Discov.* 11, 37–51. doi: 10.1038/nrd3591

Fleischmann, R. D., Adams, M. D., White, O., Clayton, R. A., Kirkness, E. F., Kerlavage, A. R., et al. (1995). Whole-genome random sequencing and assembly of *Haemophilus influenzae* Rd. *Science* 269, 496–512. doi: 10.1126/science.7542800

Fornili, S., Pizzi, R., and Rebeccani, D. (2010). Conformational analysis of a synthetic antimicrobial peptide in water and membrane-mimicking solvents: a molecular dynamics simulation study. *Int. J. Pept. Res. Ther.* 16, 223–231. doi: 10.1007/s10989-010-9211-2

Forsyth, R. A., Haselbeck, R. J., Ohlsen, K. L., Yamamoto, R. T., Xu, H., Trawick, J. D., et al. (2002). A genome-wide strategy for the identification of essential genes in *Staphylococcus aureus*. *Mol. Microbiol.* 43, 1387–1400. doi: 10.1046/j.1365-2958.2002.02832.x

Freiberg, C., Brunner, N. A., Schiffer, G., Lampe, T., Pohlmann, J., Brands, M., et al. (2004). Identification and characterization of the first class of potent bacterial acetyl-CoA carboxylase inhibitors with antibacterial activity. *J. Biol. Chem.* 279, 26066–26073. doi: 10.1074/jbc.M402989200

Freiberg, C., Fischer, H. P., and Brunner, N. A. (2005). Discovering the mechanism of action of novel antibacterial agents through transcriptional profiling of conditional mutants. *Antimicrob. Agents Chemother.* 49, 749–759. doi: 10.1128/AAC.49.2.749-759.2005

García-Quintanilla, M., Pulido, M. R., Pachón, J., and McConnell, M. J. (2014). Immunization with lipopolysaccharide-deficient whole cells provides protective immunity in an experimental mouse model of *Acinetobacter baumannii* infection. *PLoS ONE* 9:e114410. doi: 10.1371/journal.pone.01 14410

Girgis, H. S., Hottes, A. K., and Tavazoie, S. (2009). Genetic architecture of intrinsic antibiotic susceptibility. *PLoS ONE* 4:e5629. doi: 10.1371/journal.pone.0005629

Goldstein, E. J., Citron, D. M., Tyrrell, K. L., and Merriam, C. V. (2013). Comparative in vitro activities of GSK2251052, a novel boron-containing leucyl-tRNA synthetase inhibitor, against 916 anaerobic organisms. *Antimicrob. Agents Chemother.* 57, 2401–2404. doi: 10.1128/AAC.02 580-12

Gootz, T. D. (2010). The global problem of antibiotic resistance. *Crit. Rev. Immunol.* 30, 79–93. doi: 10.1615/CritRevImmunol.v30.i1.60

Gordon, Y. J., Romanowski, E. G., and McDermott, A. M. (2005). A review of antimicrobial peptides and their therapeutic potential as anti-infective drugs. *Curr. Eye Res.* 30, 505–515. doi: 10.1080/02713680590968637

Greenberg, D. E., Marshall-Batty, K. R., Brinster, L. R., Zarember, K. A., Shaw, P. A., Mellbye, B. L., et al. (2010). Antisense phosphorodiamidate morpholino oligomers targeted to an essential gene inhibit *Burkholderia cepacia* complex. *J. Infect. Dis.* 201, 1822–1830. doi: 10.1086/652807

Grossman, T. H., Starosta, A. L., Fyfe, C., O'Brien, W., Rothstein, D. M., Mikolajka, A., et al. (2012). Target- and resistance-based mechanistic studies with TP-434, a novel fluorocycline antibiotic. *Antimicrob. Agents Chemother.* 56, 2559–2564. doi: 10.1128/AAC.06187-11

Guilhelmelli, F., Vilela, N., Albuquerque, P., Derengowski Lda, S., Silva-Pereira, I., and Kyaw, C. M. (2013). Antibiotic development challenges: the various mechanisms of action of antimicrobial peptides and of bacterial resistance. *Front. Microbiol.* 4:353. doi: 10.3389/fmicb.2013.00353

Gwynn, M. N., Portnoy, A., Rittenhouse, S. F., and Payne, D. J. (2010). Challenges of antibacterial discovery revisited. *Ann. N. Y. Acad. Sci.* 213, 5–19. doi: 10.1111/j.1749-6632.2010.05828.x

Heine, H. S., Marchand, C. L., Miller, L., Halasohoris, S., Jakielaszek, C., Easom, E., et al. (2011). "Susceptibility testing of a novel mechanism antibacterial GSK2251052 against category A/B bacterial biothreat agents," in *Proceedings of the 51st Annual ICAAC, September 12–15*. Chicago, IL.

Hopkins, A. L. (2007). Network pharmacology. *Nat. Biotechnol.* 25, 1110–1111. doi: 10.1038/nbt1007-1110

Hopkins, A. L. (2008). Network pharmacology: the next paradigm in drug discovery. *Nat. Chem. Biol.* 4, 682–690. doi: 10.1038/nchembio.118

Hopkins, A. L., Mason, J. S., and Overington, J. P. (2006). Can we rationally design promiscuous drugs. *Curr. Opin. Struct. Biol.* 16, 127–136. doi: 10.1016/j.sbi.2006.01.013

Janoir, C., Zeller, V., Kitzis, M. D., Moreau, N. J., and Gutmann, L. (1996). High-level fluoroquinolone resistance in *Streptococcus pneumoniae* requires mutations in parC and gyrA. *Antimicrob. Agents Chemother.* 40, 2760–2764. PMID: 9124836

Johansen, H. K., and Gøtzsche, P. C. (2015). Vaccines for preventing infection with *Pseudomonas aeruginosa* in cystic fibrosis. *Cochrane Database Syst. Rev.* 8:CD001399. doi: 10.1002/14651858.CD001399

Jones, T. R., Carpenter, A. E., Lamprecht, M. R., Moffat, J., Silver, S. J., Grenier, J. K., et al. (2009). Scoring diverse cellular morphologies in image-based screens with iterative feedback and machine learning. *Proc. Natl. Acad. Sci. U.S.A.* 106, 1826–1831. doi: 10.1073/pnas.0808843106

Keiser, M. J., Roth, B. L., Armbruster, B. N., Ernsberger, P., Irwin, J. J., and Shoichet, B. K. (2007). Relating protein pharmacology by ligand chemistry. *Nat. Biotechnol.* 25, 197–206. doi: 10.1038/nbt1284

Khan, A. U., and Nordmann, P. (2012a). NDM-1-producing *Enterobacter cloacae* and *Klebsiella pneumoniae* from diabetic foot ulcers in India. *J. Med. Microbiol.* 61, 454–456. doi: 10.1099/jmm.0.039008-0

Khan, A. U., and Nordmann, P. (2012b). Spread of carbapenemase NDM-1 producers: the situation in India and what may be proposed. *Scand. J. Infect. Dis.* 44, 531–535. doi: 10.3109/00365548.2012.669046

Kuklin, N. A., Clark, D. J., Secore, S., Cook, J., Cope, L. D., McNeely, T., et al. (2006). A novel *Staphylococcus aureus* vaccine: iron surface determinant B induces rapid antibody responses in rhesus macques and specific increased survival in a murine model of *S. aureus* sepsis. *Infect. Immun.* 74, 2215–2223. doi: 10.1128/IAI.74.4.2215-2223.2006

Labro, M. T., and Bryskier, J. M. (2014). Antibacterial resistance: an emerging 'zoonosis?' *Expert Rev. Anti Infect. Ther.* 12, 1441–1461. doi: 10.1586/14787210.2014.976611

Lange, R. P., Locher, H. H., Wyss, P. C., and Then, R. L. (2007). The targets of currently used antibacterial agents: lessons for drug discovery. *Curr. Pharm. Des.* 13, 3140–3154. doi: 10.2174/138161207782110408

Leevy, W. M., Lambert, T. N., Johnson, J. R., Morris, J., and Smith, B. D. (2008). Quantum dot probes for bacteria distinguish *Escherichia coli* mutants and permit in vivo imaging. *Chem. Commun.* 28, 2331–2333. doi: 10.1039/b8 03590c

Levy, S. B., and Marshall, B. (2004). Antibacterial resistance worldwide: causes, challenges and responses. *Nat. Med.* 10, S122–S129. doi: 10.1038/ nm1145

Li, J. M., Wang, Y. Y., and Zhao, M. X. (2012). Multifunctional QD-based co-delivery of siRNA and doxorubicin to HeLa cells for reversal of multidrug resistance and real-time tracking. *Biomaterials* 33, 2780–2790. doi: 10.1016/j.biomaterials.2011.12.035

Lipsky, B. A., Holroyd, K. J., and Zasloff, M. (2008). Topical versus systemic antimicrobial therapy for treating mildly infected diabetic foot ulcers: a randomized, controlled, double-blinded, multicenter trial of pexiganan cream. *Clin. Infect. Dis.* 47, 1537–1545. doi: 10.1086/593185

Liu, J., Dehbi, M., Moeck, G., Arhin, F., Bauda, P., Bergeron, D., et al. (2004). Antimicrobial drug discovery through bacteriophage genomics. *Nat. Biotechnol.* 22, 185–191. doi: 10.1038/nbt932

Livermore, D. M., Mushtaq, S., Warner, M., Zhang, J. C., Maharjan, S., Doumith, M., et al. (2011). Activity of aminoglycosides, including ACHN-490, against carbapenem-resistant *Enterobacteriaceae* isolates. *J. Antimicrob. Chemother.* 66, 48–53. doi: 10.1093/jac/dkq408

Lupetti, A., Welling, M. M., Pauwels, E. K., and Nibbering, P. H. (2003). Radiolabelled antimicrobial peptides for infection detection. *Lancet Infect. Dis.* 3, 223–229. doi: 10.1016/S1473-3099(03)00579-6

Mandal, T. K., and Parvin, N. (2011). Rapid detection of bacteria by carbon quantum dots. *J. Biomed. Nanotechnol.* 7, 846–848. doi: 10.1166/jbn.2011.1344

McDevitt, D., Payne, D. J., Holmes, D. J., and Rosenberg, M. (2002). Novel targets for the future development of antibacterial agents. *Symp. Ser. Soc. Appl. Microbiol.* 31, 28S–34S. doi: 10.1046/j.1365-2672.92.5s1.16.x

Melendez-Alafort, L., Rodriguez-Cortes, J., Ferro-Flores, G., Arteaga De Murphy, C., Herrera-Rodríguez, R., Mitsoura, E., et al. (2004). Biokinetics of Tc-99m-UBI 29-41 in humans. *Nucl. Med. Biol.* 31, 373–379. doi: 10.1016/j.nucmedbio.2003.10.005

Mendes, R. E., Biedenbach, D. J., Alley, M. R. K., Sader, H. S., and Jones, R. N. (2013). Potency and spectrum of activity of AN3365, a novel boron-containing protein synthesis inhibitor, tested against clinical isolates of *Enterobacteriaceae* and nonfermentative gram-negative bacilli. *Antimicrob. Agents Chemother.* 57, 2849–2857. doi: 10.1128/AAC.00160-13

Morar, M., and Wright, G. D. (2010). The genomic enzymology of antibiotic resistance. *Annu. Rev. Genet.* 44, 25–51. doi: 10.1146/annurev-genet-102209-163517

Morphy, R., and Rankovic, Z. (2006). The physicochemical challenges of designing multiple ligands. *J. Med. Chem.* 49, 4961–4970. doi: 10.1021/jm0603015

Morphy, R., and Rankovic, Z. (2007). Fragments, network biology and designing multiple ligands. *Drug Discov. Today* 12, 156–160. doi: 10.1016/j.drudis.2006.12.006

Motter, A. E. (2010). Improved network performance via antagonism: from synthetic rescues to multi-drug combinations. *Bioessays* 32, 236–245. doi: 10.1002/bies.200900128

Murray, J. L., Kwon, T., and Marcotte, E. M. (2015). Intrinsic antimicrobial resistance determinants in the superbug *Pseudomonas aeruginosa*. *MBio* 6:e01603-15. doi: 10.1128/mBio.01603-15

Nan, Y. H., Bang, J. K., Jacob, B., Park, I. S., and Shin, S. Y. (2012). Prokaryotic selectivity and LPS-neutralizing activity of short antimicrobial peptides designed from the human antimicrobial peptide LL-37. *Peptides* 35, 239–247. doi: 10.1016/j.peptides.2012.04.004

Ng, K. P., Ebrahem, Q., Negrotto, S., Mahfouz, R. Z., Link, K. A., Hu, Z., et al. (2011). p53 independent epigenetic-differentiation treatment in xenotransplant models of acute myeloid leukemia. *Leukemia* 25, 1739–1750. doi: 10.1038/leu.2011.159

Nordmann, P., Dortet, L., and Poirel, L. (2012). Carbapenem resistance in *Enterobacteriaceae*: here is the storm! *Trends Mol. Med.* 18, 263–272. doi: 10.1016/j.molmed.2012.03.003

Nordmann, P., Poirel, L., Walsh, T. R., and Livermore, D. M. (2011). The emerging NDM carbapenemases. *Trends Microbiol.* 19, 588–595. doi: 10.1016/j.tim.2011.09.005

O'Dwyer, K., Spivak, A. T., Ingraham, K., Min, S., Holmes, D. J., Jakielaszek, C., et al. (2015). Bacterial resistance to leucyl-tRNA synthetase inhibitor GSK2251052 develops during treatment of complicated urinary tract infections. *Antimicrob. Agents Chemother.* 59, 289–298. doi: 10.1128/AAC.03774-14

Oliver, A., Cantón, R., Campo, P., Baquero, F., and Blázquez, J. (2000). High frequency of hypermutable *Pseudomonas aeruginosa* in cystic fibrosis lung infection. *Science* 288, 1251–1254. doi: 10.1126/science.288.5469.1251

Onaizi, S. A., and Leong, S. S. (2011). Tethering antimicrobial peptides: current status and potential challenges. *Biotechnol. Adv.* 29, 67–74. doi: 10.1016/j.biotechadv.2010.08.012

Otto, M. (2010). Novel targeted immunotherapy approaches for staphylococcal infection. *Expert Opin. Biol. Ther.* 10, 1049–1059. doi: 10.1517/14712598.2010.495115

Paolini, G. V., Shapland, R. H., van Hoorn, W. P., Mason, J. S., and Hopkins, A. L. (2006). Global mapping of pharmacological space. *Nat. Biotechnol.* 24, 805–815. doi: 10.1038/nbt1228

Paroo, Z., Bollinger, R. A., Braasch, D. A., Richer, E., Corey, D. R., Antich, P. P., et al. (2004). Validating bioluminescence imaging as a high-throughput, quantitative modality for assessing tumor burden. *Mol. Imaging* 3, 117–124. doi: 10.1162/1535350041464865

Pitout, J. D., and Laupland, K. B. (2008). Extended-spectrum β-lactamase-producing *Enterobacteriaceae*: an emerging public-health concern. *Lancet Infect. Dis.* 8, 159–166. doi: 10.1016/S1473-3099(08)70041-0

Probst, J., Dembski, S., Milde, M., and Rupp, S. (2012). Luminescent nanoparticles and their use for in vitro and in vivo diagnostics. *Expert Rev. Mol. Diagn.* 12, 49–64. doi: 10.1586/ERM.11.86

Roda, A., and Guardigli, M. (2012). Analytical chemiluminescence and bioluminescence: latest achievements and new horizons. *Anal. Bioanal. Chem.* 402, 69–76. doi: 10.1007/s00216-011-5455-8

Shkreta, L., Talbot, B. G., Diarra, M. S., and Lacasse, P. (2004). Immune responses to a DNA/protein vaccination strategy against *Staphylococcus aureus* induced mastitis in dairy cows. *Vaccine* 23, 114–126. doi: 10.1016/j.vaccine.2004.05.002

Smith, P. R., Le Breton, A., Horsberg, T. E., and Corsin, F. (2009). "Guidelines for antimicrobial use in aquaculture," in *Guide to Antimicrobial Use in Animals*, eds L. Guardabassi, L. B. Jensen, and H. Kruse (Oxford: Blackwell Publishing Ltd), 207–218. doi: 10.1002/9781444302639

Sommer, M. O., Dantas, G., and Church, G. M. (2009). Functional characterization of the antibiotic resistance reservoir in the human microflora. *Science* 325, 1128–1131. doi: 10.1126/science.1176950

Strebhardt, K., and Ullrich, A. (2008). Paul Ehrlich's magic bullet concept: 100 years of progress. *Nat. Rev. Cancer* 8, 473–480. doi: 10.1038/nrc2394

Sutcliffe, J. A. (2011). Antibiotics in development targeting protein synthesis. *Ann. N. Y. Acad. Sci.* 1241, 122–152. doi: 10.1111/j.1749-6632.2011.06323.x

Sutcliffe, J. A., O'Brien, W., Fyfe, C., and Grossman, T. H. (2013). Antibacterial activity of eravacycline (TP-434), a novel fluorocycline, against hospital and community pathogens. *Antimicrob. Agents Chemother.* 57, 5548–5558. doi: 10.1128/AAC.01288-13

Tacconelli, E. (2009). Antimicrobial use: risk driver of multidrug resistant microorganisms in healthcare settings. *Curr. Opin. Infect. Dis.* 22, 352–358. doi: 10.1097/QCO.0b013e32832d52e0

Tang, D., Devit, M., and Johnston, S. A. (1992). Genetic immunization is a simple method for eliciting an immune response. *Nature* 356, 152–154. doi: 10.1038/356152a0

Tavares, L. S., Silva, C. S., de Souza, V. C., da Silva, V. L., Diniz, C. G., and Santos, M. O. (2013). Strategies and molecular tools to fight antimicrobial resistance: resistome, transcriptome, and antimicrobial peptides. *Front. Microbiol.* 4:412. doi: 10.3389/fmicb.2013.00412

Tenover, F. C., Tickler, I., Armstrong, E. S., Kubo, A., Lopez, S., Persing, D. H., et al. (2011). Activity of ACHN-490 against meticillin-resistant *Staphylococcus aureus* (MRSA) isolates from patients in US hospitals. *Int. J. Antimicrob. Agents* 38, 352–354. doi: 10.1016/j.ijantimicag.2011.05.016

Thaller, M. C., Migliore, L., Marquez, C., Tapia, W., Cedeño, V., Rossolini, G. M., et al. (2010). Tracking acquired antibiotic resistance in commensal bacteria of Galápagos land iguanas: no man, no resistance. *PLoS ONE* 5:e8989. doi: 10.1371/journal.pone.0008989

Tian, X. Y., and Liu, L. (2012). Drug discovery enters a new era with multi-target intervention strategy. *Chin. J. Integr. Med.* 18, 539–542. doi: 10.1007/s11655-011-0900-2

Tossi, A., and Sandri, L. (2002). Molecular diversity in gene-encoded, cationic antimicrobial polypeptides. *Curr. Pharm. Des.* 8, 743–761. doi: 10.2174/1381612023395475

Udekwu, K. I., Parrish, N., Ankomah, P., Baquero, F., and Levin, B. R. (2009). Functional relationship between bacterial cell density and the efficacy of antibiotics. *J. Antimicrob. Chemother.* 63, 745–757. doi: 10.1093/jac/dkn554

Velden, W. J. F. M. V. D., van Iersel, T. M. P., Blijlevens, N. M. A., and Donnelly, J. P. (2009). Safety and tolerability of the antimicrobial peptide human lactoferrin 1-11 (hLF1-11). *BMC Med.* 7:44. doi: 10.1186/1741-7015-7-44

Wright, G. D. (2009). Making sense of antisense in antibiotic drug discovery. *Cell Host Microbe* 6, 197–198. doi: 10.1016/j.chom.2009.08.009

Wu, W., Huang, J., Duan, B., Traficante, D. C., Hong, H., Risech, M., et al. (2012). Th17-stimulating protein vaccines confer protection against *Pseudomonas aeruginosa* pneumonia. *Am. J. Respir. Crit. Care Med.* 186, 420–427. doi: 10.1164/rccm.201202-0182OC

Yildirim, M. A., Goh, K. I., Cusick, M. E., Barabási, A. L., and Vidal, M. (2007). Drug-target network. *Nat. Biotechnol.* 25, 1119–1126. doi: 10.1038/nbt1338

Yu, P., van der Linden, D. S., Sugiarto, H., and Anderson, R. C. (2010). Antimicrobial peptides isolated from the blood of farm animals. *Anim. Prod. Sci.* 50, 660–669. doi: 10.1071/EA07185

Zhang, W., and Sack, D. A. (2015). Current progress in developing subunit vaccines against enterotoxigenic *Escherichia coli*-associated diarrhea. *Clin. Vaccine Immunol.* 22, 983–991. doi: 10.1128/CVI.00224-15

13

Dissemination of Antimicrobial Resistance in Microbial Ecosystems through Horizontal Gene Transfer

Christian J. H. von Wintersdorff[1], John Penders[1,2], Julius M. van Niekerk[2], Nathan D. Mills[1], Snehali Majumder[2], Lieke B. van Alphen[2], Paul H. M. Savelkoul[1,2,3] and Petra F. G. Wolffs[1,2]*

[1] Department of Medical Microbiology, NUTRIM School for Nutrition and Translational Research in Metabolism, Maastricht University Medical Center+, Maastricht, Netherlands, [2] Department of Medical Microbiology, Caphri School for Public Health and Primary Care, Maastricht University Medical Center+, Maastricht, Netherlands, [3] Department of Medical Microbiology and Infection Control, VU University Medical Center, Amsterdam, Netherlands

***Correspondence:**
Petra F. G. Wolffs
p.wolffs@mumc.nl

The emergence and spread of antibiotic resistance among pathogenic bacteria has been a rising problem for public health in recent decades. It is becoming increasingly recognized that not only antibiotic resistance genes (ARGs) encountered in clinical pathogens are of relevance, but rather, all pathogenic, commensal as well as environmental bacteria—and also mobile genetic elements and bacteriophages—form a reservoir of ARGs (the resistome) from which pathogenic bacteria can acquire resistance via horizontal gene transfer (HGT). HGT has caused antibiotic resistance to spread from commensal and environmental species to pathogenic ones, as has been shown for some clinically important ARGs. Of the three canonical mechanisms of HGT, conjugation is thought to have the greatest influence on the dissemination of ARGs. While transformation and transduction are deemed less important, recent discoveries suggest their role may be larger than previously thought. Understanding the extent of the resistome and how its mobilization to pathogenic bacteria takes place is essential for efforts to control the dissemination of these genes. Here, we will discuss the concept of the resistome, provide examples of HGT of clinically relevant ARGs and present an overview of the current knowledge of the contributions the various HGT mechanisms make to the spread of antibiotic resistance.

Keywords: antibiotic resistance, resistome, transformation, conjugation, transduction, gene transfer agents, GTA, lateral gene transfer

INTRODUCTION

The ever-increasing magnitude of antimicrobial resistance (AMR) encountered in human pathogens is a huge concern for public health worldwide, limiting treatment options for bacterial infections and thereby reducing clinical efficacy while increasing treatment costs and mortality. With a lack of development of new antibiotics, and increasing resistance even to last-resort antibiotics (Nordmann et al., 2012), there is a need to conserve the ones available.

Natural antibiotics have existed for billions of years (Barlow and Hall, 2002; Hall and Barlow, 2004; Bhullar et al., 2012; Wright and Poinar, 2012), providing a selective benefit for the producing strains by inhibiting or eliminating other bacteria competing for resources (Martinez, 2008; Aminov, 2009). Additionally, their function as cell-cell signaling molecules has been described

(Davies, 2006; Linares et al., 2006). Just as antibiotics are ancient, so are antibiotic resistance genes (ARGs), as evidenced by studies identifying various ARGs in ancient permafrost samples (D'Costa et al., 2011; Perron et al., 2015) and isolated cave microbiomes (Bhullar et al., 2012). Resistance to antibiotics can occur either by mutations or by acquisition of resistance conferring genes via horizontal gene transfer (HGT), of which the latter is considered to be the most important factor in the current pandemic of AMR.

The HGT of ARGs also far predates the production and use of antibiotics by humans. For example, OXA-type β-lactamases were found to be plasmid-borne and able to transfer between bacterial species millions of years ago (Barlow and Hall, 2002). However, while antibiotic resistance and its spread by HGT are ancient mechanisms, the rate at which these processes occur and the number of resistant strains has increased tremendously over the past few decades because of selective pressure through human antibiotic use.

THE GLOBAL ANTIBIOTIC SELECTION PRESSURE

While the discovery of antibiotics revolutionized the field of medicine, their increasingly large-scale production and consumption has had widespread effects on the microbial biosphere. In their analysis, Van Boeckel et al. showed that global human antibiotic consumption amounted to 54,083,964,813 standard units (pills, capsules, or ampoules) in 2000 and had increased by 36% to 73,620,748,816 standard units by 2010 (Van Boeckel et al., 2014). The same authors estimated that antibiotic consumption in food animals, which is assumed to be larger than that of humans, was over 63 million kg in 2010 and will also drastically increase in the coming years (Van Boeckel et al., 2015) despite recent initiatives to reduce antibiotic use in animals. Such high and continuously increasing amounts of antibiotics overwhelm the natural production, causing a constantly increasing selection pressure on bacterial populations in all exposed environments.

The use and misuse of antibiotics in medicine, agriculture, and aquaculture has been linked to the emergence of resistant bacteria in these settings (Cabello, 2006; Penders and Stobberingh, 2008; Economou and Gousia, 2015). However, the impact of antibiotic usage extends further, as antibiotic residues, resistant bacteria, and genetic resistance elements subsequently spread to adjacent environments. The majority of consumed antibiotics are excreted unchanged (Sarmah et al., 2006) and are then introduced into the environment directly or through waste streams. Such waste streams, as well as wastewater treatment plants, are considered to be hotspots for the dissemination of AMR, since resistance genes, mobile genetic elements (MGEs), and (sub-inhibitory) antibiotic selection pressure from various sources are introduced to commensals and pathogens (Tennstedt et al., 2003; Martinez, 2009; Zhang et al., 2009; Graham et al., 2011). Moreover, the antibiotic compounds are often not completely removed in treatment plants (Watkinson et al., 2007; Le-Minh et al., 2010), from where they then disseminate further. A study by Larsson et al. showed that a treatment plant in India, receiving water from drug manufacturing sites, exposes its direct environment to very high levels of antibiotics, discharging ~45 kg of ciprofloxacin per day (Larsson et al., 2007), contaminating surface, ground, and drinking water in the area (Fick et al., 2009). As a result, not only were highly multiresistant bacteria found to be common within the treatment plant (Marathe et al., 2013), but high levels of ARGs and MGEs were also detected in nearby river sediments (Kristiansson et al., 2011).

How environmental exposure to antibiotics contributes to the selection of resistant strains and the increase of resistome elements is illustrated by a study comparing soil samples taken between 1940 and 2008, which shows that ARGs from all classes of antibiotics tested (β-lactams, tetracyclines, erythromycins, and glycopeptides) significantly increased since 1940, with a tetracycline ARG being over 15 times more abundant than in the 1970s (Knapp et al., 2010). Moreover, the increasing selection pressure has altered bacterial HGT processes, increasing the number of resistome elements which reside on mobile DNA compared to the pre-antibiotic era (Datta and Hughes, 1983).

RESERVOIRS OF RESISTANCE

In order to understand the dissemination of antibiotic resistance, it is necessary to map the resistome of various environments, and to unravel to what extend these environments can act as a reservoir for the dissemination of ARGs to bacterial pathogens. In recent years there has been increasing interest in this matter, as many studies have used various techniques to sample the resistome of environments such as, but not limited to, soil, wastewater, and human and animal gut microbiota (Pehrsson et al., 2013; Penders et al., 2013; Rizzo et al., 2013; von Wintersdorff et al., 2014). It has since become clear that ARGs, including clinically relevant ones, are widespread in such environments (Wright, 2010). Studies applying a metagenomic approach directly recover DNA from all micro-organisms in a biological sample, thereby avoiding the bias that is introduced when selecting certain organisms, and allowing for the investigation of the resistome of microbial ecosystems. The sequencing of metagenomes from various environments has led to a wealth of data which is often publicly available in databases. Such databases can be mined for the presence of resistance genes, even when the initial studies did not focus specifically on ARG content in these metagenomes. For example, mining such metagenomic databases for the plasmid-mediated colistin resistance gene *mcr-1*, which has recently been discovered in clinical and commensal isolates (Arcilla et al., 2015; Liu et al., 2015), has revealed that this gene had already spread to the human gut microbiome of Chinese subjects several years ago (Hu et al., 2015). While sequence based studies provide huge amounts of data, they are limited to either identifying genes that are already known, or to predicting novel sequence functions based on high homology to known sequences. Annotation by sequence-based studies will keep increasing however, as studies using functional metagenomics keep identifying novel ARGs. An increasing number of such studies have revealed a huge number of previously unknown ARGs present in environments such as soil (Riesenfeld et al., 2004; D'Costa et al., 2006; Allen et al., 2009;

Donato et al., 2010; Torres-Cortes et al., 2011; Perron et al., 2015) or activated sludge (Mori et al., 2008; Parsley et al., 2010), as well as in the microbiota of animals (Kazimierczak et al., 2009; Wichmann et al., 2014) and humans (Sommer et al., 2009; Cheng et al., 2012; Moore et al., 2013, 2015; Card et al., 2014; Fouhy et al., 2014; Clemente et al., 2015).

Recent metagenomic studies have also uncovered that ARGs predominantly cluster by ecology, implying that the resistome in soils, and wastewater treatment plants differ significantly from that of human pathogens (Gibson et al., 2015; Munck et al., 2015). Nonetheless, the authors of these works note that parts of these resistomes are shared (Forsberg et al., 2012) and stress the importance of continuing the exploration of the resistome of such environments.

That commensals and the environment are important reservoirs for resistance is supported by several examples of ARGs on MGEs in human pathogens that appear to have originated from those reservoirs. A well-known example is that of the $bla_{\text{CTX-M}}$ genes, which have become the most prevalent cause of extended-spectrum β-lactamases (ESBLs) in Enterobacteriaceae worldwide and a major cause of clinical treatment problems (Hawkey and Jones, 2009). The potential origin of these genes was identified as the chromosomal DNA of various environmental *Kluyvera* species, from where they spread very successfully to different bacterial species (Canton and Coque, 2006). *Shewanella algae*, a marine and freshwater species, was found to be the origin of plasmid-encoded *qnrA* genes, conferring quinolone resistance (Poirel et al., 2005a), and different *Vibrionaceae* species might be the reservoir for other plasmid-encoded *qnr* genes (Poirel et al., 2005b), which have disseminated globally in various Enterobacteriaceae species, with exceptionally high prevalence rates in some areas (Vien le et al., 2012). The OXA-48-type carbapenem-hydrolyzing β-lactamase genes, which are increasingly reported in enterobacterial species worldwide, were also found to originate from the chromosomes of waterborne, environmental *Shewanella* species (Poirel et al., 2012). As with these few examples, many clinically relevant resistance genes are believed to have originated from non-pathogenic bacteria, highlighting the immense potential of HGT for these pathogens in overcoming human use of antibiotics.

CONTRIBUTION OF THE VARIOUS HGT MECHANISMS TO THE SPREAD OF ARGS

Conjugation

Conjugation is the transfer of DNA through a multi-step process requiring cell to cell contact via cell surface pili or adhesins. It is facilitated by the conjugative machinery which is encoded either by genes on autonomously replicating plasmids or by integrative conjugative elements in the chromosome (Smillie et al., 2010; Wozniak and Waldor, 2010). Additionally, this conjugative machinery may enable the mobilization of plasmids that are non-conjugative, as observed for e.g., the exceptionally broad host range IncQ plasmids (Meyer, 2009). Of the various mechanisms that may facilitate HGT (**Figure 1**), conjugation is certainly the most commonly studied (Norman et al., 2009; Guglielmini et al., 2013).

ARGs are in many cases associated with conjugative elements such as plasmids or transposons. While the transfer of these elements may also occur through transformation or transduction, conjugation is often considered as the most likely responsible mechanism. This is due to the fact that it provides better protection from the surrounding environment and a more efficient means of entering the host cell than transformation, while often having a broader host range than bacteriophage transduction. Moreover, while conjugation is a process directed toward the transfer of bacterial genes, transfer of bacterial DNA by transduction is a side-effect of erroneous bacteriophage replication (Norman et al., 2009).

The conjugation of MGEs conferring AMR has been observed in many types of ecosystems, ranging from transfer between bacteria in insects, soil, and water environments to various food and healthcare associated pathogens (Davison, 1999). Importantly, transfer of plasmids and conjugative transposons, such as those of the Tn916 family, between unrelated bacteria over large taxonomic distances has been described (Shoemaker et al., 2001; Musovic et al., 2006; Roberts and Mullany, 2009; Tamminen et al., 2012), indicating that this mechanism contributes significantly to the dissemination of ARGs between different reservoirs via such broad host range MGEs.

The spread of antibiotic resistance plasmids in human pathogens is especially well studied, and shows that once resistance genes have become established on successful plasmids, they may rapidly spread across different strains, species, or even genera. This is well demonstrated by the $bla_{\text{CTX-M}}$ ESBL genes, which have disseminated to various narrow and broad host range plasmids within Enterobacteriaceae, as well as to other opportunistic human pathogens (Canton et al., 2012). These genes are now ubiquitous in humans (Woerther et al., 2013), animals, and the environment (Hartmann et al., 2012). Furthermore, the transfer of plasmids in pathogens has led to the worldwide spread of numerous ARGs encoding resistance to β-lactams, quinolones, aminoglycosides, tetracyclines, sulfonamides, and many other drug classes (Huddleston, 2014). Of particular concern is the increasingly reported spread of plasmids harboring carbapenem resistance (Carattoli, 2013) and the recent discovery of plasmid-encoded colistin resistance in China (Liu et al., 2015), which has now already been identified at multiple continents (Arcilla et al., 2015) and may cause Enterobacteriaceae to truly become pan-drug resistant. Moreover, multiple ARGs are often co-localized on the same plasmid, which allows for the relatively easy spread of multidrug resistance.

Transformation

In 1928, Griffith became the first to demonstrate direct genetic exchange between different strains of *Streptococcus pneumoniae* (Griffith, 1928). Certain bacteria appeared to be capable of uptake, integration, and functional expression of naked fragments of extracellular DNA, a process called (natural) transformation. It soon became clear that bacteria could use transformation to evade antibiotics, by exchanging ARGs. In

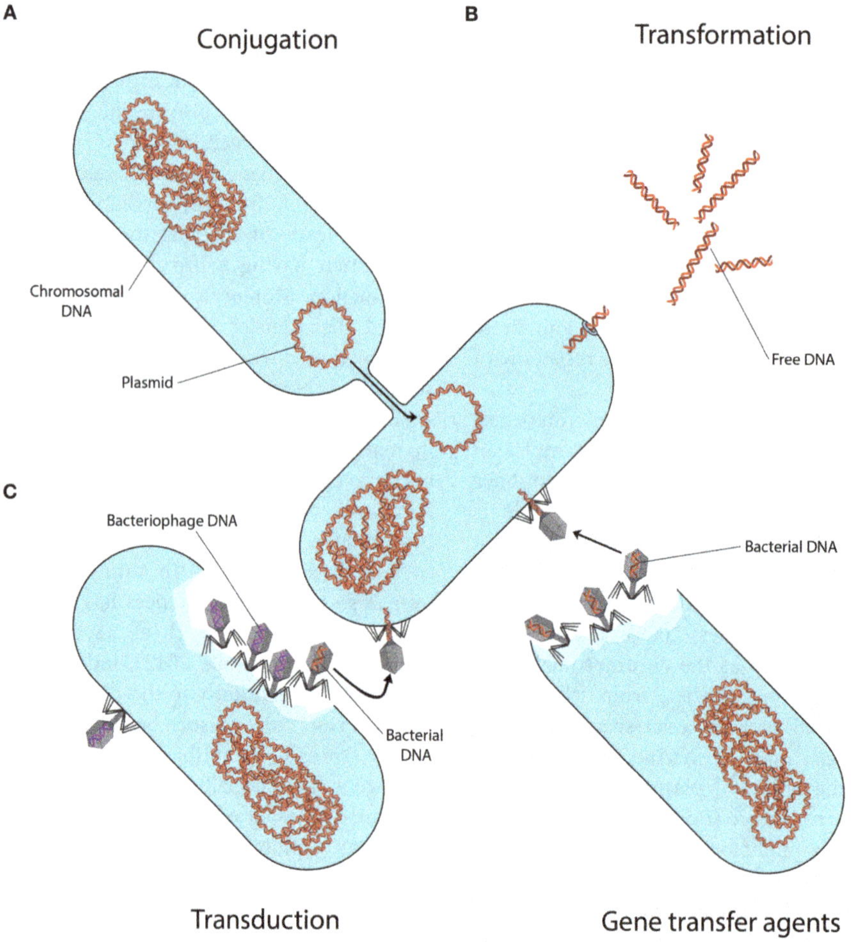

FIGURE 1 | Mechanisms of horizontal gene transfer. Each quadrant represents one different method of gene transfer. **(A)** Conjugation is a process requiring cell to cell contact via cell surface pili or adhesins, through which DNA is transferred from the donor cell to the recipient cell. **(B)** Transformation is the uptake, integration, and functional expression of naked fragments of extracellular DNA. **(C)** Through specialized or generalized transduction, bacteriophages may transfer bacterial DNA from a previously infected donor cell to the recipient cell. During generalized transduction, bacterial DNA may be accidentally loaded into the phage head (shown as a phage with a red DNA strand). During specialized transduction, genomic DNA neighboring the prophage DNA is co-excised and loaded into a new phage (not shown). **(D)** Gene transfer agents (GTAs) are bacteriophage-like particles that carry random pieces of the producing cell's genome. GTA particles may be released through cell lysis and spread to a recipient cell.

1951, Hotchkiss induced penicillin and streptomycin resistance in previously sensitive strains of *S. pneumoniae* by exposing them to DNA from resistant strains (Hotchkiss, 1951). Alexander et al. furthered this work by demonstrating intra- and inter-species transfer of streptomycin resistance between *H. influenzae*, *H. parainfluenzae*, and *H. suis* (Alexander and Leidy, 1953; Alexander et al., 1956).

In order for transformation to take place, several conditions have to be met. There must be DNA present in the extracellular environment; the recipient bacteria must be in a state of competence; and the translocated DNA must be stabilized, either by integration into the recipient genome, or by recircularisation (in the case of plasmid DNA) (Thomas and Nielsen, 2005). Whereas Neisseria spp. are considered to be constitutively competent (Sparling, 1966; Johnston et al., 2014), other bacterial species capable of natural transformation may develop competence only under certain conditions, such as the presence of peptides or autoinducers, nutritional status, or other stressful conditions, as reviewed in more detail by Johnston et al. (2014). Importantly, studies have shown that exposure to antibiotics can induce competence in many species of bacteria, meaning that antibiotics would not only select for resistant strains, but also stimulate transformation of their ARGs (Prudhomme et al., 2006; Charpentier et al., 2011, 2012).

In vitro experiments have done much to elucidate transformation of ARGs. Early work proved that ARGs could be transformed; to this end, streptomycin, rifampicin, erythromycin, nalidixic acid, and kanamycin resistance have variously been transformed into *Neisseria gonorrhoeae* (Sparling, 1966), *Bacillus* spp. (Harford and Mergeay, 1973), *Gallibacterium anatis* (Kristensen et al., 2012), and *S. pneumoniae* (Prudhomme et al., 2006). The introduction of molecular techniques allowed for the identification of the ARGs being transformed. *In vitro* studies have shown that the genes *parC* and *gyrA* are involved in the transformation of fluoroquinolone resistance between *S. pneumoniae* (Ferrandiz et al., 2000) and several viridans streptococci (Gonzalez et al., 1998; Janoir et al., 1999), and that transformation of *penA* confers penicillin resistance in commensal *Neisseria* species (*N. flavescens* and *N. cinerea*) and *N. meningitidis* (Bowler et al., 1994).

Molecular techniques have also made it possible to look for evidence of transformation outside of the laboratory. Spratt et al. identified the *penA* variant responsible for penicillin resistance in clinical isolates of *N. gonorrhoeae* (Spratt, 1988); sequence analysis revealed a mosaic structure, with blocks homologous to susceptible-type *penA* and blocks that diverge significantly (Spratt et al., 1992). These "resistant blocks" could be traced back to a strain of *N. flavescens* that had been isolated in the pre-antibiotic era, suggesting that such commensal species could have been the original source for the now ubiquitous resistance to penicillin (Spratt et al., 1989; Lujan et al., 1991). Mosaic genes are formed when sections of foreign DNA are incorporated into a recipient genome, as is the case in transformation. Their presence implies that HGT has taken place (Hakenbeck, 1998). In streptococci, the mosaic penicillin-binding protein (PBP) genes that encode PBPs with decreased affinity for β-lactam antibiotics are believed to be the result of gene transfer from related penicillin-resistant species (Sibold et al., 1994) and have disseminated penicillin resistance between various streptococci species (Dowson et al., 1990). Studies of fluoroquinolone resistance have demonstrated that mosaic variants of the genes *parC, parE,* and *gyrA* are readily transformed between *S. pneumoniae*, *Streptococcus mitis* and *Streptococcus oralis* (Balsalobre et al., 2003), and between *Streptococcus pyogenes* and *Streptococcus dysgalactiae* (Pletz et al., 2006).

Mao et al. developed a technique to extract intra- and extracellular DNA separately from environmental samples, and applied it to samples from a river basin in China. The result—a greater abundance of DNA outside of cells than inside—implies that in certain environments, extracellular DNA is a large reservoir for genes which may be accessible via transformation (Mao et al., 2014). Furthermore, Domingues et al. demonstrated that MGEs such as transposons, integrons and gene cassettes can be disseminated efficiently between species, regardless of their level of genetic relatedness (Domingues et al., 2012). Similarly, streptococcal species have been shown to exchange conjugative transposons via transformation in addition to conjugation (Chancey et al., 2015). All of this indicates that transformation provides a broad capacity for the horizontal spread of resistance elements between divergent species.

Transduction

Bacteriophages play an important role in shaping the bacterial microbiome in any environment. Through specialized or generalized transduction, bacteriophages can transfer genes that are advantageous to their microbial hosts, in turn promoting their own survival and dissemination (Modi et al., 2013). The transferable DNA sequences range from chromosomal DNA to MGEs such as plasmids, transposons and genomic islands (Brown-Jaque et al., 2015).

The mobilization or transfer of ARGs by bacteriophages has been documented for various bacterial species: the transduction of erythromycin (Hyder and Streitfeld, 1978), tetracycline or multiple resistances between strains of *S. pyogenes* (Ubukata et al., 1975); the transfer of tetracycline and gentamicin resistance between enterococci (Mazaheri Nezhad Fard et al., 2011); the carriage of β-lactamase genes by bacteriophages in *Escherichia coli* (Billard-Pomares et al., 2014) and *Salmonella* (Schmieger and Schicklmaier, 1999); or the transfer of antibiotic resistance plasmids in MRSA (Varga et al., 2012).

Recent studies applying metagenomic approaches to samples from various environments have suggested that bacteriophages may play a bigger part in the spread of ARGs than previously recognized. Colomer-Lluch et al. used qPCR to show that the β-lactam ARGs bla_{TEM}, $bla_{\text{CTX-M}}$ and *mecA* were present in bacteriophages from river and urban sewage water samples. Additionally, cloning of the phage DNA into ampicillin susceptible *E. coli* hosts resulted in resistant transformants, harboring either the bla_{TEM}, $bla_{\text{CTX-M}}$, or undetermined ARGs (Colomer-Lluch et al., 2011a). In another study, the presence of ARGs in bacteriophages was detected in respiratory tract DNA of cystic fibrosis patients (Rolain et al., 2011). Modi et al. demonstrated that treatment with antibiotics increased the number of ARGs in the intestinal phageome of mice and expanded the interactions between phage and bacterial species (Modi et al., 2013), which is an important observation considering the increased environmental exposure to antibiotics discussed earlier. Furthermore, several studies have used qPCR to detect ARGs in bacteriophages from wastewater samples (Colomer-Lluch et al., 2014a,b), animal and human fecal samples (Colomer-Lluch et al., 2011b; Quiros et al., 2014), wastewater and sludge derived from wastewater treatment plants (Calero-Caceres et al., 2014), and hospital and wastewater treatment plant effluents (Marti et al., 2014), indicating that bacteriophages are significant reservoirs of ARGs. Shousha et al. investigated bacteriophages isolated from chicken meat and found that about a quarter of the randomly isolated bacteriophages were able to transduce resistance to one or more antibiotics into an *E. coli* host. Moreover, they found a significant relationship between the presence of bacteriophages transducing kanamycin ARGs, and *E. coli* isolates resistant to kanamycin, implying a possible role of this mechanism in the spread of AMR (Shousha et al., 2015).

Considering certain bacteriophages have been reported to have a wide host range that crosses between different species (Mazaheri Nezhad Fard et al., 2011) or even different taxonomic classes (Jensen et al., 1998), the observation of the plethora of ARGs carried by bacteriophages in various bacterial communities and environments provides renewed insights into the role of transduction in the dissemination of ARGs in microbial ecosystems.

Gene Transfer Agents

Gene transfer agents (GTAs), first identified in *Rhodobacter capsulatus* (RcGTA) in 1974 (Marrs, 1974), are host-cell produced particles that resemble bacteriophage structures, capable of transferring genetic content. GTAs have several characteristic features: (i) rather than carrying DNA encoding their own machinery (as with self-propagating bacteriophages), GTAs carry random pieces of the producing cell's genome (Marrs, 1974; Humphrey et al., 1997; Stanton, 2007; Hynes et al., 2012); (ii) the amount of DNA packaged by the GTAs is insufficient to encode all of their protein components, making them unable to self-propagate (Lang and Beatty, 2000, 2001, 2007); (iii) GTA production is controlled by cell regulatory mechanisms (Lang and Beatty, 2000; Leung et al., 2012; Mercer et al., 2012; Brimacombe et al., 2014); (iv) GTA particles are released through cell lysis (Hynes et al., 2012; Westbye et al., 2013) although cultures do not display observable lysis (Marrs, 1974) as only a small subpopulation of GTA-producing cultures (~3%) is responsible for ~95% of GTA release (Fogg et al., 2012; Hynes et al., 2012); (v) recently, it has been proposed that GTAs combine key aspects of transduction and transformation for cell entry, requiring proteins involved in natural transformation (Brimacombe et al., 2015).

Although GTA particles do not necessarily carry any GTA-encoding genes (Lang et al., 2012), RcGTA-like gene clusters are widespread in alphaproteobacteria, especially in the *Rhodobacterales*: a complete set of RcGTA-like structural genes has been demonstrated in nearly every sequenced member of the *Rhodobacterales* (Lang and Beatty, 2007; Lang et al., 2012). Moreover, two species in the order of *Rhodobacterales, Roseovarius nubinhibens* and *Ruegeria mobilis,* are known to produce GTAs, and there is evidence of GTA production in *Ruegeria pomeroyi* (Biers et al., 2008; McDaniel et al., 2010; Lang et al., 2012). Other known GTAs are VSH-1 in the spirochaete *Brachyspira hyodysenteriae*, Dd1 in the deltaproteobacterium *Desulfovibrio desulfuricans*, and VTA in the archaeon *Methanococcus voltae* (Lang and Beatty, 2007; Lang et al., 2012). The genes required for GTA-production are contained within the host genome and appear to have been propagated through vertical transmission (Lang and Beatty, 2007).

It has been suggested that GTAs have several advantages over the previously described mechanisms of HGT (Stanton, 2007): GTA particles afford DNA protection from damaging environmental factors, as opposed to the naked DNA involved in natural transformation; compared to conjugation, the transfer ability of GTAs is likely maintained after conditions killing the host cell, and is moreover not constrained by cell-to-cell contact; lastly, compared to transduction, GTA particles predominantly carry random pieces of host genome, rather than mostly bacteriophage DNA. In the marine environment, GTA-mediated transfer events have been reported to be remarkably high; up to several million times higher than previous estimates of HGT in marine environments, exceeding previously described transformation and transduction frequencies (McDaniel et al., 2010). Moreover, genes can be exchanged between bacterial phyla (McDaniel et al., 2010; Lang et al., 2012), suggesting the possible widespread contribution of GTAs in shaping and driving adaptation of the natural environment.

In culture, GTA mediated transfer of antibiotic resistance markers has been readily demonstrated in *R. capsulatus* (Marrs, 1974; Solioz et al., 1975; Wall et al., 1975) and the spirochaete *Brachyspira hyodesenteriae* (Stanton et al., 2001, 2008). Moreover, GTAs have been used to transfer traits from plasmids (Scolnik and Haselkorn, 1984). In addition, the *B. hyodesenteriae* GTA VSH-1 can be induced by certain antibiotics (Stanton et al., 2008), which points out its possible impact in its natural environment, the swine intestinal tract. Other *Brachyspira* spp. occur in the intestinal tract of other species, including humans and chickens (Hampson and Ahmed, 2009), in which VSH-1 genes have been described (Motro et al., 2009). However, interspecies GTA-mediated transfer remains to be demonstrated (Motro et al., 2009).

The impact of GTAs on human health has yet to be established, but given the high frequency of transfer events in certain environments, and their ability to exchange genes between phyla, their potential to act as vehicles of resistance traits in the environment, and within the microbiota of humans and farmed animals is an area worthy of further study.

CONCLUSION

The increase in environmental levels of antibiotics, driven by medical and agricultural demand, is unprecedented and has disrupted the natural balance between microbes and antimicrobials. The effects this has on microbial communities are wide-ranging, and the result is an increasingly tangible threat to healthcare, as resistance to all known antibiotics disseminates rapidly around the globe. Our knowledge of the interactions between antimicrobials and resistance against it, observed not only in the clinic but across different ecosystems around the world, is rapidly increasing and has provided valuable insights. However, it is vital that we continue to unravel the extent of, and dissemination between resistomes of these microbial ecosystems, as any attempt at coming to terms with the AMR problem will have to account for these vast reservoirs of ARGs.

AUTHOR CONTRIBUTIONS

CW, JN, SM wrote the article. CW, JN made the Figure. JP, LA, PS, PW provided feedback and discussion on the article.

REFERENCES

Alexander, H. E., Hahn, E., and Leidy, G. (1956). On the specificity of the desoxyribonucleic acid which induces streptomycin resistance in Hemophilus. *J. Exp. Med.* 104, 305–320. doi: 10.1084/jem.104.3.305

Alexander, H. E., and Leidy, G. (1953). Induction of streptomycin resistance in sensitive *Hemophilus influenzae* by extracts containing desoxyribonucleic acid from resistant *Hemophilus influenzae. J. Exp. Med.* 97, 17–31. doi: 10.1084/jem.97.1.17

Allen, H. K., Moe, L. A., Rodbumrer, J., Gaarder, A., and Handelsman, J. (2009). Functional metagenomics reveals diverse β-lactamases in a remote Alaskan soil. *ISME J.* 3, 243–251. doi: 10.1038/ismej.2008.86

Aminov, R. I. (2009). The role of antibiotics and antibiotic resistance in nature. *Environ. Microbiol.* 11, 2970–2988. doi: 10.1111/j.1462-2920.2009.01972.x

Arcilla, M. S., van Hattem, J. M., Matamoros, S., Melles, D. C., Penders, J., de Jong, M. D., et al. (2015). Dissemination of the mcr-1 colistin resistance gene. *Lancet Infect. Dis.* 16, 147–149. doi: 10.1016/S1473-3099(15)00541-1

Balsalobre, L., Ferrandiz, M. J., Linares, J., Tubau, F., and de la Campa, A. G. (2003). Viridans group streptococci are donors in horizontal transfer of topoisomerase IV genes to *Streptococcus pneumoniae*. *Antimicrob. Agents Chemother.* 47, 2072–2081. doi: 10.1128/AAC.47.7.2072-2081.2003

Barlow, M., and Hall, B. G. (2002). Phylogenetic analysis shows that the OXA β-lactamase genes have been on plasmids for millions of years. *J. Mol. Evol.* 55, 314–321. doi: 10.1007/s00239-002-2328-y

Bhullar, K., Waglechner, N., Pawlowski, A., Koteva, K., Banks, E. D., Johnston, M. D., et al. (2012). Antibiotic resistance is prevalent in an isolated cave microbiome. *PLoS ONE* 7:e34953. doi: 10.1371/journal.pone.0034953

Biers, E. J., Wang, K., Pennington, C., Belas, R., Chen, F., and Moran, M. A. (2008). Occurrence and expression of gene transfer agent genes in marine bacterioplankton. *Appl. Environ. Microbiol.* 74, 2933–2939. doi: 10.1128/AEM.02129-07

Billard-Pomares, T., Fouteau, S., Jacquet, M. E., Roche, D., Barbe, V., Castellanos, M., et al. (2014). Characterization of a P1-like bacteriophage carrying an SHV-2 extended-spectrum β-lactamase from an *Escherichia coli* strain. *Antimicrob. Agents Chemother.* 58, 6550–6557. doi: 10.1128/AAC.03183-14

Bowler, L. D., Zhang, Q. Y., Riou, J. Y., and Spratt, B. G. (1994). Interspecies recombination between the penA genes of *Neisseria meningitidis* and commensal Neisseria species during the emergence of penicillin resistance in *N. meningitidis*: natural events and laboratory simulation. *J. Bacteriol.* 176, 333–337.

Brimacombe, C. A., Ding, H., and Beatty, J. T. (2014). *Rhodobacter capsulatus* DprA is essential for RecA-mediated gene transfer agent (RcGTA) recipient capability regulated by quorum-sensing and the CtrA response regulator. *Mol. Microbiol.* 92, 1260–1278. doi: 10.1111/mmi.12628

Brimacombe, C. A., Ding, H., Johnson, J. A., and Beatty, J. T. (2015). Homologues of genetic transformation DNA import genes are required for *Rhodobacter capsulatus* gene transfer agent recipient capability regulated by the response regulator CtrA. *J. Bacteriol.* 197, 2653–2663. doi: 10.1128/JB.00332-15

Brown-Jaque, M., Calero-Caceres, W., and Muniesa, M. (2015). Transfer of antibiotic-resistance genes via phage-related mobile elements. *Plasmid* 79, 1–7. doi: 10.1016/j.plasmid.2015.01.001

Cabello, F. C. (2006). Heavy use of prophylactic antibiotics in aquaculture: a growing problem for human and animal health and for the environment. *Environ. Microbiol.* 8, 1137–1144. doi: 10.1111/j.1462-2920.2006.01054.x

Calero-Caceres, W., Melgarejo, A., Colomer-Lluch, M., Stoll, C., Lucena, F., Jofre, J., et al. (2014). Sludge as a potential important source of antibiotic resistance genes in both the bacterial and bacteriophage fractions. *Environ. Sci. Technol.* 48, 7602–7611. doi: 10.1021/es501851s

Canton, R., and Coque, T. M. (2006). The CTX-M β-lactamase pandemic. *Curr. Opin. Microbiol.* 9, 466–475. doi: 10.1016/j.mib.2006.08.011

Canton, R., Gonzalez-Alba, J. M., and Galan, J. C. (2012). CTX-M enzymes: origin and diffusion. *Front. Microbiol.* 3:110. doi: 10.3389/fmicb.2012.00110

Carattoli, A. (2013). Plasmids and the spread of resistance. *Int. J. Med. Microbiol.* 303, 298–304. doi: 10.1016/j.ijmm.2013.02.001

Card, R. M., Warburton, P. J., MacLaren, N., Mullany, P., Allan, E., and Anjum, M. F. (2014). Application of microarray and functional-based screening methods for the detection of antimicrobial resistance genes in the microbiomes of healthy humans. *PLoS ONE* 9:e86428. doi: 10.1371/journal.pone.0086428

Chancey, S. T., Agrawal, S., Schroeder, M. R., Farley, M. M., Tettelin, H., and Stephens, D. S. (2015). Composite mobile genetic elements disseminating macrolide resistance in *Streptococcus pneumoniae*. *Front. Microbiol.* 6:26. doi: 10.3389/fmicb.2015.00026

Charpentier, X., Kay, E., Schneider, D., and Shuman, H. A. (2011). Antibiotics and UV radiation induce competence for natural transformation in *Legionella pneumophila*. *J. Bacteriol.* 193, 1114–1121. doi: 10.1128/JB.01146-10

Charpentier, X., Polard, P., and Claverys, J. P. (2012). Induction of competence for genetic transformation by antibiotics: convergent evolution of stress responses in distant bacterial species lacking SOS? *Curr. Opin. Microbiol.* 15, 570–576. doi: 10.1016/j.mib.2012.08.001

Cheng, G., Hu, Y., Yin, Y., Yang, X., Xiang, C., Wang, B., et al. (2012). Functional screening of antibiotic resistance genes from human gut microbiota reveals a novel gene fusion. *FEMS Microbiol. Lett.* 336, 11–16. doi: 10.1111/j.1574-6968.2012.02647.x

Clemente, J. C., Pehrsson, E. C., Blaser, M. J., Sandhu, K., Gao, Z., Wang, B., et al. (2015). The microbiome of uncontacted Amerindians. *Sci. Adv.* 1:e1500183. doi: 10.1126/sciadv.1500183

Colomer-Lluch, M., Calero-Caceres, W., Jebri, S., Hmaied, F., Muniesa, M., and Jofre, J. (2014a). Antibiotic resistance genes in bacterial and bacteriophage fractions of Tunisian and Spanish wastewaters as markers to compare the antibiotic resistance patterns in each population. *Environ. Int.* 73, 167–175. doi: 10.1016/j.envint.2014.07.003

Colomer-Lluch, M., Imamovic, L., Jofre, J., and Muniesa, M. (2011b). Bacteriophages carrying antibiotic resistance genes in fecal waste from cattle, pigs, and poultry. *Antimicrob. Agents Chemother.* 55, 4908–4911. doi: 10.1128/AAC.00535-11

Colomer-Lluch, M., Jofre, J., and Muniesa, M. (2011a). Antibiotic resistance genes in the bacteriophage DNA fraction of environmental samples. *PLoS ONE* 6:e17549. doi: 10.1371/journal.pone.0017549

Colomer-Lluch, M., Jofre, J., and Muniesa, M. (2014b). Quinolone resistance genes (qnrA and qnrS) in bacteriophage particles from wastewater samples and the effect of inducing agents on packaged antibiotic resistance genes. *J. Antimicrob. Chemother.* 69, 1265–1274. doi: 10.1093/jac/dkt528

Datta, N., and Hughes, V. M. (1983). Plasmids of the same Inc groups in Enterobacteria before and after the medical use of antibiotics. *Nature*. 306, 616–617. doi: 10.1038/306616a0

Davies, J. (2006). Are antibiotics naturally antibiotics? *J. Ind. Microbiol. Biotechnol.* 33, 496–499. doi: 10.1007/s10295-006-0112-5

Davison, J. (1999). Genetic exchange between bacteria in the environment. *Plasmid* 42, 73–91. doi: 10.1006/plas.1999.1421

D'Costa, V. M., King, C. E., Kalan, L., Morar, M., Sung, W. W., Schwarz, C., et al. (2011). Antibiotic resistance is ancient. *Nature* 477, 457–461. doi: 10.1038/nature10388

D'Costa, V. M., McGrann, K. M., Hughes, D. W., and Wright, G. D. (2006). Sampling the antibiotic resistome. *Science* 311, 374–377. doi: 10.1126/science.1120800

Domingues, S., Harms, K., Fricke, W. F., Johnsen, P. J., da Silva, G. J., and Nielsen, K. M. (2012). Natural transformation facilitates transfer of transposons, integrons and gene cassettes between bacterial species. *PLoS Pathog.* 8:e1002837. doi: 10.1371/journal.ppat.1002837

Donato, J. J., Moe, L. A., Converse, B. J., Smart, K. D., Berklein, F. C., McManus, P. S., et al. (2010). Metagenomic analysis of apple orchard soil reveals antibiotic resistance genes encoding predicted bifunctional proteins. *Appl. Environ. Microbiol.* 76, 4396–4401. doi: 10.1128/AEM.01763-09

Dowson, C. G., Hutchison, A., Woodford, N., Johnson, A. P., George, R. C., and Spratt, B. G. (1990). Penicillin-resistant viridans streptococci have obtained altered penicillin-binding protein genes from penicillin-resistant strains of *Streptococcus pneumoniae*. *Proc. Natl. Acad. Sci. U.S.A.* 87, 5858–5862. doi: 10.1073/pnas.87.15.5858

Economou, V., and Gousia, P. (2015). Agriculture and food animals as a source of antimicrobial-resistant bacteria. *Infect. Drug Resist.* 8, 49–61. doi: 10.2147/IDR.S55778

Ferrandiz, M. J., Fenoll, A., Linares, J., and De La Campa, A. G. (2000). Horizontal transfer of parC and gyrA in fluoroquinolone-resistant clinical isolates of *Streptococcus pneumoniae*. *Antimicrob. Agents Chemother.* 44, 840–847. doi: 10.1128/AAC.44.4.840-847.2000

Fick, J., Soderstrom, H., Lindberg, R. H., Phan, C., Tysklind, M., and Larsson, D. G. (2009). Contamination of surface, ground, and drinking water from pharmaceutical production. *Environ. Toxicol. Chem.* 28, 2522–2527. doi: 10.1897/09-073.1

Fogg, P. C., Westbye, A. B., and Beatty, J. T. (2012). One for all or all for one: heterogeneous expression and host cell lysis are key to gene transfer agent activity in *Rhodobacter capsulatus*. *PLoS ONE* 7:e43772. doi: 10.1371/journal.pone.0043772

Forsberg, K. J., Reyes, A., Wang, B., Selleck, E. M., Sommer, M. O., and Dantas, G. (2012). The shared antibiotic resistome of soil bacteria and human pathogens. *Science* 337, 1107–1111. doi: 10.1126/science.1220761

Fouhy, F., Ogilvie, L. A., Jones, B. V., Ross, R. P., Ryan, A. C., Dempsey, E. M., et al. (2014). Identification of aminoglycoside and β-lactam resistance genes from within an infant gut functional metagenomic library. *PLoS ONE* 9:e108016. doi: 10.1371/journal.pone.0108016

Gibson, M. K., Forsberg, K. J., and Dantas, G. (2015). Improved annotation of antibiotic resistance determinants reveals microbial resistomes cluster by ecology. *ISME J.* 9, 207–216. doi: 10.1038/ismej.2014.106

Gonzalez, I., Georgiou, M., Alcaide, F., Balas, D., Linares, J., and de la Campa, A. G. (1998). Fluoroquinolone resistance mutations in the parC, parE, and gyrA genes of clinical isolates of viridans group streptococci. *Antimicrob. Agents Chemother.* 42, 2792–2798.

Graham, D. W., Olivares-Rieumont, S., Knapp, C. W., Lima, L., Werner, D., and Bowen, E. (2011). Antibiotic resistance gene abundances associated with waste discharges to the Almendares River near Havana, Cuba. *Environ. Sci. Technol.* 45, 418–424. doi: 10.1021/es102473z

Griffith, F. (1928). The significance of pneumococcal types. *J. Hyg. (Lond.)* 27, 113–159. doi: 10.1017/S0022172400031879

Guglielmini, J., de la Cruz, F., and Rocha, E. P. (2013). Evolution of conjugation and type IV secretion systems. *Mol. Biol. Evol.* 30, 315–331. doi: 10.1093/molbev/mss221

Hakenbeck, R. (1998). Mosaic genes and their role in penicillin-resistant *Streptococcus pneumoniae*. *Electrophoresis* 19, 597–601. doi: 10.1002/elps.1150190423

Hall, B. G., and Barlow, M. (2004). Evolution of the serine β-lactamases: past, present and future. *Drug Resist. Updat.* 7, 111–123. doi: 10.1016/j.drup.2004.02.003

Hampson, D. J., and Ahmed, N. (2009). Spirochaetes as intestinal pathogens: lessons from a Brachyspira genome. *Gut Pathog.* 1:10. doi: 10.1186/1757-4749-1-10

Harford, N., and Mergeay, M. (1973). Interspecific transformation of rifampicin resistance in the genus Bacillus. *Mol. Gen. Genet.* 120, 151–155. doi: 10.1007/BF00267243

Hartmann, A., Locatelli, A., Amoureux, L., Depret, G., Jolivet, C., Gueneau, E., et al. (2012). Occurrence of CTX-M Producing *Escherichia coli* in Soils, Cattle, and Farm Environment in France (Burgundy Region). *Front. Microbiol.* 3:83. doi: 10.3389/fmicb.2012.00083

Hawkey, P. M., and Jones, A. M. (2009). The changing epidemiology of resistance. *J. Antimicrob. Chemother.* 64(Suppl. 1), i3–i10. doi: 10.1093/jac/dkp256

Hotchkiss, R. D. (1951). Transfer of penicillin resistance in pneumococci by the desoxyribonucleate derived from resistant cultures. *Cold Spring Harb. Symp. Quant. Biol.* 16, 457–461. doi: 10.1101/SQB.1951.016.01.032

Hu, Y., Liu, F., Lin, I. Y., Gao, G. F., and Zhu, B. (2015). Dissemination of the mcr-1 colistin resistance gene. *Lancet Infect. Dis.* 16, 146–147. doi: 10.1016/S1473-3099(15)00533-2

Huddleston, J. R. (2014). Horizontal gene transfer in the human gastrointestinal tract: potential spread of antibiotic resistance genes. *Infect. Drug Resist.* 7, 167–176. doi: 10.2147/IDR.S48820

Humphrey, S. B., Stanton, T. B., Jensen, N. S., and Zuerner, R. L. (1997). Purification and characterization of VSH-1, a generalized transducing bacteriophage of *Serpulina hyodysenteriae*. *J. Bacteriol.* 179, 323–329.

Hyder, S. L., and Streitfeld, M. M. (1978). Transfer of erythromycin resistance from clinically isolated lysogenic strains of *Streptococcus pyogenes* via their endogenous phage. *J. Infect. Dis.* 138, 281–286. doi: 10.1093/infdis/138.3.281

Hynes, A. P., Mercer, R. G., Watton, D. E., Buckley, C. B., and Lang, A. S. (2012). DNA packaging bias and differential expression of gene transfer agent genes within a population during production and release of the *Rhodobacter capsulatus* gene transfer agent, RcGTA. *Mol. Microbiol.* 85, 314–325. doi: 10.1111/j.1365-2958.2012.08113.x

Janoir, C., Podglajen, I., Kitzis, M. D., Poyart, C., and Gutmann, L. (1999). *In vitro* exchange of fluoroquinolone resistance determinants between *Streptococcus pneumoniae* and viridans streptococci and genomic organization of the parE-parC region in *S. mitis*. *J. Infect. Dis.* 180, 555–558. doi: 10.1086/314888

Jensen, E. C., Schrader, H. S., Rieland, B., Thompson, T. L., Lee, K. W., Nickerson, K. W., et al. (1998). Prevalence of broad-host-range lytic bacteriophages of *Sphaerotilus natans*, *Escherichia coli*, and *Pseudomonas aeruginosa*. *Appl. Environ. Microbiol.* 64, 575–580.

Johnston, C., Martin, B., Fichant, G., Polard, P., and Claverys, J. P. (2014). Bacterial transformation: distribution, shared mechanisms and divergent control. *Nat. Rev. Microbiol.* 12, 181–196. doi: 10.1038/nrmicro3199

Kazimierczak, K. A., Scott, K. P., Kelly, D., and Aminov, R. I. (2009). Tetracycline resistome of the organic pig gut. *Appl. Environ. Microbiol.* 75, 1717–1722. doi: 10.1128/AEM.02206-08

Knapp, C. W., Dolfing, J., Ehlert, P. A., and Graham, D. W. (2010). Evidence of increasing antibiotic resistance gene abundances in archived soils since 1940. *Environ. Sci. Technol.* 44, 580–587. doi: 10.1021/es901221x

Kristensen, B. M., Sinha, S., Boyce, J. D., Bojesen, A. M., Mell, J. C., and Redfield, R. J. (2012). Natural transformation of *Gallibacterium anatis*. *Appl. Environ. Microbiol.* 78, 4914–4922. doi: 10.1128/AEM.00412-12

Kristiansson, E., Fick, J., Janzon, A., Grabic, R., Rutgersson, C., Weijdegard, B., et al. (2011). Pyrosequencing of antibiotic-contaminated river sediments reveals high levels of resistance and gene transfer elements. *PLoS ONE* 6:e17038. doi: 10.1371/journal.pone.0017038

Lang, A. S., and Beatty, J. T. (2000). Genetic analysis of a bacterial genetic exchange element: the gene transfer agent of *Rhodobacter capsulatus*. *Proc. Natl. Acad. Sci. U.S.A.* 97, 859–864. doi: 10.1073/pnas.97.2.859

Lang, A. S., and Beatty, J. T. (2001). The gene transfer agent of *Rhodobacter capsulatus* and "constitutive transduction" in prokaryotes. *Arch. Microbiol.* 175, 241–249. doi: 10.1007/s002030100260

Lang, A. S., and Beatty, J. T. (2007). Importance of widespread gene transfer agent genes in alpha-proteobacteria. *Trends Microbiol.* 15, 54–62. doi: 10.1016/j.tim.2006.12.001

Lang, A. S., Zhaxybayeva, O., and Beatty, J. T. (2012). Gene transfer agents: phage-like elements of genetic exchange. *Nat. Rev. Microbiol.* 10, 472–482. doi: 10.1038/nrmicro2802

Larsson, D. G., de Pedro, C., and Paxeus, N. (2007). Effluent from drug manufactures contains extremely high levels of pharmaceuticals. *J. Hazard. Mater.* 148, 751–755. doi: 10.1016/j.jhazmat.2007.07.008

Le-Minh, N., Khan, S. J., Drewes, J. E., and Stuetz, R. M. (2010). Fate of antibiotics during municipal water recycling treatment processes. *Water Res.* 44, 4295–4323. doi: 10.1016/j.watres.2010.06.020

Leung, M. M., Brimacombe, C. A., Spiegelman, G. B., and Beatty, J. T. (2012). The GtaR protein negatively regulates transcription of the gtaRI operon and modulates gene transfer agent (RcGTA) expression in *Rhodobacter capsulatus*. *Mol. Microbiol.* 83, 759–774. doi: 10.1111/j.1365-2958.2011.07963.x

Linares, J. F., Gustafsson, I., Baquero, F., and Martinez, J. L. (2006). Antibiotics as intermicrobial signaling agents instead of weapons. *Proc. Natl. Acad. Sci. U.S.A.* 103, 19484–19489. doi: 10.1073/pnas.0608949103

Liu, Y. Y., Wang, Y., Walsh, T. R., Yi, L. X., Zhang, R., Spencer, J., et al. (2015). Emergence of plasmid-mediated colistin resistance mechanism MCR-1 in animals and human beings in China: a microbiological and molecular biological study. *Lancet Infect. Dis.* 16, 161–168. doi: 10.1016/S1473-3099(15) 00424-7

Lujan, R., Zhang, Q. Y., Saez Nieto, J. A., Jones, D. M., and Spratt, B. G. (1991). Penicillin-resistant isolates of Neisseria lactamica produce altered forms of penicillin-binding protein 2 that arose by interspecies horizontal gene transfer. *Antimicrob. Agents Chemother.* 35, 300–304. doi: 10.1128/AAC.35.2.300

Mao, D., Luo, Y., Mathieu, J., Wang, Q., Feng, L., Mu, Q., et al. (2014). Persistence of extracellular DNA in river sediment facilitates antibiotic resistance gene propagation. *Environ. Sci. Technol.* 48, 71–78. doi: 10.1021/es404280v

Marathe, N. P., Regina, V. R., Walujkar, S. A., Charan, S. S., Moore, E. R., Larsson, D. G., et al. (2013). A treatment plant receiving waste water from multiple bulk drug manufacturers is a reservoir for highly multi-drug resistant integron-bearing bacteria. *PLoS ONE* 8:e77310. doi: 10.1371/journal.pone.0077310

Marrs, B. (1974). Genetic recombination in *Rhodopseudomonas capsulata*. *Proc. Natl. Acad. Sci. U.S.A.* 71, 971–973. doi: 10.1073/pnas.71.3.971

Marti, E., Variatza, E., and Balcazar, J. L. (2014). Bacteriophages as a reservoir of extended-spectrum β-lactamase and fluoroquinolone resistance genes in the environment. *Clin. Microbiol. Infect.* 20, O456–O459. doi: 10.1111/1469-0691.12446

Martinez, J. L. (2009). Environmental pollution by antibiotics and by antibiotic resistance determinants. *Environ. Pollut.* 157, 2893–2902. doi: 10.1016/j.envpol.2009.05.051

Martinez, J. L. (2008). Antibiotics and antibiotic resistance genes in natural environments. *Science* 321, 365–367. doi: 10.1126/science.1159483

Mazaheri Nezhad Fard, R., Barton, M. D., Heuzenroeder, M. W. (2011). Bacteriophage-mediated transduction of antibiotic resistance in enterococci. *Lett. Appl. Microbiol.* 52, 559–564. doi: 10.1111/j.1472-765X.2011.03043.x

McDaniel, L. D., Young, E., Delaney, J., Ruhnau, F., Ritchie, K. B., and Paul, J. H. (2010). High frequency of horizontal gene transfer in the oceans. *Science* 330, 50. doi: 10.1126/science.1192243

Mercer, R. G., Quinlan, M., Rose, A. R., Noll, S., Beatty, J. T., and Lang, A. S. (2012). Regulatory systems controlling motility and gene transfer agent production and release in *Rhodobacter capsulatus*. *FEMS Microbiol. Lett.* 331, 53–62. doi: 10.1111/j.1574-6968.2012.02553.x

Meyer, R. (2009). Replication and conjugative mobilization of broad host-range IncQ plasmids. *Plasmid* 62, 57–70. doi: 10.1016/j.plasmid.2009.05.001

Modi, S. R., Lee, H. H., Spina, C. S., and Collins, J. (2013). Antibiotic treatment expands the resistance reservoir and ecological network of the phage metagenome. *Nature* 499, 219–222. doi: 10.1038/nature12212

Moore, A. M., Ahmadi, S., Patel, S., Gibson, M. K., Wang, B., Ndao, M. I., et al. (2015). Gut resistome development in healthy twin pairs in the first year of life. *Microbiome* 3:27. doi: 10.1186/s40168-015-0090-9

Moore, A. M., Patel, S., Forsberg, K. J., Wang, B., Bentley, G., Razia, Y., et al. (2013). Pediatric fecal microbiota harbor diverse and novel antibiotic resistance genes. *PLoS ONE* 8:e78822. doi: 10.1371/journal.pone.0078822

Mori, T., Mizuta, S., Suenaga, H., and Miyazaki, K. (2008). Metagenomic screening for bleomycin resistance genes. *Appl. Environ. Microbiol.* 74, 6803–6805. doi: 10.1128/AEM.00873-08

Motro, Y., La, T., Bellgard, M. I., Dunn, D. S., Phillips, N. D., and Hampson, D. (2009). Identification of genes associated with prophage-like gene transfer agents in the pathogenic intestinal spirochaetes *Brachyspira hyodysenteriae*, *Brachyspira pilosicoli* and *Brachyspira intermedia*. *Vet. Microbiol.* 134, 340–345. doi: 10.1016/j.vetmic.2008.09.051

Munck, C., Albertsen, M., Telke, A., Ellabaan, M., Nielsen, P. H., and Sommer, M. O. (2015). Limited dissemination of the wastewater treatment plant core resistome. *Nat. Commun.* 6, 8452. doi: 10.1038/ncomms9452

Musovic, S., Oregaard, G., Kroer, N., and Sorensen, S. J. (2006). Cultivation-independent examination of horizontal transfer and host range of an IncP-1 plasmid among gram-positive and gram-negative bacteria indigenous to the barley rhizosphere. *Appl. Environ. Microbiol.* 72, 6687–6692. doi: 10.1128/AEM.00013-06

Nordmann, P., Dortet, L., and Poirel, L. (2012). Carbapenem resistance in Enterobacteriaceae: here is the storm! *Trends Mol. Med.* 18, 263–272. doi: 10.1016/j.molmed.2012.03.003

Norman, A., Hansen, L. H., and Sorensen, S. J. (2009). Conjugative plasmids: vessels of the communal gene pool. *Philos. Trans. R. Soc. Lond. B Biol. Sci.* 364, 2275–2289. doi: 10.1098/rstb.2009.0037

Parsley, L. C., Consuegra, E. J., Kakirde, K. S., Land, A. M., Harper, W. F. Jr., and Liles, M. R. (2010). Identification of diverse antimicrobial resistance determinants carried on bacterial, plasmid, or viral metagenomes from an activated sludge microbial assemblage. *Appl. Environ. Microbiol.* 76, 3753–3757. doi: 10.1128/AEM.03080-09

Pehrsson, E. C., Forsberg, K. J., Gibson, M. K., Ahmadi, S., and Dantas, G. (2013). Novel resistance functions uncovered using functional metagenomic investigations of resistance reservoirs. *Front. Microbiol.* 4:145. doi: 10.3389/fmicb.2013.00145

Penders, J., and Stobberingh, E. E. (2008). Antibiotic resistance of motile aeromonads in indoor catfish and eel farms in the southern part of The Netherlands. *Int. J. Antimicrob. Agents* 31, 261–265. doi: 10.1016/j.ijantimicag.2007.10.002

Penders, J., Stobberingh, E. E., Savelkoul, P. H., and Wolffs, P. F. (2013). The human microbiome as a reservoir of antimicrobial resistance. *Front. Microbiol.* 4:87. doi: 10.3389/fmicb.2013.00087

Perron, G. G., Whyte, L., Turnbaugh, P. J., Goordial, J., Hanage, W. P., Dantas, G., et al. (2015). Functional characterization of bacteria isolated from ancient arctic soil exposes diverse resistance mechanisms to modern antibiotics. *PLoS ONE* 10:e0069533. doi: 10.1371/journal.pone.0069533

Pletz, M. W., McGee, L., Van Beneden, C. A., Petit, S., Bardsley, M., Barlow, M., et al. (2006). Fluoroquinolone resistance in invasive *Streptococcus pyogenes* isolates due to spontaneous mutation and horizontal gene transfer. *Antimicrob. Agents Chemother.* 50, 943–948. doi: 10.1128/AAC.50.3.943-948.2006

Poirel, L., Liard, A., Rodriguez-Martinez, J. M., and Nordmann, P. (2005b). Vibrionaceae as a possible source of Qnr-like quinolone resistance determinants. *J. Antimicrob. Chemother.* 56, 1118–1121. doi: 10.1093/jac/dki371

Poirel, L., Potron, A., and Nordmann, P. (2012). OXA-48-like carbapenemases: the phantom menace. *J. Antimicrob. Chemother.* 67, 1597–1606. doi: 10.1093/jac/dks121

Poirel, L., Rodriguez-Martinez, J. M., Mammeri, H., Liard, A., and Nordmann, P. (2005a). Origin of plasmid-mediated quinolone resistance determinant QnrA. *Antimicrob. Agents Chemother.* 49, 3523–3525. doi: 10.1128/AAC.49.8.3523-3525.2005

Prudhomme, M., Attaiech, L., Sanchez, G., Martin, B., and Claverys, J. P. (2006). Antibiotic stress induces genetic transformability in the human pathogen Streptococcus pneumoniae. *Science* 313, 89–92. doi: 10.1126/science.1127912

Quiros, P., Colomer-Lluch, M., Martinez-Castillo, A., Miro, E., Argente, M., Jofre, J., et al. (2014). Antibiotic resistance genes in the bacteriophage DNA fraction of human fecal samples. *Antimicrob. Agents Chemother.* 58, 606–609. doi: 10.1128/AAC.01684-13

Riesenfeld, C. S., Goodman, R. M., and Handelsman, J. (2004). Uncultured soil bacteria are a reservoir of new antibiotic resistance genes. *Environ. Microbiol.* 6, 981–989. doi: 10.1111/j.1462-2920.2004.00664.x

Rizzo, L., Manaia, C., Merlin, C., Schwartz, T., Dagot, C., Ploy, M. C., et al. (2013). Urban wastewater treatment plants as hotspots for antibiotic resistant bacteria and genes spread into the environment: a review. *Sci. Total Environ.* 447, 345–360. doi: 10.1016/j.scitotenv.2013.01.032

Roberts, A. P., and Mullany, P. (2009). A modular master on the move: the Tn916 family of mobile genetic elements. *Trends Microbiol.* 17, 251–258. doi: 10.1016/j.tim.2009.03.002

Rolain, J. M., Fancello, L., Desnues, C., and Raoult, D. (2011). Bacteriophages as vehicles of the resistome in cystic fibrosis. *J. Antimicrob. Chemother.* 66, 2444–2447. doi: 10.1093/jac/dkr318

Sarmah, A. K., Meyer, M. T., and Boxall, A. B. (2006). A global perspective on the use, sales, exposure pathways, occurrence, fate and effects of veterinary antibiotics (VAs) in the environment. *Chemosphere* 65, 725–759. doi: 10.1016/j.chemosphere.2006.03.026

Schmieger, H., and Schicklmaier, P. (1999). Transduction of multiple drug resistance of *Salmonella enterica* serovar typhimurium DT104. *FEMS Microbiol. Lett.* 170, 251–256. doi: 10.1111/j.1574-6968.1999.tb13381.x

Scolnik, P. A., and Haselkorn, R. (1984). Activation of extra copies of genes coding for nitrogenase in *Rhodopseudomonas capsulata*. *Nature* 307, 289–292. doi: 10.1038/307289a0

Shoemaker, N. B., Vlamakis, H., Hayes, K., and Salyers, A. A. (2001). Evidence for extensive resistance gene transfer among Bacteroides spp. and among Bacteroides and other genera in the human colon. *Appl. Environ. Microbiol.* 67, 561–568. doi: 10.1128/AEM.67.2.561-568.2001

Shousha, A., Awaiwanont, N., Sofka, D., Smulders, F. J., Paulsen, P., Szostak, M. P., et al. (2015). Bacteriophages isolated from chicken meat and the horizontal transfer of antimicrobial resistance genes. *Appl. Environ. Microbiol.* 81, 4600–4606. doi: 10.1128/AEM.00872-15

Sibold, C., Henrichsen, J., Konig, A., Martin, C., Chalkley, L., and Hakenbeck, R. (1994). Mosaic pbpX genes of major clones of penicillin-resistant *Streptococcus pneumoniae* have evolved from pbpX genes of a penicillin-sensitive *Streptococcus oralis*. *Mol. Microbiol.* 12, 1013–1023. doi: 10.1111/j.1365-2958.1994.tb01089.x

Smillie, C., Garcillan-Barcia, M. P., Francia, M. V., Rocha, E. P., and de la Cruz, F. (2010). Mobility of plasmids. *Microbiol. Mol. Biol. Rev.* 74, 434–452. doi: 10.1128/MMBR.00020-10

Solioz, M., Yen, H. C., and Marris, B. (1975). Release and uptake of gene transfer agent by *Rhodopseudomonas capsulata*. *J. Bacteriol.* 123, 651–657.

Sommer, M. O., Dantas, G., and Church, G. M. (2009). Functional characterization of the antibiotic resistance reservoir in the human microflora. *Science* 325, 1128–1131. doi: 10.1126/science.1176950

Sparling, P. F. (1966). Genetic transformation of *Neisseria gonorrhoeae* to streptomycin resistance. *J. Bacteriol.* 92, 1364–1371.

Spratt, B. G. (1988). Hybrid penicillin-binding proteins in penicillin-resistant strains of Neisseria gonorrhoeae. *Nature* 332, 173–176. doi: 10.1038/332173a0

Spratt, B. G., Bowler, L. D., Zhang, Q. Y., Zhou, J., and Smith, J. M. (1992). Role of interspecies transfer of chromosomal genes in the evolution of penicillin resistance in pathogenic and commensal Neisseria species. *J. Mol. Evol.* 34, 115–125. doi: 10.1007/BF00182388

Spratt, B. G., Zhang, Q. Y., Jones, D. M., Hutchison, A., Brannigan, J. A., and Dowson, C. G. (1989). Recruitment of a penicillin-binding protein gene from *Neisseria flavescens* during the emergence of penicillin resistance in *Neisseria meningitidis*. *Proc. Natl. Acad. Sci. U.S.A.* 86, 8988–8992. doi: 10.1073/pnas.86.22.8988

Stanton, T. B. (2007). Prophage-like gene transfer agents-novel mechanisms of gene exchange for Methanococcus, Desulfovibrio, Brachyspira, and Rhodobacter species. *Anaerobe* 13, 43–49. doi: 10.1016/j.anaerobe.2007.03.004

Stanton, T. B., Humphrey, S. B., Sharma, V. K., and Zuerner, R. L. (2008). Collateral effects of antibiotics: carbadox and metronidazole induce VSH-1 and facilitate gene transfer among *Brachyspira hyodysenteriae* strains. *Appl. Environ. Microbiol.* 74, 2950–2956. doi: 10.1128/AEM.00189-08

Stanton, T. B., Matson, E. G., and Humphrey, S. B. (2001). *Brachyspira* (Serpulina) *hyodysenteriae* gyrB mutants and interstrain transfer of coumermycin A(1) resistance. *Appl. Environ. Microbiol.* 67, 2037–2043. doi: 10.1128/AEM.67.5.2037-2043.2001

Tamminen, M., Virta, M., Fani, R., and Fondi, M. (2012). Large-scale analysis of plasmid relationships through gene-sharing networks. *Mol. Biol. Evol.* 29, 1225–1240. doi: 10.1093/molbev/msr292

Tennstedt, T., Szczepanowski, R., Braun, S., Puhler, A., and Schluter, A. (2003). Occurrence of integron-associated resistance gene cassettes located on antibiotic resistance plasmids isolated from a wastewater treatment plant. *FEMS Microbiol. Ecol.* 45, 239–252. doi: 10.1016/S0168-6496(03)00164-8

Thomas, C. M., and Nielsen, K. M. (2005). Mechanisms of, and barriers to, horizontal gene transfer between bacteria. *Nat. Rev. Microbiol.* 3, 711–721. doi: 10.1038/nrmicro1234

Torres-Cortes, G., Millan, V., Ramirez-Saad, H. C., Nisa-Martinez, R., Toro, N., and Martinez-Abarca, F. (2011). Characterization of novel antibiotic resistance genes identified by functional metagenomics on soil samples. *Environ. Microbiol.* 13, 1101–1114. doi: 10.1111/j.1462-2920.2010.02422.x

Ubukata, K., Konno, M., and Fujii, R. (1975). Transduction of drug resistance to tetracycline, chloramphenicol, macrolides, lincomycin and clindamycin with phages induced from *Streptococcus pyogenes*. *J. Antibiot.* 28, 681–688. doi: 10.7164/antibiotics.28.681

Van Boeckel, T. P., Brower, C., Gilbert, M., Grenfell, B. T., Levin, S. A., Robinson, T. P., et al. (2015). Global trends in antimicrobial use in food animals. *Proc. Natl. Acad. Sci. U.S.A.* 112, 5649–5654. doi: 10.1073/pnas.1503141112

Van Boeckel, T. P., Gandra, S., Ashok, A., Caudron, Q., Grenfell, B. T., Levin, S. A., et al. (2014). Global antibiotic consumption 2000 to 2010: an analysis of national pharmaceutical sales data. *Lancet Infect. Dis.* 14, 742–750. doi: 10.1016/S1473-3099(14)70780-7

Varga, M., Kuntova, L., Pantucek, R., Maslanova, I., Ruzickova, V., and Doskar, J. (2012). Efficient transfer of antibiotic resistance plasmids by transduction within methicillin-resistant *Staphylococcus aureus* USA300 clone. *FEMS Microbiol. Lett.* 332, 146–152. doi: 10.1111/j.1574-6968.2012.02589.x

Vien le, T. M., Minh, N. N., Thuong, T. C., Khuong, H. D., Nga, T. V., Thompson, C., et al. (2012). The co-selection of fluoroquinolone resistance genes in the gut flora of Vietnamese children. *PLoS ONE* 7:e42919. doi: 10.1371/journal.pone.0042919

von Wintersdorff, C. J., Penders, J., Stobberingh, E. E., Lashof, A. M., Hoebe, C. J., Savelkoul, P. H., et al. (2014). High rates of antimicrobial drug resistance gene acquisition after international travel, the Netherlands. *Emerging Infect. Dis.* 20, 649–657. doi: 10.3201/eid2004.131718

Wall, J. D., Weaver, P. F., and Gest, H. (1975). Gene transfer agents, bacteriophages, and bacteriocins of *Rhodopseudomonas capsulata*. *Arch. Microbiol.* 105, 217–224. doi: 10.1007/BF00447140

Watkinson, A. J., Murby, E. J., and Costanzo, S. D. (2007). Removal of antibiotics in conventional and advanced wastewater treatment: implications for environmental discharge and wastewater recycling. *Water Res.* 41, 4164–4176. doi: 10.1016/j.watres.2007.04.005

Westbye, A. B., Leung, M. M., Florizone, S. M., Taylor, T. A., Johnson, J. A., Fogg, P. C., et al. (2013). Phosphate concentration and the putative sensor kinase protein CckA modulate cell lysis and release of the *Rhodobacter capsulatus* gene transfer agent. *J. Bacteriol.* 195, 5025–5040. doi: 10.1128/JB.00669-13

Wichmann, F., Udikovic-Kolic, N., Andrew, S., and Handelsman, J. (2014). Diverse antibiotic resistance genes in dairy cow manure. *MBio.* 5:e01017. doi: 10.1128/mBio.01017-13

Woerther, P. L., Burdet, C., Chachaty, E., and Andremont, A. (2013). Trends in human fecal carriage of extended-spectrum β-lactamases in the community: toward the globalization of CTX-M. *Clin. Microbiol. Rev.* 26, 744–758. doi: 10.1128/CMR.00023-13

Wozniak, R. A., and Waldor, M. K. (2010). Integrative and conjugative elements: mosaic mobile genetic elements enabling dynamic lateral gene flow. *Nat. Rev. Microbiol.* 8, 552–563. doi: 10.1038/nrmicro2382

Wright, G. D. (2010). Antibiotic resistance in the environment: a link to the clinic? *Curr. Opin. Microbiol.* 13, 589–594. doi: 10.1016/j.mib.2010.08.005

Wright, G. D., and Poinar, H. (2012). Antibiotic resistance is ancient: implications for drug discovery. *Trends Microbiol.* 20, 157–159. doi: 10.1016/j.tim.2012.01.002

Zhang, X. X., Zhang, T., Zhang, M., Fang, H. H., and Cheng, S. P. (2009). Characterization and quantification of class 1 integrons and associated gene cassettes in sewage treatment plants. *Appl. Microbiol. Biotechnol.* 82, 1169–1177. doi: 10.1007/s00253-009-1886-y

14

Mechanism and *In Vivo* Evaluation: Photodynamic Antibacterial Chemotherapy of Lysine-Porphyrin Conjugate

Zengping Xu[1], Yuxiang Gao[2], Shuai Meng[1,3], Baochen Yang[1], Liyun Pang[1], Chen Wang[3] and Tianjun Liu[1]*

[1] Tianjin Key Laboratory of Biomedical Material, Institute of Biomedical Engineering, Peking Union Medical College – Chinese Academy of Medical Sciences, Tianjin, China, [2] Department of Materials Chemistry, Nankai University, Tianjin, China, [3] Tianjin Medical University Cancer Institute and Hospital, Tianjin, China

***Correspondence:**
Tianjun Liu
liutianjun@hotmail.com

Lysine-porphyrin conjugate 4i has potent photosensitive antibacterial effect on clinical isolated bacterial strains such as Methicillin-resistant *Staphylococcus aureus* (MRSA), *Escherichia coli*, and *Pseudomonas aeruginosa*. The mechanism of photodynamic antibacterial chemotherapy of 4i (4i-PACT) *in vitro* and the treatment effect *in vivo* was investigated in this paper. Atomic force microscopy (AFM) revealed that 4i-PACT can effectively destroy membrane and wall of bacteria, resulting in leakage of its content. This was confirmed by dual fluorescent staining with acridine orange/ethidium bromide and measuring materials absorption at 260 nm. Agarose gel electrophoresis measurement showed that 4i-PACT can damage genomic DNA. Healing of wound in rat infected by mixed bacteria showed that the efficiency of 4i-PACT is dependent on the dose of light. These results showed that 4i-PACT has promising bactericidal effect both *in vitro* and *in vivo*.

Keywords: lysine-porphyrin conjugate, photodynamic antimicrobial chemotherapy, antibiotic resistance, photosensitizer, mixed bacterial-infected wounds

INTRODUCTION

The antibiotics for treating common infections have become less effective in recent years. Nearly 1000 of resistance-related β-lactamases, which inactivate the antibiotics, have been identified, a 10 times increase since 1990 (Davies and Davies, 2010; Laxminarayan et al., 2013). This situation made us at the dawn of post antibiotic era (Ryono, 2014). So, it is urgent to find alternative approaches against antibiotics-resistant bacteria. Generally, there are two solutions to this problem. One is to develop novel antibacterial agents, the other is to develop novel physical sterilization. The latter includes radiation sterilization (Nusbaum and Rose, 1979), high pressure electric field sterilization (Sasagawa et al., 2006), microwave sterilization (Dovigo et al., 2009), magnetic sterilization (Haile et al., 2008), and pulse light sterilization (Krishnamurthy et al., 2004). Chemical agents and physical approaches are combined in Photodynamic antimicrobial chemotherapy (PACT) (Wainwright, 1998), which consists of a non-toxic photosensitizer (PS), illumination light of an appropriate wavelength, and ambient molecular oxygen. However, not all of the PS can be used in PACT treatment of bactrerial infection. Only special designed PS can match the PACT demand (Meng et al., 2015). So from this point of view, PACT falls between novel antibacterial agents and novel physical sterilization approaches, namely, a physicochemical treatment. With the advantage of circumventing the bacterial multidrug resistance in the treatment of infection, PACT has received great attention in recent years.

The PS is the crutial element in PACT. In the past few decades, several types of PSs have been reported, such as porphyrin, heme, phthalocyanine, phenothiazinium dyes, BODIPY, methylene blue, conjugated polyelectrolytes, cationic functionalized fullerene, as well as nanoparticals (Wainwright and Crossley, 2004; Wainwright, 2010; Fu et al., 2013; Sperandio et al., 2013). As an ideal PS candidate for photodynamic therapies (Stojiljkovic et al., 2001), Porphyrin can efficiently kill Gram-positive bacteria. Meanwhile, in combination with agents that permeabilize the highly organized outer membrane of Gram-negative bacteria, only cationic PSs, or noncationic PSs are able to kill Gram-negative species (Mbakidi et al., 2013; Prasanth et al., 2014).

In a previous paper, we have reported the synthesis, characterization, and *in vitro* photodynamic antimicrobial activity of basic amino acid-porphyrin conjugates (Meng et al., 2015), a new class of PSs. Among them, compared with other PSs, 4i exhibits a broader spectrum of photoinactivation *in vitro*, improved biocompatibility and stability (Bertolini et al., 1990; Nitzan et al., 1992; Tomé et al., 2004; Liu et al., 2012; Gomes et al., 2013; Mbakidi et al., 2013; Prasanth et al., 2014). This paper reported the mechanism of bacterial inactivation by 4i-PACT and its effectiveness *in vivo* on experimental mixed bacterial infected rat wounds. The results showed that 4i-PACT had potent bactericidal effect both *in vitro* and *in vivo*.

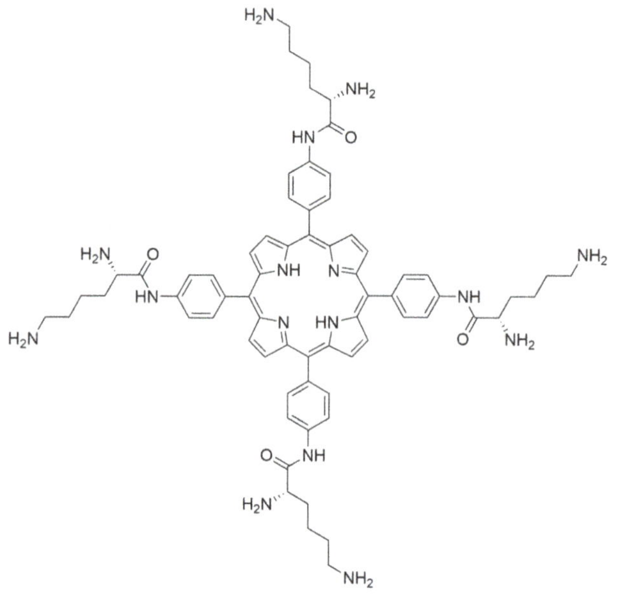

4i

FIGURE 1 | Structure of 5,10,15,20-trakis(4-((S)-2,6-diaminohexanamido)-phenyl) porphyrin (4i).

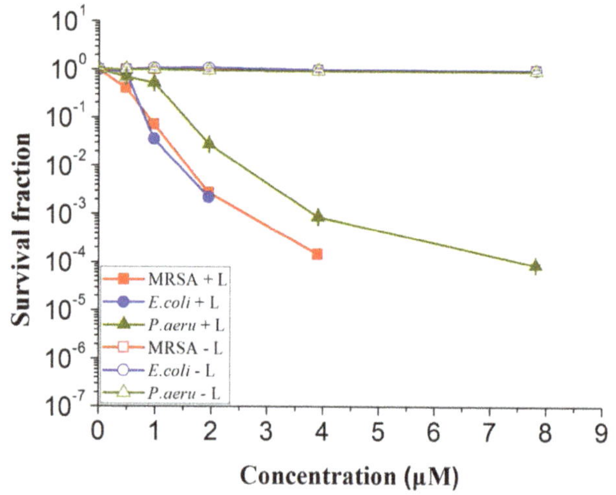

FIGURE 2 | Survival fraction of three bacterial strains treated by different concentration of 4i with and without illumination. Light toxicity marked by MRSA + L, *Escherichia coli* + L, *Pseudomonas aeruginosa* + L and dark toxicity marked by MRSA – L, *E. coli* – L, *P. aeruginosa* – L respectively.

MATERIALS AND METHODS

Bacterial Culture

In this experiment, three clinical bacterial strains, MRSA, *Escherichia Coli,* and *Pseudomonas aeruginosa* were isolated at the Tianjin Armed Police Hospital. These bacterial strains were cultured in Luria Bertani (LB) medium. A single colony was used to inoculate 10 mL of liquid medium. The bacteria was grown under aerobic condition at 37°C in a shaking incubator (200 rpm) for 18 h. The bacteria was then collected by centrifugation and resuspended in an equal volume of PBS (Zhao et al., 2014).

Chemicals and Instruments

Porphyrin derivative 4i was synthesized and characterized with the procedure reported by Meng et al. (2015). For clarity, synthetic procedure and characterization detail are omitted. The chemical structure of porphyrin derivative 4i is shown in **Figure 1**.

Light from a semiconductor laser (7404, Intense, USA) with a wavelength of 650 nm was delivered on the sample via an optic fiber. The energy density of light spot was measured by a light power meter (LM1; Carl Zeiss).

MIC and MBC Determinations

Three bacterial strains were treated with the same procedure. As an example of all of the strains, the treatment of MRSA is described in detail. Experiments were performed in 96-well flat bottom plates. Twenty microliter of MRSA suspension and 180 μL of the compounds were added to each well. The final concentration of the bacterial in the mixture was 10^6 colony-forming units/mL (CFU/mL). 4i with different mole concentrations were prepared, e.g., 0.98, 1.95, 3.91, 7.8, 15.6,

31.25, 62.5, 125, 250, and 500 μM, respectively. Plates were kept in the dark for 30 min at 37°C and then exposed to light illumination for 30 min or kept in the dark to provide dark control samples. After light exposure, the samples were incubated in dark at 37°C and CFU was evaluated after 18 h. Three sets of independent experiments were performed (Rodrigues et al., 2013).

Dose-Dependent Photoinactivation Effects

Suspensions of bacteria (10^7 CFU/mL) were incubated at 37°C for 30 min in the dark with 4i (3.91, 7.81, 15.63, 31.25, and 62.50 μM). The suspensions were then loaded into a 96-well plate and illuminated with light with energy density of 6 J/cm^2 for the photoreaction. After illumination, 100 μL mixture from each well was taken to determine the CFU. The mixtures were serially diluted to 10^1, 10^2, 10^3, 10^4, and 10^5 times of the initial concentrations using PBS. 100 μL of each dilution was plated onto LB agar plates and incubated for 18 h at 37°C in dark. The CFUs were counted, and each experiment was performed in triplicate. The surviving fractions of bacteria were expressed as ratios of CFU produced by bacteria treated with PSs and light (Grinholc et al., 2008).

Atomic Force Microscopy (AFM) Imaging

The bacteria were examined with atomic force microscope (Veeco Multi Mode 8/B0021, Veeco German) equipped with Antimony doped silicon of conical shape (Veeco). The force constant is 3 N/m. Bacterial samples in a concentration of 10^7 CFU/mL were dropped on to the mica plate surface (about 0.5 cm^2), naturally dried at ambient temperature, then were scanned in intelligent mode (Wu et al., 2014).

Fluorescence Imaging

In order to study 4i-PACT effect on the permeability of the bacterial membrane, the samples after 4i-PACT treatment were stained with 4 μL of the acridine orange/ethidium bromide (AO/EB) double fluorescent dyes mixture (100 mg/L of AO and 100 mg/L of EB) for 5 min in dark. Then 5 μL of the stained mixture was dropped on a microscopic glass slide with cover glass and immediately checked by the fluorescent microscope (Nikon Eclipse Ti/B0004, Nikon, Japan) at 200× magnification (Sui et al., 2013).

Genomic DNA Extraction and Electrophoresis

Bacterial suspensions (1 × 10^7 CFU/mL) were treated with 10 μM 4i as mentioned in experiment 2.4 above. After exposing to the laser light, the genomic DNA was extracted from bacteria immediately using a Genomic DNA Purification Kit (Solarbio, Beijing). DNA samples were gently mixed with 6x loading buffer (Solarbio, Beijing). DNA was analyzed by electrophoresis with 0.8% agarose gel in 1x TAE buffer at 70 V for 30 min. DNA green was incorporated into the agarose gel. The 15000 bp DNA Marker (TAKARA) was used as a molecular weight marker with DNA fragments between 250 and 15000 bp. The light dose had been optimized *in vitro* in our experiments. Light dose higher than 6 J/cm^2 did not improve the efficacy, while the light with lower dose results in a lower bactericidal ability. Without PS 4i, light exposure alone on bacteria *in vitro* did not have significant bactericidal effect.

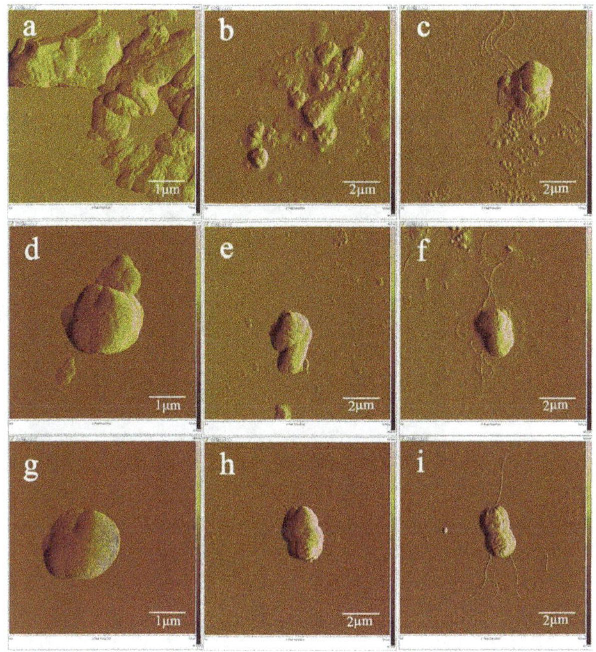

FIGURE 3 | Fluorescence microscopy image of three bacterial strains treated by 10 μM 4i with and without illumination. (a) MRSA treated by 4i-PACT, **(d)** 4i with no light, **(g)** control; **(b)** *P. aeruginosa* treated by 4i-PACT, **(e)** 4i with no light, **(h)** control; **(c)** *E. coli* treated by the 4i-PACT, **(f)** 4i with no light, **(i)** control.

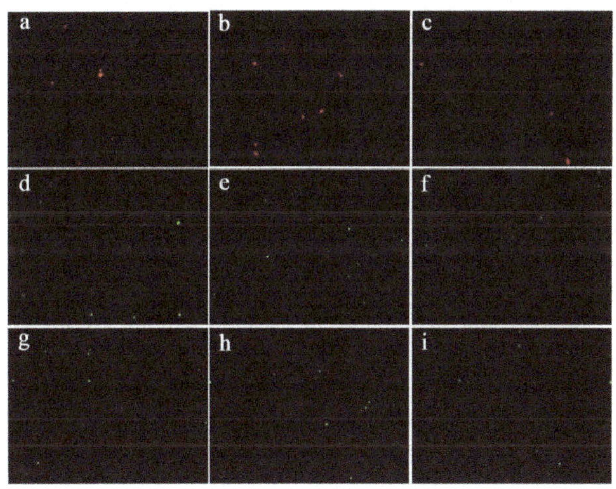

FIGURE 4 | AFM image of three bacterial strains treated by 10 μM 4i with and without illumination. (a) MRSA treated by 4i-PACT, **(d)** 4i with no light, **(g)** control; **(b)** *P. aeruginosa* treated by 4i-PACT, **(e)** 4i with no light, **(h)** control; **(c)** *E. coli* treated by 4i-PACT, **(f)** 4i with no light, **(i)** control.

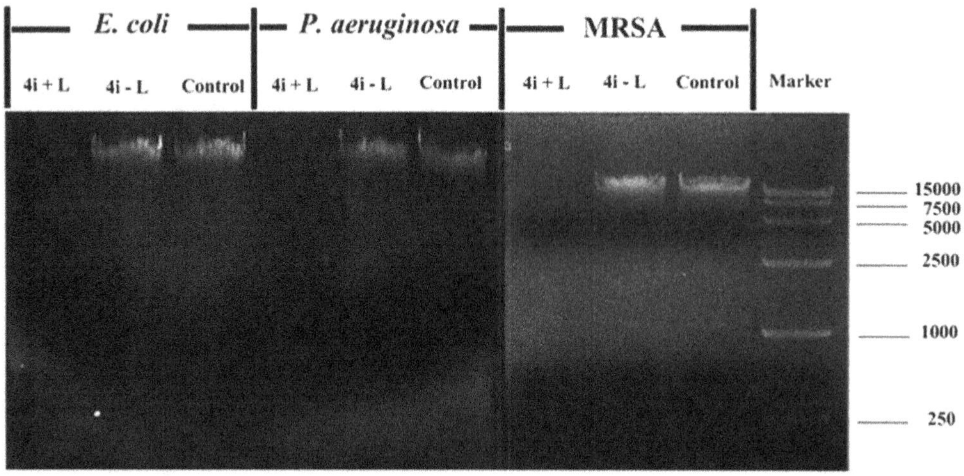

FIGURE 5 | Agarose gel electrophoresis of three bacterial strains after treated by 10 μM 4i with and without illumination. Bacteria treated with 4i-PACT (4i + L), treated with 4i in the dark (4i–L) and no treatment (control).

Exudation Study for Measuring Materials Absorption at 260 nm

DNA and RNA have absorbance at 260 nm, so exudation study was conducted by measuring the materials absorption at 260 nm for bacteria treated by 10 μM 4i-PACT, 10 μM 4i alone, and PBS, respectively. After treatment, 400 μL of the bacterial suspensions (1×10^8) were filtered to remove the bacteria. OD at 260 nm (OD_{260}) of the supernatant was recorded for treated and pre-treatment control groups.

Excisional Wound Model and Establishment of Infection

The wound healing characteristic of the 4i-PACT was evaluated using a rat model (Dash et al., 2001). **The Animal Care and Use Committee of PUMC approved all experimental protocols involving rats.** Sprague–Dawley rats from Beijing HFK Bioscience CO.,LTD, weighing about 220 g, were housed at one rat one cage and maintained in dark except PACT treatment. The rats were first anesthetized via intraperitoneal injection of chloral hydrate (300 mg/kg). Then their back was shaved with an electric razor, followed by a depilatory agent. Four circular wounds (1.5 cm in diameter) with a depth of the skin layers were prepared along both sides of the spine. Immediately after that, suspension (50 μL) of mixed bacteria (10^9 CFU/mL MRSA, 5×10^8 CFU/mL *E. coli*, 5×10^8 CFU/mL *P. aeruginosa*) in sterile PBS was inoculated onto the surface of each wound with a pipet tip and then smeared onto the wound surface with an inoculating loop. Next, a bandage was wrapped around each rat to protect the shaved skin and the wounds from other harm. This state was kept for 1 day. Then these rats were used as the wounds model for mixed bacterial infection.

4i-PACT *In Vivo*

Thirty rats with wound infected by mixed bacteria were divided into five groups: (A) no treatment control; (B) 4i + 100 J/cm^2 Light; (C) 4i + 50 J/cm^2 Light; (D) 4i + 25 J/cm^2 Light; (E) 4i + 12.5 J/cm^2 Light. Since light illumination doses alone in this study do not have significant effect on the wound healing, we did not provide light illumination doses alone groups.

Twenty four hours after infection, 50 μL of 4i solution (40 μM in PBS) was injected under eschar of the wound of groups B–E. Then after 30 min for the PS uptaken by the bacteria, rats in groups B–E were illuminated with 650 nm laser (100 mW/cm^2), the light dose was kept at 100, 50, 25, 12.5 J/cm^2 for group B–E, respectively. On the next day, the same light dose was given to increase the antibacterial effect of 4i-PACT. The above treatment was repeated three times.

The day, on which rats were infected, was regarded as day 1, the widths and lengths of the wounds were measured using a vernier caliper on days 1, 2, 3, 4, 5, 6, 7, 8, 10, and 12. The viability of each group of rats after infection was recorded, respectively. Meanwhile bacterial CFUs in the wound were calculated in the following ways. Swabs collected from the rat wounds were cultured in PBS. Viable bacteria in the PBS were counted by making 10-fold serial dilutions and culturing the dilutions on LB agar for 18 h at 37°C. Then CFUs were counted manually (Kumar et al., 2011; Sudheesh Kumar et al., 2012).

Statistical Analysis

All data are presented as mean ± SEM. The significance of differences between sample means was determined by Student's *t*-test using SPSS 19.0.

RESULTS AND DISCUSSION

MIC and MBC Determinations

The minimum inhibitory and bactericidal concentration (MIC and MBC) of 4i toward bacteria was studied. Bacterial suspensions (10^6 CFU/mL) were incubated with the 4i in dark for 30 min at 37°C and then exposed to light illumination

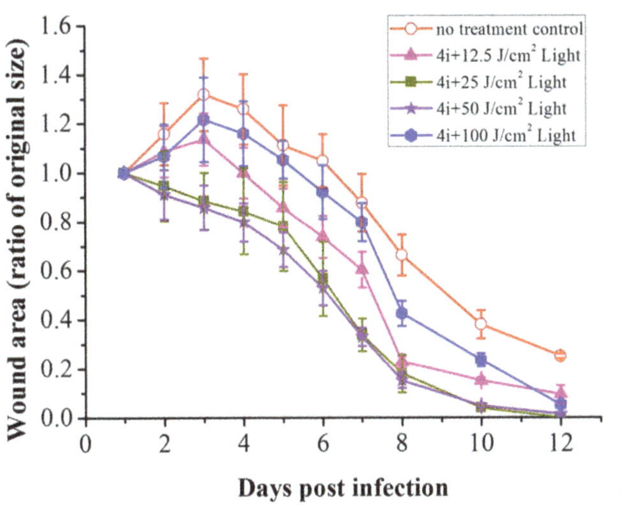

FIGURE 6 | Wound healing ratio over time in bacterial infected rats with and without 4i-PACT. Each point represents the mean ratio of the area of the original wound. Data is expressed as mean ± SEM. $N = 6$ in each group.

(650 nm, 6 J/cm^2). The concentration of 4i required to make the suspensions (10^6 CFU/mL) change visibly from turbid to clear was regarded as the minimum inhibitory concentration (MIC), while the concentration at which no more than five colonies were observed on the plates was regarded as the minimum bactericidal concentration (MBC). As shown in **Table 1**, compound 4i had high bacterial photoinactivation ability with MIC values of 3.91 μM against MRSA, 1.95 μM against *E. coli*, and 7.81 μM against *P. aeruginosa*, respectively; MBC values of 7.81 μM against MRSA, 3.91 μM against *E. coli*, and 15.60 μM against *P. aeruginosa*. Meanwhile the dark toxicity of the 4i is relatively weak, with MIC > 62.5 μM, MBC > 125 μM for these three strains. From the values of MBC, it can be concluded that 4i-PACT is very effective toward *E coli*, *P. aeruginosa* is the most resistant strain and MRSA is at the middle of them. So 4i-PACT seemly shows higher bactericidal activity toward Gram-negative strains than that of Gram-positive strains. This trend is different from the PACT of other positive charged PS (Sahu et al., 2009; Kharkwal et al., 2011; Ke et al., 2014), which show higher photoinactivation toward the Gram-positive strains than the Gram-negative counterparts. The latter possess a highly organized outer membrane which imparts a higher permeability barrier for the PSs to penetrate into the bacteria. In this study, 4i-PACT shows higher bactericidal effect toward *E. coli* than MRSA and *P. aeruginosa*. This unexpected result can be interpreted based upon the chemical structure of 4i, π−π interaction of large planar porphyrin rings, hydrogen bonding interaction and charge interaction from four lysine moieties. The ensemble interaction and difference of the outside membrane structure of these strains lead to the unexpected bactericidal effect of 4i-PACT.

TABLE 1 | Minimal inhibitory concentration (MIC, μM) and minimal bactericidal concentration (MBC, μM) of 4i against MRSA, *Pseudomonas aeruginosa*, *Escherichia coli*.

Clinical bacterial strain	Light toxicity		Dark toxicity	
	MIC	MBC	MIC	MBC
MRSA	3.91	7.81	62.50	125.00
P. aeruginosa	7.81	15.60	250	> 500
E. coli	1.95	3.91	62.50	125.00

TABLE 2 | Bacterial content exudation in the control (PBS), 4i alone, and 4i-PACT treatment groups ($n = 4$, mean ± SD) measured at 260 nm.

Clinical bacterial strain	Increase in OD_{260} relative to pre-treatment (%)		
	Control	4i alone	4i-PACT
MRSA	2.86 ± 0.34	10.98 ± 0.41	247.87 ± 17.87
P. aeruginosa	2.04 ± 0.29	9.54 ± 0.28	188.98 ± 19.32
E. coli	2.98 ± 0.33	13.31 ± 0.38	336.67 ± 28.08

Dose-Dependent Photoinactivation Effects

The photoinactivation effect of 4i against MRSA, *E. coli* and *P. aeruginosa* strains was dose-dependent (**Figure 2**). A sharp decrease in bacterial survival fraction with increase of the concentration was observed. These three strains were incubated with 3.9 μM 4i in the dark for 30 min at 37°C, then illuminated by the 650 nm laser with power of 6 J/cm^2. 4.35, 6.96, and 3.56 $\log_{10}$ reduction in bacterial survival fraction was observed for the clinical isolated MRSA, *E. coli* and *P. aeruginosa*, respectively. As a control, 4i did not show any bactericidal effect to these strains in dark at less than 10 μM.

Morphology Changes

Changes of the bacterial structure can be clearly revealed at morphological level by AFM. The representative results are shown in **Figure 3**. The normal ball shape structure of MRSA (**Figure 3g**), the rod-like shape of *P. aeruginosa* (**Figure 3h**) and *E. coli* (**Figure 3i**) was observed without any treatment. The size and shape of the bacteria agree with that reported in previous study (Eaton et al., 2008). For these three strains treated by 4i in the dark (**Figures 3d-f**), it can be seen that the bacterial structure is complete. Particles scattered at the surface of bacteria may be the aggregates of 4i. In the groups treated by 4i-PACT (**Figures 3a–c**), it was found that bacteria is damaged and fragmented. Some irregular aggregation of the dead corpse was detected. Researchers have found that the roughness, size and shape of bacterial strains are slightly altered after PACT treatment with Toluidine Blue O (Sahu et al., 2009; Jin et al., 2010; Lin et al., 2012). The leakage from *Staphylococcus aureus* cell suspension is greatly increased (Sahu et al., 2009), suggesting that cytoplasmic materials are lost through the damaged bacterial membrane. Results in this study showed that bacterial strains are completely broken into pieces. Thus, 4i-PACT treatment appeared to have potent effect on the bacterial envelope, including damaging the bacterial wall and membrane.

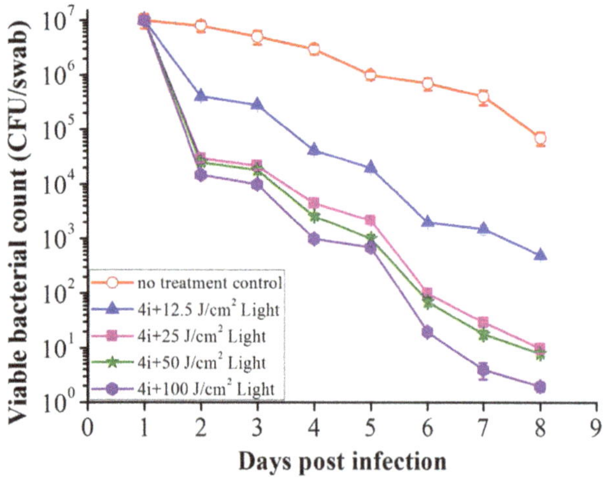

FIGURE 7 | The mean bacterial counts of the swabs collected from the rat wounds during the 8 days post infection. Data is expressed as mean ± SEM. $N = 6$ in each group.

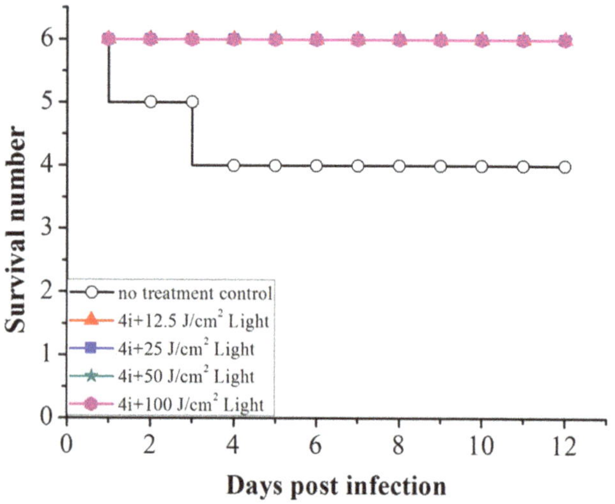

FIGURE 8 | The viability of rats against days post infection for treated versus not treated.

Membrane Integrity

The fluorescence microscopy was used to investigate the permeability of bacterial membrane before and after 4i-PACT. Fluorescent dyes (AO/EB), as the indicator of cell membrane damage, were used to assess the antibacterial activity of 4i-PACT. Living bacteria was observed as green and dead as red, respectively. **Figures 4g–i** show fluorescence microscopy images of the control samples, where no 4i was added, the bacteria is dispersed and alive with green color. **Figures 4a–c** are the fluorescence microscopy images of MRSA, *P. aeruginosa* and *E. coli* treated by 4i-PACT (10 μM, 6J/cm^2, 650 nm), respectively, where most of the bacteria is dead with red color. On the other hand, fluorescence microscopy images of MRSA (**Figure 4d**), *P. aeruginosa* (**Figure 4e**), and *E. coli* (**Figure 4f**) treated by10 μM 4i without illumination showed little bactericidal effect. The above results mean that 4i-PACT can damage the membrane of bacteria and change the permeability of the bacterial membrane. This again explains why the antimicrobial effect of 4i-PACT is so strong.

Photodynamic Effect on Genomic DNA

The influence of 4i-PACT on bacteria was further studied from a genomic point of view such as DNA leakage or damage. The electrophoresis graph (**Figure 5**) shows that the DNA bands, extracted from the processed bacterial cells, disappear after 4i-PACT (10 μM, 6 J/cm^2, 650 nm), while a clear DNA band is detected in the control groups with no 4i-PACT or treated by 4i alone. This result is consistent with the AFM morphological study as well as the fluorescent staining, which reveal that the 4i-PACT breaks the bacterial membrane and wall and causes the leakage of genomic DNA. The absence of DNA bands can be attributed to either the leakage of bacteria membrane or the break of the DNA. So we conducted another independent experiment. The naked DNA extracted from each strains was treated by 4i-PACT. The agarose gel electrophoresis graph still shows no DNA bands. This result indicated that 4i-PACT can break DNA into pieces. This phenomenon is consistent with the previous results (Menezes et al., 1990; Choi et al., 2010; Lin et al., 2012). Generally, the reason for multidrug resistance in cellular level is due to the drug only blocked or weakened the partial binding site or signal pathway, while the whole cellular bodies were kept, so it is easy to develop multidrug resistance. Double effects of 4i-PACT, destroying bacterial membrane and damaging the DNA, can account for the vanish of DNA band in electrophoresis graph. This is the reason why bacterial strains have no resistant to 4i-PACT.

Bacterial Content Exudation

Release of intracellular components is a good indicator of membrane integrity. Small ions such as potassium and phosphate tend to exude first, followed by large molecules such as DNA, RNA, and other materials. Since these nucleotides have strong UV absorption at 260 nm, measuring the absorbance at 260 nm can reveal the information of membrane integrity (Denyer and Hugo, 1991; Chen and Cooper, 2002). As shown in **Table 2**, after 10 μM 4i-PACT, the bacterial content exudation from MRSA, *P. aeruginosa*, and *E. Coli* are increased by 247.87, 188.98, 336.67%, respectively, compared with pre-treatment samples, while changes less than 10% was observed in the control or 4i group. This result is consistent with that of AFM and fluorescent images. These data are larger than that reported by Sahu et al. (2009), which were only 20–60% increase compared with the control groups.

In Vivo Antibacterial Activity and Wound-Healing Effect

In vivo antibiotics experiment, generally 5 or 10 times MIC was chosen as the working concentration. 40 μM of 4i, five times of MIC (Singh et al., 2006; Dai et al., 2009) was chosen as the working dose. The antibacterial effect of 4i-PACT with different light dose was studied. The wound healing rate is highly light dose dependent (**Figure 6**). Control group A, with no treatment, showed less wound healing at each observation time point. A rapid wound healing was observed in the treatment of groups C (50 J/cm^2) and D (25 J/cm^2) during the day 4 to 8 after infection ($p < 0.05$). After day 8, wound healing became slow till completely healed on day 12. However, in the groups B (100 J/cm^2) and E (12.5 J/cm^2), rapid wound closure happened from day 7 to 10. On the day 8, mean wound area ratios of B–E were 0.4252 ± 0.0512, 0.1515 ± 0.0312, 0.1823 ± 0.0777, and 0.2273 ± 0.0239, respectively, but in the control group wound area ratio was 0.6619 ± 0.0834, indicating B–E groups had better wound healing ratio compared with the control group. Almost total wound closure was observed by the day 12 post infection in all treated groups.

The viable bacteria in wound tissue were counted as an index of the bactericidal effect of 4i-PACT. On days 1, 2, 3, 4, 5, 6, 7, 8 post infection, PACT-treated groups exhibited obvious reduction in bacterial viability compared with the no treatment control group (**Figure 7**). At the same time point, the decrease of viable bacterial count is in the order of light illumination dose, B > C > D > E. This suggests that 4i-PACT accelerates wound healing via bactericidal effect against MRSA, *P. aeruginosa*, and *E. coli*. However, the wound healing ratio is in the order of C > D > E > B, instead of paralleling of the bactericidal effect. This indicates that 4i-PACT effect on normal tissue should be considered. A rationalized interpretation can be given based upon the multiple function of 4i-PACT *in vivo*: 4i-PACT not only photoinactivates bacteria, but also causes the normal tissue damaged and repaired. The observed effect is the balance of the ensemble results. For either a weaker 4i-PACT with a lower illumination dose (12.5 J/cm^2 in group E), or a stronger 4i-PACT with a higher illumination dose (100 J/cm^2 in group B), the total results are not good. The best result is from treatment with medium light dose like group C (50 J/cm^2). So for the practical application of PACT further study is requires.

In the no treatment control group, two rats died on day 2 and day 4, rats in other groups all survived the experiment. Therefore, the viability of rats post treatment indicates that 4i-PACT is more efficient in the treatment of mixed bacterial infection (**Figure 8**).

CONCLUSION

This paper studied the photoinactivation mechanism of 4i-PACT *in vitro* and its wound healing effect on wound rat model infected by mixed bacteria. 4i-PACT (3.91 μM, 6J/cm^2, 650 nm) had a broad potent antibacterial spectrum: 4.35, 6.96, and 3.56 log_{10} reduction in bacterial survival for MRSA, *E. coli*, and *P. aeruginosa*, respectively. AFM revealed that 4i-PACT can destroy bacterial wall and membrane. This is further confirmed by Dual fluorescent staining with AO/EB. Agarose gel electrophoresis indicated that 4i-PACT can damage the genomic DNA of bacteria. Absorbance at 260 nm reveals that 4i-PACT could cause bacterial content leakage. 4i-PACT breaks not only bacterial wall but also the genomic DNA. That is why the bacterial strains have no resistance to 4i-PACT. Wound healing effect on mixed bacterial infected rat model revealed that 4i-PACT *in vivo* is highly potent and light-dose dependent. The ensemble effect is the balanced effect of 4i-PACT both to normal tissue and bacterial strains. The best light dose is 50 J/cm^2. Overall, 4i-PACT is a highly efficient treatment modality for bacterial infection *in vitro* or *in vivo*.

AUTHOR CONTRIBUTIONS

TL designed experiments; SM, ZX, LP, and YG carried out experiments; YG and ZX analyzed experimental results, CW analyzed sequencing data. TL, ZX, and YG wrote the manuscript. TL designed experiments; SM, ZX, LP, and YG carried out experiments; YG and ZX analyzed experimental results, CW analyzed sequencing data. TL, ZX, and YG wrote the manuscript.

ACKNOWLEDGMENTS

This work was supported by the key technologies R & D program of Tianjin (12ZCDZSY11900), Peking Union Medical College Peking Union Youth Fund grant to ZX (NO.3332015030) and the National Natural Science Foundation of China (81202415).

REFERENCES

Bertolini, G., Rossi, F., Valduga, G., Jori, G., and Van Lier, J. (1990). Photosensitizing activity of water-and lipid-soluble phthalocyanines on *Escherichia coli*. *FEMS Microbiol. Lett.* 71, 149–155. doi: 10.1111/j.1574-6968.1990.tb03814.x

Chen, C. Z., and Cooper, S. L. (2002). Interactions between dendrimer biocides and bacterial membranes. *Biomaterials* 23, 3359–3368. doi: 10.1016/S0142-9612(02)00036-4

Choi, S. S., Lee, H. K., and Chae, H. S. (2010). In vitro photodynamic antimicrobial activity of methylene blue and endoscopic white light against *Helicobacter pylori* 26695. *J. Photochem. Photobiol. B Biol.* 101, 206–209. doi: 10.1016/j.jphotobiol.2010.07.004

Dai, T., Tegos, G. P., Lu, Z., Huang, L., Zhiyentayev, T., Franklin, M. J., et al. (2009). Photodynamic therapy for *Acinetobacter baumannii* burn infections in mice. *Antimicrob. Agents Chemother.* 53, 3929–3934. doi: 10.1128/AAC.00027-09

Dash, G., Suresh, P., and Ganapaty, S. (2001). Studies on hypoglycaemic and wound healing activities of *Lantana camara* Linn. *J. Nat. Remedies* 1, 105–110.

Davies, J., and Davies, D. (2010). Origins and evolution of antibiotic resistance. *Microbiol. Mol. Biol. Rev.* 74, 417–433. doi: 10.1128/MMBR.00016-10

Denyer, S. P., and Hugo, W. B. (1991). *Mechanisms of Action of Chemical Biocides. Their Study and Exploitation.* Oxford: Blackwell Scientific Publications.

Dovigo, L. N., Pavarina, A. C., Ribeiro, D. G., De Oliveira, J. A., Vergani, C. E., and Machado, A. L. (2009). Microwave disinfection of complete dentures contaminated in vitro with selected bacteria. *J. Prosthodont.* 18, 611–617. doi: 10.1111/j.1532-849X.2009.00489.x

Eaton, P., Fernandes, J. C., Pereira, E., Pintado, M. E., and Malcata, F. X. (2008). Atomic force microscopy study of the antibacterial effects of chitosans on *Escherichia coli* and *Staphylococcus aureus*. *Ultramicroscopy* 108, 1128–1134. doi: 10.1016/j.ultramic.2008.04.015

Fu, X.-J., Fang, Y., and Yao, M. (2013). Antimicrobial photodynamic therapy for methicillin-resistant *Staphylococcus aureus* infection. *Biomed Res. Int.* 2013, 159157. doi: 10.1155/2013/159157

Gomes, M. C., Silva, S., Faustino, M. A., Neves, M. G., Almeida, A., Cavaleiro, J. A., et al. (2013). Cationic galactoporphyrin photosensitisers against UV-B resistant bacteria: oxidation of lipids and proteins by 1 O 2. *Photochem. Photobiol. Sci.* 12, 262–271. doi: 10.1039/c2pp25149c

Grinholc, M., Szramka, B., Kurlenda, J., Graczyk, A., and Bielawski, K. P. (2008). Bactericidal effect of photodynamic inactivation against methicillin-resistant and methicillin-susceptible *Staphylococcus aureus* is strain-dependent. *J. Photochem. Photobiol. Biol.* 90, 57–63. doi: 10.1016/j.jphotobiol.2007.11.002

Haile, M., Pan, Z., Gao, M., and Luo, L. (2008). Efficacy in microbial sterilization of pulsed magnetic field treatment. *Int. J. Food Eng.* 4, 1–14. doi: 10.2202/1556-3758.1177

Jin, H., Huang, X., Chen, Y., Zhao, H., Ye, H., Huang, F., et al. (2010). Photoinactivation effects of hematoporphyrin monomethyl ether on Gram-positive and-negative bacteria detected by atomic force microscopy. *Appl. Microbiol. Biotechnol.* 88, 761–770. doi: 10.1007/s00253-010-2747-4

Ke, M.-R., Eastel, J. M., Ngai, K. L. K., Cheung, Y.-Y., Chan, P. K. S., Hui, M., et al. (2014). Photodynamic inactivation of bacteria and viruses using two monosubstituted zinc (II) phthalocyanines. *Eur. J. Med. Chem.* 84, 278–283. doi: 10.1016/j.ejmech.2014.07.022

Kharkwal, G. B., Sharma, S. K., Huang, Y. Y., Dai, T., and Hamblin, M. R. (2011). Photodynamic therapy for infections: clinical applications. *Lasers Surg. Med.* 43, 755–767. doi: 10.1002/lsm.21080

Krishnamurthy, K., Demirci, A., and Irudayaraj, J. (2004). Inactivation of *Staphylococcus aureus* by pulsed UV-light sterilization. *J. Food Prot.* 67, 1027–1030.

Kumar, A., Srivastava, K., Kumar, S. R., Siddiqi, M., Puri, S. K., Sexana, J. K., et al. (2011). 4-Anilinoquinoline triazines: a novel class of hybrid antimalarial agents. *Eur. J. Med. Chem.* 46, 676–690. doi: 10.1016/j.ejmech.2010.12.003

Laxminarayan, R., Duse, A., Wattal, C., Zaidi, A. K., Wertheim, H. F., Sumpradit, N., et al. (2013). Antibiotic resistance—the need for global solutions. *Lancet Infect. Dis.* 13, 1057–1098. doi: 10.1016/S1473-3099(13)70318-9

Lin, S. L., Hu, J. M., Tang, S. S., Wu, X. Y., Chen, Z. Q., and Tang, S. Z. (2012). Photodynamic inactivation of methylene blue and tungsten-halogen lamp light against food pathogen *Listeria monocytogenes*. *Photochem. Photobiol.* 88, 985–991. doi: 10.1111/j.1751-1097.2012.01154.x

Liu, F., Soh Yan Ni, A., Lim, Y., Mohanram, H., Bhattacharjya, S., and Xing, B. (2012). Lipopolysaccharide neutralizing peptide–porphyrin conjugates for effective photoinactivation and intracellular imaging of Gram-negative bacteria strains. *Bioconjug. Chem.* 23, 1639–1647. doi: 10.1021/bc300203d

Mbakidi, J.-P., Herke, K., Alvès, S., Chaleix, V., Granet, R., Krausz, P., et al. (2013). Synthesis and photobiocidal properties of cationic porphyrin-grafted paper. *Carbohydr. Polym.* 91, 333–338. doi: 10.1016/j.carbpol.2012.08.013

Menezes, S., Capella, M., and Caldas, L. (1990). Photodynamic action of methylene blue: repair and mutation in *Escherichia coli*. *J. Photochem. Photobiol. B Biol.* 5, 505–517. doi: 10.1016/1011-1344(90)85062-2

Meng, S., Xu, Z., Hong, G., Zhao, L., Zhao, Z., Guo, J., et al. (2015). Synthesis, characterization and in vitro photodynamic antimicrobial activity of basic amino acid–porphyrin conjugates. *Eur. J. Med. Chem.* 92, 35–48. doi: 10.1016/j.ejmech.2014.12.029

Nitzan, Y., Gutterman, M., Malik, Z., and Ehrenberg, B. (1992). Inactivation of gram-negative bacteria by photosensitized porphyrins. *Photochem. Photobiol.* 55, 89–96. doi: 10.1111/j.1751-1097.1992.tb04213.x

Nusbaum, H., and Rose, R. (1979). The effects of radiation sterilization on the properties of ultrahigh molecular weight polyethylene. *J. Biomed. Mater. Res.* 13, 557–576. doi: 10.1002/jbm.820130404

Prasanth, C. S., Karunakaran, S. C., Paul, A. K., Kussovski, V., Mantareva, V., Ramaiah, D., et al. (2014). Antimicrobial photodynamic efficiency of novel cationic porphyrins towards periodontal Gram-positive and Gram-negative pathogenic bacteria. *Photochem. Photobiol.* 90, 628–640. doi: 10.1111/php.12198

Rodrigues, G. B., Dias-Baruffi, M., Holman, N., Wainwright, M., and Braga, G. U. (2013). In vitro photodynamic inactivation of *Candida* species and mouse fibroblasts with phenothiazinium photosensitisers and red light. *Photodiagnosis Photodyn. Ther.* 10, 141–149. doi: 10.1016/j.pdpdt.2012.11.004

Ryono, R. (2014). Carbapenem-resistant *Enterobacteriaceae* (CRE) distribution within the veterans affairs healthcare system: 2013. *Open Forum Infect. Dis.* 1(Suppl. 1), S140–S141. doi: 10.1093/ofid/ofu052.221

Sahu, K., Bansal, H., Mukherjee, C., Sharma, M., and Gupta, P. K. (2009). Atomic force microscopic study on morphological alterations induced by photodynamic action of Toluidine Blue O in *Staphylococcus aureus* and *Escherichia coli*. *J. Photochem. Photobiol. B Biol.* 96, 9–16. doi: 10.1016/j.jphotobiol.2009.03.008

Sasagawa, A., Yamazaki, A., Kobayashi, A., Hoshino, J., Ohshima, T., Sato, M., et al. (2006). Inactivation of *Bacillus subtilis* spores by a combination of hydrostatic high-pressure and pulsed electric field treatments. *High Press. Sci. Technol.* 16, 45–53. doi: 10.4131/jshpreview.16.45

Singh, M., Govindarajan, R., Nath, V., Rawat, A. K. S., and Mehrotra, S. (2006). Antimicrobial, wound healing and antioxidant activity of *Plagiochasma appendiculatum* Lehm. et Lind. *J. Ethnopharmacol.* 107, 67–72. doi: 10.1016/j.jep.2006.02.007

Sperandio, F. F., Huang, Y.-Y., and Hamblin, M. R. (2013). Antimicrobial photodynamic therapy to kill Gram-negative bacteria. *Recent Pat. Antiinfect. Drug Discov.* 8, 108–120. doi: 10.2174/1574891X113089990012

Stojiljkovic, I., Evavold, B. D., and Kumar, V. (2001). Antimicrobial properties of porphyrins. *Expert Opin. Investig. Drugs* 10, 309–320. doi: 10.1517/13543784.10.2.309

Sudheesh Kumar, P., Lakshmanan, V.-K., Anilkumar, T., Ramya, C., Reshmi, P., Unnikrishnan, A., et al. (2012). Flexible and microporous chitosan hydrogel/nano ZnO composite bandages for wound dressing: in vitro and in vivo evaluation. *ACS Appl. Mater. Interfaces* 4, 2618–2629. doi: 10.1021/am300292v

Sui, M., Zhang, L., Sheng, L., Huang, S., and She, L. (2013). Synthesis of ZnO coated multi-walled carbon nanotubes and their antibacterial activities. *Sci. Total Environ.* 452, 148–154. doi: 10.1016/j.scitotenv.2013.02.056

Tomé, J. P., Neves, M. G., Tomé, A. C., Cavaleiro, J. A., Soncin, M., Magaraggia, M., et al. (2004). Synthesis and antibacterial activity of new poly-S-lysine-porphyrin conjugates. *J. Med. Chem.* 47, 6649–6652. doi: 10.1021/jm040802v

Wainwright, M. (1998). Photodynamic antimicrobial chemotherapy (PACT). *J. Antimicrob. Chemother.* 42, 13–28. doi: 10.1093/jac/42.1.13

Wainwright, M. (2010). 'Safe'photoantimicrobials for skin and soft-tissue infections. *Int. J. Antimicrob. Agents* 36, 14–18. doi: 10.1016/j.ijantimicag.2010.03.002

Wainwright, M., and Crossley, K. B. (2004). Photosensitising agents—circumventing resistance and breaking down biofilms: a review. *Int. Biodeterior. Biodegradation* 53, 119–126. doi: 10.1016/j.ibiod.2003.11.006

Wu, M., He, J., Ren, X., Cai, W.-S., Fang, Y.-C., and Feng, X.-Z. (2014). Development of functional biointerfaces by surface modification of polydimethylsiloxane with bioactive chlorogenic acid. *Colloids Surf. B Biointerfaces* 116, 700–706. doi: 10.1016/j.colsurfb.2013.11.010

Zhao, Z., Li, Y., Meng, S., Li, S., Wang, Q., and Liu, T. (2014). Susceptibility of methicillin-resistant *Staphylococcus aureus* to photodynamic antimicrobial chemotherapy with α-d-galactopyranosyl zinc phthalocyanines: in vitro study. *Lasers Med. Sci.* 29, 1131–1138. doi: 10.1007/s10103-013-1488-x

15

A Prescription for Resistance: Management of Staphylococcal Skin Abscesses by General Practitioners in Australia

*Christine Parrott[1,2], Gillian Wood[3,4], Ekaterina Bogatyreva[1], Geoffrey W. Coombs[5,6], Paul D. R. Johnson[7] and Catherine M. Bennett[1]**

[1] Centre for Population Health Research, School of Health and Social Development, Deakin University, Geelong, VIC, Australia, [2] Young People's Health Service, Department of Adolescent Medicine, The Royal Children's Hospital, Parkville, VIC, Australia, [3] Perinatal Medicine, Mercy Hospital for Women, Heidelberg, VIC, Australia, [4] Department of Microbiology, Dorevitch Pathology, Heidelberg, VIC, Australia, [5] School of Veterinary and Life Sciences, Murdoch University, Murdoch, WA, Australia, [6] PathWest Laboratory Medicine – Fiona Stanley Hospital, Murdoch, WA, Australia, [7] Department of Infectious Diseases, Austin Health, Heidelberg, VIC, Australia

***Correspondence:**
Catherine M. Bennett
catherine.bennett@deakin.edu.au

Objectives: We investigated the management of staphylococcal abscesses (boils) by general practitioners (GPs) in the context of rising antibiotic resistance in community strains of *Staphylococcus aureus*.

Design, Setting, Participants: We analyzed patient-reported management of 66 cases of uncomplicated skin abscesses from the frequency matched methicillin-resistant *S. aureus* (MRSA) and methicillin-sensitive *S. aureus* (MSSA) Community-Onset *Staphylococcus aureus* Household Cohort (COSAHC) study (Melbourne, Australia, 2008–2012). Susceptibilities in all cases were known: 50/66 abscesses were caused by MRSA. In order to investigate GP-reported management of staphylococcal abscesses, we surveyed a random subset of GPs, from the COSAHC study (41), and of GPs (39) who used the same community-based pathology service (December 2011–May 2012).

Main outcome measures: Patient outcomes, antibiotics prescribed, antibiotic resistance profiles of infecting strains, rates of incision and drainage (I&D), and attitudes to ordering microbiological cultures.

Results: MRSA was three times more likely to be cultured from an abscess than MSSA. Patient-reported management revealed 100% were prescribed antibiotics and only 60.6% had I&D. Of those 85% who remembered their prescription(s), 81% of MRSA cases and 23% of MSSA cases initially received inactive antibiotics. Repeat GP visits where antibiotics were changed occurred in 45 MRSA and 7 MSSA cases, although at least 33% of subsequent prescriptions were inactive for the MRSA infections.

Patients treated with I&D and antibiotics did no better than those treated with only I&D, regardless of the antibiotic activity. In the GP surveys, 89% reported I&D, with or without antibiotics, to be their preferred management. Only 29.9% of GPs would routinely swab abscesses.

Conclusion: The recommended management of uncomplicated *Staphylococcus* abscesses is I&D without antibiotics to reduce exposure to unnecessary antibiotics. In our study, I&D was performed in only 60.6% of 66 patients, and antibiotics were always prescribed. The prescribed antibiotics were frequently inactive and often changed, and did not appear to affect patient recovery. Our results show that community GPs can confidently reduce their use of antibiotics for patients with skin abscesses and should be aware that MRSA is a much more common in this type of infection.

Keywords: antibiotic resistance, *Staphylococcus aureus*, skin and soft tissue infections, community medicine, boils and abscesses

INTRODUCTION

Little is known about Australian general practitioners' (GPs) management protocols in practice for skin abscesses and how this might be evolving with the changing epidemiology of *Staphylococcus aureus*. Australian Therapeutic Guidelines: Antibiotic (version 15; Antibiotic Expert Groups, 2014) recommends *uncomplicated* abscesses should be managed with incision and drainage (I&D) alone – without antibiotics. Previous guidelines (Dermatology Expert Groups, 2009) available to GPs at the time of our study, also recommended only I&D for abscesses <5 cm. Antibiotics were only recommended if there was associated spreading cellulitis or systemic symptoms.

After a 2011 review, clinical practice guidelines from the Infectious Diseases Society of America (IDSA) continued to recommend I&D; specifically, that effective treatment requires incision, thorough evacuation of pus, and probing the cavity to break up loculations (Liu et al., 2011; Moran et al., 2013). IDSA practice guidelines are similar to the Australian Therapeutic Guidelines for primary treatment (CDC, AMA, IDSA, 2007; Lowy et al., 2008; Liu et al., 2011; Centers for Disease Control and Prevention [CDC], 2013; Moran et al., 2013). However, they differ in their recommended first line antibiotics in cases where antibiotics are indicated, due to higher rates of community-acquired MRSA (CA-MRSA) in the United States. The IDSA guidelines recommend clindamycin, trimethoprim-sulfamethoxazole, a tetracycline (doxycycline/minocycline) and linezolid (Liu et al., 2011). In contrast, the recommended antibiotics for complicated abscesses in the Australian Therapeutic Guidelines are di/flucloxacillin or, in penicillin-allergic patients, cephalexin. In penicillin hypersensitive patients, the recommendation is to use clindamycin or trimethoprim-sulfamethoxazole. Antibiotics are to be modified based on culture results (Antibiotic Expert Groups, 2014).

We have calculated that in 2006, 3–5% of patients presenting with community-onset *S. aureus* infections in Melbourne had an MRSA infection (Bennett et al., 2014). The preliminary findings of the COSAHC study suggest this has risen to 8–10% by 2010, and may be higher again when aggressive pyogenic soft tissue *S. aureus* infections have been investigated, showing MRSA the more likely causative organism (Jahamy et al., 2008; del Giudice et al., 2009; Coombs et al., 2014). This study will show that CA-MRSA is three times more likely than MSSA to be the cultured organism in skin abscesses.

With CA-MRSA increasing in prevalence in Australia and elsewhere, there may be an argument for all lesions to be swabbed for microbiological culture and sensitivity (MC&S), not only to tailor treatment (as in complicated infections) but also for MRSA surveillance (CDC, AMA, IDSA, 2007; Lowy et al., 2008; Dermatology Expert Groups, 2009; Liu et al., 2011; Centers for Disease Control and Prevention [CDC], 2013; Antibiotic Expert Groups, 2014). However, for uncomplicated abscesses, if, as is recommended, I&D is routinely and correctly used, (thorough evacuation of pus, and probing the cavity to break up loculations) and antibiotics are *not* used, then swabs may have little impact on individual care (Parnes et al., 2011). Community GPs may not realize that CA-MRSA is the most likely organism to cause uncomplicated abscesses. Further over prescription may occur with the return of a culture and sensitivity report, indicating the prescribed (unnecessary) antibiotic is inactive, which may drive an antibiotic change, resulting in even more ineffective antibiotics as well as unnecessary visits to the GP.

Our study set out to describe the management by community GPs of staphylococcal skin abscesses so we can better understand how often I&D is performed, if and what types of antibiotics are used, and whether antibiotics affect patient recovery. We also wanted to understand how often and for what reason GPs send swabs for MC&S.

MATERIALS AND METHODS

Patient Data

Community-Onset *Staphylococcus aureus* Household Cohort is a longitudinal cohort study of 291 index patients with community-onset *S. aureus* infections, and 446 household contacts. Index patients were recruited through a large private pathology provider on the basis of a positive *S. aureus* MC&S result for their infection. The pathology provider serves the entire Melbourne metropolitan area. All eligible patients with community-onset MRSA infections were invited to participate together with a frequency-matched subset of eligible patients with MSSA infections. The COSAHC project was approved by the Deakin University Human Research Ethics Committee (project number 2009-162).

Shared households (204) were followed up at 3-monthly intervals for up to 2 years (recruitment period 2008–2011). At each visit, index patients and household members had swabs obtained from nares and axillae for *S. aureus* carriage to determine the molecular epidemiology of strains circulating within households. Questionnaires were completed to provide information on the medical management and outcome of the index cases' infection as well as household interactions, infection history, new infections and risks for *S. aureus* transmission and MRSA carriage.

Of the 291 index patients, 137 had MRSA infections and 154 had MSSA infections. The majority were skin and soft tissue infections (86.2%), and 66 of the index patients had skin abscesses (50 MRSA, 16 MSSA) and are included in the present analysis. We extracted data on the doctor-reported data management (when remembered) as well as patient-reported management and outcomes for these 66 skin abscess infections; including whether I&D was performed or if and what type of antibiotics were prescribed. We also established the resistance profile of the infecting strain, and the number of days off normal activities and timing of infection resolution.

Doctor Survey Data

To understand the clinical decisions behind treatment practices, we conducted a cross-sectional survey of community GPs on their management protocols for *S. aureus* abscesses using a constructed case study (see below). Participating doctors were from one of two groups, recruited by telephone and fax from December 2011 to May 2012. The survey tool asked a series of questions on their treatment of this hypothetical case, and decisions to swab.

Case Study Extract

A patient presents to your clinic with a boil in their right armpit. Over the course of 3 days, the area has become increasingly reddened, tender and the center is raised and now forms a pus-filled head. There are no signs of systemic infection but there is evidence of localized infection. The patient has no other health problems and is not on any medication.

1. With this history, how would you treat the patient? (Select 1 or more)
   (a) No treatment
   (b) Incision and drainage (I&D)
   (c) I&D and antibiotics
   (d) Antibiotics only
   (e) Other (please specify)
2. If this boil was weeping or lanced*, would you swab this boil for culture and if so why?

Followed by a series of multiple choice and open ended questions on treatment choices and motivators for, and frequency of, collecting swabs.

**Lanced* used interchangeably with *incision*

Group 1: Doctors Who Ordered the Baseline Tests on Patients Who Were Recruited to the COSAHC Study

We surveyed a random sample of 41 doctors treating community-onset *S. aureus* infections that had previously been studied in COSAHC. A subset of these doctors had treated eight COSAHC- patients who had an abscess as their index infection, allowing us the additional opportunity to directly compare GP-reported management protocols from the survey to the real life patient-reported management in these cases.

Group 2: Comparative GP Sample

To determine how representative COSAHC doctors' patient management was, we compared their survey responses to those of a random sample of 39 GPs practicing within metropolitan Melbourne who had ordered routine blood tests (Full blood count and Urea and Electrolytes) in the same period from the same pathology provider.

Both groups of doctors were invited to return a survey tool by fax or complete over the telephone. The exclusion criteria were being on leave for more than one month at the time approached and/or no longer working at the practice. A sample size of 40 per group was recruited to provide 80% power ($\alpha = 0.05$) to detect a 30% difference in antibiotic use between GPs.

The survey tool was developed to assess management protocols and swabbing practice in the context of a short case study of a patient with an axillary skin abscess. We also asked participants to provide information on any change to their practice over the previous three years.

Analysis

Descriptive statistics were applied, including computing differences between proportions and the associated p-values and 95% confidence intervals (CIs) using StataSE12. We report median and inter-quartile range (IQR) for all non-parametric data.

RESULTS

COSAHC Participants Report of GP Management of Their Lesion

Abscess management and outcome information was obtained from the 66 index patients at the first COSAHC household visit. The susceptibilities of the organisms were known as the patients were recruited on the basis of a positive *S. aureus* MC&S result. The first household visit occurred at an average of 4 months from the onset of index infection. For the total COSAHC study, the ratio of MSSA:MRSA in the index patients' infections was 154:137. Within this abscess subset, the ratio was 16:50. This indicates that in the setting of an abscess, MRSA is much more common than background rates in community onset infections. The average age of the abscess patients was 34.4 years (95% CI 29.3, 39.5), 48% were female (95% CI 37, 60), with an average household size of 2.7 (95% CI 2.25, 3.14). Nearly half (44% (95% CI 33, 56)) reported a history of previous skin abscesses. Abscess site varied (**Table 1**), however, leg/foot was the most common (over 30%). Torso (24%) ranked second for MRSA abscesses, while torso and arm/hand were equal second for MSSA abscesses (19%).

Abscess management by the GPs, as reported by COSAHC study patients, are shown in **Table 2** with index infections stratified by methicillin resistance. I&D was performed in 60.6% of cases, but never in isolation. Antibiotics were prescribed for 100% of cases, however, two patients reported not taking the antibiotics.

Patient-reported infection resolution is shown in **Table 3**. Of those 40 patients who had I&D as part of their treatment, the

TABLE 1 | Infection sites.

Site of infection	MSSA ($n = 16$) (%, CI)	MRSA ($n = 50$) (%, CI)
Leg/foot	31% (11, 59)	34% (21, 49)
Torso (front/back)	19% (4, 46)	24% (13, 38)
Arm/hand	19% (4, 46)	12% (5, 24)
Axilla	13% (2, 38)	12% (5, 24)
Head/neck	13% (2, 38)	8% (2, 19)
Groin	6% (0.2, 30)	10% (3, 22)

TABLE 2 | Patient-reported GP abscess management by methicillin resistance (causal organism).

Treatment	MSSA ($n = 16$) (%, CI)	MRSA ($n = 50$) (%, CI)	Total ($n = 66$) (%, CI)
I&D and antibiotics	38% (15, 65)	36% (25, 53)	36% (25, 49)
I&D only	0%	0%	0%
Antibiotics only	25% (7, 52)	30% (18, 45)	29% (18, 41)
I&D, antibiotics and other*	25% (7, 52)	24% (13, 38)	24% (15, 36)
Antibiotics and other*	13% (2, 38)	10% (3, 22)	11% (4, 21)

**Other treatments include: abscess burst on its own, dressings, hospital admission, IV antibiotics, syringing, topical creams (non-antibiotic or unspecified), and surgical removal.*

infection resolved by the first home visit in 85% of cases, (95% CI 70, 94). Where I&D was not used (26) the infection was resolved in 73% of cases (95% CI 52, 88) by the first visit.

Analysis of Antibiotic Use

The antibiotics prescribed were not known for all patients, meaning the patient could recall the actual name of the antibiotic(s). However, the majority (85%) could remember the name of at least one of their prescribed antibiotics: 43 patients with MRSA and 13 patients with MSSA. We analyzed the antibiotic susceptibility profiles of the clinical isolates and the activity of the known antibiotics that were prescribed for these 56 patients (**Figures 1** and **2**). Antibiotics are described as *active* when the organism was susceptible to the prescribed antibiotic and *inactive* when the organism was resistant.

In total, over the course of their infections, there were 18 prescriptions of known antibiotics given to 13 patients with MSSA, of which three (16.7%) were inactive. Of the 81 known antibiotics prescribed for 43 patients with MRSA, 50 (62%) were

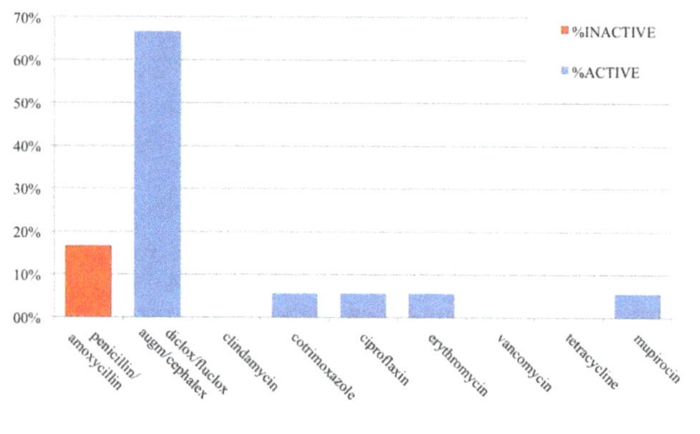

FIGURE 1 | Antibiotic susceptibility by prescription ($n = 18$) for MSSA infections.

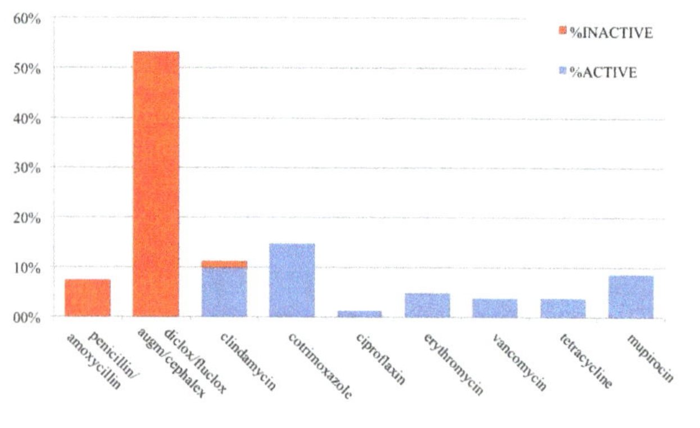

FIGURE 2 | Antibiotic susceptibility by prescription ($n = 81$) for MRSA infections.

inactive. Overall, approximately 53.5% of prescribed antibiotics were inactive: these included penicillin/amoxicillin for both MSSA and MRSA, and cephalexin, flucloxacillin, augmentin, or dicloxacillin for MRSA infections.

Prescriptions for MSSA infections were dominated by penicillin 16.7% and flucloxacillin, dicloxacillin, cephalexin, and augmentin (66.7%); However, augmentin and penicillin are not recommended first line of treatment for MSSA infections: augmentin because of its unnecessarily broad spectrum activity

TABLE 3 | Patient-reported infection resolution by first home visit (by management protocol).

	MSSA ($N = 16$)		MRSA ($N = 50$)		Total ($N = 66$)	
Treatment	Resolved	95% CI	Resolved	95% CI	Resolved	95% CI
I&D and antibiotics	5/6 (83%)	(36, 100)	15/18 (83%)	(59, 96)	20/24 (83%)	(63, 95)
I&D only	0 (0%)	–	0 (0%)	–	0 (0%)	–
Antibiotics only	3/4 (75%)	(19, 99)	12/15 (80%)	(52, 96)	15/19 (79%)	(54, 94)
I&D, antibiotics and other*	3/4 (75%)	(19, 99)	11/12 (92%)	(62, 100)	14/16 (88%)	(62, 98)
Antibiotics and other*	2/2 (100%)	(13, 99)	2/5 (40%)	(5, 85)	4/7 (57%)	(18, 90)

**Other treatments include: abscess burst on its own, dressings, hospital admission, IV antibiotics, syringing, topical creams (non-antibiotic or unspecified), and surgical removal.*

and penicillin/amoxicillin because only 5–10% of MSSA are susceptible (Turnidge et al., 2016).

Antibiotic Changes and Repeat GP Visits

Of the 43 patients with MRSA infections who recalled at least one of their specific antibiotic(s), 35 (81%) were initially prescribed an inactive drug. Of these, 23% never received an active antibiotic, whilst the rest were subsequently prescribed active (58%) or unknown (19%) antibiotic(s) at follow-up visits. Three (23.1%) of 13 patients with MSSA who recalled the specific antibiotic(s) were also prescribed an inactive drug, with one subsequently prescribed an active antibiotic.

In our study, 56 patients were able to remember a total of 99 antibiotics (an additional 19 were remembered as a prescription but not by name). Thirty-seven patients (6 with MSSA and 31 with MRSA infections) were prescribed more than one antibiotic and, of those, thirteen (1 MSSA patients and 12 MRSA) were prescribed more than two antibiotics. In addition, eight were prescribed Mupirocin (site of use unspecified but all organisms susceptible). We presume that for every new antibiotic prescribed the patients required a repeat visit to their GP for assessment, although we do not know if the subsequent prescription changes were due to treatment failure or antibiotic change based on lab results showing resistance.

GP Surveys of Abscess Management

One hundred and seventy GPs were approached and 81 completed surveys (48%; 41 COSAHC GPs, 39 comparison GP and one unlabeled form that could not be ascribed to a particular GP group). The response rate was higher in the COSAHC GP group (60% compared with 38%). The average number of years in practice of those participating was 23.1 years. No differences were found with treatment preferences between the two cohorts (**Table 4**).

Overall, GPs report 'I&D and antibiotics' as their preferred management of abscesses (70%), followed by 'I&D only' (19%) and 'Antibiotics only' (10%). Some specified I&D included additions; one would incise with review and another would prescribe antibiotic cream alongside. Other selections included 'no initial treatment, but subsequent patient review' (indicated as 'other' in **Table 4**).

Decision to Swab Wound

When we stratified treatment choices according to the GPs decision to swab, we found abscess management did not differ significantly between the two surveyed doctor groups, with 70% of both groups reporting their preferred management protocols as 'I&D and antibiotics.' This indicates we have not introduced patient-management bias via the recruitment method used, other than including a greater proportion of patients treated by GPs who swab. More COSAHC doctors did indicate they would swab if the abscess was weeping or incised (76.9% vs. 56.4%; $p = 0.049$), but this was not shown to be associated with differences in patient management, so we pooled the two GP groups for further analyses.

Overall, a minority (29.9%) of GPs reported that they would routinely swab abscesses for culture. Doctors reported they would swab for definitive diagnostic purposes (68.8%) or for persistent abscesses (97.4%). About half of doctors (48.6%) report being influenced by abscess size and a perceived increased risk of systemic infection or spread to adjacent tissues. When abscess size was identified as important, thresholds of size varied from >1 cm to >3 cm. Swabbing practice was not related to treatment choice or the commencement of antibiotics.

The rise of MRSA in the community was identified as reason for changing practice (23%). Some doctors report they are now more likely to wait for results to prescribe antibiotics and choose to swab based on clinical site and severity of abscess.

COSAHC Patient Management – GP-Reported Practice versus Actual Patient-Reported

Eight doctors of COSAHC patients with abscesses also completed the GP survey. Whilst the numbers are small, it does provide us the added opportunity of direct comparison between a patient' reported abscess treatment and their doctor's survey responses (**Table 5**).

None of the eight responded with the recommended first line treatment for an abscess, regardless of size. Two reported that they would not perform I&D and would solely prescribe antibiotics, which corresponds to the patients' report. The remaining six doctors who selected 'I&D and Antibiotics' in the survey varied in their actual clinical response – three out of six (50%) did not perform I&D and only prescribed antibiotics. Interestingly, two out of six (33%) administered an antibiotic

TABLE 4 | Self-reported management practices by doctor group.

Treatment	COSAHC GPs 41 *n* (%*)	Non-COSAHC GPs (39) *n* (%)	Total GPs (81) *n* (%)
I&D and antibiotics	29 (71%)	27 (69%)	57 (70%)
I&D	8 (20%)	7 (18%)	15 (19%)
Antibiotics only	3 (7%)	5 (13%)	8 (10%)
Other	1 (2%)	0 (0%)	1 (1%)

**All percentages are column percentages.*

TABLE 5 | Community GP-reported management for abscesses versus patient-reported management.

GP survey response	Patients' report of treatment by same GP
Treatment of patient in case study	*Treatment given for abscess*
Antibiotics	Antibiotics
Antibiotics	Antibiotics
I&D and Antibiotics	I&D and Antibiotics
I&D and Antibiotics	Self I&D, Antibiotics
I&D and Antibiotics	I&D attempt, penicillin injection, oral antibiotics
I&D and Antibiotics	I&D ×3, antibiotic injection, oral antibiotics
I&D and Antibiotics	Antibiotics (I&D of previous boil)
I&D and Antibiotics	Antibiotics

injection as well as oral antibiotics. This is particularly surprising because there are no intramuscularly injectable antibiotics that are active against most *S. aureus* organisms.

DISCUSSION

We live in an era of rising antibiotic resistance. Conservation of antibiotics is of critical importance, and in response antibiotic stewardship programs are being progressively implemented. Antibiotic stewardship originated to address the problems of antibiotic overuse in hospitals, but is now being extended to the community as it is increasingly realized most antibiotics for human use are prescribed and consumed in the community.

Australian GP compliance with clinical guidelines for abscess treatment has not previously been researched. In the US the management of community-acquired abscesses have been investigated both in general practice and in hospital emergency departments (Odenholt et al., 2002; Daly et al., 2011; Forcade et al., 2011; Kemper et al., 2011; Parnes et al., 2011; May et al., 2012; Schmitz et al., 2013). Pre/post intervention studies in primary care have been conducted to evaluate abscess management. For example, the IRENE study looked at antibiotic prescription coverage - pre-intervention cephalosporins were frequently prescribed (43%), dropping to 18% of prescriptions post-intervention. In this cohort, 84% of patients received I&D and antibiotics pre-intervention. Post-intervention, 97% received antibiotics and I&D, but there was a demonstrated increase in MRSA susceptible antibiotics. The option to not prescribe antibiotics was discussed but did not translate into practice (Daly et al., 2011).

Similarly, in the SNOCAP-USA and DARTnet study (Parnes et al., 2011), procedure rates for I&D were initially low. A practical intervention had no significant effect on the number of I&D completed or for microbiological cultures, but again, did result in increased use of MRSA-susceptible antibiotics.

STARnet (Forcade et al., 2011) conducted a prospective community based observational study of suspected MRSA abscesses. Only 7% of this cohort had I&D alone, while 64% received both antibiotics and I&D. Twenty-eight percent of the cohort received only antibiotics with trimethoprim-sulfamethoxazole used frequently as monotherapy. These studies also demonstrate the reluctance to stop providing antibiotics alongside I&D, or at all, despite recommendations.

Hospital emergency department research in the US showed only 17–19% of abscesses were treated with I&D alone and treatment with antibiotics alone ranged from 4 to 17%, while a combination of I&D and antibiotics was the most common practice (66–79.9%; Moran et al., 2006; Talan et al., 2011; May et al., 2012; Schmitz et al., 2013). A quality improvement project (Kemper et al., 2011) was conducted amongst American pediatricians to develop an intervention to increase adherence to best practice of abscesses; 83% of those interviewed responded that they *could* perform I&D, however, 34% stated it was too time consuming to perform. The challenge exists then to emphasize the importance of I&D in treating patients with abscesses and encouraging best practice.

Our study focuses on community-onset abscess infections where MRSA is over-represented as a deliberate part of our sampling strategy. The data drawn from the prospective cohort of community-onset staphylococcal infections (COSAHC) identified via a private community-based pathology service, and the cross-sectional survey of doctors ordering tests through the same pathology service, has provided the opportunity to explore doctors' attitudes and practices in the context of the changing epidemiology of *S. aureus* in an Australian urban community.

The antibiotic susceptibility of isolates for all the COSAHC participants were known and as this was the criteria for entry into the study. In the COSAHC study, we found that 85% of community-onset *S. aureus* infections were skin and soft tissue infections and in 66 the infection were skin abscesses and used in this study. In the management of the 66 participants with abscesses: 100% were prescribed antibiotics but only 60% had their abscess incised and drained. Contrary to this, a larger percentage of doctors (75%) surveyed indicated I&D with antibiotics was their management of choice for community-acquired abscesses. That is, more community GPs indicated that I&D with antibiotics was their management of choice than appeared to perform it.

Furthermore, where the antibiotic was known, the majority of patients with abscesses caused by MRSA (81%) were initially prescribed inactive antibiotics, compared with 23% of those with MSSA. Antibiotics were changed for 37 patients, resulting in nearly all MSSA (85%), but only 60.5% of MRSA infections ever being prescribed an active antibiotic. Overall, 53.5% of antibiotic choices were inactive against the targeted pathogen.

We have previously estimated that about 8% of infections caused by *S. aureus* in the community of metropolitan Melbourne are MRSA (Bennett et al., 2014), but this is likely to be much higher for abscesses based on our findings here. Given the proportion of COSAHC community-onset infections that are abscesses (66/291, 23%), and the high rate due to MRSA infections (78% compared with 47% of all infections among the frequency-matched COSAHC index cases), we estimate the prevalence of MRSA infections might be as high as 24% (three times higher) in community-onset infections presenting as abscesses in metropolitan Melbourne 2010–2012.

From our survey we found that only 30% of community GPs swab for MC&S. Therefore, many doctors would be unaware of the proportion of antibiotics prescribed that were ineffective and they are unlikely to modify their prescribing practice. According to both contemporary and Australian guidelines, almost all of the prescriptions for uncomplicated abscesses could be considered unnecessary. In support of these guidelines, our study showed there was little difference in infection resolution whether the antibiotics were active or not. This was true for 'I&D + antibiotics' and 'antibiotics' alone ($p = 0.71$), whether the antibiotics were active ($p = 1.0$) or inactive ($p = 0.84$). However, there was a trend to greater resolution at first household visit for those patients who had I&D performed, with 85% of infections resolved (95% CI 70, 94) compared with 73.1% (95%

CI 52.2, 88.4) of patients who did not have I&D performed. A 2007 literature review (Hankin and Everett, 2007) also showed that those patients treated with I&D alone had the same rate of resolution as those with I&D and antibiotics.

If an antibiotic is prescribed it is usually at first presentation. The swab will not help in the initial antibiotic prescription but a MC&S may be useful in the case of treatment failure and MRSA surveillance. If I&D is performed correctly, our findings support guidelines and no antibiotics are needed and can be stopped. Patients' expectations regarding treatment is a challenge for GPs. Patient understanding of best practice can be narrow and limited to their own situation. There is a need to increase the health literacy of patients and to make them aware of the population wider risks associated with antibiotic over prescription.

Although I&D was consistently reported by GPs to be their preferred treatment option for uncomplicated abscesses, the COSAHC study observed only 60% of patients with abscesses were treated with I&D in practice. Furthermore, I&D was always accompanied by antibiotics. This suggests that whilst there may be an understanding of the importance of I&D, there may be a lack of confidence in performing the procedure without antibiotic cover.

Given the number of antibiotic changes (37 patients requiring additional antibiotics) and therefore the presumed increased number of visits to the GP, it is clear that skin abscesses are difficult to treat and many different antibiotics are used.

Our study has a number of limitations. The response rate of 48% in the GP survey has the potential for sampling bias. However, we believe that any selection bias that may have been introduced would act to favor doctors who are more aware of community MRSA and therefore more keen to participate. Therefore, it is possible that these results underestimate the actual deviation from recommended practice in the wider GP community. If this were the case, then the true situation regarding GP practices may be even more removed from therapeutic practice guidelines than captured here. It would be useful to conduct a larger study to more comprehensively examine GP practice, and gain more detailed insight into GPs' ability to perform I&D correctly. Incision type, use of pain control, irrigation, wound cultures, and packing, would inform targeted strategies (Forcade et al., 2011; Centers for Disease Control and Prevention [CDC], 2013).

CONCLUSION

Our findings demonstrate many GPs are not following guideline recommended practice when it comes to treating patients with staphylococcal skin abscesses. Our findings support the recommendations in the current antibiotic guidelines that would act to curb this trend (Antibiotic Expert Groups, 2014). In particular:

(1) Antibiotics not indicated unless spreading cellulitis with systemic symptoms.

(2) Perform I&D correctly on all abscesses, even if antibiotic therapy is considered.

(3) Modify therapy based on clinical response to initial therapy and the results of cultures and susceptibility testing. If *S. aureus* is isolated, and lesion is responding to drainage, stop any antibiotics, inactive and active. If antibiotics are necessary: treatment for 5 days is generally sufficient, but a longer duration of therapy may be required for patients who are slow to respond or have a more severe infection.

Overall, the doctors we surveyed demonstrated awareness of the changing epidemiology of *S. aureus* infections in Melbourne. This study provides a basis for developing new programs to assist GPs to better understand and reduce their use of antibiotics, and potentially the number of return patient visits. There is also vital need to improve confidence and proficiency or surgical techniques such as I&D, which are more effective than antibiotics in such cases.

AUTHOR CONTRIBUTIONS

CP initiated this work, lead the study design and ethics approval, and managed the recruitment and oversaw the data analysis, and instigated the writing of this manuscript. GW was responsible for managing the partnership with Dorevitch laboratory and GP recruitment and contributed to the design of the survey tool, interpretation of data, and manuscript preparation. EB assisted in data analysis and preparing the figures for this paper. GC was responsible for the *S. aureus* laboratory typing and determination of resistance, and contributed to these elements of the paper. PJ also contributed to the development of the survey tool and to the writing of the manuscript, especially the clinical relevance aspects in the discussion and conclusions of this manuscript. CB developed the concept for this research with CP, lead the COSAHC study that contributed data to this work, oversaw the data analysis and data reporting processes, and contributed to the initial writing and then polishing of this manuscript.

REFERENCES

Antibiotic Expert Groups (2014). *Therapeutic Guidelines: Antibiotic, Version 15.* Melbourne, VIC: Therapeutic Guidelines Limited.

Bennett, C. M., Coombs, G. W., Wood, G. M., Howden, B. P., Johnson, L. E. A., White, D., et al. (2014). Community-onset *Staphylococcus aureus* infections presenting to general practices in South-eastern Australia. *Epidemiol. Infect.* 142, 501–511. doi: 10.1017/S0950268813001581

CDC, AMA, IDSA (2007). *CDC Outpatient Management of MRSA Skin and Soft Tissues Infections in the Era of Community-Associated MRSA [Internet].* Atlanta, GA: Centers for Disease Control and Prevention.

Centers for Disease Control and Prevention [CDC] (2013). *Treating MRSA Skin and Soft Tissue Infections in Outpatient Settings [Internet]*. Atlanta, GA: Centers for Disease Control and Prevention.

Coombs, G. W., Daley, D. A., Pearson, J. C., Nimmo, G. R., Collignon, P. J., McLaws, M.-L., et al. (2014). Community-onset *Staphylococcus aureus* surveillance Programme Annual Report 2012. *Commun. Dis. Intell. Q. Rep.* 38, E59–E69.

Daly, J. M., Levy, B. T., Ely, J. W., Swanson, K., Bergus, G. R., Jogerst, G. J., et al. (2011). Management of skin and soft tissue infections in community practice before and after implementing a "best practice" approach: an iowa Research Network (IRENE) Intervention Study. *J. Am. Board Fam. Med.* 24, 524–533. doi: 10.3122/jabfm.2011.05.110017

del Giudice, P., Blanc, V., de Rougemont, A., Bes, M., Lina, G., Hubiche, T., et al. (2009). Primary skin abscesses are mainly caused by Panton-Valentine Leukocidin-positive *Staphylococcus aureus* strains. *Dermatology* 219, 299–302. doi: 10.1159/000232391

Dermatology Expert Groups (2009). *Therapeutic Guidelines: Dermatology, Version 3*. Melbourne, VIC: Therapeutic Guidelines Limited.

Forcade, N. A., Parchman, M. I., Jorgensen, J. H., Du, L. C., Nyren, N. R., Trevino, L. B., et al. (2011). Prevalence, severity, and treatment of community-acquired methicillin-resistant *Staphylococcus aureus* (CA-MRSA) skin and soft tissue infections in 10 medical clinics in texas: a South Texas Ambulatory Research Network (STARNet) study. *J. Am. Board Fam. Med.* 24, 543–550. doi: 10.3122/jabfm.2011.05.110073

Hankin, A., and Everett, W. W. (2007). Are antibiotics necessary after incision and drainage of a cutaneous abscess? *Ann. Emerg. Med.* 50, 49–51.

Jahamy, H., Ganga, R., Al Raiy, B., Shemes, S., Nagappan, V., Sharma, M., et al. (2008). *Staphylococcus aureus* skin/soft-tissue infections: the impact of SCCmec type and Panton-Valentine leucocidin. *Scand. J. Infect. Dis.* 40, 601–606. doi: 10.1080/00365540701877312

Kemper, A. R., Dolor, R. J., and Gowler, V. G. Jr. (2011). Management of skin abscesses by primary care pediatricians. *Clin. Pediatr.* 50, 525–528. doi: 10.1177/0009922810394837

Liu, C., Bayer, A., Cosgrove, S. E., Daum, R. S., Fridkin, S. K., Gorwitz, R. J., et al. (2011). Clinical practice guidelines by the infectious diseases society of america for the treatment of methicillin-resistant *Staphylococcus aureus*. *Clin. Infect. Dis.* 52, 285–292. doi: 10.1093/cid/ciq146

Lowy, F. D., Sexton, D. J., and Baron, E. L. (2008). *Treatment of Skin and Soft Tissue Infections Due to Methicillin-Resistant Staphylococcus aureus in Adults*. Waltham, MA: UpToDate.

May, L., Harter, K., Yadav, K., Strauss, R., Abualenain, J., Keim, A., et al. (2012). Practice patterns and management strategies for purulent skin and soft-tissue infections in an urban academic ED. *Am. J. Emerg. Med.* 30, 302–310. doi: 10.1016/j.ajem.2010.11.033

Moran, G., Krishnadasan, A., Gorwitz, R., Fosheim, G. E., McDougal, L. K., Carey, R. B. et al. (2006). Methicillin-resistant *S. aureus* infections among patients in the emergency department. *New Engl. J. Med.* 355, 666–674. doi: 10.1056/NEJMoa055356

Moran, G. J., Abrahamian, F. M., LoVecchio, F., and Talan, D. A. (2013). Acute bacterial skin infections: developments since the 2005 Infectious Diseases Society of America (IDSA) guidelines. *J. Emerg. Med.* 44, e397–e412. doi: 10.1016/j.jemermed.2012.11.050

Odenholt, I., Bylander-Groth, A., Fridmodt-Moller, N., Rokstad, K. S., and Molstad, S. (2002). Differences in antibiotic prescribing patterns between general practitioners in Scandinavia: a questionnaire study. *Scand. J. Infect. Dis.* 34, 602–609.

Parnes, B., Fernald, D., Coombs, L., DeAlleaume, L., Brandt, E., Webster, B., et al. (2011). Improving the management of skin and soft tissue infections in primary care: a report from State Networks of Colorado Ambulatory Practices and Partners (SNOCAP-USA) and the Distributed Ambulatory Research in Therapeutics Network (DARTNet). *J. Am. Board Fam. Med.* 24, 534–542. doi: 10.3122/jabfm.2011.05.110018

Schmitz, G., Goodwin, T., Singer, A., Kessler, C. S., Bruner, D., Larrabee, H., et al. (2013). The treatment of cutaneous abscesses: comparison of emergency medicine providers' practice patterns. *West. J. Emerg. Med.* 14, 23–28. doi: 10.5811/westjem.2011.9.6856

Talan, D. A., Krishnadasan, A., Gorwitz, R. J.,Fosheim, G. E., Limbago, B., Albrecht, V., et al. (2011). Comparison of *Staphylococcus aureus* from skin and soft-tissue infections in US emergency department patients, 2004 and 2008. *Clin. Infect. Dis.* 53, 144–149. doi: 10.1093/cid/cir308

Turnidge, J., Rao, N., Chang, F.-Y., Fowler, V. G., Kellie, S. M., Arnold, S., et al., (2016). "*Staphylococcus aureus*: susceptibility in vitro and in vivo," in *Antimicrobial Therapy and Vaccines: Microbes*, Vol. 1. Available at: http://www.antimicrobe.org/ (accessed April 26, 2016).

16

Susceptibility of Austrian Clinical *Klebsiella* and *Enterobacter* Isolates Linked to Patient-Related Data

Alexandra Badura[1], Gudrun Pregartner[2], Judith C. Holzer[1], Gebhard Feierl[1] and Andrea J. Grisold[1]*

[1] Institute of Hygiene, Microbiology and Environmental Medicine, Medical University of Graz, Graz, Austria, [2] Institute for Medical Informatics, Statistics and Documentation, Medical University of Graz, Graz, Austria

***Correspondence:**
Alexandra Badura
alexandra.badura@medunigraz.at

The aim of the study was to analyze the antimicrobial susceptibility of Austrian clinical *Klebsiella* sp. and *Enterobacter* sp. isolates linked to patient-related data over a time period from 1998 to 2014. The main findings of this study were (i) a marked difference of antibiotic susceptibility rates between different infection sites for both *Klebsiella* sp. and *Enterobacter* sp., (ii) significantly greater percentages of resistant isolates among both *Klebsiella* sp. and *Enterobacter* sp. in male patients compared to female patients and (iii) significantly greater percentages of resistant isolates among both *Klebsiella* sp. and *Enterobacter* sp. from hospital-derived samples compared to samples from the community. In conclusion, our statistical data analysis clearly indicated a strong association of patient-related data and *Klebsiella* sp. and *Enterobacter* sp. susceptibility profiles.

Keywords: antibiotic resistance, *Klebsiella*, *Enterobacter*, Austria, statistical analysis

INTRODUCTION

Whereas the antibiotic resistance crisis in Gram-positive pathogens largely seems to be kept under control, the emergence and dissemination of antibiotic resistance in Gram-negative pathogens risk getting out of control (Arya et al., 2008; Slama, 2008; Bush et al., 2011; Livermore, 2012). To gain useful information on overall trends in a specific region and alert for more effective prevention and control measures, surveillance studies based on large data sets are of particular importance in this field (World Health Organization [WHO], 2014). Multivariate statistical analysis further allows studying possible relationships between antimicrobial resistance data and patient-related factors; however, there are only a limited number of studies up to now on that issue mainly dealing with *Escherichia coli*. The main findings of these studies are that susceptibilities to several antimicrobial agents are strongly depending on infection site as well as patient location (hospital/community), gender and age (Livermore et al., 2003; Miguel Sahuquillo-Arce et al., 2011; Badura et al., 2015). Under the hypothesis that the same is true for *Klebsiella* sp. and *Enterobacter* sp., the aim of this study is to analyze a large amount of antibiotic resistance data (almost 39.000 isolates) from our geographical region according to patient-related factors. The application of multivariate statistical analysis enables us to detect significant associations between patient's characteristics and the percentages of resistant isolates what is of key importance to further identify possible risk factors related to antibiotic-resistant *Klebsiella* and *Enterobacter* infections.

TABLE 1 | Data basis for the statistical analysis.

	Patient gender (%)		Patient location (%)		Number of isolates
	Female	Male	Community	Hospital	
Klebsiella sp.	59.4	40.5	52.3	47.7	24024
Enterobacter sp.	52.8	47.1	44.0	56.0	14969
Total					38993

TABLE 2 | Overall resistance percentages of *Klebsiella* sp. and *Enterobacter* sp.

Antibiotic	*Klebsiella* sp.		*Enterobacter* sp.	
	%R	n/total	%R	n/total
AN	3.47	366/10550	0.96	78/8094
AMC	9.44	2264/23979		
CAZ	7.19	1230/17102	20.55	2341/11389
CIP	6.43	1543/23995	5.2	778/14961
CTX	5.76	1370/23765	19.87	2943/14811
NF	24.43	2297/9404	30.71	1502/4891
GM	6.66	1458/21889	2.76	392/14216
IPM	0.89	60/6747	0.54	26/4839
MEC	3.73	120/3220		
MEM	0.67	70/10511	0.28	22/7720
PT	6.98	1270/18186	20.17	2505/12418
SXT	10.82	2595/23990	6.22	930/14958

AN, amikacin; AMC, amoxicillin-clavulanic acid; CAZ, ceftazidime; CIP, ciprofloxacin; CTX, cefotaxime; NF, nitrofurantoin; GM, gentamicin; IPM, imipenem; MEC, mecillinam; MEM, meropenem; PT, piperacillin/tazobactam; SXT, trimethoprim/sulfamethoxazole; %R, percentages of non-susceptible isolates.

MATERIALS AND METHODS

A total of 24.024 *Klebsiella* sp. and 14.969 *Enterobacter* sp. isolates were included in the present analysis. The study design of this retrospective observational study (data origin, laboratory methods, and statistical analysis) is largely similar to our previous report on *E. coli* (Badura et al., 2015). Data were retrieved from the Laboratory of Medical Bacteriology and Mycology of the Medical University of Graz, Austria from January 1998 to March 2014. In the event of multiple isolates from one person in a year, only the first one was considered. For each isolate, patient-related data (age, gender), patient location (community/hospital) and culture site were obtained. Culture sites were subdivided into the following categories: urinary tract (UT), genital tract (GT), wounds (WOU), respiratory tract (RES), and blood (BLO); patient age was categorized as follows: <1, 1–9, 10–19, 20–29, 30–39, 40–49, 50–59, 60–69, 70–79, >= 80 years.

All isolates had been tested for antibiotic susceptibilities in the routine microbiology laboratory in the same way as reported in a previous study using the disk diffusion method or a VITEK 2 system (bioMérieux, Marcy l'Etoile France) (Badura et al., 2015). From January 1st, 1998 to May 31st, 2011 results were interpreted using the criteria recommended by the Clinical and Laboratory Standards Institute (CLSI), formerly known as National Committee for Clinical Laboratory Standards (NCCLS) (CLSI, 2012). From June 1st, 2011 results were interpreted using the criteria recommended by the European Committee on Antimicrobial Susceptibility Testing (EUCAST breakpoint tables v1.2, 2011) in its respective current version. For this study, resistance to the following 12 antibiotic agents was analyzed: amikacin (AN), amoxicillin-clavulanic acid (AMC; analyzed for *Klebsiella* sp. only), ceftazidime (CAZ), ciprofloxacin (CIP), cefotaxime (CTX), nitrofurantoin (NF; analyzed for urinary tract isolates only), gentamicin (GM), imipenem (IPM), mecillinam (MEC; analyzed for *Klebsiella* sp. urinary tract isolates only); meropenem (MEM), piperacillin/tazobactam (PT), and trimethoprim/sulfamethoxazole (SXT). Resistant and intermediate resistant isolates were combined.

Statistical Analysis

For each of the two microbes and for each antibiotic under consideration, the absolute and relative frequencies of resistant samples were determined in total, per culture site, patient location, age group, gender and year of acquisition. In order to assess the influence of the covariates on antibiotic resistance, multivariable logistic regression analysis was performed. For binary covariates, odds ratios and 95% confidence intervals are presented and are adjusted for year of acquisition, patient gender, patient age, patient location and resistance phenotype; for culture site a model containing the aforementioned covariates as well as cultures site has been tested against a model without culture site and p values from the respective Chi-square test are presented. Statistical analysis was performed using the R package, version 3.1.1 and SPSS, version 21.0 (R Development Core Team, 2008; IBM Corp, 2012).

Ethics Statement

The study was approved by the Ethics Committee of the Medical University of Graz (26-502 ex 13/14); patient records were anonymized prior to analysis.

RESULTS

The underlying data basis for the present analysis is shown in **Table 1**. In total, 38.993 clinical isolates of *Klebsiella* sp. and *Enterobacter* sp. were included in the statistical analysis.

Species Distribution

Within the *Klebsiella* samples, *K. pneumoniae* (61%) and *K. oxytoca* (27.1%) were the most frequently recovered species;

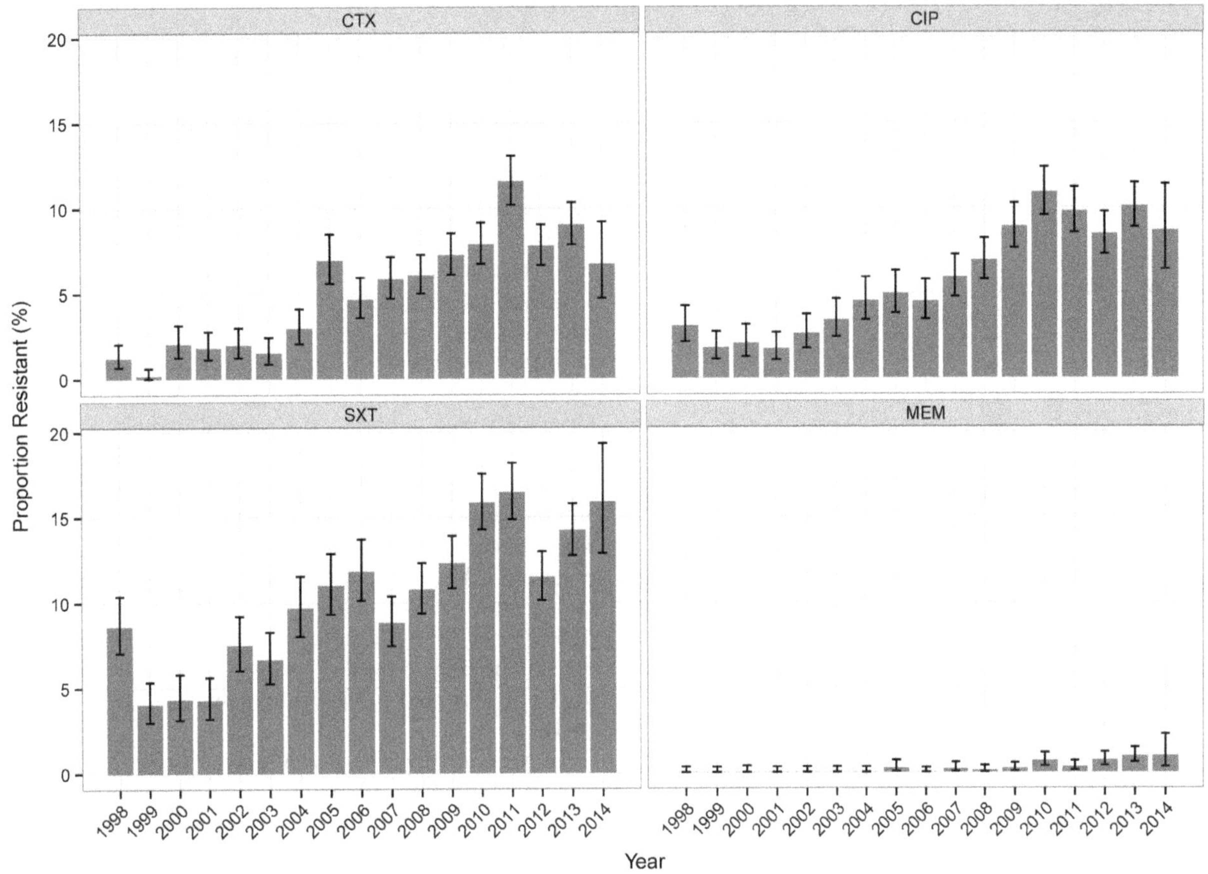

FIGURE 1 | Annual antibiotic resistance percentages of *Klebsiella* sp. for selected antibiotics.

within the *Enterobacter* samples, *E. cloacae* complex (59.2%) and *E. aerogenes* (15.4%) were the most frequently recovered species.

Overall and Annual Resistance Percentages

Table 2 shows the overall resistance percentages of all tested isolates. For *Klebsiella* sp. isolates, NF (analyzed for UT isolates only) and SXT showed the highest values, for *Enterobacter* sp. the highest values were found for NF, CAZ, PT, and CTX. For *Klebsiella* sp. isolates, most antibiotics (CAZ, CTX, NF, CIP, SXT, IPM, and MEM) showed increasing percentages of resistant isolates over time (**Figure 1**, **Supplemental Table S1**). The percentages of resistant *Enterobacter* sp. isolates did not change considerably over the investigational period for the majority of antibiotic agents (Supplemental Table S1).

Resistance Percentages According to Patient-Related Data

Results of the multivariate analysis of the antibiotic resistance patterns according to culture sites for both pathogens are presented in **Table 3**. The findings reveal the lowest resistance percentages from samples originating from the male or female genital tract (GT). For *Klebsiella* sp. isolates, the highest resistance percentages for almost all antibiotics analyzed occurred in blood infections. For *Enterobacter*, the highest resistance percentages were found in isolates originating from blood (CAZ, CTX, GM, PT, SXT), and urinary tract infections (AN, CIP) (**Table 3**).

Antibiotic resistance patterns in relation to patient gender are shown in **Table 4**. Resistance percentages for almost all antibiotic agents analyzed are higher in male patients. A significant difference can be shown for all antibiotics except for AN for *Klebsiella* sp. isolates and for AN, GM, IPM, MEM, and PT for *Enterobacter* sp., respectively. Antibiotic resistance patterns in relation to patient location are shown in **Table 5**. Resistance percentages for almost all antibiotic agents analyzed are significantly higher in hospital treated patients. This is true for both *Klebsiella* sp. and *Enterobacter* sp. isolates.

Regarding the association between antibiotic resistance percentages of *Klebsiella* sp. and *Enterobacter* sp. isolates and patient age, the majority of antibiotics show a balanced distribution except for CIP where a constant increase with age can be shown for both pathogen groups (**Figure 2**).

TABLE 3 | Resistance percentages of *Klebsiella* sp. and *Enterobacter* sp. according to culture sites.

	Klebsiella sp. %R (n/total)						*Enterobacter* sp. %R (n/total)					
	UT	GT	WOU	RES	BLO	p-value[a]	UT	GT	WOU	RES	BLO	p-value[a]
AN	4.2 (32/766)	0.1 (1/1648)	1.4 (37/2657)	1.7 (48/2867)	0 (0/103)	0.022	5.7 (22/388)	0 (0/767)	0.5 (13/2629)	0.4 (10/2467)	0 (0/68)	<0.001
AMC	6.9 (845/12264)	2.7 (63/2363)	9.7 (298/3086)	10.7 (357/3347)	14.3 (17/119)	<0.001						
CAZ	7.9 (486/6156)	0.8 (16/1893)	5.2 (152/2923)	5.9 (190/3228)	10.1 (12/119)	<0.001	21.8 (611/2806)	6.4 (56/871)	17.9 (513/2869)	19.9 (553/2778)	36 (31/86)	<0.001
CIP	7.6 (937/12262)	1.6 (39/2365)	6.9 (213/3088)	5.9 (198/3354)	10.1 (12/119)	<0.001	7.4 (436/5887)	0.7 (7/1075)	5 (153/3039)	4 (115/2874)	4.7 (4/86)	<0.001
CTX	4.3 (518/12044)	1 (24/2364)	5.2 (161/3084)	5.6 (189/3350)	10.9 (13/119)	0.011	19.3 (1111/5747)	6.8 (73/1076)	18.2 (553/3038)	19.7 (564/2865)	36 (31/86)	<0.001
GM	3.5 (351/10162)	0.7 (17/2363)	3.9 (119/3087)	5.9 (198/3352)	4.2 (5/119)	<0.001	1.7 (86/5144)	0.1 (1/1076)	1.2 (37/3039)	1.3 (36/2872)	2.3 (2/86)	<0.001
IPM	0.2 (2/1110)	0 (0/814)	0.8 (12/1495)	1.1 (20/1755)	3.7 (3/81)	0.013	0.2 (1/583)	0 (0/306)	0.5 (7/1380)	0.3 (5/1476)	0 (0/54)	0.025
MEM	0.2 (5/2101)	0 (0/1124)	0.7 (15/2286)	1 (24/2414)	3.7 (4/108)	<0.001	0.3 (3/931)	0 (0/580)	0.2 (4/2344)	0.1 (3/2076)	0 (0/80)	0.003
PT	5.9 (421/7102)	1.4 (30/2121)	7.8 (230/2948)	9.1 (288/3156)	12.7 (15/118)	<0.001	16.3 (805/4934)	22.7 (204/899)	22.6 (539/2390)	23.4 (567/2426)	38 (27/71)	<0.001
SXT	12.6 (1551/12263)	4.2 (100/2365)	8 (248/3085)	7.2 (242/3354)	9.2 (11/119)	<0.001	6 (354/5881)	6.2 (67/1076)	6 (182/3041)	6.3 (182/2873)	14 (12/86)	0.221

UT, urinary tract; GT, genital tract; WOU, wounds; RES, respiratory tract; BLO, blood; AN, amikacin; AMC, amoxicillin-clavulanic acid; CAZ, ceftazidime; CIP, ciprofloxacin; CTX, cefotaxime; NF, nitrofurantoin; GM, gentamicin; IPM, imipenem; MEM, meropenem; PT, piperacillin/tazobactam; SXT, trimethoprim/sulfamethoxazole. [a]*The p-values stem from a goodness-of-fit test comparing a model including all variables against a reduced model including all variables except for culture site.*

DISCUSSION

We here report an observational study whose aim is to analyze the susceptibility of Austrian clinical *Klebsiella* sp. and *Enterobacter* sp. isolates linked to patient-related data. The underlying database for this statistical analysis covers the period from 1998 to 2014. A major limitation of the present study is that it was not possible to link the data to severity of disease and patient outcome as these data were not available. Additionally, information about the patient's length of the hospital stay was not included in the analysis which would have been useful for the classification as hospital or community acquired infections. In the present work, infections were categorized depending on the patient's location at the moment the clinical sample was obtained. The passage from CLSI to EUCAST guidelines in 2011 in Austria may further bias data comparability. Several authors have reported an increase of antibiotic resistance rates for certain *Enterobacteriaceae* species/drug combinations following EUCAST breakpoints implementation (Hombach et al., 2012; Wolfensberger et al., 2013). However, we did not observe any artificial rise of antibiotic resistance at that time indicating that the change of interpretation criteria does not apparently impact the results of the large data set analyzed.

In general, surveillance is a substantial basis in the combat against antimicrobial resistance in both community and hospital settings; a large number of resistance surveillance reports thus exist about *Klebsiella* sp. and *Enterobacter* sp. isolates from various parts of the world describing the current resistance situation (Jones et al., 2004; Bedenic et al., 2010; Gales et al., 2012; Badal et al., 2013; Kaye and Pogue, 2015). Furthermore, studies dealing with the association of antimicrobial resistance data and specific factors depending on the host are of major importance with regard to the identification of possible risk factors related to antibiotic-resistant infections. Several studies aimed to find various patient demographics and clinical factors associated with the presence of antibiotic-resistant *Enterobacteriaceae* isolates, however, most of them involve particular infections, patient cohorts, anatomic sites or specific resistance problems. These studies thus mostly cover a small amount of isolates consequently limiting statistical data processing (O'Fallon et al., 2010; Metan et al., 2013; Ivady et al., 2015; Moini et al., 2015; Oliveira et al., 2015). Here we present a comprehensive statistical analysis on associations between patient-related data and the percentages of antibiotic resistant *Klebsiella* sp. and *Enterobacter* sp. isolates referring on a large database with almost 39.000 isolates from Austria. The main findings of this study are (i) a marked difference of antibiotic susceptibility rates between different infection sites for both *Klebsiella* sp. and *Enterobacter* sp., (ii) significantly greater percentages of resistant isolates among both *Klebsiella* sp. and *Enterobacter* sp. in male patients compared to female patients and (iii) significantly greater percentages of resistant isolates among both *Klebsiella* sp. and *Enterobacter* sp. isolates from hospital-derived samples compared to samples from the community.

TABLE 4 | Antibiotic resistance percentages of *Klebsiella* sp. and *Enterobacter* sp. according to patient gender.

	Klebsiella sp. %R (n/total)			*Enterobacter* sp. %R (n/total)		
Antibiotic	**Female**	**Male**	**OR**	**Female**	**Male**	**OR**
AN	3.2 (174/5396)	3.7 (192/5141)	1.16 [0.95, 1.44]	0.8 (28/3731)	1.1 (50/4355)	1.43 [0.89, 2.34]
AMC	7.4 (1053/14245)	12.5 (1210/9715)	1.78 [1.63, 1.94]			
CAZ	5.9 (552/9398)	8.8 (677/7688)	1.55 [1.38, 1.74]	17.7 (990/5598)	23.3 (1350/5782)	1.13 [1.03, 1.25]
CIP	4.5 (647/14248)	9.2 (895/9728)	2.13 [1.92, 2.37]	3.3 (263/7899)	7.3 (515/7050)	2.2 [1.88, 2.57]
CTX	4.3 (611/14093)	7.9 (758/9653)	1.88 [1.68, 2.1]	17.4 (1361/7812)	22.6 (1580/6987)	1.1 [1.01, 1.2]
NF	22.4 (1392/6208)	28.3 (905/3196)	1.37 [1.24, 1.51]	28.2 (837/2972)	34.7 (665/1919)	1.23 [1.09, 1.4]
GM	4.8 (613/12791)	9.3 (844/9079)	2.04 [1.83, 2.27]	2.3 (170/7416)	3.3 (222/6788)	1.11 [0.9, 1.38]
IPM	0.5 (17/3464)	1.3 (43/3273)	2.7 [1.57, 4.87]	0.5 (12/2255)	0.5 (14/2578)	0.8 [0.37, 1.76]
MEC	3 (60/2012)	5 (60/1208)	1.62 [1.11, 2.36]			
MEM	0.4 (19/5174)	1 (51/5326)	2.07 [1.24, 3.61]	0.3 (9/3509)	0.3 (13/4206)	1 [0.43, 2.43]
PT	5.3 (545/10257)	9.2 (724/7912)	1.35 [1.19, 1.52]	19.7 (1286/6523)	20.7 (1216/5887)	1.01 [0.93, 1.11]
SXT	9.3 (1321/14245)	13.1 (1273/9726)	1.3 [1.19, 1.43]	5.8 (457/7897)	6.7 (472/7049)	1.16 [1.01, 1.33]

AN, amikacin; AMC, amoxicillin-clavulanic acid; CAZ, ceftazidime; CIP, ciprofloxacin; CTX, cefotaxime; NF, nitrofurantoin; GM, gentamicin; IPM, imipenem; MEC, mecillinam; MEM, meropenem; PT, piperacillin/tazobactam; SXT, trimethoprim/sulfamethoxazole. OR, odd ratio

TABLE 5 | Antibiotic resistance percentages of *Klebsiella* sp. and *Enterobacter* sp. according to patient location.

	Klebsiella sp. %R (n/total)			*Enterobacter* sp. %R (n/total)		
Antibiotic	**Outpatient**	**Hospital**	**OR**	**Outpatient**	**Hospital**	**OR**
AN	0.3 (10/2894)	4.6 (356/7656)	4.18 [2.24, 8.71]	0.6 (11/1782)	1.1 (67/6312)	1.39 [0.74, 2.83]
AMC	4.8 (602/12557)	14.6 (1662/11422)	2.43 [2.18, 2.71]			
CAZ	4.5 (303/6703)	8.9 (927/10399)	1.32 [1.04, 1.69]	10.2 (369/3607)	25.3 (1972/7782)	2.97 [2.63, 3.37]
CIP	5.6 (700/12558)	7.4 (843/11437)	1.08 [0.96, 1.23]	4.5 (297/6587)	5.7 (481/8374)	1.22 [1.05, 1.43]
CTX	2.7 (335/12552)	9.2 (1035/11213)	2.39 [1.8, 3.18]	11.8 (775/6584)	26.4 (2168/8227)	2.67 [2.44, 2.93]
NF	21 (1376/6557)	32.3 (921/2847)	1.77 [1.59, 1.96]	26.1 (872/3339)	40.6 (630/1552)	1.82 [1.6, 2.07]
GM	2 (205/10465)	11 (1253/11424)	2.86 [2.4, 3.42]	0.7 (40/5847)	4.2 (352/8369)	4.48 [3.23, 6.39]
IPM	0.2 (4/1863)	1.1 (56/4884)	2.55 [1.01, 8.59]	0 (0/1032)	0.7 (26/3807)	*
MEC	3.3 (78/2393)	5.1 (42/827)	1.3 [0.87, 1.93]			
MEM	0.2 (4/2508)	0.8 (66/8003)	5.14 [2.09, 17.09]	0.1 (1/1534)	0.3 (21/6186)	5.79 [1.18, 104.62]
PT	3.4 (266/7892)	9.8 (1004/10294)	2.71 [2.34, 3.14]	18.3 (956/5219)	21.5 (1549/7199)	1.2 [1.09, 1.32]
SXT	9.5 (1190/12556)	12.3 (1405/11434)	0.95 [0.86, 1.05]	5.9 (387/6582)	6.5 (543/8376)	1.05 [0.91, 1.21]

*AN, amikacin; AMC, amoxicillin-clavulanic acid; CAZ, ceftazidime; CIP, ciprofloxacin; CTX, cefotaxime; NF, nitrofurantoin; GM, gentamicin; IPM, imipenem; MEC, mecillinam; MEM, meropenem; PT, piperacillin/tazobactam; SXT, trimethoprim/sulfamethoxazole. *Not estimable because of 0 resistant isolates in outpatient group. OR, odd ratio*

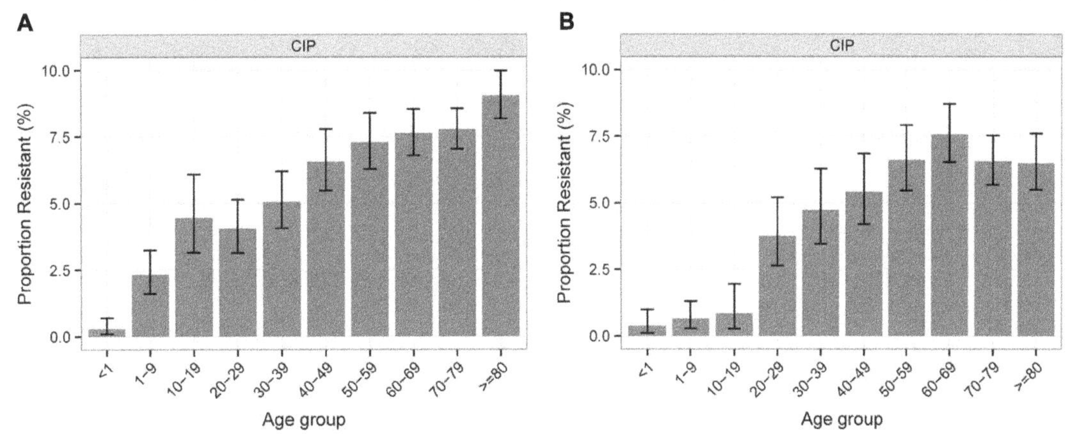

FIGURE 2 | Percentages of antibiotic resistance of *Klebsiella* sp. (A) and *Enterobacter* sp. (B) to CIP according to patient age.

To our knowledge, this is the first report to compare percentages of antibiotic resistant *Klebsiella* sp. and *Enterobacter* sp. isolates from different infection sites within a specific region. The highest resistance percentages for the majority of antibiotics analyzed can be shown for both pathogen groups originating from blood infections. This is in accordance with previous statistical analyses on the association of the infection site and *Escherichia coli* susceptibility profiles (Miguel Sahuquillo-Arce et al., 2011; Badura et al., 2015). As reported for *Escherichia coli, Klebsiella* sp. and *Enterobacter* sp. isolates originating from the GT generally show the lowest resistance percentages indicating that detection from this culture site often represents the normal patient flora. Interestingly, antibiotic-resistant *Klebsiella* sp. and *Enterobacter* sp. infections within our study collection derive mostly from men. The same association between patient sex and antibiotic resistance was previously shown for *Escherichia coli,* however, the underlying cause remains as yet largely unclear (Livermore et al., 2003; Miguel Sahuquillo-Arce et al., 2011; Badura et al., 2015). Similar to the results from several other studies dealing with antibiotic resistance percentages of *Enterobacteriaceae* in community and hospital settings we found significantly greater resistance rates for both pathogen groups amongst the hospital-derived isolates suggesting that the problem of antibiotic resistance amongst Gram-negative pathogens is still focused on hospital settings in our region (Boyd et al., 2008; Ferjani et al., 2015; McKay and Bamford, 2015).

CONCLUSION

Our statistical data analysis clearly indicates a strong association between patient characteristics (gender, localization, infection site) and *Klebsiella* sp. and *Enterobacter* sp. susceptibility profiles. To gain further insight in the correlation of bacterial antibiotic resistance and its host, additional studies analyzing large databases of microbiological information are of crucial importance ultimately influencing local antimicrobial therapy guidelines.

AUTHOR CONTRIBUTIONS

AB: general conception, study design, data acquisition, data analysis, data interpretation, writing of the manuscript; GF: data interpretation, revising of the manuscript; JH and GP: statistical analysis, data interpretation, revising of the manuscript; AG: data interpretation, revising of the manuscript.

SUPPLEMENTARY MATERIAL

TABLE S1 | Annual resistance percentages of *Klebsiella* sp. and *Enterobacter* sp.

REFERENCES

Arya, S. C., Agarwal, N., and Agarwal, S. (2008). Emerging Gram-negative antibiotic resistance: daunting challenges, declining sensitivities, and dire consequences. *Respir. Care* 53, 1749–1750; author reply 1750.

Badal, R. E., Bouchillon, S. K., Lob, S. H., Hackel, M. A., Hawser, S. P., and Hoban, D. J. (2013). Etiology, extended-spectrum beta-lactamase rates and antimicrobial susceptibility of gram-negative bacilli causing intra-abdominal infections in patients in general pediatric and pediatric intensive care units-global data from the study for monitoring antimicrobial resistance trends 2008 to 2010. *Pediatr. Infect. Dis. J.* 32, 636–640. doi: 10.1097/INF.0b013e3182886377

Badura, A., Feierl, G., Pregartner, G., Krause, R., and Grisold, A. J. (2015). Antibiotic resistance patterns of more than 120 000 clinical *Escherichia coli* isolates in Southeast Austria, 1998-2013. *Clin. Microbiol. Infect.* 21:569.e1-7. doi: 10.1016/j.cmi.2015.02.012

Bedenic, B., Goic-Barisic, I., Budimir, A., Tonkic, M., Mihajkevic, L. J., Novak, A., et al. (2010). Antimicrobial susceptibility and beta-lactamase production of selected gram-negative bacilli from two Croatian hospitals: MYSTIC study results. *J. Chemother.* 22, 147–152. doi: 10.1179/joc.2010.22.3.147

Boyd, L. B., Atmar, R. L., Randall, G. L., Hamill, R. J., Steffen, D., and Zechiedrich, L. (2008). Increased fluoroquinolone resistance with time in *Escherichia coli* from > 17,000 patients at a large county hospital as a function of culture site, age, sex, and location. *BMC Infect. Dis.* 8:4. doi: 10.1186/1471-2334-8-4.

Bush, K., Courvalin, P., Dantas, G., Davies, J., Eisenstein, B., Huovinen, P., et al. (2011). Tackling antibiotic resistance. *Nat. Rev. Microbiol.* 9, 894–896. doi: 10.1038/nrmicro2693

CLSI (2012) *Performance Standards for Antimicrobial Disk and Dilution Susceptibility Tests for Bacteria Isolated from Animals; Approved StandardCLSI Document M31-A3*, 3rd Edn. Wayne, PA: CLSI.

Ferjani, S., Saidani, M., Amine, F. S., and Boutiba Ben Boubaker, I. (2015). A comparative study of antimicrobial resistance rates and phylogenetic groups of community-acquired versus hospital-acquired invasive *Escherichia coli. Med. Mal. Infect.* 45, 133–138. doi: 10.1016/j.medmal.2015.01.012

Gales, A. C., Castanheira, M., Jones, R. N., and Sader, H. S. (2012). Antimicrobial resistance among Gram-negative bacilli isolated from Latin America: results from SENTRY Antimicrobial Surveillance Program (Latin America, 2008-2010). *Diagn. Microbiol. Infect. Dis.* 73, 354–360. doi: 10.1016/j.diagmicrobio.2012.04.007

Hombach, M., Bloemberg, G. V., and Böttger, E. C. (2012). Effects of clinical breakpoint changes in CLSI guidelines 2010/2011 and EUCAST guidelines 2011 on antibiotic susceptibility test reporting of Gram-negative bacilli. *J. Antimicrob. Chemother.* 67, 622-632 doi: 10.1093/jac/dkr524

IBM Corp (2012). *IBM SPSS Statistics for Windows, Version 21.0.* Armonk, NY: IBM.

Ivady, B., Kenesei, E., Toth-Heyn, P., Kertesz, G., Tarkanyi, K., Kassa, C., et al. (2015). Factors influencing antimicrobial resistance and outcome of Gram-negative bloodstream infections in children. *Infection* [Epub ahead of print]. doi: 10.1007/s15010-015-0857-8

Jones, M. E., Karlowsky, J. A., Draghi, D. C., Thornsberry, C, Sahm, D. F., and Bradley, J. S. (2004). Rates of antimicrobial resistance among common bacterial pathogens causing respiratory, blood, urine, and skin and soft tissue infections in pediatric patients. *Eur. J. Clin. Microbiol. Infect. Dis.* 23, 445–455. doi: 10.1007/s10096-004-1133-5

Kaye, K. S., and Pogue, J. M. (2015). Infections caused by resistant gram-negative bacteria: epidemiology and management. *Pharmacotherapy* 35, 949–962. doi: 10.1002/phar.1636

Livermore, D. M. (2012). Current epidemiology and growing resistance of gram-negative pathogens. *Korean J. Intern. Med.* 27, 128–142. doi: 10.3904/kjim.2012.27.2.128

Livermore, D. M., Nichols, T., Lamagni, T. L., Potz, N., Reynolds, R., and Duckworth, G. (2003). Ciprofloxacin-resistant *Escherichia coli* from bacteraemias in England; increasingly prevalent and mostly from men. *J. Antimicrob. Chemother.* 52, 1040–1042. doi: 10.1093/jac/dkg479

McKay, R., and Bamford, C. (2015). Community- versus healthcare-acquired bloodstream infections at Groote Schuur Hospital, Cape Town, South Africa. *S. Afr. Med. J.* 105, 363–369. doi: 10.7196/samj.8183

Metan, G., Demiraslan, H., Kaynar, L. G., Zararsiz, G., Alp, E., and Eser, B. (2013). Factors influencing the early mortality in haematological malignancy patients with nosocomial Gram negative bacilli bacteraemia: a retrospective analysis of 154 cases. *Braz. J. Infect. Dis.* 17, 143–149. doi: 10.1016/j.bjid.2012.09.010

Miguel Sahuquillo-Arce, J., Selva, M., Perpinan, H., Gobernado, M., Armero, C., Lopez-Quilez, A., et al. (2011). Antimicrobial resistance in more than 100,000 *Escherichia coli* isolates according to culture site and patient age, gender, and location. *Antimicrob. Agents Chemother.* 55, 1222–1228. doi: 10.1128/AAC.00765-10

Moini, A. S., Soltani, B., Taghavi Ardakani, A., Moravveji, A., Erami, M., Haji Rezaei, M., et al. (2015). Multidrug-resistant *Escherichia coli* and *Klebsiella* pneumonia isolated from patients in Kashan, Iran. *Jundishapur J. Microbiol.* 8:e27517.

O'Fallon, E., Kandel, R., Schreiber, R., and D'Agata, E. M. (2010). Acquisition of multidrug-resistant gram-negative bacteria: incidence and risk factors within a long-term care population. *Infect. Control Hosp. Epidemiol.* 31, 1148–1153. doi: 10.1086/656590

Oliveira, M. C., Oliveira, C. R., Goncalves, K. V., Santos, M. S., Tardelli, A. C., and Nobre, V. A. (2015). Enterobacteriaceae resistant to third generation cephalosporins upon hospital admission: risk factors and clinical outcomes. *Braz. J. Infect. Dis.* 19, 239–245. doi: 10.1016/j.bjid.2015.01.006

R Development Core Team (2008). *R: A Language and Environment Forstatistical Computing.* Vienna: R Foundation for Statistical Computing.

Slama, T. G. (2008). Gram-negative antibiotic resistance: there is a price to pay. *Crit. Care* 12(Suppl 4), S4. doi: 10.1186/cc6820

Wolfensberger, A., Sax, H., Weber, R, Zbinden, R., Kuster, S. P., and Hombach, M. (2013). Change of antibiotic susceptibility testing guidelines from CLSI to EUCAST: influence on cumulative hospital antibiograms. *PLoS ONE* 8: e79130. doi: 10.1371/journal.pone.0079130. eCollection 2013.

World Health Organization [WHO] (2014). *Antimicrobial Resistance: Global Report on Surveillance.* Available at: http://apps.who.int/iris/bitstream/10665/112642/1/9789241564748_eng.pdf

17

Development of Cefotaxime Impregnated Chitosan as Nano-Antibiotics: *De Novo* Strategy to Combat Biofilm Forming Multi-Drug Resistant Pathogens

Bushra Jamil[1], Huma Habib[2], Shahid A. Abbasi[3], Ayesha Ihsan[4], Habib Nasir[5] and Muhammad Imran[1]**

[1] Microbiology and Public Health Group, Department of Biosciences, COMSATS Institute of Information Technology, Islamabad, Pakistan, [2] Center for Micro and Nano Devices, COMSATS Institute of Information Technology, Islamabad, Pakistan, [3] Department of Pathology, Al-Sayed Hospital, Rawalpindi, Pakistan, [4] Industrial Biotechnology Division, National Institute of Biotechnology and Genetic Engineering, Faisalabad, Pakistan, [5] School of Natural Sciences, National University of Sciences and Technology, Islamabad, Pakistan

***Correspondence:**
Muhammad Imran
m.imran@comsats.edu.pk
Bushra Jamil
bushrajamil2000@gmail.com

Frequent incidents of antibiotic-resistant biofilm forming pathogens in community-associated and hospital-acquired infections have become a global concern owing to failure of conventional therapies. Nano-antibiotics (NABs) are *de novo* tools to overcome the multi-drug resistant mechanisms employed by the superbugs. Inhibition of biofilm formation is one of those strategies to curb multi drug resistance phenomenon. In the current study, the anti-biofilm and antibacterial potential of newly synthesized cefotaxime loaded chitosan based NABs have been investigated. Both bare and cefotaxime loaded NABs were prepared by ionotropic gelation method. They were found carrying positive zeta potential of more than +50 mV, indicating highly stable nano-dispersion. Moreover, microscopic studies revealed their size as less than 100 nm. NABs were tested against clinical isolates of multi drug resistant *Klebsiella pneumoniae, Pseudomonas aeruginosa, Escherichia coli, and* methicillin resistant *Staphylococcus aureus* and wherein they demonstrated broad-spectrum anti-biofilm and anti-pathogenic activity. Thus, *in vitro* synergistic action of cephalosporin drugs and chitosan polymer at nano-scale in contrast to free antibiotics can be an improved broad-spectrum strategy to thwart resistance mechanisms in both Gram-positive and Gram-negative resistant pathogens.

Keywords: biofilm, chitosan nano-carriers, cephalosporins, drug resistance, growth kinetics, zeta potential

INTRODUCTION

Though, it is a mutually agreeable fact that bacteria has no definite nervous system but it is also conceded that they evolve certain survival mechanisms that allow them to exist in any environment. Biofilm formation is one of such survival mechanisms. Most of the bacterial species prefer to live in a well-developed community (biofilm) rather than planktonic form (isolated individual cells; Dheilly et al., 2010; Sayem et al., 2011). Along with numerous other benefits, biofilms also provide the basic mechanism of resistance to antibiotics, antibodies, bacteriophages, disinfectants and other host defense systems (Dheilly et al., 2010) by constituting a multi-layered protection mechanisms (Stewart, 2002). Extracellular polymeric substance (EPS) covering the biofilms make them impermeable to many antibiotics. Likewise, in biofilms microbes exhibit slow growth rate which further makes them resistant to therapeutic agents. Furthermore, biofilm forming microbes develop adaptive stress responses which collectively evince another defense mechanism. The formation of persister cells are further addition to this menace and is the main cause of recurrent and chronic infections (Lewis, 2005). Biofilms also facilitate the horizontal or lateral gene transfer (Madsen et al., 2012) which is considered a significant feature in the evolutionary process of acquiring antibiotic resistance genes between species. Biofilms also provide a wide variety of genetic elements (plasmids) to be transferred among unrelated bacterial species including genes that promote biofilm formation and responsibles for resistance (Donlan, 2002).

Extracellular DNA (eDNA) which is formed by the autolysis of a microbial subpopulation also makes an integral part of microbial biofilms and plays a foremost role in the stability of the biofilms (Watnick and Kolter, 2000). These biofilms accumulate large quantity of antibiotic degrading enzymes too (Delcour, 2009). In addition, biofilm formation is associated with the virulence of pathogenic bacteria, and cells included within a biofilm are generally 1000 times more resistant. National Institutes of Health (NIH) has estimated that 70% of all microbial infections in the world are associated with biofilms (Perumal and Mahmud, 2013). It is, therefore, a major concern not only in health care systems but in certain other domains as well. It has also been a major source of contamination in the food industry, water supply pipes, medical implants, catheters and equipment etc (Dheilly et al., 2010; Perumal and Mahmud, 2013).

The effectiveness of many antimicrobial agents is currently decreasing owing to increasing prevalence of multidrug-resistant (MDR) pathogens (Fabbretti et al., 2011). The emergence of these MDR pathogens remains a serious challenge to medicine and healthcare systems (Carlet et al., 2012). One of the mechanisms for such resistance is the formation of biofilms. If antibiotics cannot traverse the biofilm they fail to eradicate other defense strategies. Therefore, it is important to search for alternative therapeutics to control biofilm-associated MDR infections (Perumal and Mahmud, 2013; Kirker et al., 2015).

The development of anti-biofilm and anti-MDR strategies is therefore a major area of interest and currently constitutes an important field of investigation. Albeit, various naturally occurring compounds (including plant extracts) have been investigated in this regard (Salta et al., 2013). However, nano-antimicrobials (NAMs) are offering more promising future to beat MDR phenomenon (Allaker and Memarzadeh, 2014; Jamil et al., 2015). NAMs can also overcome resistance caused by biofilm formation and can prevent biofilm's further growth as well (Jamil et al., 2015). Recently, various NAMs have displayed their anti-biofilm potential to combat resistance mechanisms. Liposomes help thrashing biofilms by promoting adsorption at the outer surfaces of biofilms (Smith, 2005). Besides, silica nano-particles (NPs) act by releasing large amount of Nitric oxide (NO; Hetrick et al., 2009). Analogously, ZnO, TiO_2, MgF_2 NPs and super paramagnetic iron oxide NPs (SPIONs) have also inhibited biofilm formation (Pelgrift and Friedman, 2013). The rationale behind successful eradication of biofilms lies in strong interaction between biofilms and NAMs. The majority of NAMs bear positive charge that attaches firmly to biofilm matrixes carrying negative charge (Hajipour et al., 2012). However, due to metallic NPs associated toxicity issues, nano-medicine research focus has been shifted toward bio-based NPs or nano-carrier systems (NCS). In general, NCS protects the drug from both endogenous and exogenous factors and provide a sustained release and more enhanced bioactivity.

Cefotaxime is a third generation broad spectrum cephalosporins for parenteral administration with a short half-life of 0.8–1.4 h, it is bactericidal and mainly used in the treatment of infections caused by Gram-positive and Gram-negative microorganisms. Very recent and frequent emergence of extended spectrum beta lactamases (ESBL) and metallo beta lactamases (MBL) are reducing the susceptibility of all cephalosporins including cefotaxime. Therefore, present investigation has been carried out in an attempt to enhance the bactericidal activity of this β-lactam antibiotic synergistically with antimicrobial bio polymer chitosan to render it more effective against biofilm producing MDR pathogens.

MATERIALS AND METHODS

Chitosan-medium molecular weight was purchased from Sigma–Aldrich (Product number 448877, 75–85% deacetylation, 200–800 cP viscosity of 1% w/v in 1% v/v acetic acid). Pentasodium triphosphate (TPP) and glacial acetic acid were also procured from Sigma–Aldrich. All antibiotic disks were obtained from Oxoid. Nutrient agar and nutrient broth were purchased from Oxoid. Cefotaxime sodium for injection (0.5 g) was procured from Sanofi Aventis Pakistan Limited. Standard stock solution of cefotaxime sodium was prepared by dissolving 1 mg/mL in sterilized water.

Culture Collection

The clinical isolates were obtained from Al-Sayed Hospital (Pvt) Ltd, Rawalpindi and stored at −80°C in nutrient broth containing 20% glycerol. Their identities were confirmed by biochemical test using API (analytical profile index) kits. For the purpose of this study, we had collected pathogenic bacteria which were capable of biofilm formation and were documented as causative agents for severe infections. Clinically resistant pathogens used in this study includes *Klebsiella pneumoniae* (KP), *Pseudomonas aeruginosa, Escherichia coli* (*E. coli*), *and* Methicillin resistant *Staphylococcus aureus* (MRSA). We could not get clinical isolates of *Listeria monocytogenes,* so *L. monocytogenes* ATCC 13932 had been employed for this study.

Inoculum was prepared by the method described in literature with slight modifications. All the bacterial strains were recovered on a fresh nutrient agar (Oxoid) plate 24 h prior to antimicrobial test. To prepare the inoculum, colonies from fresh agar were transferred into sterile Mueller Hinton (MH) liquid growth medium and incubated at 37°C overnight. The optical density was adjusted to 0.1 at 600 nm wavelength (Perumal and Mahmud, 2013).

Resistance Spectra by Disk Diffusion Method

Selected microbes were subjected to antibiotic disks by standard Kirby Bauer method and their resistance patterns were studied and compared to CLSI guidelines. Following antibiotic disks were used including Ceftazidime (CAZ), Cefotaxime (CTX), Imipenem (IPM), Cefepime (FEP), Ceftriaxone (CRO), Aztreonam (ATM), Ampicillin (AMP), Vancomycin (VA), Augmentin (AMC), Colistin (CT), Cefoxitin (FOX), and Minocycline (MH). All selected bacterial cultures were marked as resistant or susceptible based upon their zones of inhibition.

Quantification of Antibiotics by Nanophotometer

UV-Vis spectrophotometer (Nanophotometer Implen) was used for this purpose (El-Shaboury et al., 2007; Bushra et al., 2014). Volumetric dilutions of cefotaxime were prepared in triplicate from stock solution. λ_{max} was obtained after the wave scan for 200–900 nm range. Calibration curve was constructed with the average absorbance of three replicates. The trend line was obtained by linear regression with standard equation and R squared value.

Chitosan Nanoparticles (CSNPs) Fabrication

Ionotropic gelation method was used to fabricate Chitosan Nanoparticles (CSNPs; Du et al., 2009; Jamil et al., 2016). Ionotropic gelation is based on the ability of poly electrolytes to cross link in the presence of counter-ions to form hydrogel beads also called as gelispheres (Patil et al., 2012). These gelispheres have the ability to control the release of drug. Cefotaxime solution was prepared in tripolyphosphate (TPP) and it was then added dropwise in chitosan (CS) solution with constant stirring. The TPP diffuses slowly into the CS solution forming a three dimensional lattice of ionically crosslinked moiety that has entrapped drug in it (Patil et al., 2012). It was then subjected to sonication for another 30 min by using Sonozap ultrasonic homogenizer 25 kHz. These NPs were then centrifuged at 12000 *g* for 10 min.

Nanoparticles Characterizations

The detection and characterization of nanoparticles entail particular challenges. As particle size is a key criterion in nanotechnology, maintaining particle size both *in vitro* and *in vivo* is crucial. Stability of NPs is determined mainly by their size maintenance. Flocculation and aggregation due to van der Waals forces should be avoided as the behavior of NPs is remarkably different from the bulk material of the same matter. Bulk material does not change its physical properties as the size of matter changes, while the NCS display size dependent properties. As a general rule, extent of size reduction is directly proportional to the surface area. Increased surface area contributes toward greater activity.

Scanning Electron Microscopy (SEM)

Scanning electron microscopy uses electrons instead of light to form an image and is one of the most widely used techniques for the characterization of nanostructures. Jeol JSM 6490A analytical scanning electron microscope was used for this purpose. Sample was prepared by placing a small drop of formulation on glass slide. Gold coating by Jeol Quick Auto Coater (JFC-1500) ion sputtering device was done for 6 s only. Analyses of both empty and drug loaded nanoparticles were carried out at the resolution of 20 kV and 3000–50000× magnification by the procedure already published (Jamil et al., 2016).

Atomic Force Microscopy (AFM)

SEM gives a 2D image while AFM can provide a 3D topographic picture of prepared nano-systems. Agilent Pico Plus was used for this purpose. The AFM probe has a very sharp tip, often less than 100 Å diameter, at the end of a small cantilever beam. The probe is attached to a piezoelectric scanner tube. Inter-atomic forces between the probe tip and the sample surface cause the cantilever to deflect as the sample's surface topography or other properties change. A laser light reflected from the back of the cantilever measures the deflection of the cantilever. Based on the type of application, different operation modes of AFM are used like the contact mode, semi contact mode and tapping mode (Suresh, 2015). However, for this study, all the images were taken in tapping mode at ambient conditions.

Fourier Transform Infrared Spectroscopy (FTIR) Spectra

Fourier Transform Infrared Spectroscopy was done for qualitative analysis of prepared formulations. Infrared spectroscopy is associated with vibrational energy of atoms or group of atoms in a material. It gives peaks for each functional groups and also gives a clue about bonding and interactions. Perkin Elmer FTIR spectroscope was used to analyze dry sample after preparing their pallet with KBr (FTIR grade Merck) while liquids were analyzed directly. The spectral resolution was 4 cm^{-1}, with 96 scans, and an aperture of 4 mm. The optimum beam incidence angle was 45° and all the spectra were acquired in a range between 4000 and 600 cm^{-1}.

Determination of Zeta Potential

Zeta potential was measured to get an indication about long term stability of nano-formulations. Zetasizer Nano ZS (Malvern Instruments, UK) using Doppler electrophoresis as the basic principle of operation was used in this study. The data collected were then imported to Excel and the means and standard deviations of the replicate measurements were calculated.

Determination of Encapsulation Efficiency

The encapsulation efficiency (EE) of nanoparticles was calculated by the method earlier mentioned (Rotar et al., 2014). Drug loaded CSNPs were isolated from the free drug by centrifugation (12,000 *g* for 15 min, Eppendorf 5415D, Germany). Free drug in the supernatant was quantified by spectrophotometer at λ_{max}

(298) obtained from wave scan. The concentration of drug in the supernatant was estimated by the equation obtained from standard curve. Experiments were performed in triplicate and the EE was calculated as follows:

$$EE = (\text{total drug} - \text{un encapsulated drug}) \div \text{total drug} \times 100$$

Antimicrobial Potential of the Prepared Nano-antibiotics (NABs)

Antibacterial activity of blank and β-lactam antibiotic loaded CSNPs were evaluated according to standard liquid micro-dilution susceptibility assays. To this aim, selected microbes were grown in nutrient broth until the exponential growth phase at 37°C while shaking. Bacterial turbidity was compared to Mc-Farland solution. Ten microliters of the bacterial suspension were added to 9 mL broth and similar concentration of antibiotic and drug loaded CSNP were added in inoculated broth. Test tubes were incubated in shaker incubator at 37°C overnight. Optical densities values were taken after every 24 h for 144 h at 595 nm on Elisa Multi-plate reader (Jamil et al., 2016). Both positive and negative controls were added in this assay. Negative control contains only the nutrient broth without culture and served as control of any possible contamination while the positive control contains nutrient broth and inoculum to serve as a control of cell-viability.

At the end of experiment colony forming unit (CFU) assay was done to confirm the results. Serially diluted bacterial suspensions were plated on Nutrient agar surface and incubated for 48 h at 37°C. Results were expressed as log10 CFU/ml.

Anti-Biofilm Potential of the Prepared Nano-antibiotics

To assess the anti-biofilm activity of cephalosporin loaded CSNPs against clinically important pathogens; MicroTiter Plate (MTP) assay was carried out using 96-well flat bottom polystyrene titer plates (Kirker et al., 2015).

Biofilms were formed on ELISA plate by the method of George with few modifications (George, 2011). Briefly, all selected pathogens were cultured on fresh Petri plate from stocks preserved at −80°C and from that pure media inoculum was prepared. Turbidity was compared to that of McFarland turbidity standard and 10 μL inoculum was added in test tube containing 9 mL of freshly sterilized nutrient broth. Nano-antibiotic and simple antibiotic solution prepared at same concentration were then added in each test tube. Approximately 200 μL of each sample was added in each well of 96 well ELISA dish. Each sample was prepared in triplicate and incubated at 37°C. After incubation, planktonic cells were removed by turning the plate upside down. It was then submerge gently in a small tub of water and water was removed. Washing was done thrice to remove all the unattached cells and also to lower background staining. Afterwards 200 μL of a 0.1% solution of crystal violet was added to each well of the microtiter plate. It was left in incubator for 10–15 min. Crystal violet solution was removed by tilting the plate and by rinsing with water 3–4 times. It was then blot dried.

To quantify the biofilms, 200 μL of 30% v/v acetic acid solution was added to each well to completely solubilize the crystal violet. The microtiter plate was incubated at room temperature for 10-15 min. The resultant solution was transferred to a new microtiter dish and absorbance reading was taken in a micro-plate reader at 595 nm (George, 2011; Perumal and Mahmud, 2013).

RESULTS

Resistance Spectra by Disk Diffusion Method

Resistance spectra of selected microbes were determined by standard disk diffusion method. Results were compared to CLSI guidelines to categorize organisms either as susceptible or resistant. Cefoxitin was used as an indicator of methicillin susceptibility disks and an inhibition zone diameter of ≤14 mm was reported as methicillin resistant. According to our results, *S. aureus* was resistant to cefoxitin (FOX) that is why we marked it as Methicillin Resistant *S. aureus* (**Figure 1**). It was also resistant to whole range of tested cephalosporins (**Table 1**). Likewise, *K. pneumoniae* was also resistant to all cephalosporins and augmentin as well, but was susceptible to Imipenem (IPM), Colistin (CT) and Minocycline (MH). *E. coli* was found to be ESBL positive as the inhibition zone expansion was observed with Augmentin (**Figure 1C**). In case of *P. aeruginosa,* it was susceptible to Colistin (CT) only otherwise it was observed to be highly resistant to all other tested antibiotics. So all the clinical pathogens were found to be highly resistant to the available therapeutic options. However, *L. monocytogenes* (ATCC 13932) was susceptible to all tested antibiotic disks except vancomycin.

Characterization of Nano-Particles

Ultramicroscopic characterization of nanoparticles was done to gather a firsthand information on particles morphology, size and distribution. AFM was performed to get surface topography and size distribution images of nano-formulations. 3D AFM images of both nano-systems revealed that both nano-formulations were homogeneously dispersed and a maximum height of 50 nm was observed for empty CSNPs and 51 nm for cefotaxime loaded CSNPs (**Figure 2**). Both empty and loaded nano-formulations were found to be quite uniform. However, cefotaxime loaded CSNPs were displaying more dense population. SEM results revealed that empty and cefotaxime loaded NPs were in the size range of less than 100 nm. Both AFM and SEM analysis demonstrated that there was more concentrated and more dense population of drug loaded NPs as compare to blank NPs (**Figure 3**).

FTIR Spectra

Fourier Transform Infrared Spectroscopy analysis of chitosan raw material, cefotaxime powder empty CSNPs and drug loaded CSNPs are shown in **Figure 4**. FTIR spectra of CS raw material revealed major peaks at 3401, 2878, 1651, 1380, 1080, and at 607 cm^{-1} that corresponded to O-H stretching peak, C-H stretching, N-H stretch, CH_2 bending, C-O-C stretch and $-C \equiv C-H$, respectively (**Figure 4A**).

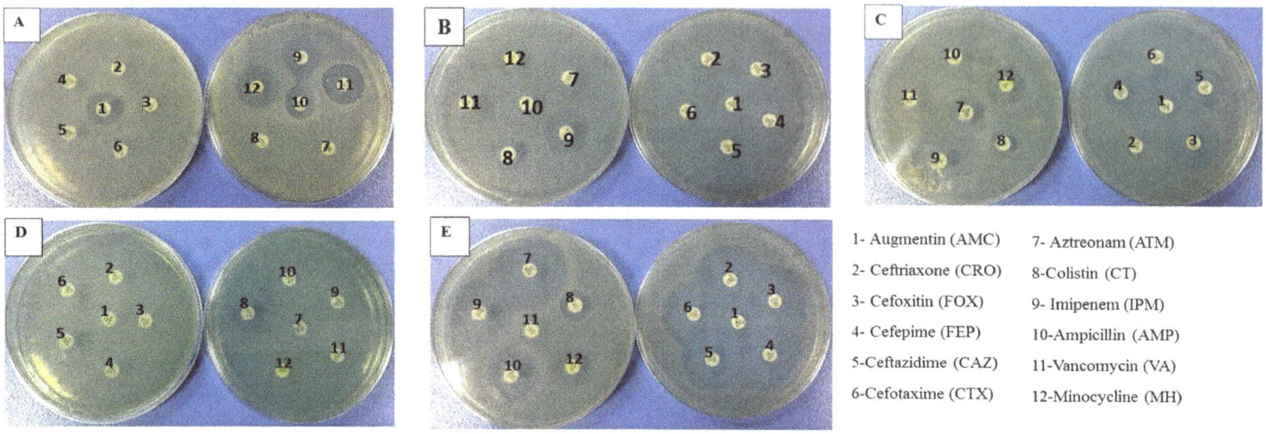

FIGURE 1 | Zones of Inhibitions formed on nutrient agar surface by different antibiotic disks against (A) Methicillin-resistant *Staphylococcus aureus* (MRSA), (B) *Klebsiella pneumoniae* (C) *Escherichia coli* displaying extended spectrum beta lactamases (ESBL) phenomenon exhibited by extension in zone of inhibition formed between augmentin and cephalosporins (D) *Pseudomonas aeruginosa* and (E) *Listeria monocytogenes,* after incubation at 37°C after 24 h.

In case of CSNPs more broad, strong and characteristic peak for CS was observed at 3406 cm^{-1} representing 0-H stretching or H-bonding for alcohol or phenols instead of 3401 cm^{-1} (for CS) indicating that H bonding is enhanced during NPs formation while the amide peak shifted from 1651 to 1644 cm^{-1}. A new sorption bands at 2089 cm^{-1} appear, which shows that the ammonium groups are crosslinked with tripolyphosphate molecules.

Analysis of FTIR spectra of CSNPs showed that it was very similar to that of cefotaxime loaded CSNPs (**Figures 4C,D**). This fact was predictable because the amount of drug loaded in nano-scaffold was very small as compare to the amount of building blocks of nano-structures, that is why no peaks of cefotaxime was observed in the drug loaded nanoparticles.

Determination of Zeta Potential

According to our results, both the blank CSNPs and drug loaded CSNPs had demonstrated a zeta potential of more than +50 mV (**Figures 5A,B**). This can be predicted from the data that β-lactam loaded nano-sytems are offering long term stability.

Determination of Encapsulation Efficiency

Encapsulation efficiency was determined at different drug concentrations. It was observed that EE augmented with increase in concentration of drug. It was calculated to be 60% at 100 μg/mL; 71% at 800 μg/mL and 90% at 2000 μg/mL concentration.

Antimicrobial Potential of the Prepared Nano-antibiotics

Drug loaded CSNPs were prepared with 1000 μg/mL of drug concentration and tested against above-mentioned pathogens by broth dilution assay (**Figure 6**). It was compared to both plain antibiotic solution and bare CSNPs for 7 days (144 h). It was observed that nano-cefotaxime was highly effective against all MDR pathogens while the simple antibiotic could not control them at all. However, when we compare efficiency of drug loaded CSNPs to bare CSNPs, the difference seems to be low. In case of *P. aeruginosa* the activity was equal. However, for other pathogens bare nano-systems were effective till first 48 h.

TABLE 1 | Zones of Inhibition formed by clinical isolates against different tested antibiotic disks.

Pathogens	AMC	CRO	FOX	FEP	CAZ	CTX	ATM	CT	IPM	AMP	VA	MH
	Zones of inhibition (mm)											
MRSA	18	–	–	–	–	–	–	–	17	15	20	20
Klebsiella pneumoniae	–	–	–	–	–	–	–	15	23	–	–	15
Escherichia coli	–	–	24*	16*	19*	–	15	14	28	–	–	18
Pseudomonas aeruginosa	–	–	–	–	–	–	–	16	12	–	–	–
Listeria monocytogenes (ATCC 13932)	30	29	26	29	29	30	33	15	30	25	–	16

Where Augmentin (AMC), Ceftriaxone (CRO), Cefoxitin (FOX) Cefepime (FEP), Ceftazidime (CAZ), Cefotaxime (CTX), Aztreonam (ATM), Colistin (CT), Imipenem (IPM), Ampicillin (AMP), Vancomycin (VA), and Minocycline (MH). ESBL phenomenon exhibited by increase in zone of inhibition. Whereas (–) means 'no zone of inhibition.
**indicates ESBL phenomenon marked by increase in zone of inhibition caused by AMC and cephalosporin discs.*

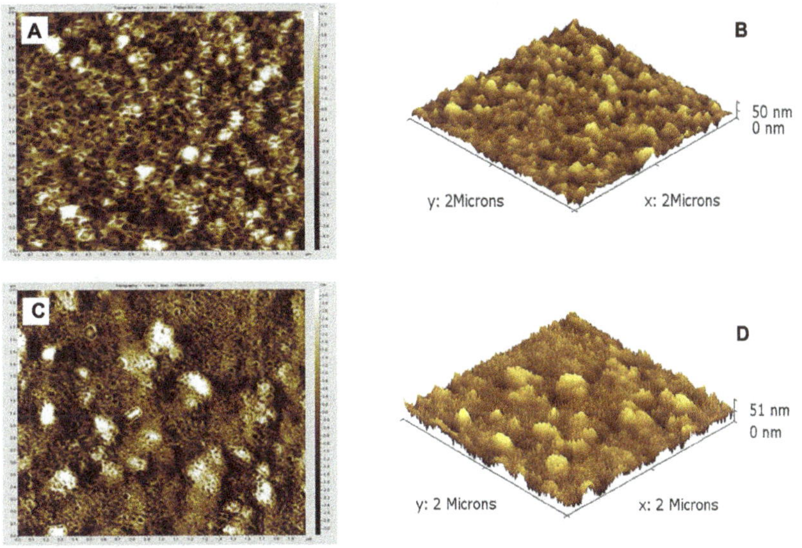

FIGURE 2 | Atomic force microscopic images of surface topography and 3-Dimensional (3D) structures of empty CSNPs (A,B) and cefotaxime loaded CSNPs (C,D) respectively. A small drop of sample was dried on glass slide and all images were taken at room temperature without any sample treatment. Results obtained depict height of 50 and 51 nm.

Nonetheless, the drug loaded CSNPs were proved to be more effective in contending the other four pathogens including ATCC *L. monocytogenes* for more prolonged period of time. At the end of experiment CFU count was done to confirm the hypothesis (**Figure 7**). It also endorse the above statement as no colonies were observed in case of *P. aeruginosa,* however, in other pathogens growth was observed only in case of CSNPs.

Anti-Biofilm Activity of the Fabricated Nano-antibiotics

It was observed from the present study that the formation and intensity of biofilm increase with the intensity of pathogenicity and resistance spectrum of pathogens. The most resistant Gram-negative pathogens were *K. pneumoniae* and *P. aeruginosa* and they formed more intense biofilms. Whereas, *L. monocytogenes* (ATCC) was most susceptible to antibiotic disks and was the weakest in term of biofilm intensity. Antibiotic alone fails to eradicate the biofilm, however, nano-cefotaxime was found to be highly effective in controlling the formation of biofilms (**Figure 8**). CSNPs were also found to be efficient in controlling the biofilms but the drug loaded CSNPs were more effective in every case. It may be concluded that bare CSNPs can effectively kill the planktonic cells, however, cannot efficiently control biofilm formation. Whereas drug loaded CSNPs were more

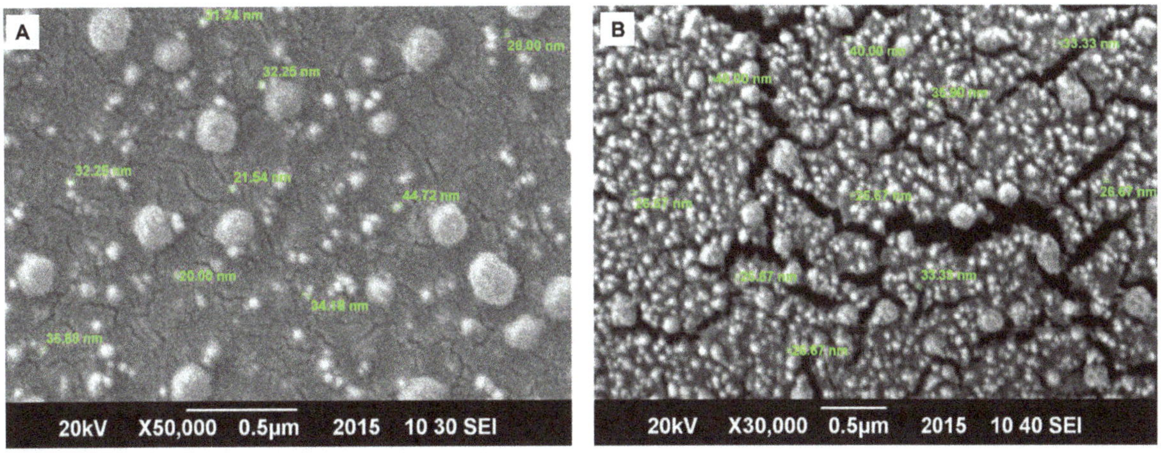

FIGURE 3 | Scanning electron microscopy (SEM) of bare (A) and drug loaded CSNPs (B). SEM images were taken by placing a tiny droplet of sample on I × I cm glass slide and it was spreaded evenly. After gold sputtering, images were taken at ambient conditions. SEM images depicted spherical particles having diameter of less than 100 nm.

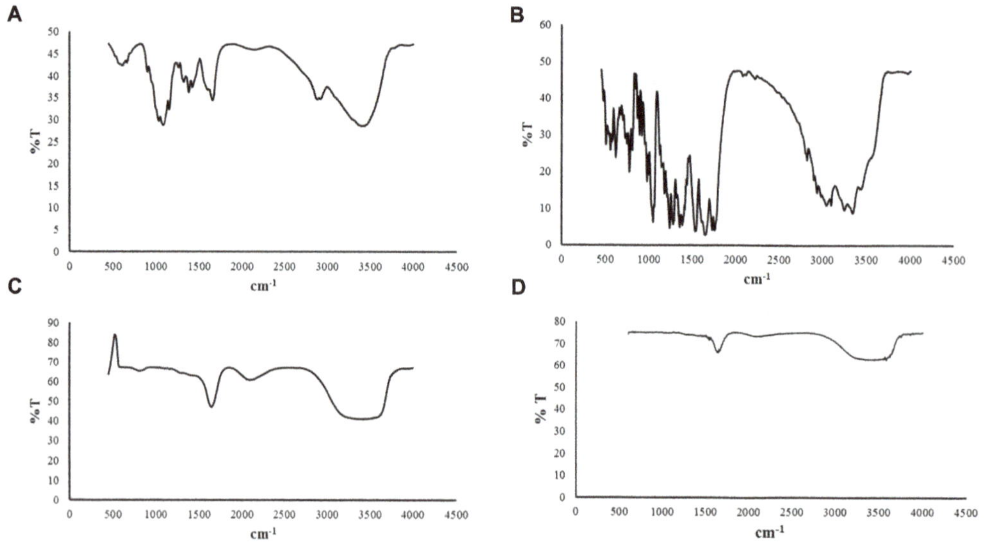

FIGURE 4 | Fourier Transform Infrared Spectroscopy spectra (A) Chitosan raw material (B) Cefotaxime raw material (C) bare CSNPs (D) cefotaxime loaded CSNPs. FTIR spectrum of powders were taken after mixing raw material with KBr. Whereas liquid samples were analyzed directly by palcing a tiny drop over glass assembly. FTIR spectra indicated no new bond formation so the drug is not reacting chemically with nano-scaffolds.

effective as a therapeutic agent to prevent the formation of biofilm and also in terms of killing pathogens for prolonged period of time.

DISCUSSION

Biofilms are defined as microbial communities of cells that are irreversibly attached to a substratum or to an interface or to each other, and are embedded into a matrix of EPSs that they have produced. There are as many different types of biofilms as are bacteria, and that a single bacterium may even make several different types of biofilms under different environmental conditions (Karatan and Watnick, 2009). These biofilms are offering inherent barrier to the penetration of conventional antibiotics. Though anti-biofilm potential of plant extracts was reported by many others (Perumal and Mahmud, 2013), yet this study has been designed to sort out the potential of antibiotic loaded chitosan NPs as an antibacterial and anti-biofilm agents. Cefotaxime has been used for this purpose. Albeit, numerous methods are available for qualitative and quantitative assays of antibiotics, nevertheless the UV-Vis Spectrophotometric method has proved to be simple, effective, fast, economical and reproducible for quantification of cefotaxime sodium in pharmaceutical form powder for injectable solution. Resultantly, λ_{max} was obtained at 298 nm. Similar method was also employed by other authors though different λ_{max} values were achieved by them. According to Bushra et al. (2014) λ_{max} value for cefotaxime was obtained at 260 nm, at 228 nm (El-Shaboury et al., 2007), and 253 nm (Hammood et al., 2011). NPs were formulated by ionic gelation method that has proved to be most efficient

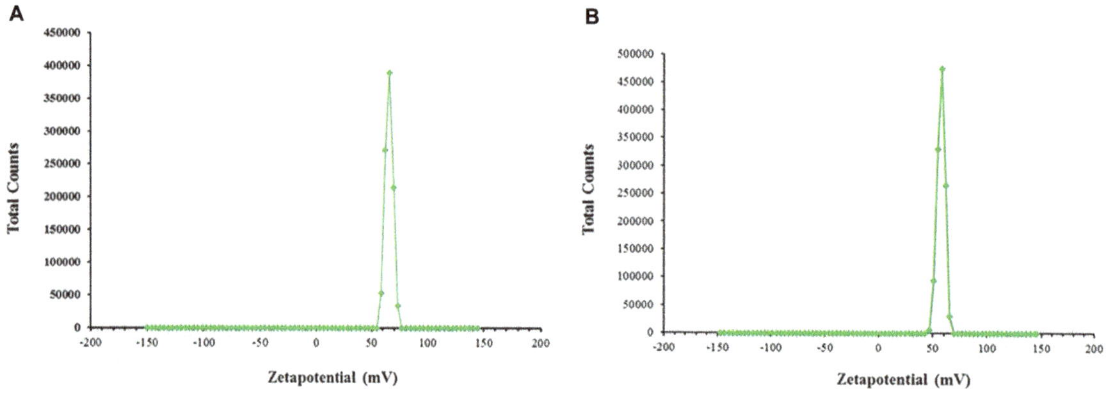

FIGURE 5 | Zeta potential. Measured by Malvern Zeta sizer at ambient conditions **(A)** empty CSNPs **(B)** β-lactam drug loaded CSNPs. Both empty and drug loaded CSNPs are displaying zeta potential values greater than 50 mV. It indicates highly stable colloidal dispersion.

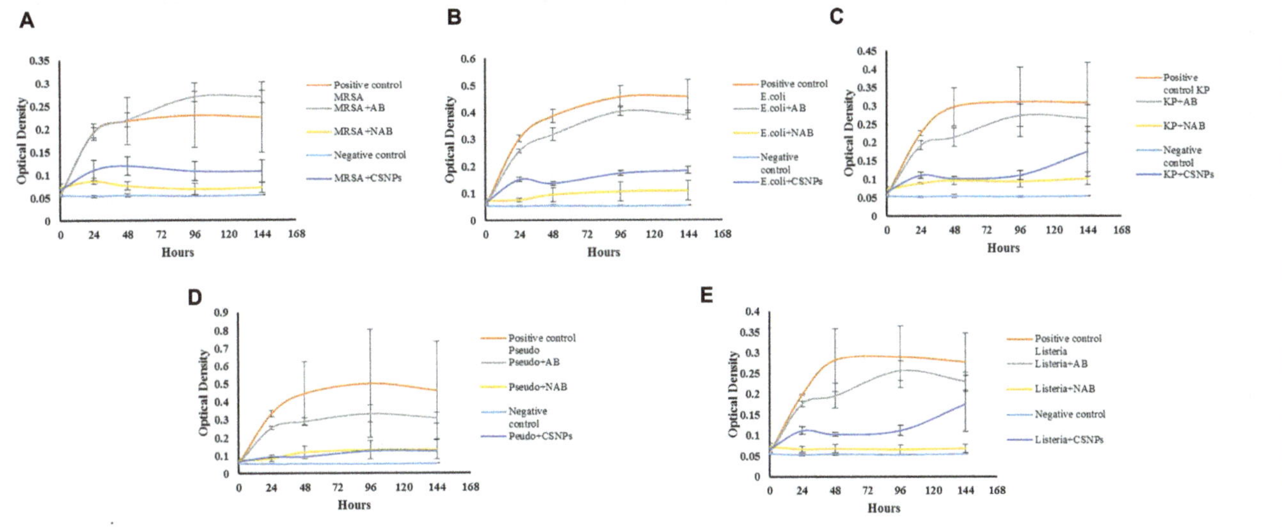

FIGURE 6 | Comparative Anti-pathogenic ability of Aqueous solution of Antibiotic and Antibiotic loaded CSNPs against pathogens (A) Methicillin-resistant *Staphylococcus aureus* (MRSA), (B) *Escherichia coli* (*E. coli*) (C), *Klebsiella pneumoniae* (KP), (D) *Pseudomonas aeruginosa* (Pseudo) and (E) *Listeria monocytogenes* (Listeria). Pathogens were exposed to Antibiotic solution (AB), blank chitosan nano-particles (CSNPs), and antibiotic loaded CSNPs (NAB). All samples were incubated at 37°C for 144 h and after every 24 h reading were taken on ELISA plate reader at 595 nm. Negative control contains only the media and no inoculum where as positive control contain inoculated media.

and convenient method. Engineered and naturally forming NPs can vary widely in their physicochemical characteristics such as shape, size, and charge. These characteristics have been reported to impact their interactions with biofilm-coated surfaces (Ikuma et al., 2015). Microscopic attributes were studied via AFM and SEM wherein the results displayed much smaller size of NPs as compared to previous studies. Previous studies have reported the size of CSNPs in the range of 140–250 nm (Gan et al., 2005; Nesalin and Smith, 2013; Chaubey and Mishra, 2014; Miladi et al., 2015) while in this research size less than 100 nm was achieved.

Fourier Transform Infrared Spectroscopy spectroscopic studies were carried out in order to confirm the formation of NPs and type of interactions between antibiotic and polymer. FTIR has proved to be a powerful and useful characterization

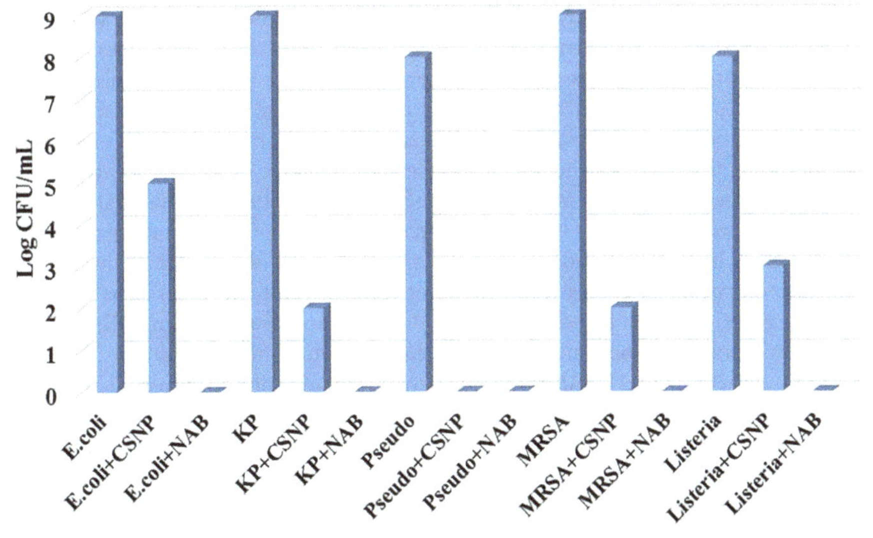

FIGURE 7 | Colony forming unit (CFU) assay. CFU assay was performed to count the viable bacteria after reaction of CSNPs and drug loaded CSNPs with pathogens. CFU was done by plating 10μL of sample from each test tube after serial dilutions in normal saline (0.9% NaCl). All plates were then incubated for 48 h and colonies were counted manually. CSNP, Chitosan nano-particles, NAB, Nano-antibiotic; KP, *Klebsiella pneumoniae*; *Pseudo*, *Pseudomonas aeruginosa* and MRSA for Methicillin-resistant *S. aureus*.

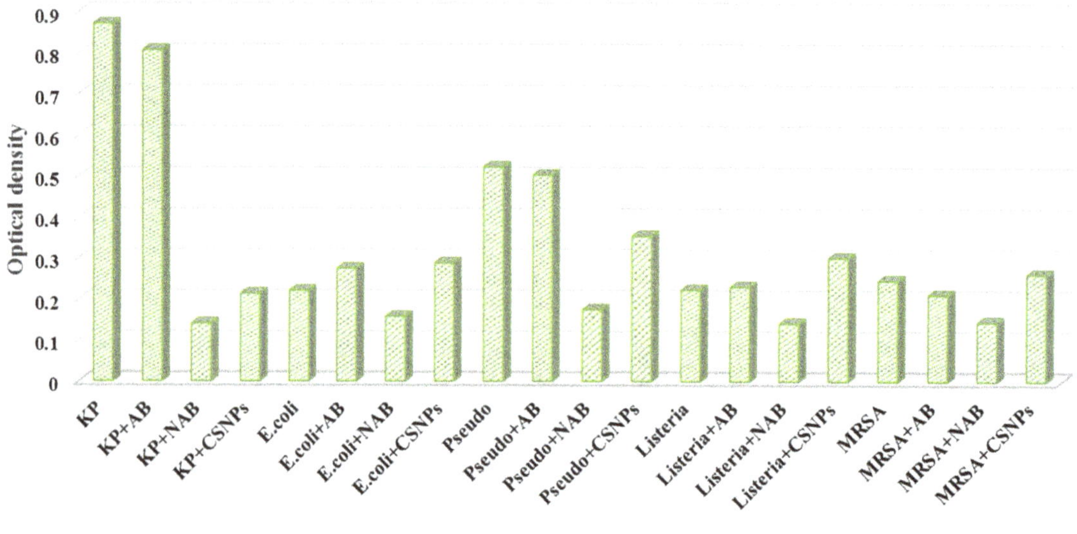

FIGURE 8 | Anti-biofilm activity of antibiotic suspension (AB) Chitosan nano-particles (CSNPs) and Cefotaxime loaded CSNPs (NAB) against pathogens. Methicillin-resistant *S. aureus* (MRSA), *Klebsiella pneumoniae* (KP), *Escherichia coli (E. coli), Pseudomonas aeruginosa (Pseudo),* and *Listeria monocytogenes (Listeria)* were incubated on ELISA plates at 37°C for 24 h. Biofilms were stained by crystal violet stain and removed by 30% acetic acid solution. This solution was then measured on ELISA plate reader at 595 nm.

method for polymers, and materials in general. This is quite an economical, short time characterization that allows to establish the chemical composition, microstructure, chemical interactions and follow variation of specific functional groups with the passage of time during reactions (Barrios et al., 2012).

Fourier Transform Infrared Spectroscopy spectrum of chitosan showed resemblance with an already reported spectra for this biopolymer (Khan et al., 2002; Qi et al., 2004; Vitali et al., 2006). Spectrum of cefotaxime raw material was also in accordance with previously reported spectrum for this cephalosporin drug (Hammood et al., 2011). Likewise, FTIR spectrum of empty CSNPs was similar to already reported spectra, however, it was quite different from the spectrum of bulk material that indicated the formation of NPs (Hosseini et al., 2013; de Pinho Neves et al., 2014; Antoniou et al., 2015). The spectrum for drug loaded NPs was almost superimposable to that of empty nano-formlation indicating that there was no chemical bonding between the drug and polymers (**Figures 4C** and **3B**).

Zeta potential is an indicator of long term stability of colloidal dispersions. Nanoparticles with a zeta potential between −10 and +10 mV are considered approximately neutral, while nanoparticles with zeta potentials of greater than +30 mV or less than −30 mV are considered strongly cationic and strongly anionic, respectively (Clogston and Patri, 2011) and represent a stable formulation as there would be less aggregation and flocculation as the repulsive forces become more strong (Gazori et al., 2009). According to results, both the blank CSNPs and drug loaded CSNPs were displaying highly positive zeta potential of more than +50 mV (**Figures 5A,B**). This can be predicted from the data that β-lactam loaded nano-systems are offering long term stability. Positive zeta potential in the range of 21–45 was already reported by many authors (De Campos et al., 2001; Miladi et al., 2015; Zhang et al., 2016).

Encapsulation efficiency was determined at various concentrations of cefotaxime to check the influence of drug concentration on EE. It was observed that EE augmented with increase in concentration of drug. However, the findings indicated that if the drug was dissolved in CS solution and TPP was added afterward it had resulted in very low EE (<3%). Honary et al. (2014) encapsulated vancomycin in CSNPs and reported 60–69% EE (Honary et al., 2014) while 42–55% after encapsulation of 5-Fluorouracil. The well -characterized CSNPs were further investigated for their antipathogenic and anti-biofilm potential.

Bacterial biofilms were first described in 1943. Biofilm formation is an intricate process and colloquially the biofilms are also referred to as microbial cities. Preliminary step to this phenomenon is the attachment to any solid surface termed as 'adsorption.' These biofilms are sheltered by a self-secretory matrix called EPS. This EPS hold the cells organized and safeguard them against extraneous agents because of its composition. Biofilms also aid in quorum sensing thus facilitating microbes to communicate with each other. The composition of EPS is protein, polysaccharides and extracellular DNA. Biofilms can ensure maximum intake of nutrients from outside environment. The organization of microbes in these biofilms is such that ancient and dead cell recline in the center where the metabolites get accumulated while the fresh and new cells lie near the outer surface where the flow of materials is maximum. These biofilms are offering an innate resistance mechanism to conventional antibiotics, however, NAMs can encounter biofilms successfully.

The interactions between NPs and the biofilm can be viewed as a three-step process: (1) transport of NPs to the vicinity of the biofilm; (2) attachment to the biofilm surface; and (3) migration within the biofilms (Ikuma et al., 2015).

It has been observed from the present study that the nano-cefotaxime was highly effective in controlling the formation of biofilms (**Figure 8**). Though anti-biofilm potential of plant extracts has been reported by many others (Perumal and Mahmud, 2013), however, this is the first report to prove the anti-biofilm activity of cefotaxime loaded CSNPs. It has been mentioned earlier that more than 70% pathogenic microbes are biofilm forming and that is the main mechanism of resistance in pathogens. Blank CSNPs also exhibited good potential in lowering the biofilm formation intensity but fails to eradicate it completely. Therefore it can be concluded that chitosan NPs causes the clumping of bacterial mass and help to slow the growth of pathogens, however, cannot control the biofilm formation efficiently. Less intensity of biofilm is the direct result of less number of pathogens in culture media. The drug loaded CSNPs totally eradicated the pathogens and therefore biofilm formation.

CONCLUSION

Foregoing in view, it can be positively concluded that the main mechanism of action by which NAMs control MDR pathogens is inhibition of biofilm formation. The results in this research have confirmed that chitosan can be a potential carrier system for cefotaxime to target Gram-negative and Gram-positive multi drug resistant microorganisms that have the tendency to form microbial biofilms. The prepared NPs have been perceived to be stable as carrying positive zeta of more than +50 mV and were displaying homogeneity in both size and shape.

AUTHOR CONTRIBUTIONS

BJ designed, developed, and performed all the experimental work, analysed and interpreted the data and wrote the manuscript. HH performed and helped in analyzing the Atomic Force Microscopy (AFM) Assays. SA helped in collection of clinical isolates and their characterization. AI provided technical assistance for Zeta sizer analysis. HN done the FTIR analysis and its interpretation. MI supervised the work at each step, provided the budget and scientific assistance for the manuscript write-up.

REFERENCES

Allaker, R. P., and Memarzadeh, K. (2014). Nanoparticles and the control of oral infections. *Int. J. Antimicrob. Agents* 43, 95–104. doi: 10.1016/j.ijantimicag.2013.11.002

Antoniou, J., Liu, F., Majeed, H., Qi, J., Yokoyama, W., and Zhong, F. (2015). Physicochemical and morphological properties of size-controlled chitosan–tripolyphosphate nanoparticles. *Colloids Surf. A Physicochem. Eng. Asp.* 465, 137–146. doi: 10.1016/j.colsurfa.2014.10.040

Barrios, V. A. E., Espinosa, G. A., Rodríguez, J. L. D., Méndez, J. R. R., and Aguilar, N. V. P. (2012). *FTIR-An Essential Characterization Technique for Polymeric Materials.* Rijeka: InTech Open Access Publisher.

Bushra, M. U., Akter, N., Hassan, M. R., Islam, A., and Hossain, M. R. (2014). Development and validation of a simple UV spectrophotometric method for the determination of cefotaxime sodium in bulk and pharmaceutical formulation. *IOSR J. Pharm.* 4, 74–77.

Carlet, J., Jarlier, V., Harbarth, S., Voss, A., Goossens, H., and Pittet, D. (2012). Ready for a world without antibiotics? The pensières antibiotic resistance call to action. *Antimicrob. Resist. Infect. Control* 1, 1–13.

Chaubey, P., and Mishra, B. (2014). Mannose-conjugated chitosan nanoparticles loaded with rifampicin for the treatment of visceral leishmaniasis. *Carbohydr. Polym.* 101, 1101–1108. doi: 10.1016/j.carbpol.2013.10.044

Clogston, J. D., and Patri, A. K. (2011). "Zeta potential measurement," in *Characterization of Nanoparticles Intended for Drug Delivery*, ed. S. E. McNeil (New York, NY: Humana Press), 63–70.

De Campos, A. M., Sánchez, A., and Alonso, M. J. (2001). Chitosan nanoparticles: a new vehicle for the improvement of the delivery of drugs to the ocular surface. Application to cyclosporin A. *Int. J. Pharm.* 224, 159–168. doi: 10.1016/S0378-5173(01)00760-8

de Pinho Neves, A. L., Milioli, C. C., Müller, L., Riella, H. G., Kuhnen, N. C., and Stulzer, H. K. (2014). Factorial design as tool in chitosan nanoparticles development by ionic gelation technique. *Colloids Surf. A Physicochem. Eng. Asp.* 445, 34–39. doi: 10.1016/j.colsurfa.2013.12.058

Delcour, A. H. (2009). Outer membrane permeability and antibiotic resistance. *Biochim. Biophys. Acta* 1794, 808–816. doi: 10.1016/j.bbapap.2008.11.005

Dheilly, A., Soum-Soutéra, E., Klein, G. L., Bazire, A., Compère, C., Haras, D., et al. (2010). Antibiofilm activity of the marine bacterium *Pseudoalteromonas* sp. strain 3J6. *Appl. Environ. Microbiol.* 76, 3452–3461. doi: 10.1128/AEM.02632-09

Donlan, R. M. (2002). Biofilms: microbial life on surfaces. *Emerg. Infect. Dis.* 8, 881–890. doi: 10.3201/eid0809.020063

Du, W. L., Niu, S. S., Xu, Y. L., Xu, Z. R., and Fan, C. L. (2009). Antibacterial activity of chitosan tripolyphosphate nanoparticles loaded with various metal ions. *Carbohydr. Polym.* 75, 385–389. doi: 10.1016/j.carbpol.2008.07.039

El-Shaboury, S. R., Saleh, G. A., Mohamed, F. A., and Rageh, A. H. (2007). Analysis of cephalosporin antibiotics. *J. Pharm. Biomed. Anal.* 45, 1–19. doi: 10.1016/j.jpba.2007.06.002

Fabbretti, A., Gualerzi, C. O., and Brandi, L. (2011). How to cope with the quest for new antibiotics. *FEBS Lett.* 585, 1673–1681. doi: 10.1016/j.febslet.2011.04.029

Gan, Q., Wang, T., Cochrane, C., and McCarron, P. (2005). Modulation of surface charge, particle size and morphological properties of chitosan–TPP nanoparticles intended for gene delivery. *Colloids Surf. B Biointerfaces* 44, 65–73. doi: 10.1016/j.colsurfb.2005.06.001

Gazori, T., Khoshayand, M. R., Azizi, E., Yazdizade, P., Nomani, A., and Haririan, I. (2009). Evaluation of Alginate/Chitosan nanoparticles as antisense delivery vector: formulation, optimization and in vitro characterization. *Carbohydr. Polym.* 77, 599–606. doi: 10.1016/j.carbpol.2009.02.019

George, A. (2011). Microtiter dish biofilm formation assay. *J. Vis. Exp.* 47, 2437. doi: 10.3791/2437

Hajipour, M. J., Fromm, K. M., Ashkarran, A. A., Jimenez de Aberasturi, D., de Larramendi, I. R., Rojo, T., et al. (2012). Antibacterial properties of nanoparticles. *Trends Biotechnol.* 30, 499–511. doi: 10.1016/j.tibtech.2012.06.004

Hammood, M. K., Qasim, A. W., and Jasim, F. (2011). An indirect atomic absorption spectrophotometric determination of cefotaxime in pharmaceutical formulations by using rhodium (II) as a mediating metal. *Nat. J. Chem.* 41, 27–37.

Hetrick, E. M., Shin, J. H., Paul, H. S., and Schoenfisch, M. H. (2009). Anti-biofilm efficacy of nitric oxide-releasing silica nanoparticles. *Biomaterials* 30, 2782–2789. doi: 10.1016/j.biomaterials.2009.01.052

Honary, S., Ebrahimi, P., and Hadianamrei, R. (2014). Optimization of particle size and encapsulation efficiency of vancomycin nanoparticles by response surface methodology. *Pharm. Dev. Technol.* 19, 987–998. doi: 10.3109/10837450.2013.846375

Hosseini, S. F., Zandi, M., Rezaei, M., and Farahmandghavi, F. (2013). Two-step method for encapsulation of oregano essential oil in chitosan nanoparticles: preparation, characterization and in vitro release study. *Carbohydr. Polym.* 95, 50–56. doi: 10.1016/j.carbpol.2013.02.031

Ikuma, K., Decho, A. W., and Lau, B. L. (2015). When nanoparticles meet biofilms-Interactions guiding the environmental fate and accumulation of nanoparticles. *Front. Microbiol.* 6:591. doi: 10.3389/fmicb.2015.00591

Jamil, B., Bokhari, H., and Imran, M. (2015). Mechanism of action: how nano-antimicrobials act? *Curr. Drug Targets* doi: 10.2174/138945 0116666151019101826 [Epub ahead of print].

Jamil, B., Habib, H., Abbasi, S., Nasir, H., Rahman, A., Rehman, A., et al. (2016). Cefazolin loaded chitosan nanoparticles to cure multi drug resistant Gram-negative pathogens. *Carbohydr. Polym.* 136, 682–691. doi: 10.1016/j.carbpol.2015.09.078

Karatan, E., and Watnick, P. (2009). Signals, regulatory networks, and materials that build and break bacterial biofilms. *Microbiol. Mol. Biol. Rev.* 73, 310–347. doi: 10.1128/MMBR.00041-08

Khan, T. A., Peh, K. K., and Chang, H. S. (2002). Reporting degree of deacetylation values of chitosan: the influence of analytical methods. *J. Pharm. Pharm. Sci.* 5, 205–212.

Kirker, K. R., Fisher, S. T., and James, G. A. (2015). Potency and penetration of telavancin in staphylococcal biofilms. *Int. J. Antimicrob. Agents* 46, 451–455. doi: 10.1016/j.ijantimicag.2015.05.022

Lewis, K. (2005). Persister cells and the riddle of biofilm survival. *Biochemistry (Mosc.)* 70, 267–274. doi: 10.1007/s10541-005-0111-6

Madsen, J. S., Burmølle, M., Hansen, L. H., and Sørensen, S. J. (2012). The interconnection between biofilm formation and horizontal gene transfer. *FEMS Immunol. Med. Microbiol.* 65, 183–195. doi: 10.1111/j.1574-695X.2012.00960.x

Miladi, K., Sfar, S., Fessi, H., and Elaissari, A. (2015). Enhancement of alendronate encapsulation in chitosan nanoparticles. *J. Drug Deliv. Sci. Technol.* 30, 391–396. doi: 10.1016/j.jddst.2015.04.007

Nesalin, J. A. J., and Smith, A. A. (2013). Preparation and evaluation of stavudine loaded chitosan nanoparticles. *J. Pharm. Res.* 6, 268–274. doi: 10.1016/j.jopr.2013.02.004

Patil, P., Chavanke, D., and Wagh, M. A. (2012). Review on ionotropic gelation method: novel approach for controlled gastroretentive gelispheres. *Int. J. Pharm. Pharm. Sci.* 4, 27–32.

Pelgrift, R. Y., and Friedman, A. J. (2013). Nanotechnology as a therapeutic tool to combat microbial resistance. *Adv. Drug Deliv. Rev.* 65, 1803–1815. doi: 10.1016/j.addr.2013.07.011

Perumal, S., and Mahmud, R. (2013). Chemical analysis, inhibition of biofilm formation and biofilm eradication potential of *Euphorbia hirta* L. against clinical isolates and standard strains. *BMC Complement. Altern. Med.* 13:346. doi: 10.1186/1472-6882-13-346

Qi, L., Xu, Z., Jiang, X., Hu, C., and Zou, X. (2004). Preparation and antibacterial activity of chitosan nanoparticles. *Carbohyd. Res.* 339, 2693–2700. doi: 10.1016/j.carres.2004.09.007

Rotar, O. V., Tenedja, K., Arkhelyuk, A. D., Rotar, V. I., Davidencko, I. S., and Fediv, V. I. (2014). Preparation of chitosan nanoparticles loaded with glutathione for diminishing tissue ischemia-reperfusion injury. *Int. J. Adv. Eng. Nano Technol.* 1, 19–23.

Salta, M., Wharton, J. A., Dennington, S. P., Stoodley, P., and Stokes, K. R. (2013). Anti-biofilm performance of three natural products against initial bacterial attachment. *Int. J. Mol. Sci.* 14, 21757–21780. doi: 10.3390/ijms1411 21757

Sayem, S. M., Manzo, E., Ciavatta, L., Tramice, A., Cordone, A., Zanfardino, A., et al. (2011). Anti-biofilm activity of an exopolysaccharide from a sponge-associated strain of *Bacillus licheniformis*. *Microb. Cell Fact.* 10, 74. doi: 10.1186/1475-2859-10-74

Smith, A. W. (2005). Biofilms and antibiotic therapy: is there a role for combating bacterial resistance by the use of novel drug delivery systems? *Adv. Drug Deliv. Rev.* 57, 1539–1550. doi: 10.1016/j.addr.2005.04.007

Stewart, P. S. (2002). Mechanisms of antibiotic resistance in bacterial biofilms. *Int. J. Med. Microbiol.* 292, 107–113. doi: 10.1078/1438-4221-00196

Suresh, A. K. (2015). "Analytical and physical characterization techniques employed to assess microbial toxicity of nanoparticles," in *Co-Relating Metallic Nanoparticle Characteristics and Bacterial Toxicity*, ed. A. K. Suresh (New York, NY: Springer International Publishing), 15–26.

Vitali, L., Justi, K. C., Laranjeira, M., and Fávere, V. T. (2006). Impregnation of chelating agent 3, 3-bis-N, N bis-(carboxymethyl) aminomethyl-o-cresolsulfonephthalein in biopolymer chitosan: adsorption equilibrium of Cu (II) in aqueous medium. *Polímeros* 16, 16–122. doi: 10.1590/S0104-14282006000200011

Watnick, P., and Kolter, R. (2000). Biofilm, city of microbes. *J. Bacteriol.* 182, 2675–2679. doi: 10.1128/JB.182.10.2675-2679.2000

Zhang, H., Jung, J., and Zhao, Y. (2016). Preparation, characterization and evaluation of antibacterial activity of catechins and catechins-Zn complex loaded β-chitosan nanoparticles of different particle sizes. *Carbohydr. Polym.* 137, 82–91. doi: 10.1016/j.carbpol.2015.10.036

18

Serotypes and Antimicrobial Susceptibility of *Salmonella* spp. Isolated from Farm Animals in China

Xiuhua Kuang[1,2], *Haihong Hao*[1,2,3*], *Menghong Dai*[2,3], *Yulian Wang*[2,3], *Ijaz Ahmad*[3], *Zhenli Liu*[1,3] *and Zonghui Yuan*[1,2,3*]

[1] *MOA Laboratory for Risk Assessment of Quality and Safety of Livestock and Poultry Products, Huazhong Agricultural University, Wuhan, China,* [2] *Hubei Collaborative Innovation Center for Animal Nutrition and Feed Safety, Huazhong Agricultural University, Wuhan, China,* [3] *National Reference Laboratory of Veterinary Drug Residues and MOA Key Laboratory for Detection of Veterinary Drug Residues, Huazhong Agricultural University, Wuhan, China*

Correspondence:
Haihong Hao,
National Reference Laboratory of Veterinary Drug Residues and MOA Laboratory for Risk Assessment of Quality and Safety of Livestock and Poultry Products, Huazhong Agricultural University, No. 1, Shizhishan Street, Hongshan District, 430070 Wuhan, China
haohaihong@mail.hzau.edu.cn;
Zonghui Yuan,
National Reference Laboratory of Veterinary Drug Residues and MOA Key Laboratory for Detection of Veterinary Drug Residues, Huazhong Agricultural University, No. 1, Shizhishan Street, Hongshan District, 430070 Wuhan, China
yuan5802@mail.hzau.edu.cn

Salmonella spp. can indirectly infect humans via transfer from animals and animal-derived food products, and thereby cause potentially fatal diseases. Therefore, gaining an understanding of *Salmonella* infection in farm animals is increasingly important. The aim of this study was to identify the distribution of serotypes in *Salmonella* samples isolated from chickens ($n = 837$), pigs ($n = 930$), and dairy cows ($n = 418$) in central China (Henan, Hubei, and Hunan provinces) in 2010–2011, and investigate the susceptibility of strains to antimicrobial agents. *Salmonella* isolates were identified by PCR amplification of the *invA* gene, serotypes were determined by using a slide agglutination test for O and H antigens, and susceptibility to 24 antimicrobials was tested using the agar dilution method. In total, 248 *Salmonella* strains were identified: 105, 105, and 38 from chickens, dairy cows, and pigs, respectively. Additionally, 209 strains were identified in diseased pigs from the Huazhong Agricultural University veterinary hospital. Among these 457 strains, the dominant serotypes were Typhimurium in serogroup B, IIIb in serogroup C, and Enteritidis in serogroup D. In antimicrobial susceptibility tests, 41.14% of *Salmonella* spp. were susceptible to all antimicrobial agents, 48.14% were resistant to at least one, and 34.72% were resistant to more than three classes. Strains were highly resistant to sulfamethoxazole-trimethoprim (39.61%), nalidixic acid (39.17%), doxycycline (28.22%), and tetracycline (27.58%). Resistance to cephalosporins and fluoroquinolones ranged from 5.25 to 7.44% and 19.04 to 24.51%, respectively. Among penicillin-resistant and cephalosporin-resistant strains, 25 isolates produced extended-spectrum β-lactamases (ESBLs). The multidrug-resistant and ESBL-producing *Salmonella* strains identified in healthy animals here will present a challenge for veterinary medicine and farm animal husbandry, and could also pose a threat to public health. The level of antibiotic resistance observed in this study further highlights the need for careful and selective use of antibiotics.

Keywords: *Salmonella,* farm animals, serotype, antibiotics, antimicrobial resistance

Introduction

Salmonella spp. are a common source of foodborne diseases that cause morbidity and mortality worldwide (Chiu et al., 2010). Treating *Salmonella* infection in humans is expensive; for example, in the USA, it causes illness in ~1.2 million patients annually, resulting in estimated medical costs of $365 million (Centers for Disease Control and Prevention, 2014). In the European Union (EU), salmonellosis is the second most commonly reported gastrointestinal infection, with a confirmed case rate of 20.4 cases per 100,000 individuals in 2011 (European Centre for Disease Prevention and Control, 2013). In China, *Salmonella* causes an estimated 22.2% of foodborne diseases (Wang et al., 2007), and salmonellosis ranks fourth among the most prevalent foodborne diseases caused by microbial agents (Zhu et al., 2012). Many *Salmonella* serotypes exist, with >2600 serovars classified based on the reactivity of antisera to O and H antigens (Stevens et al., 2009), and ~292 identified in China between the 1980s and the end of 2000 (Yang, 2010). *Salmonella* also affects farm animals, and infections on farms can cause substantial economic damage in relation to, for example, loss of poultry stocks and costly animal husbandry. Numerous serotypes of isolated *Salmonella* have been found to overlap between farm animals and humans (Alcaine et al., 2006). Indeed, *Salmonella* not only directly infects humans but also causes indirect infections via transfer from animals and animal-derived food products such as pork and milk.

The use of antimicrobials is important for the control and treatment of *Salmonella*. However, since the early 1990s, antimicrobial- and multidrug-resistant *Salmonella* strains have emerged, leading to treatment failure. Researchers have reported a link between the use of antimicrobials in food animals and the emergence of antimicrobial resistance in pathogenic bacteria (Gong et al., 2013). Multidrug-resistant bacteria pose a severe threat to public health, particularly those that are resistant to β-lactams and fluoroquinolones (Lai et al., 2014). The increasing number of multidrug-resistant *Salmonella* strains is a global concern, with some countries and international organizations creating surveillance systems which include collaboration between human health, veterinary, and food-related sectors to monitor the spread of these and other foodborne bacteria. Examples include the Danish Integrated Antimicrobial Resistance Monitoring and Research Program, the European Food Safety Authority, the National Antimicrobial Resistance Monitoring System in the USA, and the Global Foodborne Infections Network run by the World Health Organization. These surveillance systems are also employed to monitor antimicrobial resistance, antimicrobial consumption in livestock, and serotype distribution, and data describing the current trend of increasing resistance to multiple drugs has been made available (European Centre for Disease Prevention and Control, 2013). In contrast, surveillance reports are unavailable in China; however, the National Monitoring Network for Bacteria of Animal Origin was launched as a surveillance system in 2008. Travel, migration, and the distribution of food between countries can also contribute to the spread of foodborne diseases and multidrug-resistant bacteria. Therefore, monitoring the distribution of *Salmonella* serotypes and levels of antibiotic resistance in animals and animal-food products is also important for maintaining safe travel and the commercial trade in food animals (Lai et al., 2014; Russell et al., 2014).

In central China, Henan, Hubei, and Hunan provinces are important residential and trade centers. These three areas are also the main producers of animal-derived foods in China; in 2012, their output of meat, eggs, and milk accounted for 19.14%, 19.45%, and 9.17% of total Chinese production, respectively (China Agriculture Statistical Report, 2012). Previous studies documented a phenotype for *Salmonella* serovars that was discovered in chickens and pigs, and in animal-derived foods, in China (Gong et al., 2013; Li et al., 2013; Lai et al., 2014; Wang et al., 2014). However, specific knowledge of the *Salmonella* serovars that exist in dairy cows and other farm animals in central China is currently lacking. Therefore, the aim of this study was to evaluate the prevalence of *Salmonella* in chickens, pigs, and dairy cows on farms in central China. Additionally, the diversity of *Salmonella* serovars on these farms was identified, and their susceptibility and resistance to antimicrobial agents was investigated. A diverse range of serotypes was observed in healthy and diseased farm animals, and several multidrug-resistant and extended-spectrum β-lactamase (ESBL)-producing *Salmonella* strains were identified.

Materials and Methods

Samples and *Salmonella* Isolation

Cloacal and anal swabs were collected from healthy animals on farms in Henan, Hubei, and Hunan provinces between March 2010 and July 2011. Each sampling site was visited only once. In total, 2185 samples were collected in a random manner from chickens ($n = 837$), pigs ($n = 930$), and dairy cows ($n = 418$). Farms were chosen based on their scale with the following requirements: for pigs, annual sales were >10,000 heads; for chickens, the breeding stock was >100,000 heads; and for dairy cows, the breeding stock was >1000 heads. The owners of each farm gave permission for swab samples to be to collected. The animals from which samples were extracted remained alive, did not undergo any surgery, and were not administered any drugs. Therefore, ethical approval was not required for the study because the sampling process did not harm the animals; however, their distress was considered and minimized at all times. All collected samples were stored at 4 °C and cultured at least 24 h before the isolation experiments were conducted.

The procedure for culture and isolation was based on standard laboratory protocol (WHO Global Foodborne Infections Network, 2010). Briefly, the samples were mixed with 5 mL of 0.85% saline solution for 30 min, and 1 mL of this mixture solution was added to buffered peptone water (BPW; Hopebiol, Qingdao, China) at a volume ratio of 1:10. The resultant mixture was incubated for 10 h at 37 °C for pre-enrichment. Approximately 500 μL of this BPW mixture was then added to 5 mL selenite cystine broth (Hopebiol, Qingdao, China) and incubated at 37 °C for 20 h. The broth was streaked onto CHROMagar *Salmonella* (CHROMagar, France) and incubated at 37 °C for 24–48 h. Potential *Salmonella* colonies were transferred into Luria–Bertani agar for purification and enrichment, and then incubated for 20 h at 37 °C to facilitate identification.

Additionally, 209 strains of *Salmonella* were isolated from samples collected from diseased pigs in the Huazhong Agricultural University veterinary hospital (HAUvh) between 2008 and 2010.

Salmonella Identification

Biochemical testing and the *invA* gene were used to confirm the identity of isolates with typical *Salmonella* phenotypes. Biochemical testing was performed using a biochemical tube (Hangzhou Microbe Reagent Co., Ltd., China), and the results were interpreted based on Bergey's Manual of Systematic Bacteriology (Garrity et al., 2004). The *invA* gene was amplified by polymerase chain reaction (PCR) (Malorny et al., 2003). Positive results were randomly selected for sequencing. The obtained sequences were compared with the same gene registered in GenBank by using BLAST.

Determination of *Salmonella* Serogroup and Serotype

The serogroup and serovars of the *Salmonella* isolates were determined by slide agglutination tests with O antigen and H antigen antiserums obtained from Lansheng, Lanzhou Institute of Biology, China. The results were interpreted according to the Kauffmann-White scheme (Grimont and Weill, 2007).

Antimicrobial Susceptibility Testing

The agar dilution method with Mueller-Hinton agar (Oxoid Ltd., England) was used to test the susceptibility of *Salmonella* to 24 antibiotics (**Table 1**). These antimicrobials were classified based on their importance to human medicine (Government of Canada, 2005). *Escherichia coli* ATCC 25922 was used as the control microorganism. The results of the tests for ampicillin (AMP), amoxicillin (AMX), amoxicillin-clavulanic acid (AMC), ceftriaxone (CRO), imipenem (IPM), aztreonam (ATM), gentamicin (GEN), amikacin (AMK), tetracycline (TET), doxycycline (DOX), ciprofloxacin (CIP), levofloxacin (LEV), nalidixic acid (NAL), sulfamethoxazole-trimethoprim (SXT), chloramphenicol (CHL), and fosfomycin (FOS) were interpreted based on CLSI M100-S22 (Clinical and Laboratory Standards Institute, 2012), whereas those for ceftiofur (CEF), enrofloxacin (ENO), and florfenicol (FFC) were interpreted based on CLSI M31-A3 (Clinical and Laboratory Standards Institute, 2008). Interpretive CLSI criteria were not available for cefquinome (CEQ), polymyxin B (PB), azithromycin (AZM), olaquindox (OLA), and mequindox (MEQ); therefore, results with the following minimum inhibitory concentration (MIC) values were considered resistant for these antibiotics: CEQ $\geq$8 μg/mL (using CEF as a reference); PB $\geq$4 μg/mL (Kwa et al., 2007); AZM $\geq$16 μg/mL (Sjölund-Karlsson et al., 2011); OLA and MEQ $\geq$64 μg/mL (Sørensen et al., 2003).

Strains that were resistant to AMP, AMX, ATM, and/or CRO were examined for ESBLs by using the MIC values of ceftazidime, ceftazime-clavulanic acid, cefotaxime, and cefotaxime-clavulanic acid. Results were interpreted based on CLSI M100-S22 (Clinical and Laboratory Standards Institute, 2012), and *Klebsiella pneumoniae* ATCC 700603 and *E. coli* ATCC 25922 were used as the control organisms.

TABLE 1 | Antibiotics and the range of concentrations tested.

Antibiotic	Abbreviation	Concentration range (μg/mL)
Ampicillin	AMP	0.06 ~ 256
Amoxicillin	AMX	0.06 ~ 256
Amoxicillin-clavulanic acid	AMC	0.06/0.03 ~ 128/256
Ceftriaxone	CRO	0.06 ~ 512
Ceftiofur	CEF	0.06 ~ 512
Cefquinome	CEQ	0.015 ~ 256
Imipenem	IPM	0.03 ~ 128
Aztreonam	ATM	0.06 ~ 512
Gentamicin	GEN	0.5 ~ 512
Amikacin	AMK	0.5 ~ 512
Tetracycline	TET	0.5 ~ 512
Doxycycline	DOX	0.5 ~ 512
Ciprofloxacin	CIP	0.015 ~ 512
Enrofloxacin	ENO	0.06 ~ 512
Levofloxacin	LEV	0.06 ~ 512
Nalidixic acid	NAL	0.06 ~ 512
Sulfamethoxazole-trimethoprim	SXT	0.25/4.75 ~ 128/2432
Chloramphenicol	CHL	0.5 ~ 512
Florfenicol	FFC	0.5 ~ 512
Fosfomycin	FOS	1 ~ 2,048
Polymyxin B	PB	0.5 ~ 512
Azithromycin	AZM	0.5 ~ 512
Olaquindox	OLA	0.25 ~ 128
Mequindox	MEQ	0.25 ~ 128

Statistical Analysis

The isolated strains were categorized as sensitive (S), intermediary (I), or resistant (R) based on the MIC values and the CLSI interpretive criteria. MIC_{50} and MIC_{90} were calculated using previously described methods (Schwarz et al., 2010), and 95% confidence intervals were calculated using SPSS 16.0 software (IBM, USA).

Results

Salmonella Isolates and Serotypes

In total, 248 bacterial isolates taken from healthy chickens, pigs, and dairy cows, and 209 isolates from diseased pigs, were verified as *Salmonella* spp., and 457 strains identified as serotypes were tested for antimicrobial susceptibility. In all samples taken from healthy animals, the prevalence of *Salmonella* spp. was 11.35% (248/2185). The specific prevalence of *Salmonella* spp. in chickens, pigs, and dairy cows was 12.55% (105/837), 4.09% (38/930), and 25.12% (105/418), respectively.

After serotyping, all isolates were divided into three groups (**Table 2**). Thirty-four isolates did not cluster for

TABLE 2 | Serovar distribution of isolated *Salmonella* (n = 457).

Serotype (N)[a]	Serovars	Chicken (n[b])	Pig (n[b])	Dairy cow (n[b])
Unable to self- agglutination (34)		6	28	0
Group A (3)	Unidentified types	3	0	0
Group B (205)	Unidentified subtypes	31	19	45
	Typhimurium	20	11	26
	Agona	3	0	12
	Derby	1	2	6
	II	1	1	4
	Kunduchi	0	0	4
	Schwarzenground	0	3	0
	Lagos	0	2	1
	Fyris	0	0	2
	Agama	1	1	0
	Farsta	1	0	0
	Gloucester	1	0	0
	Kingston	0	0	1
	Kubacha	1	0	0
	Saintpaul	1	0	0
	Stanley	0	1	0
	Travis	0	1	0
	Tumodi	0	0	1
	Uppsala	0	1	0
Group C1 (141)	Unidentified subtypes	0	90	1
	IIIb	0	22	0
	Typhisuis	0	7	0
	II	0	6	0
	Schwabach	0	5	0
	Irumu	0	3	0
	Kaduna	0	2	0
	Birkenhead	0	1	0
	Cotonou	0	1	0
	Hissar	0	1	0
	Paratyphic	0	1	0
	Thompson	0	1	0
Group C2-C3 (5)	Unidentified subtypes	0	4	0
	Quiniela	0	1	0
Group D1 (16)	Unidentified subtypes	4	0	0
	Enteritidis	9	0	1
	II	1	0	0
	Berta	1	0	0
Group D3 (1)	II	0	1	0
Group E1 (4)	Meleagridis	1	0	0
	Newlands	0	2	0
	Simi	1	0	0
Group E4 (20)	Unidentified subtypes	2	9	0
	Kouka	4	0	0
	Gnesta	0	3	0
	Visby	0	1	0
	Rideau	1	0	0
Unidentified subgroups (28)		11	16	1

[a]*N, the total number of Salmonella isolates per serogroup.*
[b]*n, number of isolates with a given serotype of animals.*

self-agglutination in sterile saline. Twenty-eight isolates could self-agglutination in sterile saline, but such activity was not observed with O antigen. The serogroups of the remaining 395 strains were determined. Eight distinct serogroups and 41 distinct serotypes were identified, as shown in **Table 2**. Group B (n = 205, 44.86%) and group C1 (n = 141, 30.85%) were identified as the dominant serogroups. Typhimurium 12.47% (n = 57) and IIIb 4.81% (n = 22) were the dominant serovars. Detailed serotypes could not be determined for 208 *Salmonella* isolates using the available H antigen in the different serogroups. According to the species of animal tested, the dominant serotypes were Typhimurium and Enteritidis in chickens, IIIb and Typhimurium in pigs, and Typhimurium and Agona in dairy cows (**Table 2**).

Antimicrobial Susceptibility Testing

Results of antimicrobial susceptibility testing are summarized in **Table 3**. Among the 457 isolates, 188 (41.14%) were susceptible to all tested antimicrobials and 220 (48.14%) were resistant to at least one antibiotic. All strains showed susceptibility or intermediate susceptibility to imipenem. Strains were most commonly resistant to nalidixic acid (39.17%), sulfamethoxazole-trimethoprim (39.61%), doxycycline (28.22%), and tetracycline (27.58%). They also showed resistance to all specialist drugs used only in veterinary medicine, including enrofloxacin (24.51%), florfenicol (20.13%), ceftiofur (7.44%), and cefquinome (5.25%), and to drugs used in both veterinary and human medicine, such as ciprofloxacin (24.07%), gentamicin (19.69%), ceftriaxone (6.34%), and amoxicillin/clavulanate (4.38%). Resistance to azithromycin, which is one of the macrolides often used against gram-positive bacteria, was expressed at 16.19%. Although they are rarely used in clinical applications, resistance to polymyxin B (18.82%) and fosfomycin (12.04%) was also observed.

When antibiotic resistance was analyzed according to animal species, the resistance rates of *Salmonella* were different for the majority of the drugs tested (**Table 4**). Excluding imipenem, resistance to the other 23 drugs ranged from 1.90 to 49.52% in chickens and 0.40 to 48.18% in pigs. In comparison, *Salmonella* from dairy cows showed resistance to 12 types of drug, and resistance rates ranged from 0.95 to 10.48%.

In total, 159 strains (34.72%) exhibited varying degrees of multidrug resistance (MDR) (**Table 5**), defined as resistance to at least three different classes of antimicrobials. The *Salmonella* spp. that exhibited MDR consisted of 104 strains from pigs (including 15 and 89 strains from healthy and diseased pigs, respectively), 51 strains from healthy chickens, and 4 strains from healthy dairy cows. MDR isolates showed diverse resistance to different classes of antibiotics, but were most frequently resistant to penicillins, fluoroquinolones, and quinolones (each occurring 11 times). β-lactam/β-lactamase inhibitor combinations appeared with the lowest frequency (five times) in *Salmonella* strains with MDR.

Based on analysis of MIC values and CLSI, 25 of the 457 isolates (5.47%) were confirmed as ESBL producers, with three suspected strains (**Table 6**). The ESBL-producing strains were obtained from different animals and areas as follows: two strains from chickens in Hubei, 15 strains from chickens in Henan, and eight strains from diseased pigs. Because the differences in MIC values between CAZ, CAZ/C and/or CTX, and CTX/C were not =3-fold based on CLSI, three strains from diseased pigs were suspected to be ESBL-producing strains.

The *Salmonella* serotypes of isolates differed in terms of their sensitivity to drugs (**Table 7**). Among all drug-sensitive isolates (n = 188), 80 isolates were identified in 17 specific serotypes. Typhimurium (n = 28) was the major serotype. Isolates of *Salmonella* strains with MDR showed 26 specific serotypes and the major serotypes were Enteritidis and IIIb (both n = 10). All serotypes were resistant to nalidixic acid, but differences were observed in the resistance profiles of *Salmonella* serotypes that exhibited MDR. The most common resistance profiles in *Salmonella* IIIb (n = 10) and Enteritidis isolates (n = 10) were AMP-AMX-SXT-NAL and SXT-OLA-MEQ-NAL, respectively. The resistance profile was AMP-AMX-TET-DOX-ENO-SXT-CHL-NAL in Typhimurium (n = 6), TET-DOX-CIP-ENO-SXT-CHL-FFC-NAL in Schwabach (n = 4), and PB-OLA-MEQ-NAL in Kouka (n = 4).

Discussion

The prevalence of *Salmonella* spp. in the center of China were in agreement with those obtained from Sichuan province farm animals (Li et al., 2013), but differed from other areas. The results were higher than in EU (European Food Safety Authority, 2014), where chicken 2.7%, pig 6.3%, cattle 2.4%, but were lower than in USA (National Antimicrobial Resistance Monitoring System, 2011), where chicken 52.56% ~ 47.95%, pig 10.34% ~ 8.79%, cattle 23.02% ~ 33.20%. Differences in isolation rates can be interpreted based on differences in region, sample types, collection seasons, culture methods, isolation methodologies, culture media, and local environmental conditions. For example, salmonellosis cases increased over the summer months, peaking in August and September, began decreasing thereafter (European Centre for Disease Prevention and Control, 2013). Therefore, a global perspective should ideally be adopted during sample collection, isolate separation, and, in particular, long-term monitoring.

The prevalence of *Salmonella* serotypes differed among animals and regions. Serogroup B and C1 were dominant, this result was consistent with in USA (Antunes et al., 2011). Serotype differ from other study. The dominant in chicken, pig, dairy cattle were Typhimurium and Enteritidis, IIIb and Typhimurium, Typhimurium and Agona in this study, respectively. The dominant serotype from chicken were Derby and Typhimurium in Sichuan province (Li et al., 2013), from pig were Enteritidis Indianain in Shandong province (Lai et al., 2014). The dominant from chicken, pig, cattle were Kentucky and Enteritidis, Adelaide and Johannesburg, Montevideo and Dublin in USA (National Antimicrobial Resistance Monitoring System, 2011); and from chicken, pig, cattle were Enteritidis and Infantis, Typhimurium and Typhimurium (monophasic), Typhimurium and Dublin in EU (European Food Safety Authority, 2014). This difference suggests serogroups and serotypes are varying according to geographical regions, and diversities and complexities. Certain serovars can emerge within a country or region for a certain period and then disappear with no evident cause or intervention.

TABLE 3 | Susceptibility of *Salmonella* isolates (n = 457) to antimicrobials.

Drug	Distribution of MICs (μg/mL)[a]																		S(%)	I(%)	R(%)	MIC_{50}	MIC_{90}	95%CI	Category[d]
	2048[b]	1024	512[b]	256[b]	128	64	32	16	8	4	2	1	0.5[c]	0.25[c]	0.125	0.06[c]	0.03[c]	0.015[c]							
AMP				95	15	7	4	3	2	3	34	163	4			127			72.87	0.67	26.46	1	>256	59.40–79.42	II
AMX				99	15	2	2	5	1	3	1	64	137	1	1	126			73.09	1.09	25.82	0.5	>256	64.55–85.37	II
AMC					11	1	6	13	61	18	14	5	198	3	127				92.78	2.84	4.38	0.5/0.25	128/64	12.07–19.39	I
CRO				8	9	5	1	4	2		1		1		26	400			93.44	0.22	6.34	<0.06	2	7.60–16.82	I
CEF			9	6	10	4	1	0	3	21	47	106	132	4	1	113			87.96	4.60	7.44	0.5	8	14.46–29.93	I
CEQ[e]					2		6	13	3	1	3	15	10	34	35	190	37	108	94.53	0.22	5.25	0.06	1	1.03–2.82	I
IPM											13	3	40	226	48	8	119		97.16	2.84	0	0.25	1	0.34–0.44	I
ATM			1				2		10	8	4		11	3	17	401			97.15	2.18	0.67	<0.06	0.125	0.11–7.73	I
GEN			7	1	16	18	33	15	0	3	47	169	148						80.31	0	19.69	1	64	19.25–32.35	II
AMK			7				1	8	41	38	200	17	145						98.25	0.22	1.53	2	8	4.84–16.36	II
TET			5	38	55	27	0	1	5	92	120	16	98						71.33	1.09	27.58	4	128	40.65–57.47	III
DOX			6	14	37	42	16	14	54	131	13		130						59.96	11.82	28.22	4	128	30.16–44.54	III
CIP						6	60	9	10	2	9	14	9	14	28	20	5	271	64.77	11.16	24.07	<0.015	32	4.48–6.83	I
ENR				45	4	3	28	8	5	9	10	19	32	12	8	274			64.33	11.16	24.51	<0.06	128	22.29–36.35	I
LEV						46	6	11	23	6	16	8	26	30	11	274			79.65	1.31	19.04	<0.06	64	6.10–9.65	I
NA			165	4	4	5	1	2	64	97	7	1	1	4	79	23			60.83	–	39.17	8	>512	1.68–2.13	III
SXT					127	15	3	22	5	9	90	69	5	112					60.39	–	39.61	2/38	>128/2432	34.26–44.60	III
CHL			26	73	7	5	3	2	1	21	179	42	98						74.62	0.44	24.94	2	256	59.68–85.76	III
FFC			38	18	21	11	2	2	4	27	141	66	127						78.99	0.88	20.13	2	256	48.66–75.67	III
FOX	24	18	12		5	6		1	2	1	30	358							86.87	1.09	12.04	<1	512	1.19–2.10	–
PB[f]			56	1			1		10	18	5	161	205								18.82	1	>512	48.86–79.73	III
AZM[g]			22		14		28	11	2	13	24	56	287								16.19	<0.5	32	21.44–41.77	II
OLA[h]					80	41	28	107	114	8				79							26.48	16	128	31.84–40.25	IV
MEQ[h]					76	39	26	61	159	13	2			81							25.38	8	128	29.94–38.35	IV

AMP, Ampicillin; AMX, Amoxicillin; AMC, Amoxicillin-clavulanic acid; CRO, Ceftriaxone; CEF, Ceftiofur; CEQ, Cefquinome; IPM, Imipenem; ATM, Aztreonam; GEN, Gentamicin; AMK, Amikacin; TET, Tetracycline; DOX, Doxycycline; CIP, Ciprofloxacin; ENO, Enrofloxacin; LEV, Levofloxacin; NAL, Nalidixic acid; SXT, Sulfamethoxazole-trimethoprim; CHL, Chloramphenicol; FFC, Florfenicol; FOS, Fosfomycin; PB, Polymyxin B; AZM, Azithromycin; OLA, Olaquindox; MEQ, Mequindox.

[a] *Susceptibility breakpoints are indicated by black vertical bars and resistance breakpoints are double vertical bars. CLSI breakpoints used when available. CLSI breakpoints do not exist for cefquinome, polymyxin B, azithromycin, olaquindox, and mequindox.*

[b] *Including higher than this tested MIC value.*

[c] *Including lower than this tested MIC value.*

[d] *Category I: antimicrobials of very high importance in human medicine, essential to the treatment of serious bacterial infections, no alternatives for resistant infections; Category II: antimicrobials of high importance in human medicine, used to treat a variety of infections, alternatives for resistance to category III antimicrobials; Category III: antimicrobials of medium importance in human medicine, used as first-line drugs, alternatives for resistance are generally available; Category IV: antimicrobials that are currently of limited use in human medicine.*

[e] *CLSI interpretative criteria for this bacterium/antimicrobial combination are not currently available. Reference R breakpoint of Ceftiofur.*

[f] *CLSI interpretative criteria for this bacterium/antimicrobial combination are not currently available. Isolates with an MIC ≥4 μg/mL were reported as resistant.*

[g] *CLSI interpretative criteria for this bacterium/antimicrobial combination are not currently available. Isolates with an MIC ≥16 μg/mL were reported as resistant.*

[h] *CLSI interpretative criteria for this bacterium/antimicrobial combination are not currently available. Isolates with an MIC ≥64 μg/mL were reported as resistant.*

TABLE 4 | Antibiotic resistance of *Salmonella* isolated from different food-producing animals unit: %.

Drug	Total (n = 457)	Chicken (n = 105)	Pig (n = 247)	Dairy cow (n = 105)
AMP	26.46	31.43	35.22	0.95
AMX	25.82	30.48	34.41	0.95
AMC	4.38	2.86	6.88	0
CRO	6.34	20.00	3.24	0
CEF	7.44	20.95	4.45	0.95
CEQ	5.25	15.24	3.24	0
IPM	0	0	0	0
ATM	0.67	1.90	0.40	0
GEN	19.69	17.14	29.15	0
AMK	1.53	6.67	0	0
TET	27.58	22.86	41.30	0
DOX	28.22	23.81	42.11	0
CIP	24.07	25.71	32.39	2.86
ENO	24.51	26.67	32.79	2.86
LEV	19.04	19.04	27.13	0
NA	39.17	46.67	48.18	10.48
SXT	39.61	49.52	47.77	10.48
CHL	24.94	26.67	34.41	0.95
FFC	20.13	20.95	27.94	0.95
FOS	12.04	6.67	19.43	0
PB	18.82	23.81	24.70	0
AZM	16.19	15.24	23.08	0.95
OLA	26.48	40.00	30.77	2.86
MEQ	25.38	40.95	28.34	2.86

AMP, Ampicillin; AMX, Amoxicillin; AMC, Amoxicillin-clavulanic acid; CRO, Ceftriaxone; CEF, Ceftiofur; CEQ, Cefquinome; IPM, Imipenem; ATM, Aztreonam; GEN, Gentamicin; AMK, Amikacin; TET, Tetracycline; DOX, Doxycycline; CIP, Ciprofloxacin; ENO, Enrofloxacin; LEV, Levofloxacin; NAL, Nalidixic acid; SXT, Sulfamethoxazole-trimethoprim; CHL, Chloramphenicol; FFC, Florfenicol; FOS, Fosfomycin; PB, Polymyxin B; AZM, Azithromycin; OLA, Olaquindox; MEQ, Mequindox.

TABLE 5 | The number of multidrug-resistance *Salmonella* strains identified in sampled animals unit: strain.

Resistance pattern	Chickens	Pigs	Dairy cows
3	3	6	1
4	16	7	2
5	1	4	0
6	3	7	1
7	6	13	0
8	7	18	0
9	4	3	0
10	9	13	0
11	2	22	0
12	0	7	0
13	0	4	0
Total	51	104	4

For instance, compared with data in 2010, the number of Enteritidis and Typhimurium decreased by 6% and 9% in 2011, respectively, (European Centre for Disease Prevention and Control, 2013); similar, compared with results in 2009, Enteritidis decreased, even disappeared from chicken and pig in 2012 from Shandong province (Lai et al., 2014).

The *Salmonella* serotypes isolated from farm animals overlapped with those that cause illnesses in humans, further highlighting the fact that *Salmonella* could be transmitted from animals to humans via the food chain (Alcaine et al., 2006; de Jong et al., 2009), such as Typhimurium and Enteritidis had identified from human in Henan and Hubei provinces (Cui et al., 2009; Xia et al., 2009). Some researchers have suggested that the differences in the dominant serotypes between animals and humans might be due to variations in their pathogenicity and corresponding resistance profiles (Volf et al., 2010), the strain containing Typhimurium and Enteritidis could acquired resistance to a large number of different antimicrobial compounds. At least two different serotypes existed from multiple-two strains to multiple-eleven strains, especially Enteritidis and Typhimurium, which were similar with other study from animals (Li et al., 2013; European Food Safety Authority, 2014; Lai et al., 2014), also with human (Cui et al., 2009; Xia et al., 2009). This may be related to the presence of the genetic structure known as *Salmonella* genomic island 1 (SGI1) and resistance genes (European Food Safety Authority, 2014). Therefore, monitoring of *Salmonella* should preferably focus more strongly on serovars that could, for example, be involved in a large outbreak.

Based on our MIC analysis, antibiotic-resistant bacteria, including multidrug-resistant bacteria, appeared in both healthy and diseased farm animals. These results were similar with other study (Gong et al., 2013; Li et al., 2013; Lai et al., 2014). One potential explanation is the use of antibiotics during breeding. Disease control and prevention in China during the breeding process mainly depends on the use of antibiotics (Gong et al., 2013). This arguably irrational use of antibiotics has contributed to the emergence of multidrug-resistant bacteria under selective antimicrobial pressure. Huazhong area (Henan, Hubei, and Hunan provinces) is one of the more concentrated areas of farm animals (China Agriculture Statistical Report, 2012), the demands and uses of drugs are huge, then inevitable there would be unreasonable use of drugs. These drugs, or the raw materials of the drugs, are inexpensive and easy to obtain; they have been widely used on animals in China. However, some steps have been taken to prevent the emergence of drug-resistant bacteria and promote food safety and public health with the Ministry of Agriculture of the People's Republic of China having formulated plans to ban or reduce the use of specific antimicrobials (Ministry of Agriculture of the People's Republic of China, 2002).

After the therapeutic effects of antimicrobials were confirmed in humans in the mid-1940s, they were soon introduced to veterinary medicine (McEwen, 2006). Even though some drugs were exclusively designed for veterinary use, the compounds administered are identical or very similar to those used in human medicine because they belong to the same antimicrobial classes (Heuer et al., 2009) such as β-lactams, cephalosporins, aminoglycosides, macrolides, tetracycline, sulfonamides, fluoroquinolones. Most of the antibiotic resistance to different classes has appeared in humans, animals, and/or animal

TABLE 6 | MICs used to verify ESBL-producing *Salmonella*.

Sample code	Ceftazidime (μg/mL)	Ceftazidime-clavulanic acid (μg/mL)	Cefotaxime (μg/mL)	Cefotaxime-clavulanic acid (μg/mL)	Source
147	2	0.5	64	<0.25	Chicken/Henan
151	4	0.5	>64	<0.25	Chicken/Henan
157	2	0.25	64	<0.25	Chicken/Henan
165	4	0.5	>64	<0.25	Chicken/Henan
171	4	0.5	>64	<0.25	Chicken/Henan
173	4	0.5	>64	<0.25	Chicken/Henan
174	4	0.5	>64	<0.25	Chicken/Henan
175	2	0.25	64	<0.25	Chicken/Henan
176	4	0.25	64	<0.25	Chicken/Henan
199	4	0.5	>64	<0.25	Chicken/Hubei
209	2	<0.25	32	<0.25	Chicken/Henan
211	2	<0.25	32	<0.25	Chicken/Henan
216	64	0.5	>64	<0.25	Chicken/Henan
217	2	<0.25	64	<0.25	Chicken/Henan
218	64	0.5	>64	<0.25	Chicken/Henan
264	2	0.5	32	<0.25	Chicken/Henan
268	128	2	32	1	Chicken/Hubei
4p	0.5	<0.25	16	<0.25	Pig/HAUvh
78p	0.5	<0.25	32	<0.25	Pig/HAUvh
127p	0.5	0.5	4	0.25	Pig/HAUvh
128p	0.5	0.5	64	4	Pig/HAUvh
151p	>128	128	16	8	Pig/HAUvh (suspected)
153p	4	0.5	64	<0.25	Pig/HAUvh
159p	4	0.5	>64	<0.25	Pig/HAUvh
167p	4	0.5	>64	<0.25	Pig/HAUvh
187p	>128	>128	16	8	Pig/HAUvh (suspected)
201p	128	64	>64	>64	Pig/HAUvh (suspected)
212p	0.5	0.5	64	0.5	Pig/HAUvh
212p	0.5	0.5	64	0.5	Pig/HAUvh

HAUvh, Huazhong Agricultural University veterinary hospital.

products. Ceftriaxone had showed resistance rates ≤13% and 4% from imported foods and humans (Akiyama and Khan, 2012; Wong et al., 2014). Similar, gentamicin had shown resistance in animals and humans (Lai et al., 2014; Wong et al., 2014). Overlapping resistance not only can lead to treatment failure, but also have negative consequences in both humans and animals.

ESBL-producing *Salmonella* strains were isolated from chickens and pigs in different areas in this study. Currently, the resistance genes were still on attempting to identify and sequencing from the samples. The emergence of producing-ESBLs bacteria in animals and animal products is of particular concern to public health, it allow bacteria to become resistant to a wide variety of penicillins and cephalosporins. ESBL-producing bacteria have appeared in poultry, pig, and cattle farms (Horton et al., 2011; European Food Safety Authority, 2014). In *Salmonella,* acquisition of resistance genes was likely to have occurred by conjugation, usually with other Enterobacteriaceae through the transfer of plasmids (European Food Safety Authority, 2014). Bacteria that develop resistance via ESBLs could become a reservoir of resistance genes, which may enter the food chain (European Food Safety Authority, 2012). When antibiotic resistance occurs during infection, the remaining treatment option is usually an antibiotic from the carbapenem family. While carbapenems were previously drugs of last resort, their use is now also contributing to resistance (Centers for Disease Control and Prevention, 2014). They are used to treat highly resistant infections in humans, and are not used in food-producing animals. However, carbapenemase-producing organisms have been isolated from farm animals (Fischer et al., 2012). In China, monitoring strategies do not currently contain testing and identification of ESBL- or AmpC-producing organisms in isolates from animals and/or animal-derived food products. It suggest that this should be established within surveillance procedures to anticipate possible changes in the status of ESBL enzymes.

Salmonella isolates showed multiple-resistance in results, it suggested the emergence of co-resistance and/or cross-resistance (Cantón and Ruiz-Garbajosa, 2011). For example, amikacin had showed low levels of resistance (0.67%); this may be due to cross-resistance among aztreonam, ciprofloxacin, and β-lactams (Livermore, 2002). Co-resistance to fluoroquinolones and third- and fourth-generation cephalosporins has also been identified in *Salmonella* isolated from humans (Zhang et al., 2014). Considering these results, the prudent use of antibacterial

TABLE 7 | Distribution of resistant *Salmonella* isolates according to serovars unit: strain.

Serogroup, serotype	Pan-susceptible	Intermediary	Number of antimicrobial classes in resistance pattern						Total
			1~2	3~4	5~6	7~8	9~10	11~13	
B, Typhimurium	28	18	5	0	0	5	1	0	57
B, Agona	13	0	1	1	0	0	0	0	15
B, Derby	5	0	2	2	0	0	0	0	9
B, II	4	0	1	0	0	0	0	1	6
B, Kunduchi	4	0	0	0	0	0	0	0	4
B, Schwarzenground	0	0	0	0	0	1	1	1	3
B, Lagos	1	0	0	0	0	1	0	1	3
B, Agama	0	1	0	0	0	0	0	1	2
B, Fyris	2	0	0	0	0	0	0	0	2
B, Farsta	1	0	0	0	0	0	0	0	1
B, Gloucester	0	1	0	0	0	0	0	0	1
B, Kingston	1	0	0	0	0	0	0	0	1
B, Kubacha	0	0	0	0	0	1	0	0	1
B, Saintpaul	0	1	0	0	0	0	0	0	1
B, Stanley	0	0	0	0	0	0	1	0	1
B, Travis	0	0	0	0	0	0	1	0	1
B, Tumodi	0	0	1	0	0	0	0	0	1
B, Uppsala	0	0	0	0	0	0	1	0	1
C1, III b	7	0	5	5	1	0	2	2	22
C1, Typhisuis	6	0	1	0	0	0	0	0	7
C1, II	3	0	1	0	0	1	1	0	6
C1, Schwabach	0	0	1	0	0	3	1	0	5
C1, Irumu	1	0	0	0	0	1	0	1	3
C1, Kaduna	0	0	0	0	0	0	2	0	2
C1, Birkenhead	0	0	1	0	0	0	0	0	1
C1, Cotonou	0	0	0	0	0	1	0	0	1
C1, Hissar	0	0	0	0	1	0	0	0	1
C1, Paratyphic	1	0	0	0	0	0	0	0	1
C1, Thompson	1	0	0	0	0	0	0	0	1
C2-C3, Quiniela	1	0	0	0	0	0	0	0	1
D1, Enteritidis	0	0	0	7	2	1	0	0	10
D1, Berta	0	0	0	1	0	0	0	0	1
D1, II	0	0	0	0	0	1	0	0	1
D3, II	1	0	0	0	0	0	0	0	1
E1, Newlands	0	0	0	0	0	2	0	0	2
E1, Meleagridis	0	0	0	0	0	1	0	0	1
E1, Simi	0	0	0	0	0	0	1	0	1
E4, Gnesta	0	0	3	0	0	0	0	0	3
E4, Kouka	0	0	0	3	0	1	0	0	4
E4, Rideau	0	0	0	1	0	0	0	0	1
E4, Visby	0	0	1	0	0	0	0	0	1
A, Unidentified subtypes	0	0	0	0	0	1	1	1	3
B, Unidentified subtypes	43	23	6	2	4	12	2	3	95
C1, Unidentified subtypes	39	3	14	6	5	5	4	15	91
C2-C3, Unidentified subtypes	2	0	0	0	0	0	1	1	4
D1, Unidentified subtypes	0	0	0	1	0	2	1	0	4
E4, Unidentified subtypes	0	1	8	2	0	0	0	0	11
Unidentified subgroup	10	0	2	3	1	2	6	4	28
Without-self-curing	14	1	8	1	1	3	2	4	34
Total	188	49	61	35	15	45	29	35	457

agents should be strongly recommended in clinical, veterinary, and agricultural settings in order to preserve antibiotic activity and avoid the development of cross-resistance.

In previous studies, researchers have demonstrated the relationship between the increased prevalence of antimicrobial-resistant bacteria and (a) the increased use of antimicrobials in human and veterinary medicine, (b) greater movement of people and animals, and (c) increased industrialization (Cheng et al., 2012). Huazhong is central to China; this area not only meets the needs of its own people via the production of animals and food but also supplies other areas and imports animals and food from other regions. This movement is a potential contributor to the spread of antibiotic-resistant bacteria. The environment itself also contains a variety of bacteria that potentially represent an immense pool of antibiotic-resistance genes, which if transferred between bacteria could cause human and animal disease (D'Costa et al., 2006). For example, wild animals that are carriers of antimicrobial-resistant bacteria could pass on colonies of resistant strains when they encounter humans, farming areas, and/or waste (Literak et al., 2011). A limitation of our study was that the samples were only collected from farm animals. For complete consideration in a surveillance system, samples should also be collected from, for example, the farm environment and farm workers.

Despite bans and legislation, some antibiotics are still routinely fed to livestock prophylactically to increase profits and to limit potential bacterial infections in stressed and crowded livestock (Ndi and Barton, 2011). Antibiotic-resistant bacteria will inevitably follow wherever antimicrobials are used; therefore, a coordinated multi-disciplinary approach will be required to address this issue (Smith et al., 2009). Various programs around the world have been established to monitor and control antibiotic-resistant bacteria. Recently, an official document, "National Medium- and Long-Term Planning for Prevention and Control of Animal Epidemics (2012 to 2020)," (General Office of State Council of China, 2012) was issued in China. The government outlined plans to control diseases by detection and purification using a medium- or long-term program, with the aim of reducing the antimicrobials used in animals and in symptomatic treatment. In future, the safest way to prevent the problem may be reducing antimicrobial usage with strict policies and legislation to control the development and spread of resistant bacteria in animals.

Funding

This research is supported by the Ministry of Science and Technology of the People's Republic of China (2012 BAK01B02), National Natural Science Foundation of China (31101856/31302143), Grants from National Basic Research program of China (2013CB127200), National Key Technology R&D Program (2012BAK01B00), Fundamental Research Funds for the Central Universities (2662015PY035) and project supported by the morning program of Wuhan in China (2015070404010191).

Author Contributions

XK, HH, MD, YW, and ZY designed the study. XK, HH, IA, and ZL collected the antimicrobial susceptibility data. XK, HH, YW, and ZL collected the serotype data. XK, HH, MD, and ZY analyzed the data. XK, HH, IA, and YW wrote the manuscript. XK, HH, MD, and ZY revised manuscript.

Acknowledgments

We thank Professor Aizhen Guo, who provided some of the *Salmonella* spp. isolates from diseased pigs.

References

Akiyama, T., and Khan, A. A. (2012). Molecular characterization of strains of fluoroquinolone-resistant *Salmonella enterica* serovar Schwarzengrund carrying multidrug resistance isolated from imported foods. *J. Antimicrob. Chemother.* 67, 101–110. doi: 10.1093/jac/dkr414

Alcaine, S. D., Soyer, Y., Wamick, L. D., Su, W. L., Sukhnanand, S., Richards, J., et al. (2006). Multilocus sequence typing supports the hypothesis that cow-and human-associated *Salmonella* isolates represent distinct and overlapping populations. *Appl. Environ. Microbiol.* 72, 7575–7585. doi: 10.1128/AEM.01174-06

Antunes, P., Mourao, J., Pestana, N., and Peixe, L. (2011). Leakage of emerging clinically relevant multidrug-resistant *Salmonella* clones from pig farms. *J. Antimicrob. Chemother.* 66, 2028–2032. doi: 10.1093/jac/dkr228

Cantón, R., and Ruiz-Garbajosa, P. (2011). Co-resistance: an opportunity for the bacteria and resistance genes. *Curr. Opin. Pharmacol.* 11, 477–485. doi: 10.1016/j.coph.2011.07.007

Centers for Disease Control and Prevention (CDC). (2014). *Antibiotic Resistance Threats in the United States*, 2013. 73. Available online at: http://www.cdc.gov/drugresistance/threat-report-2013/pdf/ar-threats-2013-508.pdf

Cheng, A. C., Turnidge, J., Collignon, P., Looke, D., Barton, M., and Gottlieb, T. (2012). Control of fluoroquinolone resistance through successful regulation, Australia. *Emerg. Infect. Dis.* 18, 1453–1460. doi: 10.3201/eid1809.111515

China Agriculture Statistical Report. (2012). *Ministry of Agriculture*. Beijing: PRC. China Agriculture Press.

Chiu, L. H., Chiu, C. H., Horn, Y. M., Chiou, C. S., Lee, C. Y., Yeh, C. M., et al. (2010). Characterization of 13 multi-drug resistant *Salmonella* serovars from different broiler chickens associated with those of human isolates. *BMC Microbiol.* 10:86. doi: 10.1186/1471-2180-10-86

Clinical and Laboratory Standards Institute. (2008). *Performance Standards for Antimicrobial Disk and Dilution Susceptibility Tests for Bacteria Isolated from Animals; Approved Standard-Third Edition.* Wayne, PA: CLSI (Informational Supplement, M31-A3).

Clinical and Laboratory Standards Institute. (2012). *Performance Standards for Antimicrobial Susceptibility Testing; Twenty-second Informational Supplement.*Wayne, PA: CLSI (Twenty-Two Informational Supplement M100-S22).

Cui, S., Li, J., Sun, Z., Hu, C., Jin, S., Li, F., et al. (2009). Characterization of *Salmonella* enterica isolates from infants and toddlers in Wuhan, China. *J. Antimicrob. Chemother.* 63, 87–94. doi: 10.1093/jac/dkn452

D'Costa, V. M., McGrann, K. M., Hughes, D. W., and Wright, G. D. (2006). Sampling the antibiotic resistome. *Science* 311, 374–377. doi: 10.1126/science.1120800

de Jong, A., Bywater, R., Butty, P., Deroover, E., Godinho, K., Klein, U., et al. (2009). A pan-European survey of antimicrobial susceptibility towards human-use antimicrobial drugs among zoonotic and commensal enteric bacteria isolated from healthy food-producing animals. *J. Antimicrob. Chemother.* 63, 733–744. doi: 10.1093/jac/dkp012

European Centre for Disease Prevention and Control. (2013). *Annual Epidemiological Report Reporting on 2011 Surveillance Data and 2012 Epidemic Intelligence Data.* 103–108. Available online at: http://www.ecdc.

europa.eu/en/publications/_layouts/forms/Publication_DispForm.aspx?List=4f55ad51-4aed-4d32-b960-af70113dbb90&ID=989

European Food Safety Authority. (2012). Technical specifications on the harmonised monitoring and reporting of antimicrobial resistance in *Salmonella*, *Campylobacter* and indicator *Escherichia coli* and *Enterococcus* spp. bacteria transmitted through food. *EFSA J.* 10:2742. doi: 10.2903/j.efsa.2012.2742

European Food Safety Authority. (2014). The European Union summary report on antimicrobial resistance in zoonotic and indicator bacteria from humans, animals and food in 2012. *EFSA J.* 12:3590. doi: 10.2903/j.efsa.2014.3590

Fischer, J., Rodriguez, I., Schmoger, S., Friese, A., Roesler, U., Helmuth, R., et al. (2012). *Escherichia coli* producing VIM-1 carbapenemase isolated on a pig farm. *J. Antimicrob. Chemother.* 67, 1793–1795. doi: 10.1093/jac/dks108

Garrity, G. M., Bell, J. A., and Lilburn, T. G. (2004). *Bergey's Manual of Systematic Bacteriology,* 2nd Edn. New York, NY: Springer.

General Office of State Council of China. (2012). *National Medium and Long-term Planning for Prevention and Control of Animal Epidemics* (2012-2020), notice no 31. Available online at: http://www.gov.cn/gongbao/content/2012/content_2152427.htm

Gong, J., Xu, M., Zhu, C., Miao, J., Liu, X., Xu, B., et al. (2013). Antimicrobial resistance, presence of integrons and biofilm formation of *Salmonella* Pullorum isolates from eastern China (1962-2010). *Avian Pathol.* 42, 290–294. doi: 10.1080/03079457.2013.788129

Government of Canada. (2005). *Current Thinking on Risk Management Measures to Address Antimicrobial Resistance Associated with the Use of Antimicrobial Agents in Food-producing Animals.* ON: Health Canada, Veterinary Drugs Directorate. Available online at: http://www.hc-sc.gc.ca/dhp-mps/alt_formats/hpfb-dgpsa/pdf/vet/amr-ram_rep-rap_06_05-eng.pdf

Grimont, P. A. D., and Weill, F.-X. (2007). *Antigenic Formulae of the Salmonella Serovars* 9th Edn. Paris: WHO collaborating Centre for Reference and Research on *Salmonella*, Institut Pasteur.

Heuer, O. E., Kruse, H., Grave, K., Collignon, P., Karunasagar, I., and Angulo, F. J. (2009). Human health consequences of use of antimicrobial agents in aquaculture. *Clin. Infect. Dis.* 49, 1248–1253. doi: 10.1086/605667

Horton, R. A., Randall, L. P., Snary, E. L., Cockrem, H., Lotz, S., Wearing, H., et al. (2011). Fecal carriage and shedding density of CTX-M extended-spectrum beta-lactamase-producing *Escherichia coli* in cattle, chickens, and pigs: implications for environmental contamination and food production. *Appl. Environ. Microbiol.* 77, 3715–3719. doi: 10.1128/AEM.02831-10

Kwa, A., Kasiakou, S. K., Tam, V. H., and Falagas, M. E. (2007). Polymyxin B: similarities to and differences from colistin (polymyxin E). *Expert. Rev. Anti. Infect. Ther.* 5, 811–821. doi: 10.1586/14787210.5.5.811

Lai, J., Wu, C., Wu, C., Qi, J., Wang, Y., Wang, H., et al. (2014). Serotype distribution and antibiotic resistance of *Salmonella* in food-producing animals in Shandong province of China, 2009-2012. *Int. J. Food Microbiol.* 180, 30–38. doi: 10.1016/j.ijfoodmicro.2014.03.030

Li, R., Lai, J., Wang, Y., Liu, S., Li, Y., Liu, K., et al. (2013). Prevalence and characterization of *Salmonella* species isolated from pigs, ducks and chickens in Sichuan Province, China. *Int. J. Food Microbiol.* 163, 14–18. doi: 10.1016/j.ijfoodmicro.2013.01.020

Literak, I., Petro, R., Dolejska, M., Gruberova, E., Dobiasova, H., Petr, J., et al. (2011). Antimicrobial resistance in fecal *Escherichia coli* isolates from healthy urban children of two age groups in relation to their antibiotic therapy. *Antimicrob. Agents Chemother.* 55, 3005–3007. doi: 10.1128/AAC.01724-10

Livermore, D. M. (2002). Multiple mechanisms of antimicrobial resistance in *Pseudomonas aeruginosa*: our worst nightmare? *Clin. Infect. Dis.* 34, 634–640. doi: 10.1086/338782

Malorny, B., Hoorfar, J., Bunge, C., and Helmuth, R. (2003). Multicenter validation of the analytical accuracy of *Salmonella* PCR: towards an international standard. *Appl. Environ. Microbiol.* 69, 290–296. doi: 10.1128/AEM.69.1.290-296.2003

McEwen, S. A. (2006). Antibiotic use in animal agriculture: what have we learned and where are we going? *Anim. Biotechnol.* 17, 239–250. doi: 10.1080/10495390600957233

Ministry of Agriculture of the People's Republic of China. (2002). *List of Bans for Veterinary Drugs and Other Compounds in Animal Food.* Available online at: http://www.moa.gov.cn/zwllm/tzgg/gg/201104/t20110422_1976324.htm

National Antimicrobial Resistance Monitoring System. (2011). *Animal Arm Annual Report.* Available online at: http://ars.usda.gov/SP2UserFiles/Place/60400520/NARMS/NARMS2009/NARMSAnimalArm2009.pdf

Ndi, O., and Barton, M. (2011). "Antibiotic resistance in animals—The Australian perspective," in *Antimicrobial Resistance in the Environment,* eds P. L. Keenand and M. H. M. M. Montforts (New York, NY: Wiley-Blackwell), 265–290.

Russell, S. B., Emilio, E. D., Kevin, L., Winthrop, J. A., Lapidus, R. V., and Paul, R. C. (2014). Travel-associated antimicrobial drug-resistant nontyphoidal Salmonellae, 2004-2009. *Emerg. Infect. Dis.* 20, 603–611. doi: 10.3201/eid2004.131063

Schwarz, S., Silley, P., Simjee, S., Woodford, N., van Duijkeren, E., Johnson, A. P., et al. (2010). Assessing the antimicrobial susceptibility of bacteria obtained from animals. *Vet. Microbiol.* 141, 1–4. doi: 10.1016/j.vetmic.2009.12.013

Sjölund-Karlsson, M., Joyce, K., Blickenstaff, K., Ball, T., Haro, J., Medalla, F. M., et al. (2011). Antimicrobial susceptibility to azithromycin among *Salmonella enterica* isolates from the United States. *Antimicrob. Agents Chemother.* 55, 3985–3989. doi: 10.1128/AAC.00590-11

Smith, P. R., LeBreton, A., Horsberg, T. E., and Corsin, F. (2009). "Guidelines for antimicrobial use in aquaculture," in *Guide to Antimicrobial Use in Animals,* eds L. Guardabassi, L. B. Jensen, and H. Kruse (Oxford: Blackwell Publishing Ltd), 207–218.

Sørensen, A. H., Hansen, L. H., Johannesen, E., and Sørensen, S. J. (2003). Conjugative plasmid conferring resistance to olaquindox. *Antimicrob. Agents Chemother.* 47, 798–799. doi: 10.1128/AAC.47.2.798-799.2003

Stevens, M. P., Humphrey, T. J., and Maskell, D. J. (2009). Molecular insights into farm animal and zoonotic *Salmonella* infections. *Philos. Trans. R. Soc. Lond B Biol. Sci.* 364, 2709–2723. doi: 10.1098/rstb.2009.0094

Volf, J., Havlickova, H., Hradecka, H., Ondrackova, P., Matiasovic, J., Faldyna, M., et al. (2010). Epidemiology and interaction of *Salmonella enterica* serovar Derby, Infantis and Typhimurium with porcine alveolar macrophages. *Vet. Microbiol.* 146, 105–110. doi: 10.1016/j.vetmic.2010.04.031

Wang, S. J., Duan, H. L., Zhang, W., and Li, J. (2007). Analysis of bacterial foodborne disease outbreaks in China between 1994 and 2005. *FEMS Immunol. Med. Microbiol.* 51, 8–13. doi: 10.1111/j.1574-695X.2007.00305.x

Wang, Y., Chen, Q., Cui, S. H., Xu, X., Zhu, J., Luo, H., et al. (2014). Enumeration and characterization of *Salmonella* isolates from retail chicken carcasses in Beijing, China. *Foodborne Pathog Dis.* 11, 126–132. doi: 10.1089/fpd.2013.1586

WHO Global Foodborne Infections Network. (2010). *Laboratory Protocol, Isolation of Salmonella spp. from Food and Animal Faeces,* 5th Edn. Available online at: http://www.antimicrobialresistance.dk/232-169-215-protocols.htm

Wong, M. H. Y., Yan, M., Chan, E. W. C., Biao, K., and Chen, S. (2014). Emergence of clinical *Salmonella* Typhimurium with concurrent resistance to ciprofloxacin, ceftriaxone and azithromycin. *Antimicrob. Agents Chemother.* 58, 3752–3756. doi: 10.1128/AAC.02770-13

Xia, S., Hendriksen, R. S., Xie, Z., Huang, L., Zhang, J., Guo, W., et al. (2009). Molecular characterization and antimicrobial susceptibility of *Salmonella* isolates from infections in humans inHenan Province, China. *J. Clin. Microbiol.* 47, 401–409. doi: 10.1128/JCM.01099-08

Yang, B. W. (2010). *Prevalence and Characterization of Chicken Borne Salmonella Serovars in Eight Provinces and Cities of China.* Ph.D. Master's Thesis. Northwest A&F University. 5. Available online at: http://210.27.80.82/opac/item.php?marc_no=0000477458

Zhang, J., Jin, H., Hu, J., Yuan, Z., Shi, W., Ran, L., et al. (2014). Serovars and antimicrobial resistance of non-typhoidal *Salmonella* from human patients in Shanghai, China, 2006–2010. *Epidemiol Infect.* 142, 826–832. doi: 10.1017/S0950268813001659

Zhu, M., Cui, S., Lin, L., Xu, B., Zhao, J., Xia, S., et al. (2012). Analysis of the aetiology of diarrhea in outpatients in 2007, Henan province, China. *Epidemiol. Infect.* 7, 540–548. doi: 10.1017/S0950268812000970

19

Characterization of Antibiotic Resistance in Commensal Bacteria from an Aquaculture Ecosystem

*Ying Huang[1], Lu Zhang[1], Laura Tiu[2] and Hua H. Wang[1,3,4]**

[1] Department of Food Science and Technology, The Ohio State University, Columbus, OH, USA, [2] South Centers, The Ohio State University, Piketon, OH, USA, [3] Department of Microbiology, The Ohio State University, Columbus, OH, USA, [4] School of Biological Sciences, Fudan University, Yangpu, Shanghai, China

***Correspondence:**
Hua H. Wang,
Department of Food Science and Technology, The Ohio State University, 2015 Fyffe Court, Columbus, OH 43210, USA
wang.707@osu.edu

The objective of the study was to improve the understanding of antibiotic resistance (AR) ecology through characterization of antibiotic-resistant commensal isolates associated with an aquaculture production system. A total of 4767 isolates non-susceptible to sulfamethoxazole/trimethoprim (Sul/Tri), tetracycline (Tet), erythromycin (Erm), or cefotaxime (Ctx), originated from fish, feed, and environmental samples of an aquaculture farm with no known history of antibiotic applications were examined. Close to 80% of the isolates exhibited multi-drug resistance in media containing the corresponding antibiotics, and representative AR genes were detected in various isolates by PCR, with feed isolates had the highest positive rate detected. Identified AR gene carriers involved 18 bacterial genera. Selected AR genes led to acquired resistance in other bacteria by transformation. The AR traits in many isolates were stable in the absence of selective pressure. AR-rich feed and possibly environmental factors may contribute to AR in the aquaculture ecosystem. For minimum inhibitory concentration test, brain heart infusion medium was found more suitable for majority of the bacteria examined than cation-adjusted Mueller Hinton broth, with latter being the recommended medium for clinical isolates by standard protocol. The data indicated a need to update the methodology due to genetic diversity of microbiota for better understanding of the AR ecology.

Keywords: antibiotic resistance, aquaculture ecosystem, multiple risk factors, commensal bacteria

Introduction

The rapid emergence of antibiotic resistance (AR) in the global ecosystem has become a major public health concern. In the past decade, with a broadened scope of investigation, both population- and organism-based studies have illustrated that commensal bacteria likely have played a key role in AR ecology (Andremont, 2003; Wang et al., 2006; Wang and Schaffner, 2011). With the expansion of research territory, AR has been found prevalent across the ecosystem, from clinical samples, animal and human hosts, retail foods, to waste water, soil, and other natural environment (Zhanel et al., 2000; Österblad et al., 2001; Aubry-Damon et al., 2004; Wang et al., 2006; Koike et al., 2007; Sommer et al., 2009; Li and Wang, 2010; D'Costa et al., 2011; Zhang, 2011; Ye et al., 2013). For instance, using non-specific culturing methods and culture-independent real-time PCR, the abundance of AR in the food chain was revealed and a broad-spectrum of non-pathogenic and even beneficial bacteria were found carrying transmissible AR genes (Duran and Marshall, 2005; Wang et al., 2006; Manuzon et al., 2007). Characterization of antibiotic-resistant (ART) isolates associated with food animals, ready-to-eat food products, human, and environmental samples has led to the discovery of various mechanisms involved in AR evolution (Sommer et al., 2009; Bhullar et al., 2012), enrichment (Zhang et al., 2011), and persistence (Sørum et al., 2006; Rosvoll et al., 2010; Li et al., 2011). It becomes evident that commensal flora provides a particular window of vulnerability of AR in the ecosystem, and prompt response to the early indication can be critically important for preventive AR management (Andremont, 2003; Wang et al., 2006; Wang and Schaffner, 2011). Due to the advancement in metagenomics and other molecular techniques, the complexity of microbiome associated with both hosts and environment has been gradually uncovered (Venter et al., 2004; Sommer et al., 2009; Zhang et al., 2011). However, the extremely large size and diverse distribution of the commensal population, as well as genetic diversity of the subpopulations presented several major challenges to researchers. There is no single way of recovering, culturing, or characterizing all the cultures, making proper interpretation of data a daunting task.

Aquatic creatures are susceptible to infectious diseases. Use of antibiotics in aquaculture production systems is considered a major risk factor contributing to AR in aquaculture products and the ecosystem. ART pathogens, such as *Aeromonas* (Akinbowale et al., 2007; Penders and Stobberingh, 2008), *Vibrio* (Oh et al., 2011; Rebouças et al., 2011), and *Salmonella* (Ribeiro et al., 2010; Budiati et al., 2013), have been reported to be associated with the aquaculture system. Particularly, certain AR determinants have been found in both aquaculture and clinical isolates, indicating potential AR dissemination between food and humans. For instance, one gene cassette containing bla_{CMY-2}, *sugE*, and *blc* detected in *Aeromonas salmonicida* ssp. *salmonicida* isolates from Atlantic Canadian salmon farm was identical to a transponson-like element widely distributed among clinical and food-borne *Salmonella* and other Enterobacteriaceae throughout Asia and the United States (McIntosh et al., 2008). Rhodes et al. (2000) reported the dissemination of *tet*(A)-associated Tn*1721* and Tn*1721*-like elements among different *Aeromonas* species and *Escherichia coli*, and between the human and aquaculture environment in distinct geographical locations (including Norway, Scotland, England, and Germany). In addition, various AR genes were found in a broad spectrum of commensal bacteria associated with aquaculture products and the environment (Ye et al., 2013; Shah et al., 2014). However, these data are still insufficient in elucidating AR risk factors in the aquaculture ecosystem.

In a recent study, we have uncovered a rich profile of ART bacteria in samples from a domestic aquaculture farm with no known history of antibiotic application, by culture-dependent and -independent methods (Huang, 2014). The objective of this study was to characterize the genotypic and phenotypic features of the corresponding ART isolates, as well as AR persistence and dissemination, for an improved understanding of the AR ecology associated with aquaculture production. During the evaluation of minimum inhibitory concentration (MIC) for representative antibiotics of the isolates, we have compared the data using both standard approach for pathogens (CLSI, 2013) and a modified method (Wang et al., 2006), to collect baseline information for further methodology improvement, to address the needs for proper assessment of commensal bacteria.

Materials and methods

Bacterial Strains and Culture Condition

A total of 4767 isolates recovered from Sul/Tri-, Tet-, Erm-, or Ctx-containing agar plates were examined in the study. These isolates originated from fish intestine (1045 isolates), fish surface rinsing water (850 isolates), fish feed (150 isolates), pond mud (1293 isolates), and pond water (1429 isolates) from an aquaculture farm with no known history of antibiotic applications. All isolates were cultured in brain heart infusion (BHI) media containing the corresponding antibiotics, including 152 μg/ml of sulfamethoxazole (Sigma-Aldrich, St. Louis, MO, USA) with 8 μg/ml of trimethoprim (Sigma-Aldrich), 16 μg/ml of tetracycline (Sigma-Aldrich), 100 μg/ml of erythromycin (Fisher Scientific, Waltham, MA, USA), or 4 μg/ml of cefotaxime (Sigma-Aldrich; Ye et al., 2013).

Determination of Drug Resistance Profiles, AR Genes, and Identification of AR Gene Carriers

Recovered Sul/Tri^r, Tet^r, Erm^r, and Ctx^r isolates were spotted on BHI agar plates containing each of the four antibiotics for rapid assessment of their phenotypic resistance profile.

Approximately one-fourth of the ART isolates were randomly selected for conventional PCR screening for representative AR genes (Li and Wang, 2010). AR gene primers used in the study were listed in **Table 1**. Approximately 10% of the positive PCR products were confirmed by DNA sequence assessment using an ABI Prism 3700 sequencer (Applied Biosystems, Foster City, CA, USA) at the Plant Microbe Genomics Facility, The Ohio State University, and the obtained DNA sequences were compared with published AR gene sequences deposited in the NCBI database. Approximately 50% of the AR gene carriers were further identified by PCR and partial 16S rRNA gene sequence analysis, as described previously (Wang et al., 2006).

MIC Assessments

Twenty-nine ART isolates carrying AR genes were subjected to the MIC test. The assessments were conducted using microbroth dilution method as suggested by CLSI (2013) protocol. BHI and cation-adjusted Mueller Hinton (CAMH) broth were employed as basic medium independently. ART isolates were grown in the broth containing the corresponding antibiotic (including up to 608 μg/ml Sul with 32 μg/ml Tri, 512 μg/ml Tet, 512 μg/ml Erm, or 512 μg/ml Ctx). Reference strains *Staphylococcus aureus* ATCC®29213, *Enterococcus faecalis* ATCC®29212, *E. coli* ATCC®25922, and *Pseudomonas aeruginosa* ATCC®27853 were examined in parallel as controls.

TABLE 1 | Primers used for conventional PCR.

Primer	Sequence (5′–3′)	Reference
*sul*1 F	CGGCGTGGGCTACCTGAACG	Kerrn (2002)
*sul*1 R	GCCGATCGCGTGAAGTTCCG	
*sul*2 F	GCAGGCGCGTAAGCTGA	Zhang et al. (2011)
*sul*2 R	GGCTCGTGTGTGCGGATG	
*tet*S F	GAACGCCAGAGAGGTATT	Zhang et al. (2011)
*tet*S R	TACCTCCATTTGGACCTCAC	
*tet*L F	TTGGATCGATAGTAGCC	Zhang et al. (2011)
*tet*L R	GTAACCAGCCAACTAATGAC	
*tet*M F	CGAACAAGAGGAAAGCATAAG	Zhang et al. (2011)
*tet*M R	CAATACAATAGGAGCAAGC	
*erm*B F	TGGTATTCCAAATGCGTAATG	Zhang et al. (2011)
*erm*B R	CTGTGGTATGGCGGGTAAGT	
*erm*C F	GCTAATATTGTTTAAATCGTCAAT	Wang et al. (2006)
*erm*C R	TCAAAACATAATATAGATAAA	
bla_{TEM} F	CATTTCCGTGTCGCCCTTATTC	Dallenne et al. (2010)
bla_{TEM} R	CGTTCATCCATAGTTGCCTGAC	
bla_{SHV} F	AGCCGCTTGAGCAAATTAAAC	Dallenne et al. (2010)
bla_{SHV} R	ATCCCGCAGATAAATCACCAC	
bla_{OXA} F	GGCACCAGATTCAACTTTCAAG	Dallenne et al. (2010)
bla_{OXA} R	GACCCCAAGTTTCCTGTAAGTG	
bla_{CMY-2} F	GACAGCCTCTTTCTCCACA	Zhang et al. (2011)
bla_{CMY-2} R	TGGAACGAAGGCTACGTA	
$bla_{CTX\,MU1}$	ATGTGCAGYACCAGTAARGT	Zhang et al. (2011)
$bla_{CTX\,MU2}$	TGGGTRAARTARGTSACCAGA	

Persistence of AR

AR stability in resistant isolates was determined according to the published procedures (Li et al., 2011) with slight modifications. Basically, after consecutive transfer every 12 h for 30 days, the cultures were serially diluted and plated on BHI agar plates. One hundred colonies were randomly picked from each sample, and spotted onto BHI agar plates with and without the corresponding antibiotic. The ratio of resistant to total colonies was used to describe the resistance persistence in ART isolates at the absence of the antibiotic selective pressure.

Transformation

Chemical transformation was conducted using plasmids from nine Gram-negative ART isolates carrying AR genes and *E. coli* DH5α as a recipient by the calcium chloride transformation method (Dagert and Ehrlich, 1979). Meanwhile, electroporation was employed when introducing plasmids from five Gram-positive ART isolates carrying AR genes to *Lactococcus lactis* LM 2301 following the procedures described previously (Mcintyre and Harlander, 1989).

Results

MIC Assessment

MIC analysis showed that the MIC results of Tet, Erm, or Ctx for the four reference strains were comparable in BHI and CAMH broth. However, culture medium had varied but clear impact on MIC results of Sul/Tri. For instance, while the MIC values of Sul/Tri for *P. aeruginosa* ATCC®27853 in both media were comparable (608/32 μg/ml), the other three reference strains showed 4- to 64-fold higher MIC values in BHI than that of in CAMH. It is worth noting that *E. faecalis* ATCC®29212 didn't grow as well in CAMH as in BHI broth.

As illustrated in **Table 2**, twenty-nine isolates used in the MIC assessment were identified and they belonged to 15 genera. MIC values for Tet, Erm, or Ctx in BHI were the same as, or twofold to fourfold higher than the results from CAMH. Among the strains examined, 9 out of 20 (45%) Ter^r, 6 out of 6 (100%) Erm^r, and 2 out of 5 (40%) Ctx^r isolates exhibited high and consistent MIC values (no less than 128 μg/ml) in both BHI and CAMH for Tet, Erm, or Ctx, respectively. But the MIC values for Sul/Tri in BHI and CAMH varied significantly in close to 70% of the isolates (21 out of 29). Some Sul/Tri^r isolates showed very high value (no less than 608/32 μg/ml) in both BHI and CAMH, including *Plesiomonas* sp., *Aeromonas* sp., and *Psychrobacter* sp. Bacteria from genera such as *Enterobacter* sp., *Bacillus* sp., and *Kurthia* sp. showed higher MIC value in BHI (no less than 304/16 μg/ml) than that in CAMH (no more than 9.5/0.5 μg/ml). Moreover, isolates of *Vagococcus* sp., *Aerococcus* sp., *Corynebacterium* sp., and *Enterococcus* sp. didn't grow or had poor growth in CAMH, but exhibited higher MIC value in BHI (no less than 608/32 μg/ml).

Phenotypic-Resistant Profiles of the ART Isolates

Of the recovered Sul/Tri^r, Tet^r, Erm^r, and Ctx^r isolates (from BHI plates) associated with fish intestine, surface rinsing water, fish feed, pond mud, and pond water samples, 3772 of 4767 total isolates (79.1%) showed resistance to more than one antibiotic, and 824 isolates (17.4%) were resistant to all four antibiotics tested. As shown in **Table 3**, multi-drug-resistant bacteria were common in all samples.

Prevalence of the AR Genes and Identification of the Isolates

As shown in **Table 4**, more AR genes were detected in isolates associated with fish feed and fish intestine than surface rinsing water, pond mud, and pond water samples. For instance, a high percentage and broad spectrum of AR genes were found in isolates from fish feed samples, including *sul*1 (10.2%), *sul*2 (2.0%), *tet*L (13.3%), *tet*M (9.2%), *tet*S (6.1%), and *erm*B (1.0%). Within the 13 AR determinants examined, *tet*M had the highest detection rate (8.1%) in the isolates.

As illustrated in **Table 4**, identified AR gene carriers belonged to 18 genera. *Aeromonas* sp., *Enterococcus* sp., *Enterobacter* sp., and *Plesiomonas* sp. identified in fish intestine samples were commonly isolated from fish (Austin, 2002). Some of the isolates examined, including *Bacillus* sp., *Carnobacterium* sp., *Corynebacterium* sp., *Enterococcus* sp., *Plesiomonas* sp., *Lactococcus* sp., and *Psychrobacter* sp. were found to carry multiple resistance encoding genes. Fish feed contained various AR genes in a broad spectrum of organisms, though total count of ART bacteria was relatively low.

TABLE 2 | Comparison of MIC results between BHI and CAMH medium.

Isolates	Identity	AR genes carried	Resistance phenotype and MIC (μg/ml)							
			Sul/Tri^r		Tet^r		Erm^r		Ctx^r	
			BHI	CAMH	BHI	CAMH	BHI	CAMH	BHI	CAMH
17iT21	*Plesiomonas* sp.	*sul*1	>608/32	>608/32	256	128	–	–	–	–
17wT9	*Plesiomonas* sp.	*tet*M	–	–	256	128	–	–	–	–
18iS4	*Plesiomonas* sp.	*sul*2	>608/32	>608/32	–	–	–	–	–	–
18iS31	*Plesiomonas* sp.	*sul*2	>608/32	>608/32	–	–	–	–	–	–
17fS1	*Enterococcus* sp.	*tet*M, *tet*L	>608/32	Weak growth ≤9.5/0.5	256	128	–	–	–	–
17fS3	*Enterococcus* sp.	*sul*1	>608/32	Weak growth ≤9.5/0.5	16	16	–	–	–	–
18iX15	*Enterococcus* sp.	*tet*S, *tet*L	>608/32	Weak growth ≤9.5/0.5	256	128	–	–	512	512
18fT19	*Enterococcus* sp.	*tet*S	>608/32	Weak growth ≤9.5/0.5	256	128	–	–	–	–
17iE3	*Enterobacter* sp.	*sul*2	304/16	≤9.5/0.5	–	–	512	256	–	–
17iE10	*Enterobacter* sp.	*sul*2	>608/32	≤9.5/0.5	–	–	512	256	–	–
17iE11	*Enterobacter* sp.	*sul*2	304/16	≤9.5/0.5	–	–	512	256	16	8
17iE26	*Enterobacter* sp.	*sul*2	>608/32	≤9.5/0.5	–	–	512	256	–	–
17fT6	*Kocuria* sp.	*sul*1	>608/32	≤9.5/0.5	64	64	–	–	–	–
17fT2	*Corynebacterium* sp.	*sul*1	>608/32	Weak growth	256	128	–	–	–	–
18fT26	*Corynebacterium* sp.	*tet*L	–	–	32	32	–	–	–	–
18fT27	*Corynebacterium* sp.	*tet*L	–	–	32	32	–	–	–	–
18iS7	*Aeromonas* sp.	*sul*1	>608/32	>608/32	–	–	–	–	–	–
18fE1	*Bacillus* sp.	*erm*B	>608/32	≤9.5/0.5	256	256	512	512	4	4
17fT12	*Aerococcus* sp.	*tet*M	>608/32	Weak growth	256	128	–	–	–	–
17fS5	*Aerococcus* sp.	*tet*M	>608/32	Weak growth	32	32	–	–	–	–
18fS13	*Psychrobacter* sp.	*sul*2	>608/32	>608/32	32	32	–	–	–	–
18fS19	*Psychrobacter* sp.	*sul*1, *sul*2	>608/32	>608/32	32	32	–	–	–	–
18pwE5	*Staphylococcus* sp.	*erm*C	>608/32	≤9.5/0.5	–	–	>512	>512	>512	>512
18fT47	*Carnobacterium* sp.	*tet*S, *tet*L	–	–	64	64	–	–	–	–
18fT5	*Kurthia* sp.	*tet*M	>608/32	≤9.5/0.5	256	256	–	–	64	16
18fT29	*Lactobacillus* sp.	*tet*L	–	–	32	32	–	–	–	–
18fS10	*Pseudoclavibacter* sp.	*sul*1	608/32	608/32	32	32	-	–	–	–
18fT12	*Vagococcus* sp.	*tet*L	>608/32	No growth	128	No growth	–	–	–	–

BHI, Brain heart infusion; CAMH, cation-adjusted Mueller Hinton.

TABLE 3 | Multi-drug-resistant isolates from aquaculture samples.

Sample	Isolates resistant to antibiotic			
	1AR[a]	2AR	3AR	4AR
Surface rinsing water (*n* = 850)	18.7% (159/850)	35.6% (303/850)	32.2% (274/850)	13.4% (114/850)
Fish intestine (*n* = 1045)	19.8% (207/1045)	58.5% (611/1045)	12.1% (126/1045)	9.7% (101/1045)
Pond mud (*n* = 1293)	13.4% (173/1293)	34.9% (451/1293)	34.0% (440/1293)	17.7% (229/1293)
Pond water (*n* = 1429)	8.7% (125/1429)	15.2% (217/1429)	50.6% (723/1429)	25.5% (364/1429)
Fish feed (*n* = 150)	36.0% (54/150)	31.3% (47/150)	22.0% (33/150)	10.7% (16/150)

[a]*Number of antibiotic(s) the isolates were resistant to.*

Stability of the AR

Results of persistence assessment showed that 90–100% of the progenies from nine ART isolates examined retained their original AR traits, indicating that the AR determinants are generally stable in the resistant isolates without the corresponding antibiotic selective pressure. Progenies of an *Enterococcus* strain from the intestine sample retained resistance to Sur/Tri but became susceptible to Tet and Ctx.

Functionality of the AR Determinants

Plasmids from two out of nine Gram-negative isolates (*sul*1$^+$ *Aeromonas* sp. from the fish intestine and *sul*2$^+$ *Psychrobacter* sp. from the fish feed) and one out of five Gram-positive isolate (*tet*L$^+$ *Vagococcus* sp. from fish feed) were successfully transferred to *E. coli* and *L. lactis,* respectively, resulting in acquired resistance in transformants. The transformants exhibited comparable MIC for the corresponding antibiotic with

TABLE 4 | The identity of AR gene carriers.

Sample (# isolates tested)	Detected AR genes (# positive isolates)	Gene carrier [AR gene (#isolates identified)]
Surface rinsing water (209)	*sul*1 (8), *sul*2 (1), *tet*M (30), *sul*1+*tet*M (5)	*Plesiomonas* sp. [*sul*1 (3), *sul*2 (1), *tet*M(3), *sul1*+*tet*M (2)]
Fish intestine (357)	*sul*1 (7), *sul*2 (15), *tet*L (1), *tet*M (9), *sul*1+*tet*M (1), *tet*L+ *tet*S(1),	*Aeromonas* sp. [*sul*1 (1)]; *Enterobacter* sp., [*sul*2 (7)]; *Enterococcus* sp. [*tet*L (1), *tet*L+ *tet*S (1)]; *Plesiomonas* sp. [*sul*1 (3), *sul*2 (6), *sul*1+ *tet*M (1)];
Pond Mud (269)	*sul*1 (3), *sul*2 (1)	*Aeromonas* sp. [*sul*1 (1)]; *Plesiomonas* sp. [*sul*1 (1)]
Pond water (244)	*sul*1 (5), *tet*S (1), *tet*L+*tet*S (3), *erm*C(1)	*Exiguobacterium* sp. [*sul*1 (2)]; *Staphylococcus* sp. [*erm*C (1)]; *Lactococcus* sp. [*tet*S (1), *tet*L+*tet*S (2)];
Fish feed (98)	*sul*1 (9), sul2 (1), *sul*1+*sul*2 (1), *tet*L (4), *tet*M (2), *tet*S (3), *tet*L+ *tet*M (6), *tet*L+ *tet*S (2), *tet*L+*tet*M+*tet*S (1), *erm*B (1)	*Aerococcus* sp. [*tet*M (2)]; *Bacillus* sp. [*tet*S (1), *erm*B (1)]; *Carnobacterium* sp. [*tet*L+*tet*S (1)]; *Corynebacterium* sp. [*sul*1 (1), *tet*L (2)]; *Kurthia* sp. [*tet*M (1)]; *Enterococcus* sp. [*sul*1 (1), *tet*S (2), *tet*L+*tet*M (5), *tet*L+*tet*S (1), *tet*L+*tet*M+*tet*S (1)]; *Kocuria* sp. [*sul*1 (4)]; *Lactobacillus* sp. [*tet*L (1)]; *Pseudoclavibacter* sp. [*sul*1 (1)]; *Psychrobacter* sp. [*sul*2 (1), *sul*1+*sul*2 (1)]; *Staphylococcus* sp. [*sul*1 (1)]; *Vagococcus* sp. [*tet*L (1)]

the donors, indicating the resistance genes were functional in other bacteria if acquired via horizontal gene transfer events.

Discussion

It is recognized that AR ecology, of the emergence, persistence, and dissemination of ART bacteria and AR genes in the microbial ecosystem, is much more complicated than previously thought. Up to 10^7 CFU/g ART bacteria, representing about 1% of the total bacterial population, were detected in the samples from this aquaculture farm, despite that the farm has no known history of antibiotic applications during production (Huang, 2014). Here, we report that majority of the ART isolates from the fish and aquaculture environment were resistant to two or more antibiotics.

MIC is a relatively precise measure of resistance to antibiotics. The measurement is essential for AR assessment not just because of the need to measure resistance trend, but more importantly, the MIC value is correlated to the dosage required for effective therapy. It is important to recognize that bacterial strains carrying the same resistance gene may have different MIC values, even for those from the same genus (Miranda et al., 2003). Understanding the molecular mechanisms contributing to the phenotype would be of great value to properly evaluate AR risk and control its dissemination. However, it has been difficult to compare antibiotic susceptibility results because of variation in testing methods in published studies. Most studies in the United States used CAMH broth, following NCCLS-recommended procedure (now it is CLSI), while Iso-Sensitest broth is widely used in Europe (Koeth et al., 2000). Koeth et al. (2000) conducted a study using 124 Centers for Disease Control and Prevention (CDC) reference strains compared the medium effect on MIC results, and concluded that data from the above two broth were comparable.

Due to genetic diversity of microbiota associated with both host and natural environment, bacterial media used in the studies likely have an impact on the results. Sul/Tri^r population was found abundant in microbiota across the host and environmental samples. Considering the potential effect of cultural medium on MIC results, in this study we have examined MIC for representative strains in both CAMH and BHI. The isolates had different MIC values in the two media, especially for Sul/Tri^r isolates. Approximately 67% Sul/Tri^r isolates recovered from BHI medium exhibited resistance against Sul/Tri in CAMH medium (data no shown), and some of them had much higher MIC values in BHI than that in CAMH. As shown in **Table 2**, some isolates such as *Enterococcus* sp. (17fS1, 17fS3, 18iX15, and 18fT19) and *Enterobacter* sp. (17iE3, 17iE10, 17iE11, and 17iE26) were classified as susceptible to Sul/Tri using CAMH, but showed high MIC values in BHI. In fact, the corresponding resistance determinants *sul*1 or *sul*2 were identified in the above strains with positive detection rate comparable to other AR genes, suggesting their MIC results in CAMH-Sul/Tri broth cannot represent their real resistance status against the antibiotics. As a matter of fact, CLSI has acknowledged the mismatch between MIC results of *Enterococcus* sp. using CAMH-Sul/Tri medium and resistant patterns in clinical treatments (CLSI, 2013). Moreover, although CAMH medium is widely used for MIC test, bacteria from certain genera didn't grow well in CAMH. As shown in **Table 2**, one *tet*L bearing isolate *Vagococcus* sp. could not grow in CAMH-Tet, but showed high MIC value (128 μg/ml) in BHI-Tet. These data indicated the limitations of CAMH as the medium for MIC assessment. While we have found that BHI serves the need for MIC analysis for most of the commensal isolates in this study, further validation using more reference strains and supplementation of media for cultures discriminated by BHI will be essential for methodology improvement. Moreover, ART isolates with higher MIC values are more difficult to eliminate with antibiotics. Whether the high MICs of the above strains are due to new molecular determinants or established resistance genes but with additional enhancement mechanisms are worth further investigation.

As illustrated in **Table 4**, 30 of 98 ART isolates (30.6%) from fish feed samples were found to carry one or more of the 12 AR genes examined, and the positive detection rate was much higher than those of the ART isolates from other samples, being 9.5% (34 of 357) in fish intestine, 21% (44 of 209) in surface rinsing water associated with skin microbiota, 4.1% (10 of 244) in pond water, and 1.5% (4 of 269) in pond mud sample. This result was consistent with the finding that multiple AR gene pools in high levels were detected in fish feed samples by real-time PCR (Huang, 2014). In addition, fish skin and intestine samples also contained a large number of ART bacteria and AR genes which also is in agreement with the results reported by Ye et al. (2013). Because animal and fish by-products, often rich in ART bacteria, are used in fish feed as an important protein source, it is inevitable that there is a large pool of AR genes and potentially AR gene carrying bacteria in fish feed. ART bacteria even multi-drug-resistant bacteria were reported in various types of animal feeds, such as poultry feeds (Schwalbe et al., 1999), cattle feed ingredients (Dargatz et al., 2005), and rendered animal protein products originating from poultry, cattle, and fish (Hofacre et al., 2001). Without proper treatment, fish feed rich in AR gene-carrying bacteria survived the feed manufacturing process could be a potential risk factor spreading ART bacteria in the aquaculture production system and subsequently the food chain. In fact, several genera of ART bacteria were found in multiple types of samples. For example, *Plesiomonas* sp. were detected in surface rinsing water, fish intestine, and pond mud samples, while *Aeromonas* sp. were present in fish intestine and pond mud samples. The data suggested that these microorganisms were present in both the host and farm environment, and may have been circulating within the aquaculture ecosystem.

As illustrated in **Table 4**, there was no significant correlation of the types of AR encoding genes and their carriers between fish intestine and feed, indicating that hosts (fish) potentially also have a role in the selective enrichment of or breeding certain resistant bacteria in the population. In this study, the *sul*1 gene of *Aeromonas* sp. from the fish intestine, the *sul*2 gene of *Psychrobacter* sp. and the *tet* (L) gene of *Vagococcus* sp. from the fish feed were found functional after being transferred to the corresponding recipients, suggesting that they can serve as a source of AR genes if involved in horizontal gene transfer events. Finally, representative AR genes were only found in a small percent of the ART isolates. A functional genomic analysis has already discovered a new Tet^r-encoding gene, *tet*47, from a Tet^r isolate associated with a fish intestine sample (Huang et al., 2015).

In summary, ART commensal bacteria associated with this aquaculture system with no known history of antibiotics application exhibited multi-drug-resistance (MDR). Various AR determinants were detected and 18 bacterial genera were identified among those AR gene carrying isolates. The data suggested that the aquaculture system is a rich reservoir of AR, risk factors other than direct antibiotic application, such as AR-rich feed or even environmental factors, may have played important role(s) disseminating AR in this ecosystem. Follow-up studies are needed to reveal a more comprehensive picture of AR in aquaculture production, and for targeted and effective AR mitigation in the ecosystem. Moreover, BHI medium was found more suitable for majority of the commensal bacteria examined than CAMH broth for MIC assessment.

Acknowledgments

This study is supported by Ohio Soybean Council (RF project 60031678), U.S.-UK Global Innovation Initiative Award by Institute of International Education, U.S. Department of State (RF project 60043259), and State and federal funds appropriated to The Ohio State University, Ohio Agricultural Research and Development Center (project OHOA1006). Chinese Scholarship Council provided stipend support for YH.

References

Akinbowale, O. L., Peng, H., Grant, P., and Barton, M. D. (2007). Antibiotic and heavy metal resistance in motile aeromonads and pseudomonads from rainbow trout (*Oncorhynchus mykiss*) farms in Australia. *Int. J. Antimicrob. Agents* 30, 177–182. doi: 10.1016/j.ijantimicag.2007.03.012

Andremont, A. (2003). Commensal flora may play key role in spreading antibiotic resistance. *ASM News* 69, 601–607.

Aubry-Damon, H., Grenet, K., Sall-Ndiaye, P., Che, D., Cordeiro, E., Bougnoux, M. E., et al. (2004). Antimicrobial resistance in commensal flora of pig farmers. *Emerg. Infect. Dis.* 10, 873–879. doi: 10.3201/eid1005.030735

Austin, B. (2002). The bacterial microflora of fish. *Sci. World J.* 2, 558–572. doi: 10.1100/tsw.2002.137

Bhullar, K., Waglechner, N., Pawlowski, A., Koteva, K., Banks, E. D., Johnston, M. D., et al. (2012). Antibiotic resistance is prevalent in an isolated cave microbiome. *PLoS ONE* 7:e34953. doi: 10.1371/journal.pone.0034953

Budiati, T., Rusul, G., Wan-Abdullah, W. N., Arip, Y. M., Ahmad, R., and Thong, K. L. (2013). Prevalence, antibiotic resistance and plasmid profiling of *Salmonella* in catfish (*Clarias gariepinus*) and tilapia (*Tilapia mossambica*) obtained from wet markets and ponds in Malaysia. *Aquaculture* 37, 127–132. doi: 10.1016/j.aquaculture.2012.11.003

CLSI. (2013). *Perfomance Standards for Antimicrobial Susceptibility Testing; Twenty-Third Informational Supplement.* Wayne, PA: Clinical and Laboratory Standards Institue.

Dagert, M., and Ehrlich, S. D. (1979). Prolonged incubation in calcium chloride improves the competence of *Escherichia coli* cells. *Gene* 6, 23–28. doi: 10.1016/0378-1119(79)90082-9

Dallenne, C., Da Costa, A., Decré, D., Favier, C., and Arlet, G. (2010). Development of a set of multiplex PCR assays for the detection of genes encoding important β-lactamases in Enterobacteriaceae. *J. Antimicrob. Chemother.* 65, 490–495. doi: 10.1093/jac/dkp498

Dargatz, D. A., Strohmeyer, R. A., Morley, P. S., Hyatt, D. R., and Salman, M. D. (2005). Characterization of *Escherichia coli* and *Salmonella enterica* from cattle feed ingredients. *Foodborne Pathog. Dis.* 2, 341–347. doi: 10.1089/fpd.2005.2.341

D'Costa, V. M., King, C. E., Kalan, L., Morar, M., Sung, W. W., Schwarz, C., et al. (2011). Antibiotic resistance is ancient. *Nature* 477, 457–461. doi: 10.1038/nature10388

Duran, G. M., and Marshall, D. L. (2005). Ready-to-eat shrimp as an international vehicle of antibiotic-resistant bacteria. *J. Food Prot.* 68, 2395–2401.

Hofacre, C. L., White, D. G., Maurer, J. J., Morales, C., Lobsinger, C., and Hudson, C. (2001). Characterization of antibiotic-resistant bacteria in rendered animal products. *Avian Dis.* 45, 953–961. doi: 10.2307/1592874

Huang, Y. (2014). *Antibiotic Resistance in Aquaculture Production.* Ph.D. dissertation, The Ohio State University, Columbus, OH.

Huang, Y., Zhang, L., and Wang, H. H. (2015). Identification of a new tetracycline resistance determinant *tet47* from fish intestine. *J. Food Prot.* 78, 1581–1585. doi: 10.4315/0362-028X.JFP-15-025

Kerrn, M. B. (2002). Susceptibility of Danish *Escherichia coli* strains isolated from urinary tract infections and bacteraemia, and distribution of sul genes conferring sulphonamide resistance. *J. Antimicrob. Chemother.* 50, 513–516. doi: 10.1093/jac/dkf164

Koeth, L. M., King, A., Knight, H., May, J., Miller, L. A., Phillips, I., et al. (2000). Comparison of cation-adjusted Mueller-Hinton broth with Iso-Sensitest broth for the NCCLS broth microdilution method. *J. Antimicrob. Chemother.* 46, 369–376. doi: 10.1093/jac/46.3.369

Koike, S., Krapac, I. G., Oliver, H. D., Yannarell, A. C., Chee-Sanford, J. C., Aminov, R. I., et al. (2007). Monitoring and source tracking of tetracycline resistance genes in lagoons and groundwater adjacent to swine production facilities over a 3-year period. *Appl. Environ. Microbiol.* 73, 4813–4823. doi: 10.1128/AEM.00665-07

Li, X., Alvarez, V., Harper, W. J., and Wang, H. H. (2011). Persistent, toxin-antitoxin system-independent, tetracycline resistance-encoding plasmid from a dairy *Enterococcus faecium* isolate. *Appl. Environ. Microbiol.* 77, 7096–7103. doi: 10.1128/AEM.05168-11

Li, X., and Wang, H. H. (2010). Tetracycline resistance associated with commensal bacteria from representative ready-to-consume deli and restaurant foods. *J. Food Prot.* 73, 1841–1848.

Manuzon, M. Y., Hanna, S. E., Luo, H., Yu, Z., Harper, W. J., and Wang, H. H. (2007). Quantitative assessment of the tetracycline resistance gene pool in cheese samples by real-time TaqMan PCR. *Appl. Environ. Microbiol.* 73, 1676–1677. doi: 10.1128/AEM.01994-06

McIntosh, D., Cunningham, M., Ji, B., Fekete, F. A., Parry, E. M., Clark, S. E., et al. (2008). Transferable, multiple antibiotic and mercury resistance in Atlantic Canadian isolates of *Aeromonas salmonicida* subsp. salmonicida is associated with carriage of an IncA/C plasmid similar to the Salmonella enterica plasmid pSN254. *J. Antimicrob. Chemother.* 61, 1221–1228. doi: 10.1093/jac/dkn123

Mcintyre, D. A., and Harlander, S. K. (1989). Improved electroporation efficiency of intact *Lactococcus lactis subsp. lactis* cells grown in defined mediat. *Appl. Environ. Microbiol.* 55, 2621–2626.

Miranda, C. D., Kehrenberg, C., Ulep, C., Schwarz, S., and Roberts, M. C. (2003). Diversity of tetracycline resistance genes in bacteria from Chilean salmon farms. *Appl. Environ. Microbiol.* 47, 883–888.

Oh, E. G., Son, K. T., Yu, H., Lee, T. S., Lee, H. J., Shin, S., et al. (2011). Antimicrobial resistance of *Vibrio parahaemolyticus* and *Vibrio alginolyticus* strains isolated from farmed fish in Korea from 2005 through 2007. *J. Food Prot.* 74, 380–386. doi: 10.4315/0362-028X.JFP-10-307

Österblad, M., Norrdahl, K., Korpimäki, E., and Huovinen, P. (2001). How wild are wild mammals? *Nature* 409, 37–38. doi: 10.1038/35051173

Penders, J., and Stobberingh, E. E. (2008). Antibiotic resistance of motile aeromonads in indoor catfish and eel farms in the southern part of the Netherlands. *Int. J. Antimicrob. Agents* 31, 261–265. doi: 10.1016/j.ijantimicag.2007.10.002

Rebouças, R. H., de Sousa, O. V., Lima, A. S., Vasconcelos, F. R., de Carvalho, P. B., Vieira, R. H. S., et al. (2011). Antimicrobial resistance profile of *Vibrio* species isolated from marine shrimp farming environments (*Litopenaeus vannamei*) at Ceará, Brazil. *Environ. Res.* 111, 21–24. doi: 10.1016/j.envres.2010.09.012

Rhodes, G., Huys, G., Swings, J., Mcgann, P., Hiney, M., Smith, P., et al. (2000). Distribution of oxytetracycline resistance plasmids between aeromonads in hospital and aquaculture environments: implication of Tn 1721 in dissemination of the tetracycline resistance determinant Tet A. *Appl. Environ. Microbiol.* 66, 3883–3890. doi: 10.1128/AEM.66.9.3883-3890.2000

Ribeiro, R. V., Reis, E. M. F., Reis, C. M. F., Freitas-Almeida, A. C., and Rodrigues, D. P. (2010). Incidence and antimicrobial resistance of enteropathogens isolated from an integrated aquaculture system. *Lett. Appl. Microbiol.* 51, 611–618. doi: 10.1111/j.1472-765X.2010.02946.x

Rosvoll, T. C. S., Pedersen, T., Sletvold, H., Johnsen, P. J., Sollid, J. E., Simonsen, G. S., et al. (2010). PCR-based plasmid typing in *Enterococcus faecium* strains reveals widely distributed pRE25-, pRUM-, pIP501- and pHTbeta-related replicons associated with glycopeptide resistance and stabilizing toxin-antitoxin systems. *FEMS Immunol. Med. Microbiol.* 58, 254–268. doi: 10.1111/j.1574-695X.2009.00633.x

Schwalbe, R. S., McIntosh, A. C., Qaiyumi, S., Johnson, J. A., and Morris, J. G. (1999). Isolation of vancomycin-resistant enterococci from animal feed in USA. *Lancet* 353, 722. doi: 10.1016/S0140-6736(98)05441-5

Shah, S. Q. A., Cabello, F. C., L'abée-Lund, T. M., Tomova, A., Godfrey, H. P., Buschmann, A. H., et al. (2014). Antimicrobial resistance and antimicrobial resistance genes in marine bacteria from salmon aquaculture and non-aquaculture sites. *Environ. Microbiol.* 16, 1310–1320. doi: 10.1111/1462-2920.12421

Sommer, M. O. A., Dantas, G., and Church, G. M. (2009). Functional characterization of the antibiotic resistance reservoir in the human microflora. *Science* 325, 1128–1131. doi: 10.1126/science.1176950

Sørum, M., Johnsen, P. J., Aasnes, B., Rosvoll, T., Kruse, H., Sundsfjord, A., et al. (2006). Prevalence, persistence, and molecular characterization of glycopeptide-resistant enterococci in Norwegian poultry and poultry farmers 3 to 8 years after the ban on avoparcin. *Appl. Environ. Microbiol.* 72, 516–521. doi: 10.1128/AEM.72.1.516-521.2006

Venter, J. C., Remington, K., Heidelberg, J. F., Halpern, A. L., Rusch, D., Eisen, J. A., et al. (2004). Environmental genome shotgun sequencing of the Sargasso Sea. *Science* 304, 66–74. doi: 10.1126/science.1093857

Wang, H. H., Manuzon, M., Lehman, M., Wan, K., Luo, H., Wittum, T. E., et al. (2006). Food commensal microbes as a potentially important avenue in transmitting antibiotic resistance genes. *FEMS Microbiol. Lett.* 254, 226–231. doi: 10.1111/j.1574-6968.2005.00030.x

Wang, H. H., and Schaffner, D. W. (2011). Antibiotic resistance: how much do we know and where do we go from here? *Appl. Environ. Microbiol.* 77, 7093–7095. doi: 10.1128/AEM.06565-11

Ye, L., Lu, Z., Li, X., Shi, L., Huang, Y., and Wang, H. H. (2013). Antibiotic-resistant bacteria associated with retail aquaculture products from Guangzhou, China. *J. Food Prot.* 76, 295–301. doi: 10.4315/0362-028X.JFP-12-288

Zhanel, G. G., Karlowsky, J. A., Harding, G. K. M., Carrie, A., Mazzulli, T., Low, D. E., et al. (2000). A Canadian national surveillance study of urinary tract isolates from outpatients: comparison of the activities of trimethoprim-sulfamethoxazole, ampicillin, mecillinam, nitrofurantoin, and ciprofloxacin. *Antimicrob. Agents Chemother.* 44, 1089–1092. doi: 10.1128/AAC.44.4.1089-1092.2000

Zhang, L. (2011). *Establishment and Development of Antibiotic Resistant Bacteria in Host Gastrointestinal Tract—Food, Drug, or are We Born with It?* Ph.D. dissertation, The Ohio State University, Columbus, OH.

Zhang, L., Kinkelaar, D., Huang, Y., Li, Y., Li, X., and Wang, H. H. (2011). Acquired antibiotic resistance: are we born with it? *Appl. Environ. Microbiol.* 77, 7134–7141. doi: 10.1128/AEM.05087-11

20

$bla_{CTX-M-152}$, a Novel Variant of CTX-M-group-25, Identified in a Study Performed on the Prevalence of Multidrug Resistance among Natural Inhabitants of River Yamuna, India

Mudsser Azam[1†], Arif T. Jan[2†] and Qazi M. R. Haq[1*]

[1] Microbiology Research Laboratory, Department of Biosciences, Jamia Millia Islamia, New Delhi, India, [2] Molecular Biology Laboratory, School of Biotechnology, Yeungnam University, Gyeongsan, South Korea

***Correspondence:**
Qazi M. R. Haq
haqqmr@gmail.com

† These authors have contributed equally to this work.

Natural environment influenced by anthropogenic activities creates selective pressure for acquisition and spread of resistance genes. In this study, we determined the prevalence of Extended Spectrum β-Lactamases producing gram negative bacteria from the River Yamuna, India, and report the identification and characterization of a novel CTX-M gene variant $bla_{CTX-M-152}$. Of the total 230 non-duplicate isolates obtained from collected water samples, 40 isolates were found positive for ESBL production through Inhibitor-Potentiation Disc Diffusion test. Based on their resistance profile, 3% were found exhibiting pandrug resistance (PDR), 47% extensively drug resistance (XDR), and remaining 50% showing multidrug resistant (MDR). Following screening and antimicrobial profiling, characterization of ESBLs (bla_{TEM} *and* bla_{CTX-M}), and mercury tolerance determinants (*mer*P, *mer*T, *and mer*B) were performed. In addition to abundance of $bla_{TEM-116}$ (57.5%) and $bla_{CTX-M-15}$ (37.5%), bacteria were also found to harbor other variants of ESBLs like $bla_{CTX-M-71}$ (5%), $bla_{CTX-M-3}$ (7.5%), $bla_{CTX-M-32}$ (2.5%), $bla_{CTX-M-152}$ (7.5%), $bla_{CTX-M-55}$ (2.5%), along with some non-ESBLs; bla_{TEM-1} (25%) and bla_{OXY} (5%). Additionally, co-occurrence of mercury tolerance genes were observed among 40% of isolates. *In silico* studies of the new variant, $bla_{CTX-M-152}$ were conducted through modeling for the generation of structure followed by docking to determine its catalytic profile. CTX-M-152 was found to be an out-member of CTX-M-group-25 due to Q26H, T154A, G89D, P99S, and D146G substitutions. Five residues Ser70, Asn132, Ser237, Gly238, and Arg273 were found responsible for positioning of cefotaxime into the active site through seven H-bonds with binding energy of -7.6 Kcal/mol. Despite small active site, co-operative interactions of Ser237 and Arg276 were found actively contributing to its high catalytic efficiency. To the best of our knowledge, this is the first report of $bla_{CTX-M-152}$ of CTX-M-group-25 from Indian subcontinent. Taking a note of bacteria harboring such high proportion of multidrug and mercury resistance determinants, their presence in natural water resources employed for human consumption increases the chances of potential risk to human health. Hence, deeper insights into mechanisms pertaining to resistance development are required to frame out strategies to tackle the situation and prevent acquisition and dissemination of resistance determinants so as to combat the escalating burden of infectious diseases.

Keywords: antibiotics, ESBL, mechanisms of resistance, polluted environment, resistance genes

INTRODUCTION

Extended spectrum β-lactamases (ESBLs), which have emerged in response to the widespread use of cephalosporins, represent the most diverse group of class A β-lactamases. With more than 220 variants of bla_{TEM} and 172 different bla_{CTX-M} variants reported to date, these active site serine β-lactamases (bla_{TEM} and bla_{CTX-M}) represent the most prevalent β-Lactamases among members of Enterobacteriaceae (http://www.lahey.org/studies). By conferring higher hydrolytic activity, ESBLs exhibit a high level of resistance toward aminopenicillins (ampicillin or amoxicillin), carboxypenicillins (carbenicillin or tricarcillin), ureidopenicillins (piperacillin), cephalosporins (cephalothin, cephaloridine, and cefuroxime), oxi-imino cephalosporins (cefotaxime and ceftriaxone), cefepime, and cefpirome. Based on the broad host range and efficiency of conjugation, bla_{TEM} and bla_{CTX-M}genes after several mobilization events via horizontal gene transfer, have now became part of plasmids among different bacterial species (Thomas and Nielsen, 2005; Barlow et al., 2008; Woodford et al., 2009).

The emergence of ESBL producing isolates have been often studied in clinics because they are commonly associated with outbreaks or sporadic infections (Kohlenberg et al., 2012; Walsh, 2013). However, a lot of studies have also been dedicated toward investigation of ESBL producers among microbial inhabitants of aquatic environments that receive a continuous influx of treated and untreated sewage (Prado et al., 2008; Chagas et al., 2011; Korzeniewska and Harnisz, 2013; Wellington et al., 2013). There are reports that suggest an additional selection effect by partially metabolized (10–90%) antibiotics used for human and animal health care in aquatic ecosystems (Kummerer, 2009; Harnisz, 2013). Concomitantly, the persistence of mercury in sewage has enabled bacteria to develop an array of resistance mechanisms based on clustering of genes either on the chromosome or plasmids (Jan et al., 2009; Jackson et al., 2011). Co-selection for metal and drug resistance determinants has resulted in conferring an advantage to bacteria that helps their survival in heavily polluted environments (Seiler and Berendonk, 2012; Zhou et al., 2015). Taken together, these findings highlight the necessity for controlling the emergence, and therefore, the dissemination of multi-drug and mercury resistance in bacteria through aquatic environments.

Antibiotic resistance has worsened in developing countries owing to compromised sanitary conditions, which exacerbate movement of genes via mobile genetic elements (Schlüter et al., 2007; Kelly et al., 2009; Knapp et al., 2010). The disease burden of India is highest among different countries of the world (GARP-India, 2011). In this regard, Study of the Monitoring of Antimicrobial Resistance Trends (SMART) revealed *E. coli* in being the most prevalent pathogen among the top five resistant gram-negative bacteria, causing 47.8% of intra-abdominal and 44.3% of urinary tract infections worldwide (Morrissey et al., 2013). In another resistance surveillance program carried out in India, Mendes et al. (2013) found that nearly 78% of *E. coli* and 64% of *Klebsiella spp.* carry ESBL determinants imparting resistance (Mendes et al., 2013). Despite these studies, there still lies paucity in the available information regarding prevalence of resistance determinants among bacteria and the pattern of antimicrobial resistance they exhibit. Hence, it becomes necessary to have an understanding of potential genetic variables that lead to acquisition of resistance and information regarding ESBL producers ($ESBL^+$) among the microbial inhabitants of aquatic environments. The present study was conducted to investigate the prevalence of ESBL genes (bla_{TEM} and bla_{CTX-M}) and the pattern of antimicrobial resistance among the natural inhabitants of river Yamuna, India, in order to have an insight of the resistance mechanisms that operate against β-lactam antibiotics. A novel variant of bla_{CTX-M} gene identified in the study was characterized to unravel its catalytic profile through *in silico* studies. As the river receives higher amount of discharges (both treated and untreated), it raises serious concerns as water from the River Yamuna after passing through different stages of treatment processes, is used for several domestic, industrial and agricultural purposes. In studies of Sehgal et al. (2012) and Malik et al. (2014), they report presence of higher amount of mercury along with other metals in the samples collected from river Yamuna, India (Sehgal et al., 2012; Malik et al., 2014). Taking this into account, an investigation of *mer* operon genes as a representation of tolerance to metals was carried out to determine its role in the selection and survival of these isolates in polluted environments. The present study provides useful information regarding occurrence of multidrug resistance among bacterial inhabitants of aquatic environment that exhibit broader risk for community infections. From the study, it becomes evident that polluted water bodies acts as a pool for the emergence of new variants; thereby highlights the need to carry out in depth studies preferably toward understanding the factors that led to transfer and as such acquisition of different determinants among bacteria in their natural habitats.

METHODOLOGY

Sample Collection and Screening for Identification of Bacteria

Water samples were collected from the 22 km Delhi stretch of the Yamuna River, starting from upstream of the Wazirabad barrage to downstream of the Okhla barrage. The Yamuna River primarily receives sewage (treated, partially treated, or untreated) from domestic and industrial settings. For this study, samples were collected aseptically during March 2012–August 2014 from 13 different sites ~100–150 m downstream of major drains discharging into the river. Soon after collection, samples were screened for the presence of bacterial isolates using nutrient agar and nutrient broth. Lactose fermenting Gram negative bacterial colonies were initially assessed based on their characteristic growth on MacConkey agar and Eosin Methylin Blue (EMB) agar followed by the IMViC standard biochemical tests (Clinical and Laboratory Standards Institute, 2010). Isolates from single site that were found to have same phenotypes such as growth characteristics, colony morphology, and resistance phenotypes, were excluded from the study. Further confirmation of all non-duplicate phenotypically identified bacterial isolates was carried out through analysis of the 16S rRNA gene. Subsequent to amplification of the desired (~685 bp) fragment that exhibit maximum variability across different groups of bacteria, sequencing reaction was carried out to get isolates correctly annotated with their respective group members. In case, similarity with more than one group was observed, they were re-sequenced for larger (~1250 bp) fragment size of the 16S rRNA gene for identification.

Antibiotic Susceptibility Tests

After identification, screening for ESBL production was performed against third generation cephalosporins (ceftazidime, cefotaxime, and ceftriaxone) by the Kirby Bauer disc diffusion method using Mueller Hinton Agar (MHA) plates. Isolates with a zone diameter of ≤22, ≤27, and ≤25 mm corresponding to ceftazidime, cefotaxime, and ceftriaxone, respectively, were considered ESBL producers. An Inhibitor-Potentiation Disc Diffusion (IPDD) test was then performed by placing discs containing ceftazidime (30 μg) and cefotaxime (30 μg) alone and in combination with clavulanic acid (10 μg) 30 mm apart on MHA plates. A ≥5 mm increase in zone diameter around the disc with antibiotic plus clavulanic acid relative to the discs with antibiotics alone was considered positive for ESBL production (Clinical and Laboratory Standards Institute, 2012). *K. pneumonia* ATCC 700603 and *E. coli* ATCC 25922 were used as ESBL positive and negative controls, respectively.

The *in vitro* antimicrobial susceptibilities against 21 antibiotics belonging to 13 different classes (β-lactam, aminoglycosides, fluoroquinolones, polymixins, rifampicins, tetracyclines, and trimethoprim from HiMedia labs., India) were then investigated according to the Clinical Laboratory Standards Institute guidelines (Clinical and Laboratory Standards Institute, 2012). The minimum inhibitory concentrations (MICs) against ceftazidime (CAZ), ceftazidime + clavulanic acid (CAC), cefotaxime (CTX), and cefotaxime + clavulanic acid (CEC) were determined for all ESBL-producing isolates by the broth micro-dilution method using Luria Bertania broth. Results were interpreted according to the CLSI guidelines (Clinical and Laboratory Standards Institute, 2012).

Determination of Mercury Tolerance among Bacterial Isolates

Screened isolates were checked for tolerance to mercury by streaking on luria agar plates containing 0.02 mg/L mercuric chloride ($HgCl_2$). This value was ~10 times higher than its permissible limit of 0.002 mg/L for drinking water (US-EPA, http://water.epa.gov/drink/). Isolates showing tolerance to mercury were selected for MIC determination against various concentrations of mercuric chloride (0.02–20 mg/L) by the broth micro-dilution method using Luria Bertania broth. The MIC was defined as the lowest concentration of $HgCl_2$ at which no growth was seen for the isolates in the culture media. *E. coli* ATCC 25922 was used as negative control.

Detection of Genes Imparting Resistance to Bacteria

Screened bacterial isolates were analyzed for the presence of ESBLs (*bla*$_{TEM}$ and *bla*$_{CTX\text{-}M}$) and *mer* operon determinants (*mer*P, *mer*T, and *mer*B) conferring resistance to a broad range of antibiotics and mercury. Overnight grown cultures were used for isolation of genomic DNA by phenol-chloroform-isoamyl (PCI) method and plasmid DNA by alkaline lysis method using Qiagen kit. After retrieving information from NCBI, multiple sequence alignment using ClustalW option of the BioEdit program, was performed for selection of region to design gene specific primers. After procurement of gene specific primers (**Table 1**), amplification corresponding to full or partial length (*bla*$_{TEM}$, *bla*$_{CTX\text{-}M\text{-}1}$, *bla*$_{CTX\text{-}M\text{-}25}$, *mer*B, *mer*T, and *mer*P) gene sequences were accomplished under the following cycle conditions: 94°C for 5 min (initial denaturation) followed by 30 cycles of denaturation at 94°C for 1 min, annealing at temperatures specific for each primer set (54.5–62°C) for 30 s and extension at 72°C for 1 min followed by final extension at 72°C for 10 min. Following purification using a QIA quick spin column (Qiagen Inc.), samples corresponding to different gene products were sequenced using an automated sequencer (ABI 1377) at Xcelris Lab (Gujarat, India). Additionally, isolates harboring the new identified variant (*bla*$_{CTX\text{-}M\text{-}152}$) were analyzed for localization of the gene on chromosomal DNA and/or plasmid DNA by PCR. A reaction of 16S rRNA gene was used as control in case plasmid DNA was used as template for PCR to minimize chances of contamination of chromosomal DNA.

In silico Analysis of Variants

Sequences of different genes were analyzed for genetic relatedness corresponding to their respective group members followed by identification of variations using ClustalW in the BioEdit 5.0.9 sequence analysis software and the MEGA6 software program. The complete coding sequence (CDS) of novel variant represented here as *bla*$_{CTX\text{-}M\text{-}152}$ of *Kluyvera georgiana* was translated using the Expasy translation tool (www.expasy.org/translate). However, to obtain insight into the relationship between amino acid substitutions and affinity for the substrate (cefotaxime), we conducted modeling and docking studies of the variant *bla*$_{CTX\text{-}M\text{-}152}$with respect to its ligand, cefotaxime.

Analysis of Deleterious Substitution by SIFT

Sorting Intolerant from Tolerant (SIFT), which predicts the phenotypic effect of amino acid substitutions on a protein, works

TABLE 1 | Sequences of primers used for the detection of different genes among ESBL^{+} isolates.

Gene type	Primer	Sequence	Product size (bp)	Reference
16S rDNA	ID-F	5′-GGCGGACGGGTGAGTAATG- 3′	685	Designed primers for this study.
	ID-R	5′-ATCCTGTTTGCTCCCCACG- 3′		
	RRF	5′-GGCGGACGGGTGAGTAATG-3′	1250	
	RRR	5′-GAAGTCGGAATCGCTAGTAATCG-3′		
TEM	TEM-F	5′-ATGAGTATTCAACATTTCCGTGT- 3′	861	
	TEM-R	5′-TTA CCA ATG CTT AAT CAG TGA GG- 3′		
CTX-M	CTX-MF	5′-SCVATGTGCAGYACCAGTAA- 3′	480	
	CTX-MR	5′-GCTGCCGGTYTTATCVCC- 3′		
CTX-M-1	CM1F	5′-ATGGTTAAAAAATCACTGCGYCAGTTCACGC- 3′	875	
	CM1R	5′-TTACAAACCGTYGGTGACGATTTTAGCCG- 3′		
CTX-M-2	CM2F	5′-ATGATGACTCAGAGCATTCGCC- 3′	742	
	CM2R	5′-TCGTTGGTGGTGCCATAATCTCC- 3′		
CTX-M-8	CM8F	5′-AACGCACAGACGCTCTACC- 3′	517	
	CM8R	5′-GGGTAGCCCAGCCTGAAT- 3′		
CTX-M-9	CM9F	5′-ATGGTGACAAAGAGAGTGCAACGG- 3′	875	
	CM9R	5′-TTACAGCCCTTCGGCGATGATTC- 3′		
CTX-M-25	CM25F	5′-ATGATGAGAAAAAGCGTAAGGCGGG- 3′	876	
	CM25R	5′-TTAATAACCGTCGGTGACAATTCTGGC- 3′		
merP	merP-F	5′-ATGAAGAAACTGTTTGCCTCC- 3′	276	
	merP-R	5′-TCACTGCTTGACGCTGGACG- 3′		
merT	merT-F	5′-TTAATAGAAAAATGGAACGAC- 3′	351	
	merT-R	5′-ATGTCTGAACCACAAAACGGG- 3′		
merB	merB-F	5′-ATGAAGCTCGCCCCATATATTTTAG- 3′	667	
	merB-R	5′-TCACGGTGTCCTAGATGACATGG- 3′		

on the principle of correlation of protein evolution with protein function (Ng and Henikoff, 2001, 2003). Here, we submitted a query in the form of protein sequences to detect the nature of substitutions. SIFT analysis was conducted by allowing the algorithm to search for homologous sequences using the default settings (SWISS-PROT 45 and TrEMBL 28 databases, median conservation score 3.00, remove sequences >90% identical to query sequence). This generated alignments with homologous sequences and assigned scores to each residue between 0 and 1 for evolutionary conservation and intolerance and tolerance to substitution. SIFT scores <0.05 are predicted by the algorithm to be intolerant (deleterious amino acid substitutions), whereas scores >0.05 are considered tolerant (Ng and Henikoff, 2003). A higher tolerance index of a particular amino acid substitution is associated with a lower probable impact.

Homology Modeling for Structure Prediction of CTX-M-152

To retrieve potential structural templates for homology modeling of *bla*$_{\text{CTX-M-152}}$, *bla*$_{\text{CTX-M}}$ sequences were searched using the protein data bank (PDB). Rather than finding a close associate, we found that crystal structures for PDB ID 1YLJ (CTX-M-9) and 1IYQ (Toho-1) showed the highest homology (85 and 86%) with that of *bla*$_{\text{CTX-M-152}}$. Using these as a template for modeling of our protein (KJ461948) by I-TASSER (an online server for modeling), the best model was selected based on the highest C-score and lowest Z-score. Simultaneously, protein modeling was conducted manually using Modeller version 9.12. Upon selection of the best model with the lowest DOPE score, a comparative study of both models (obtained from I-TASSER and Modeller 9.12) with our template was performed. The model with the lowest RMSD was then selected for further studies. Verification of the selected model for structural constrains was conducted using a Ramachandran plot generated with the Rampage server tool (http://mordred.bioc.cam.ac.uk/~rapper/rampage). Prior to docking studies, the verified structure was submitted to the Dogsite Server (http://dogsite.zbh.uni-hamburg.de/) for potential active site prediction. This tool predicted the existence of 10 different pockets, and the one with the highest P score was selected as the most reliable active site pocket and considered to have potential active site residues.

Docking of Cefotaxime with CTX-M-152

Following retrieval of the cefotaxime structure from Drug Bank (Accession no. DB00493), it was docked against the modeled structure of CTX-M-152 using Autodock 4.2. Before docking, the ligand was prepared by adding partial Gasteiger charges and defining free rotatable bonds. Simultaneously, the target structure (CTX-M-152) was prepared by removing solvent (water) molecules and adding non-polar hydrogen atoms. An affinity grid was generated using the Autogrid program of the Autodock package with a defined spacing of 1 Å and grid size of 50 × 50 × 50 Å. pI was calculated using the Compute pI/Mw tool provided by Expasy and crosschecked by ProtParam.

RESULTS

Screening for ESBL Producing Bacterial Isolates

Of the total 230 non-duplicate bacterial isolates, 40 isolates belonging to different groups of Gram negative bacteria were found to be ESBL producers based on the Kirby Bauer disc diffusion (**Table S1**) and IPDD tests (**Table S2**). Subsequent analysis of sequences corresponding to 16S rRNA genes from all 40 isolates for their correct representation revealed 34 to be *E. coli*, while the remaining isolates were *Klebsiella pneumonia* (1), *Aeromona sps.* (2), *Klebsiella oxytoca* (1), *K. georgiana* (1), and *Acinetobacter junii* (1) (**Table 2**). Screening of ESBL$^+$ isolates revealed MIC values ≥512 mg/L for 25 (63%) isolates against cefotaxime, 17 (43%) isolates against ceftazidime, and 28 (70%) isolates against ceftriaxone (**Table 2**). Among the ESBL$^+$ isolates, five (MRA11, MRC17, MRE18, MRE31, and MRE44) were resistant to a combination of ceftazidime + clavulanic acid and cefotaxime + clavulanic acid, and showed the highest resistance toward third generation cephalosporins. Resistance to fluoroquinolones was found to be increased with 55% (22/40) of isolates being resistant to ciprofloxacin and 28% (11/40) for levofloxacin and ofloxacin among ESBL$^+$ isolates. The test isolates were reported to have high resistance level for ampicillin (100%) and rifampicin (93%), while on other hand, the resistance level was low for amikacin (5%) and imipenem (8%) (**Figure 1**).

Based on European Centre for Disease Prevention and Control (ECDC) and the Centre for Disease Control and Prevention (CDC) categorization, 3% of the 40 isolates investigated in this study were PDR, 47% XDR and 50% MDR. Regardless of the origin or mode of action, resistance was observed for all classes of antibiotics among all isolates, with susceptibility slightly higher for polymixin B and tobramycin. Information regarding patterns of resistance for these isolates against different classes of antibiotics is summarized in **Tables S3A,B**. All bacterial isolates in the test library were multidrug resistant against at least four classes of antibiotics, with one strain represented as PDR being resistant to at least one agent of all 13 categories.

Mercury Tolerance among ESBL$^+$ Isolates

Screening of ESBL$^+$ isolates for their ability to tolerate various concentrations of mercury revealed that 40% of isolates were tolerant to 2 mg/L (10^3 times higher than its permissible limit of 0.002 mg/L for drinking water), while the rest were tolerant to 0.2 mg/L of mercury. Around, 23% isolates tolerating high concentrations of mercuric chloride (2 mg/L), were found positive for presence of all three (*mer*T, *mer*P, and *mer*B) *mer* operon genes. Presence of *mer* operon genes are believed for attributing bacterial isolates with the resistance phenotype. To our surprise, an *E. coli* isolate (MRC3) that tested negative for all three *mer* operon genes, was also found to tolerate high concentration of mercury (2 mg/L), attributed to the presence of resistance determinants other than that used in the study.

Screening for Determinants Imparting Dual Resistance to Bacteria

β-lactamase genes detected more often among the ESBL$^+$ isolates include $bla_{TEM-116}$ (23, 57.5%) and $bla_{CTX-M-15}$ (15, 37.5%). Additionally, they were found to harbor $bla_{CTX-M-71}$ (2, 5%), $bla_{CTX-M-3}$ (3, 7.5%), $bla_{CTX-M-32}$ (1, 2.5%), $bla_{CTX-M-152}$ (3, 7.5%), $bla_{CTX-M-55}$ (1, 2.5%), and some non-ESBL genes like bla_{TEM-1} (10, 25%) and bla_{OXY} (2, 5%) (**Table 2**). All of the CTX-M encoding isolates harbored genes with sequence homology to members of group 1 (i.e., CTX-M-15, 3, 32, 55, and 71), except for one sequence [later denoted $bla_{CTX-M-152}$ by lahey's organization (www.lahey.org)] that showed maximum similarity to a CTX-M-group-25 member, $bla_{CTX-M-78}$ (Rodríguez et al., 2010). The *mer* operon consist of genes mostly associated with functions such as transport (*mer*T and *mer*P), regulation (*mer*R and *mer*D), and reduction (*mer*A and *mer*B; Jan et al., 2009). Of 40 ESBL$^+$ isolates, 26 (65%) and 28 (70%) were positive for *mer*P and *mer*T genes respectively that encodes for membrane transport proteins. The *mer*B gene encoding organomercurial lyase, which catalyzes protonolytic cleavage of the carbon-mercury bond of organomercurials, was amplified from 20 (50%) isolates (**Table 2**). Taken together, 14 bacterial isolates were found harboring broad spectrum *mer* operon genes (*mer*T, *mer*P, and *mer*B), known for their significant contribution in achieving tolerant phenotype against mercury. One isolate was found to have only *mer*B gene. In comparison to isolate MRC24 which was found negative for all genes, five isolates were found to harbor both ESBL genes (bla_{TEM} and bla_{CTX-M}) and determinants of the *mer* operon (*mer*P, *mer*T, and *mer*B) responsible for imparting resistance to a broad range of antibiotics and mercury.

Comparative Studies of CTX-M Variants

Sequences of bla_{TEM} were found to be highly homologous to TEM-1 and TEM-116, while those corresponding to the bla_{CTX-M} gene displayed a disparity in their homology with five different members of the CTX-M-group-1 viz. CTX-M-3, CTX-M-15, CTX-M-32, CTX-M-55, and CTX-M-71 (**Figure 2**). The conserved motifs involved in cefotaxime hydrolysis found in CTX-M-1, were also conserved among variants obtained in the study (**Figure S1**). The nucleotide sequence of one variant of CTX-M gene denoted CTX-M-152 was found to be highly homologous with members of the CTX-M-group-25. Unlike CTX-M-1, CTX-M-25 like β-lactamases has been observed less frequently worldwide. Similar to our study, two other novel variants, CTX-M-94 and CTX-M-100 belonging to group-25 were reported in Israel (Vervoort et al., 2012). The $bla_{CTX-M-152}$ variant identified in *K. georgiana* isolate was found localized on chromosomal DNA while those identified

TABLE 2 | Characterization of gene sequences along with their MIC values for different antibiotics and heavy metals among ESBL^{+} bacterial isolates.

	β -Lactamases genes		GenBank Accession nos.		*mer* operon genes			MIC values (μg/ml)					
	ESBL	Non-ESBL	16S rRNA gene	β-lactamases genes	*mer*P	*mer*T	*mer*B	CAZ	CAC	CTX	CEC	CTR	$HgCl_2$
Klebsiella pneumoniae MRA3	TEM-116	–	KJ906614		–	+	–	>512	0.38	512	0.125	>512	2
Aeromonas sps MRA5	TEM-116, CTX-M-15	–	KJ957158	KJ923000, KM873149	+	+	+	>512	0.75	512	0.25	128	20
Aeromonas sps MRA10	TEM-116, CTX-M-15	–	KJ957159	KJ923001, KM873161	–	–	–	4	1	16	0.75	4	2
E. coli MRA11	TEM-116	TEM-1	KJ957160	KJ923003, KJ923002	+	+	+	512	>4	512	>1	>512	2
Klebsiella oxytoca MRA13	TEM-116	–	KJ957161	KJ923004	+	+	+	64	1.5	32	0.25	4	20
E. coli MRB2	TEM-116	–	KJ906615	KJ923005	+	+	–	256	2	64	0.5	64	2
E. coli MRB6	TEM-116, CTX-M-71	–	KJ906619	KJ923006, KM873170	+	+	+	32	0.5	>512	0.75	>512	20
E. coli MRC2	TEM-116, CTX-M-15	–	KJ906616	KJ923008, KM873150	+	+	–	16	2	128	0.5	512	20
E. coli MRC3	TEM-116, CTX-M-15	–	KJ906617	KJ923009, KM873151	–	–	–	32	1	512	0.5	>512	20
E. coli MRC6	TEM-116, CTX-M-71	–	KJ906618	KJ939551, KM873171	+	+	+	16	3	512	0.75	>512	2
E. coli MRC7	–	–	KM822763		+	–	–	32	0.25	16	0.125	16	2
E. coli MRC13	TEM-116	–	KM822764	KM873145	–	–	–	4	2	512	0.094	>512	2
E. coli MRC17	CTX-M-55	TEM-1	KJ906623	KM873174, KJ939552	+	+	–	256	>4	128	>1	256	20
E. coli MRC24	–	–	KM822765		–	–	–	>512	0.125	>512	0.094	128	2
E. coli MRE2	TEM-116, CTX-M-15	–	KC963022	KJ939553, KM873162	+	+	–	512	3	>512	0.125	512	2
E. coli MRF6	–	TEM-1	KC963027	KJ939560	+	+	+	>512	0.25	>512	0.032	512	20
Acinetobacter junii MRH8	CTX-M-15	TEM-1	KC963028	KM873163, KM593699	–	–	+	>512	3	256	0.023	16	2
E. coli MRK28	TEM-116	OXY	KJ923019	KM593700	+	+	–	512	1	128	0.125	512	2
E. coli MROB6	CTX-M-3	TEM-1	KC963015	KM873169, KM593701	–	+	+	64	0.5	16	0.125	16	20
E. coli MROB11	CTX-M15	TEM-1	KC963018	KM873164, KM593702	+	+	+	512	0.5	128	0.125	16	20
E. coli MROB16	CTX-M-15	TEM-1	KC963017	KM873165, KM593703	–	–	+	256	0.38	128	0.19	64	20
E. coli MRAE2	TEM-116, CTX-M-32	–	KM822766	KM593704, KR560052	–	–	–	16	2	>512	0.25	>512	2
E. coli MRAE5	TEM-116, CTX-M-15	–	KJ906620	KJ939554, KM873152	–	–	+	8	0.5	512	0.032	>512	2
E. coli MRAE6	TEM-116, CTX-M-15	–	KJ906624	KJ939555, KM873153	–	+	–	16	3	>512	0.19	>512	2
E. coli MRAE9	CTX-M-15	–	KJ923010	KM873154	+	+	–	16	0.5	128	0.094	>512	20
E. coli MRAE14	TEM-116	–	KM822767	KM873146	+	–	–	16	0.75	512	0.125	>512	2
E. coli MRAE17	CTX-M-3	–	KJ906621	KM873166	+	+	+	16	2	512	0.094	>512	2
E. coli MRAE18	TEM-116, CTX-M-3	–	KJ906622	KJ939556, KM873167	+	+	+	>512	>4	>512	>1	>512	2

(Continued)

TABLE 2 | Continued

	β -Lactamases genes		GenBank Accession nos.		*mer* operon genes			MIC values (μg/ml)					
	ESBL	**Non-ESBL**	**16S rRNA gene**	**β-lactamases genes**	***mer*P**	***mer*T**	***mer*B**	**CAZ**	**CAC**	**CTX**	**CEC**	**CTR**	**$HgCl_2$**
E. coli MRAE21	TEM-116, CTX-M-152	–	KJ923011	KM873147, KM873172	+	+	–	>512	2	>512	0.064	>512	2
E. coli MRAE23	CTX-M-15	TEM-1	KJ923012	KM873155, KM593705	–	+	+	>512	0.38	>512	0.125	>512	20
E.coli MRAE25	–	–	KJ923013		+	+	+	>512	1	>512	0.094	>512	2
E. coli MRAE26	TEM-116	–	KJ923014	KJ939557	+	+	+	>512	0.094	>512	0.125	>512	20
E. coli MRAE27	TEM-116, CTX-M-15	–	KJ923015	KJ939558, KM873156	–	+	–	512	0.38	256	0.125	512	2
E. coli MRAE31	CTX-M-15	–	KJ923016	KM873157	+	+	+	>512	>4	>512	>1	>512	20
E. coli MRAE32	TEM-116, CTX-M-3, CTX-M-15	–	KJ923017	KJ939559, KM873168, KM873158	+	+	+	8	0.5	512	0.125	>512	2
E. coli MRAE33	TEM-116	–	KM822768	KM873148	+	+	+	64	0.38	512	0.047	>512	20
E. coli MRAE36	CTX-M-15	–	KJ957162	KM873159	+	+	+	16	0.25	256	0.125	>512	20
E. coli MRAE42	CTX-M-15	–	KJ957163	KM873160	–	–	–	64	1	512	0.094	>512	2
E. coli MRAE44	TEM-116, CTX-M-152	–	KJ923018	KM593706, KM873173	+	+	–	512	>4	256	>1	512	2
Kluyvera georgiana MRB7	TEM-116, CTX-M-152	–	KM822769	KJ923007, KJ461948	+	–	–	256	1.5	>512	0.38	256	2
Klebsiella pneumoniae ATCC 700603	–	–	–	–	–	–	–	>32	2	8	0.75	16	0.02
E. coli ATCC 25922	–	–	–	–	–	–	–	2	0.094	1	0.023	0	0.02

CAZ, Ceftazidime; CAC, Ceftazidime + clavulanic acid; CTX, Cefotaxime; CEC, Cefotaxime + clavulanic acid; CTR, Ceftriaxone; $HgCl_2$, Mercuric chloride.

in *E. coli* isolates screened from samples collected from downstream region of river Yamuna were found localized on plasmid. It strongly depicts their mobilization in the aquatic habitat. *K. georgiana* isolate harboring $bla_{CTX\text{-}M\text{-}152}$ was found to have high MIC values against penicillins, cephalosporins, monobactams, and rifampicins (**Table 3**).

Sequence of $bla_{CTX\text{-}M\text{-}152}$ was found to be 98.6% similar with $bla_{CTX\text{-}M\text{-}78}$ (CTX-M-group-25 member first identified in *K. georgiana*; Rodríguez et al., 2010). $bla_{CTX\text{-}M\text{-}152}$ also showed 97.3% homology with the $bla_{CTX\text{-}M\text{-}25}$ and $bla_{CTX\text{-}M\text{-}94}$ sequences, 97.5% homology with $bla_{CTX\text{-}M\text{-}39}$, and 97.4% homology with $bla_{CTX\text{-}M\text{-}26}$, $bla_{CTX\text{-}M\text{-}89}$, and $bla_{CTX\text{-}M\text{-}100}$. Both variants (CTX-M-152 and CTX-M-78) differed from other members of the CTX-M-group-25 by amino acids substitutions M7I, C24Y, G81D, P99S, and G146D. CTX-M-152 is the only variant in the CTX-M-group-25 with a T154A substitution. This is the first report of any CTX-M variant containing histidine substituted with glutamine at position 26 (**Figure S1**). The genetic relatedness of the identified variant to members of group-25 obtained by MEGA6 suggests earlier branching of CTX-M-152, possibly due to Q26H, T154A, G89D, P99S, and D146G amino acid substitutions.

SIFT Analysis for Deleterious Substitutions

A homology check of the sequence revealed 10 individual substitutions (Q26H, Q89D, N92S, P99S, V103I, A120G, T189A, H197N, T209M, P266S) in sequence of CTX-M-152 in comparison to the most relevant CTX-M-9 with respect to sequence homology. To predict the functional importance of amino acid substitutions, all 10 substitutions were submitted independently to the SIFT programme to check their tolerance index with respect to CTX-M-9. Of the 10 substitutions, one having the T189A substitution was found to be deleterious, with a tolerance index score of 0.02, while others nine viz. Q29H,

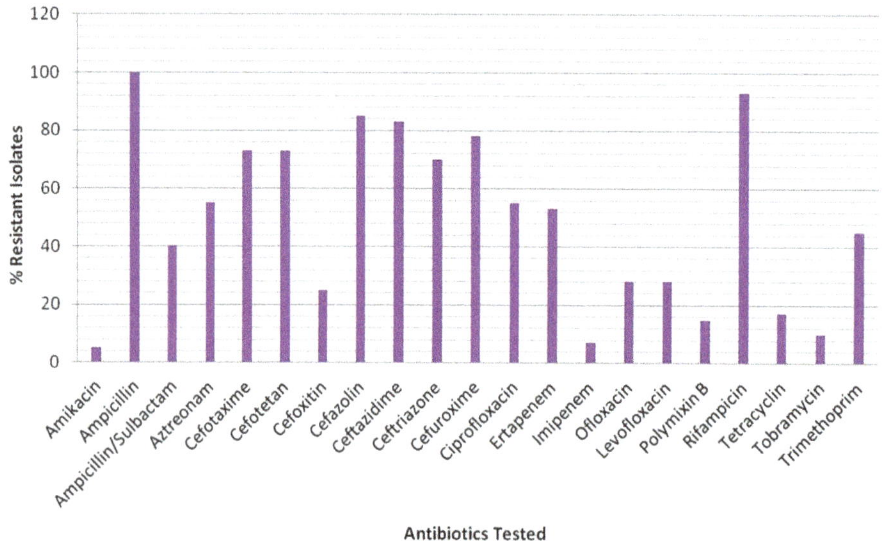

FIGURE 1 | Percentage of resistant isolates against the β-lactam and non β-lactam classes of antibiotics.

Q92D, N95S, P102S, V106I, A123G, H200N, T212M, and P269S are tolerable having tolerance index score of 0.12, 0.32, 0.64, 0.08, 0.17, 0.15, 0.50, 0.10, and 0.37, respectively.

Homology Modeling of CTX-M-152

When compared to the well-studied TEM, SHV and CTX-M-1 group members, there have been no structural studies of CTX-M-group-25 members to best of our knowledge. The nucleotide sequence of $bla_{\text{CTX-M-152}}$ contains several point mutations (87G→C, 368C→G, 369A→G, 574A→G, and 576G→T), which lead to Q26H, A120G, and T189A amino acid substitutions, respectively. Upon finding close relatedness to CTX-M-9 (PDB 1YLJ), the backbone was used to generate the structural model of CTX-M-152. The structure generated by I-TASSER was monitored for stereochemical quality of the models using the PROCHECK and Rampage programs. As revealed by the Ramachandran contour plot obtained using the Rampage software, over 84% of the amino acid residues in the modeled structure were present in the most favored region, while another 10% were in the allowed region. The modeled structure contains an α and α/β domain, with the active site residing at the interface of two domains. Despite differences in orientation that include length of the helix and pleated regions, resemblance in the backbone structure of the two variants (CTX-M-9 and -152) shows an RMSD value (C^{α}) of 0.412 Å (**Figure 3**). The pI value as calculated by Expasy tool was reported to be 8.81.

Docking with Cefotaxime

For docking purpose, a maximum of nine different conformations corresponding to cefotaxime (DB00497) were taken into account to estimate ligand binding conformations using the Lamarckian Genetic Algorithm (LGA) in the Auto dock. The conformation of the ligand with least binding energy indicates high affinity of β-lactamases for cefotaxime. Therefore, ligands showing a binding energy of -7.6 Kcal/mol that depict a more stable and effective interaction for facilitating the enzyme activity, was selected for further analysis. Although the docking results revealed interactions via seven H-bonds with five proposed active site residues (Ser70, Asn132, Ser237, Gly238, and Arg273), there were other surrounding residues that were also found to contribute toward hydrophobicity at the active site (**Figures 4, 5**). The active sites residues in association with the surrounding interacting residues are known to have four conserved regions that are critical to catalyze the substrate. The first conserved element (Ser70-Xxx-Xxx-Lys73) contains active serine70 and one helix turn with downstream Lys73, pointing to the bottom of the active site. Accordingly, we found that residues were similar, even in the structure of CTX-M-152. Drawz and Bonomo (2010) showed that CTX-M enzymes use this reactive serine (Ser70), a catalytic water molecule and an activator residue (Glu166) to hydrolyze the β-lactam ring through an acid-base catalytic mechanism (Drawz and Bonomo, 2010). Complying with the results of Chen et al. (2005a) regarding substitution of histidine for proline at position 99 in CTX-M-27, Pro99Ser substitution in CTX-M-152 was found to be in the tolerable range, thereby conferring no change in stability and function of CTX-M-152 (Chen et al., 2005a). The second motif, Ser130-Asp131-Asn132 situated on the short loop in the alpha domain forms the left side of the catalytic cavity. Among Ser130, Asp131, and Asn132 residues in the structure of CTX-M-152, only Asn132 interacted with cefotaxime. These findings are in accordance with studies suggesting residues in helixes and pleated regions (in the case of CTX-M-9) are favored over linker region residues for interaction with the substrate. Similarly, residue Asn104 and Tyr105 forms a bend in the binding site as observed in the structure of both CTX-M-9 and CTX-M-152. While working with the Toho-1-cefotaxime complex, Shimamura et al. (2002) reported involvement of the N104 side chain residue in hydrogen bonding with the side chain carbonyl of cefotaxime (Shimamura et al., 2002). However,

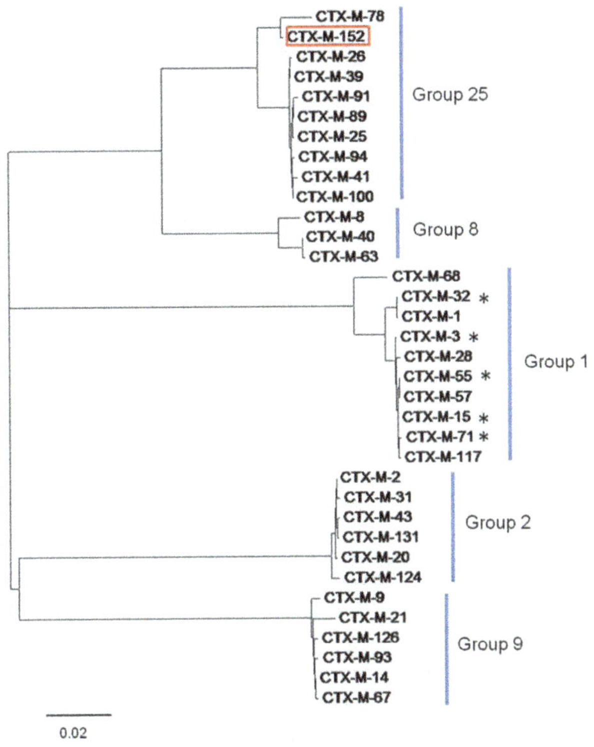

FIGURE 2 | Tree diagram showing similarity among the CTX-M lineage enzymes and clustering of different CTX-M group members. The tree was constructed with the MEGA6 software. The variant CTX-M-152 is highlighted red and variants identified in this study are marked by asterisk.

TABLE 3 | MIC values corresponding to different antibiotics for *K. georgiana* MRB7 isolate.

Antibiotic(s)	MIC (mg/L)
Amikacin	0.5
Amoxycillin	>240
Aztreonam	120
Carbenicillin	>512
Cefotaxime	>512
Cefotaxime + Clavulanic Acid	0.38
Ceftazidime	256
Ceftazidime + Clavulanic Acid	1.5
Ceftriaxon	256
Ciprofloxacin	2
Kanamycin	3
Ofloxacin	0.1
Rifampicin	32
Tetracycline	12

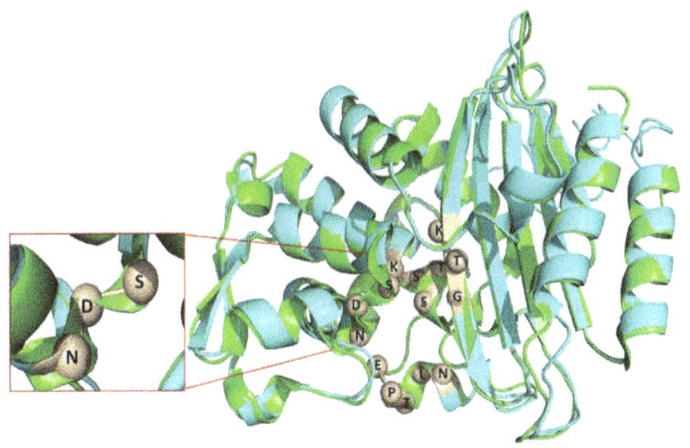

FIGURE 3 | Superimposed image of CTX-M-152(blue) and CTX-M-9 (green). The conserved element number 1 (S70-T71-S72-K73), conserved element number 2 (S130-D131-N132), conserved element number 3 (K234-T235-G236) and conserved element number 4 (E166-P167-T168-L169-N170) are labeled to show the active site.

changes in the hydrolytic pocket resulting from substitution of isoleucine for valine (V103I) render N104 residue out of range to form a hydrogen bond. The V103 residue conserved in CTX-M-1, -2, and -14 was replaced by isoleucine among members of CTX-M-group-25 in a similar method as reported for CTX-M-group-8. The conformational change influencing the positioning of Asn104 and/or Tyr105 greatly affects the interaction between enzymes and substrates. Based on the location of the third conserved element (Lys234-Thr235-Gly236) on the β3 strand of the β-sheet in the α/β domain, it forms the opposite wall of the catalytic cavity. Shakil and Khan (2010) reported the same type of interaction between side chains of cefotaxime and the backbone oxygen of Ser237 (Shakil and Khan, 2010). Upon docking of cefotaxime against the modeled CTX-M-152, only Ser237 of the Ser237 and Asn104 residues was found to interact with the carboxylate group of cefotaxime. This interaction might induce rotation of the carboxylate group in the acyl-intermediate structure of CTX-M, bringing the carbonyl group of β-lactam to a suitable position in the oxyanion hole, thereby promoting drug-hydrolysis. The last conserved element (Glu166-Pro167-Thr168-Leu169-Asn170) located on the 19-residue loop (positions 161–179), which is referred to as the omega (Ω) loop, forms the floor of active site. Both the β3 strand and the Ω-loop are important constituents of the active site cleft.

Among other residues that contribute to effective interaction between enzymes and antibiotics, Asn104, Ser237, Asp240, and Arg276, which form the flexible arms of the β3 strand and Ω-loop, were found to be involved in cefotaxime hydrolysing activity of CTX-M enzymes. As reported by Perez-Llarena et al. (2011), Ala219 in the loop that connects α and α/β domains (occupying top of active site), and are critical to the flexibility and breathing dynamics of β-lactamases, was also found conserved in CTX-M-152 (Perez-Llarena et al., 2011). In another study, Delmas et al. (2008) found that Val180, Arg191, Ala247, and Val260 constituted different hydrophobic clusters, thereby affecting the dynamics and flexibility of enzymes important to the hydrolysis of substrates (Delmas et al., 2008). Frequent among class A members, Arg274 residue increase substrate specificity because the side chain point toward the active site cavity. Similarly, residues Cys69, Ser72, Met135, Phe160 Thr165, and Ser237, which were conserved in CTX-M-152, are considered important with respect to substrate specificity (Péduzzi et al.,

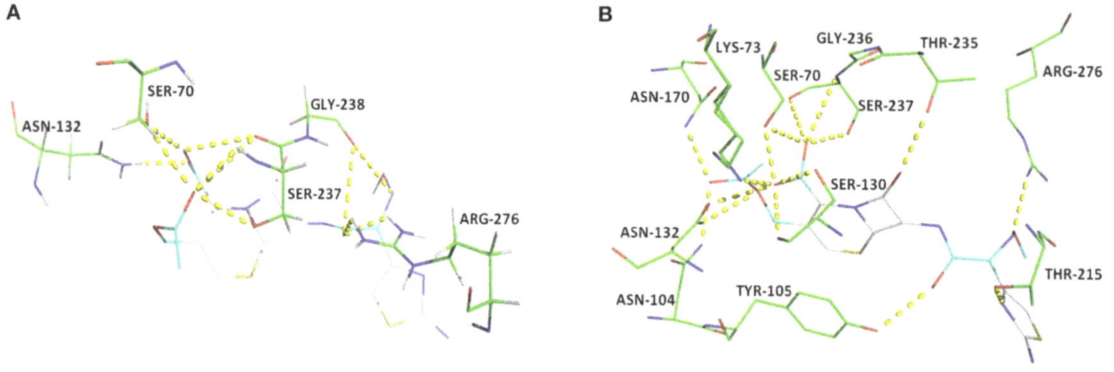

FIGURE 4 | Key polar interactions observed between enzyme CTX-M-152 (A) or CTX-M-9 (B) and Cefotaxime. The broken lines represent hydrogen bonds and interacting amino acid residues are labeled. The cefotaxime is shown in stick form; oxygen atoms are red, nitrogen atoms in blue, carbon atoms white, and sulfur atoms in yellow.

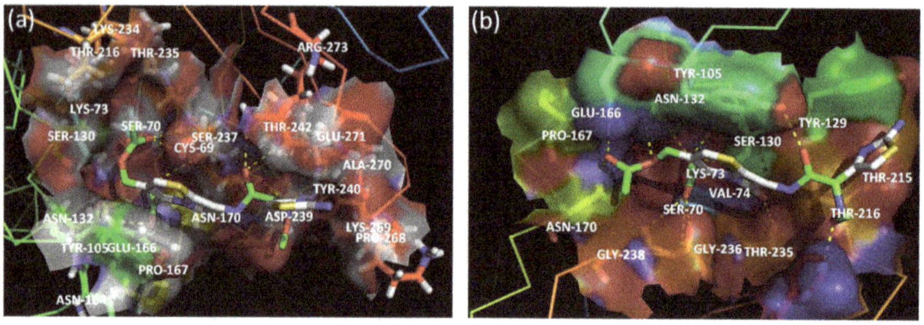

FIGURE 5 | Active site of CTX-M-152 (A) and CTX-M-9 (B) with substrate cefotaxime. Residues around the binding pocket of substrate are depicted in transparent cloud form. The cefotaxime is presented in stick form; oxygen atoms are red, nitrogen atoms in blue, carbon atoms white, and sulfur atoms in yellow.

1997). In comparison to Asn270 residue of CTX-M-14 (along with other members of group-9) involved in establishing hydrogen bond with Asp240, CTX-M-152 similar to other members of group-25 possesses Lys270 to interact with residue Asp240 for correct positioning of β3 strand residues during catalytic process. CTX-M-152 containing Asp240 rather than Gly240 that increases its catalytic efficacy against ceftazidime, helped the variant to retain the high stability of the enzyme in the activity stability trade-off.

DISCUSSION

The escalating problem of multidrug resistance among infection causing organisms represents one of the greatest challenges worldwide. With increased antimicrobial usage, complexities in the resistance mechanisms have become more advanced. Densely populated centers with improper water supplies and inconsistent sanitation contribute significantly to acquisition and dissemination of resistance determinants among microbial inhabitants of water bodies. The Yamuna River, which originates from the Yamnotri glacier in the lower Himalayas (38°59′N 78°27′E), is the major source of water to urban areas in Delhi. Although the proportion of the river catchment area in Delhi is small (~2%), this area contributes more than 50% of pollutants that it receives through sewage from urban effluents, with high levels of antimicrobials in addition to toxic compounds being discharged by industries (Sharma and Kansal, 2011; Sehgal et al., 2012; Mutiyar and Mittal, 2014). The acquisition and transmission of resistance genes from microflora of human and animal origin discharged as part of sewage can substantially influence the pattern of resistance among the microbial inhabitants of the aquatic ecosystem (Amos et al., 2014).

Increasing incidences of ESBL-producing bacteria that showed a drastic shift in recent years in environmental settings are of serious concern. Contribution of selection to acquisition and as such spread of resistance among bacteria against major classes of antibiotics is alarming due to their higher dissemination rate. As such, high prevalence of ESBL producing isolates in natural water bodies like ponds, lakes, rivers, and tap water has drawn concern regarding increased spread of resistance in the environment (Upadhyay and Joshi, 2015). Recently, Bajaj et al. (2015) and Ahammad et al. (2014) also reported high prevalence of the several β-lactamase genes (TEM, SHV, CTX-M, AmpC, and NDM-1) among *E. coli* and other coliform bacterial species screened in collected water samples from upper ranges of Ganges River till its tributary Yamuna that stretches in Delhi and beyond. In our study, 93% of ESBL$^+$ Gram negative isolates were observed to harbor bla_{TEM}, $bla_{CTX\text{-}M}$, and/or bla_{OXY}. These variants were showing similarity to those reported by Wattal et al. (2010) and Rastogi et al. (2010), during their studies on ESBL production among clinical isolates (Rastogi et al., 2010; Wattal et al., 2010). In our study, we found ESBL producing bacterial isolates to have co-resistance to five others non-β-lactam classes of antibiotics in addition of exhibiting resistant phenotype to aztreonam (55%), ceftazidime (83%), cefazolin (85%), cefotaxime (73%), cefotetan (73%), and ertapenem (53%). The resistance of 21 isolates to ertapenem alerts for the decrease of carbapenem activity in the treatment of potential infections caused by these bacteria. These results are in concordance with the study of Datta et al. (2012), which reported steady increase in the percentage of carbapenem resistance among *E. coli* (40% in 2002 to 61% in 2009) and *K. pneumonia* (2% in 2002 to 52% in 2009) in a span of 10 years in tertiary-care hospital in New Delhi. In an another study, Center for Disease Dynamics, Economics & Policy (CDDEP) reported an increase in the percentage of carbapenems resistance from 10% in 2008 to 13% in 2013 among *E. coli* and 29% in 2008 to 57% in 2014 in *isolates of K. pneumonia* from India (Datta et al., 2012; Center for Disease Dynamics Economics and Policy (CDDEP), 2015). Besides strengthening the existing knowledge of their prevalence, presence of MDR, XDR, and PDR bacteria in the natural environment endorses them for the potent threat that they posses for the mankind. Mercury tolerance among the tested isolates appears to be an adaptation of bacteria that is correlated with their ability to live in mercury polluted environments. Accordingly, investigations of ESBL genes (bla_{TEM} and $bla_{CTX\text{-}M}$) among bacteria that harbor both multidrug resistance and mercury tolerance are thought to provide useful information regarding their epidemiology in human influenced polluted environments.

Identification of $bla_{CTX\text{-}M\text{-}152}$ in *K. georgiana* as part of this study is the first report of identification of any CTX-M-group-25 member from India. Docking studies of cefotaxime against modeled CTX-M-152 revealed that formation of a hydrogen bond between Ser237 and a carboxylate oxygen of cefotaxime induced rotation of the carboxylate group in the acyl-intermediate structure of CTX-M. Interaction of Ser237 with cefotaxime helps bring the carbonyl group of β-lactam to a suitable position in the oxyanion hole, thereby promoting hydrolysis of the drug. This was confirmed by the mutant S70G:S237A:R276A-cefotaxime complex, which displayed a significant loss of activity as a cefotaximase (Adamski et al., 2015). Simultaneously, Ser237 and Arg276, which are responsible for high substrate specificity, act cooperatively to promote cefotaxime hydrolysis through structural alterations in the active site to accommodate the larger cefotaxime molecule (Delmas et al., 2008, 2010). In a recent study, Adamski et al. (2015) revealed that co-operative interactions of Ser237 and Arg276 for cefotaxime enhance hydrolysis (~30-fold) relative to TEM-1/SHV-1 (Adamski et al., 2015). Hence, the presence of Ser237 and Arg276 in CTX-M-152 supports its high catalytic efficacy, even though it has a small active site similar to classical TEM-1 and SHV-1. Amino acid substitutions are of considerable significance in that they have direct or indirect involvement in changing enzyme activity. The hydrogen bond between side chains of Lys234 and Ser130 connecting α domain and α/β domain in class A enzymes was not observed in CTX-M-152. Conversely, substitutions such as N92S, P99S, A121G, and H197N, which represent changes with bulkier to light side chains, are thought to be involved in increasing the flexibility of protein, which is responsible for its high catalytic efficiency.

Delmas et al. (2008, 2010) reported binding of cefotaxime to CTX-M-9 that results in conformational changes at active sites though breakage of the hydrogen bond between Asn170 and Asp240 connecting the omega loop to the β3 strand (Delmas et al., 2008, 2010). This expands the active site to allow adequate positioning of the cefotaxime substrate for catalysis. The Asp240Gly substitution, which is known to increase the activity toward ceftazidime, was missing in CTX-M-152. Similar to Asp240Gly, the Val231Ala substitution on the β3 strand responsible for the stability-activity trade-off in the evolution of resistance enzymes, was absent from CTX-M-152. Although the two substitutions (Val231Ala and Asp240Gly) in the CTX-M enzymes did not alter the active site configuration, both have been reported to cause decreased protein stability, presumably through loss of favorable packing and polar interactions (Chen et al., 2005b). Hence, CTX-M-152 with residues having higher stability obtained from the Yamuna River isolate of *K. georgiana* is believed to be the progenitor of CTX-M genes. It is in concordance with the previous reports that documented the possible emergence of $bla_{CTX\text{-}M}$ genes from *Kluyvera sp.* (Sarria et al., 2001; Humeniuk et al., 2002; Bonnet, 2004; Munday et al., 2004; McGettigan et al., 2009; Zhang et al., 2009).

Continuous threat posed by resistant organisms to human health has necessitated the need for further studies to improve understanding of their resistance mechanisms. Presence of CTX-M-152 with high stability and hydrolytic efficacy in an isolate of *K. georgiana* from the river Yamuna goes hand-on-hand with the generalization regarding natural environment acting as a source of resistance genes from which newer variants of enzymes evolve. Alongside, the presence of CTX-M-152 variant on the plasmid of *E. coli* isolates collected from downstream region of river Yamuna possibly demonstrate the mobilization of resistance genes through recombination events in bacteria. High incidence of CTX-M family member's warrant additional studies to be performed that might provide deeper insight into prevalence and information about the factors that led to spread of the resistant determinants, thereby can help in adopting strategies that can prevent selection, expansion, and transmission of resistance genes among bacteria associated with multiple human complications.

AUTHOR CONTRIBUTIONS

QH conceived the topic. MA and AT contributed equally to this work. MA, AJ, and QH together contributed equally to the writing.

ACKNOWLEDGMENTS

Mudsser Azam acknowledge Council of Scientific & Industrial Research (**CSIR**), India for financial support as Senior Research Fellowship (09/466(0136)/2011-EMR-I).

SUPPLEMENTARY MATERIAL

Table S1 | *In vitro* susceptibility of ESBL$^+$ bacterial isolates to 3rd generation cephalosporins.

Table S2 | Phenotypic disc confirmatory test of ESBL$^+$ bacterial isolates.

Table S3 | (A) Susceptibilities of ESBL$^+$ isolates to β-lactam class of antibiotics. **(B)** Susceptibilities of ESBL$^+$ isolates to non-β-lactam classes of antibiotics.

Figure S1 | Multiple sequence alignment of CTX-M β-lactamases. Amino acid sequences of representative members from five different groups of CTX-M ESBLs are aligned using CLUSTAL W program. Asterisks indicate identical amino acids. The four conserved domains of class A β-lactamases are marked with red line.

REFERENCES

Adamski, C. J., Cardenas, A. M., Brown, N. G., Horton, L. B., Sankaran, B., Prasad, B. V. V, et al. (2015). Molecular basis for the catalytic specificity of the ctx-m extended spectrum β-lactamases. *Biochemistry* 54, 447-457. doi: 10.1021/bi501195g

Ahammad, Z. S., Sreekrishnan, T. R., Hands, C. L., Knapp, C. W., and Graham, D. W. (2014). Increased waterborne blaNDM-1 resistance gene abundances associated with seasonal human pilgrimages to the upper ganges river. *Environ. Sci. Technol.* 48, 3014–3020. doi: 10.1021/es405348h

Amos, C. A., Hawkey, P. M., Gaze, W. H., and Wellington, E. M. (2014). Waste water effluent contributes to the dissemination of CTX-M-15 in the natural environment. *J. Antimicrob. Chemother.* 69, 1785–1791. doi: 10.1093/jac/dku079

Bajaj, P., Singh, N. S., Kanaujia, P. K., and Virdi, J. S. (2015). Distribution and molecular characterization of genes encoding CTX-M and AmpC β-lactamases in *E. coli* isolated from an Indian urban aquatic environment. *Sci. Total Environ.* 505, 350–356. doi: 10.1016/j.scitotenv.2014.09.084

Barlow, M., Reik, R. A., Jacobs, S. D., Medina, M., and Meyer, M. P. (2008). High rate of mobilization for *bla*CTX-Ms. *Emerg. Infect. Dis.* 14, 423–428. doi: 10.3201/eid1403.070405

Bonnet, R. (2004). Growing group of extended-spectrum β-lactamases: the CTX-M enzymes. *Antimicrob. Agents Chemother.* 48, 1–14. doi: 10.1128/AAC.48.1.1-14.2004

Center for Disease Dynamics Economics and Policy (CDDEP) (2015). *State of the World's Antibiotics, 2015.* Washington, DC: CDDEP.

Chagas, T. P. G., Seki, L. M., Cury, J. C., Oliveira, J. A. L, Davila, A. M. R, Silva, D. M., et al. (2011). Multiresistance, beta-lactamase-encoding genes and bacterial diversity in hospital wastewater in Rio de Janeiro. *Brazil. J. Appl. Microbiol.* 111, 572–581. doi: 10.1111/j.1365-2672.2011.05072.x

Chen, Y., Delmas, J., Sirot, J., Shoichet, B., and Bonnet, R. (2005a). Atomic resolution structures of CTX-M β-lactamases: extended spectrum activities from increased mobility and decreased stability. *J. Mol. Biol.* 348, 349–362. doi: 10.1016/j.jmb.2005.02.010

Chen, Y., Shoichet, B., and Bonnet, R. (2005b). Structure, function, and inhibition along the reaction co-ordinate of CTX-M β-lactamases. *J. Am. Chem. Soc.* 127, 5423–5434. doi: 10.1021/ja042850a

Clinical and Laboratory Standards Institute (2010). *Performance Standards For Antimicrobial Susceptibility Testing. CLSI M100 S20 Ed. 20.* Wayne, PA.

Clinical and Laboratory Standards Institute (2012). *Performance Standards For Antimicrobial Susceptibility Testing. M100 S22.* Wayne, PA.

Datta, S., Wattal, C., Goel, N., Oberoi, J. K., Raveendran, R., and Prasad, K. J. (2012). A ten year analysis of multi-drug resistant blood stream infections caused by *Escherichia coli* and *Klebsiella pneumoniae* in a tertiary care hospital. *Indian J. Med. Res.* 135, 907–912.

Delmas, J., Chen, Y., Prati, F., Robin, F., Shoichet, B. K., and Bonnet, R. (2008). Structure and dynamics of CTX-M enzymes reveal insights into substrate accommodation by extended-spectrum β-lactamases. *J. Mol. Biol.* 375, 192–201. doi: 10.1016/j.jmb.2007.10.026

Delmas, J., Leyssene, D., Dubois, D., Birck, C., Vazeille, E., Robin, F., et al. (2010). Structural insights into substrate recognition and product expulsion in CTX-M enzymes. *J. Mol. Biol.* 400, 108–120. doi: 10.1016/j.jmb.2010.04.062

Drawz, S. M., and Bonomo, R. A. (2010). Three decades of β-lactamase inhibitors. *Clin. Microbiol. Rev.* 23, 160–201. doi: 10.1128/CMR.000 37-09

GARP-India (2011). *Situation Analysis, Antibiotic Use and Resistance in India.* Available online at: http://www.resistancestrategies.org/wp-content/Uploads/2011/03/India-report

Harnisz, M. (2013). Total resistance of native bacteria as an indicator of changes in the water environment. *Environ. Pollut.* 174, 85–92. doi: 10.1016/j.envpol.2012.11.005

Humeniuk, C., Arlet, G., Gautier, V., Grimont, P., Labia, R., and Philippon, A. (2002). β-Lactamases of *Kluyvera ascorbata*, probable progenitors of some plasmid-encoded CTX-M types. *Antimicrob. Agents Chemother.* 46, 3045–3049. doi: 10.1128/AAC.46.9.3045-3049.2002

Jackson, R. W., Vinatzer, B., Arnold, D. L., Dorus, S., and Murillo, J. (2011). The influence of the accessory genome on bacterial pathogen evolution. *Mob. Genetic Elements.* 1, 55–65. doi: 10.4161/mge.1.1.16432

Jan, A. T., Murtaza, I., Ali, A., and Haq, Q. M. R. (2009). Mercury pollution: an emerging problem and potential bacterial remediation strategies. *World J. Microbiol. Biotech.* 25, 1529–1537. doi: 10.1007/s11274-009-0050-2

Kelly, B. G., Vespermann, A., and Bolton, D. J. (2009). Gene transfer events and their occurrence in selected environments. *Food Chem. Toxicol.* 47, 978–983. doi: 10.1016/j.fct.2008.06.012

Knapp, C. W., Zhang, W., Sturm, B. S. M., and Graham, D. W. (2010). Differential fate of erythromycin and beta-lactam resistance genes from swine lagoon waste under different aquatic conditions. *Environ. Pollut.* 158, 506–1512. doi: 10.1016/j.envpol.2009.12.020

Kohlenberg, A., Schwab, F., and Ruden, H. (2012). Wide dissemination of extended spectrum beta-lactamase (ESBL)-producing *Escherichia coli* and *Klebsiella spp.* in acute care and rehabilitation hospitals. *Epidemiol. Infect.* 140, 528–534. doi: 10.1017/S0950268811000781

Korzeniewska, E., and Harnisz, M. (2013). Beta-lactamase-producing Enterobacteriaceae in hospital effluents. *J. Environ. Manage.* 123, 1–7. doi: 10.1016/j.jenvman.2013.03.024

Kummerer, K. (2009). Antibiotics in the aquatic environment: a review- Part, I. *Chemosphere* 75, 417–434. doi: 10.1016/j.chemosphere.2008.11.086

Malik, D., Singh, S., Thakur, J., Singh, R. K., Kaur, A., and Nijhawan, S. (2014). Heavy metal pollution of the yamuna river: an introspection. *Int. J. Curr. Microbiol. Appl. Sci.* 3, 856–863.

McGettigan, S. E., Hu, B., Andreacchio, K., Nachamkin, I., and Edelstein, P. H. (2009). Prevalence of CTX-M β-lactamases in philadelphia, pennsylvania. *J. Clin. Microbiol.* 47, 2970–2974. doi: 10.1128/JCM.00319-09

Mendes, R. E., Mendoza, M., Singh, K. K. B., Castanheira, M., Bell, J. M., Turnidge, J. D., et al. (2013). Regional resistance surveillance program results for 12 Asia-Pacific nations (2011). *Antimicrob. Agents Chemother.* 57, 5721–5726. doi: 10.1128/AAC.01121-13

Morrissey, I., Hackel, M., Badal, R., Bouchillon, S., Hawser, S., and Biedenbach, D. (2013). A review of ten years of the study for Monitoring Antimicrobial Resistance Trends (SMART) from 2002 to 2011. *Pharmaceuticals* 6, 1335–1346. doi: 10.3390/ph6111335

Munday, C. J., Boyd, D. A., and Brenwald, N. (2004). Molecular and kinetic comparison of the novel extended-spectrum beta-lactamases CTX-M-25 and CTX-M-26. *Antimicrob. Agents Chemother.* 48, 4829–4834. doi: 10.1128/AAC.48.12.4829-4834.2004

Mutiyar, P. K., and Mittal, A. K. (2014). Occurrences and fate of selected human antibiotics in influents and effluents of sewage treatment plant and effluent-receiving river Yamuna in Delhi (India). *Environ. Monit. Assess.* 186, 541–557. doi: 10.1007/s10661-013-3398-6

Ng, P. C., and Henikoff, S. (2001). Predicting deleterious amino acid substitutions. *Genome Res.* 11, 863–874. doi: 10.1101/gr.176601

Ng, P. C., and Henikoff, S. (2003). SIFT: predicting amino acid changes that affect protein function. *Nucleic Acids Res.* 31, 3812–3814. doi: 10.1093/nar/gkg509

Péduzzi, J., Farzaneh, S., Reynaud, A., Barthelemy, M., and Labia, R. (1997). Characterization and amino acid sequence analysis of a new oxyimino cephalosporin-hydrolyzing class A beta-lactamase from *Serratia fonticola* CUV. *Biochim. Biophys. Acta* 1341, 58–70. doi: 10.1016/S0167-4838(97)00020-4

Perez-Llarena, F. J., Kerff, F., Abian, O., Mallo, S., Fernandez, M. C., Galleni, M., et al. (2011). Distant and new mutations in CTX-M-1 β-lactamase affect cefotaxime hydrolysis. *Antimicrob. Agents Chemother.* 55, 4361–4368. doi: 10.1128/AAC.00298-11

Prado, T., Pereira, W. C., Silva, D. M., Seki, L. M., Carvalho, A. P., and Asensi, M. D. (2008). Detection of extended-spectrum β-lactamase-producing *Klebsiella pneumonia* in effluents and sludge of a hospital sewage treatment plant. *Lett. Appl. Microbiol.* 46, 136–141. doi: 10.1111/j.1472-765X.2007.02275.x

Rastogi, V., Nirwan, P. S., Jain, S., and Kapil, A. (2010). Nosocomial outbreak of septicaemia in neonatal intensive care unit due to extended spectrum β-lactamase producing *Klebsiella pneumoniae* showing multiple mechanisms of drug resistance. *Indian J. Med. Microbial.* 28, 380–384. doi: 10.4103/0255-0857.71834

Rodríguez, M. M., Power, P., Sader, H., Galleni, M., and Gutkind, G. (2010). Novel chromosome-encoded CTX- M-78 β-lactamase from a *Kluyvera georgiana* clinical isolate as a putative origin of CTX-M-25 subgroup. *Antimicrob. Agents Chemother.* 54, 3070–3071. doi: 10.1128/AAC.01615-09

Sarria, J. C., Vidal, A. M., and Kimbrough, R. C. (2001). Infections caused by *Kluyvera* species in humans. *Clin. Infect. Dis.* 33, 69–74. doi: 10.1086/322686

Schlüter, A., Szczepanowski, R., Puhler, A., and Top, E. M. (2007). Genomics of IncP-1antibiotic resistance plasmids isolated from wastewater treatment plants provides evidence for a widely accessible drug resistance gene pool. *FEMS Microbiol. Rev.* 31, 449–477. doi: 10.1111/j.1574-6976.2007.00074.x

Sehgal, M., Garg, A., Suresh, R., and Dagar, P. (2012). Heavy metal contamination in the Delhi segment of Yamuna basin. *Environ. Monit. Assess.* 184, 1181–1196. doi: 10.1007/s10661-011-2031-9

Seiler, C., and Berendonk, T. U. (2012). Heavy metal driven co-selection of antibiotic resistance in soil and water bodies impacted by agriculture and aquaculture. *Front. Microbiol.* 3:399. doi: 10.3389/fmicb.2012.00399

Shakil, S., and Khan, A. U. (2010). Infected foot ulcers in male and female diabetic patients: a clinico-bioinformative study. *Ann. Clin. Microbiol. Antimicrob.* 9, 1–10. doi: 10.1186/1476-0711-9-2

Sharma, D., and Kansal, A. (2011). *Current Condition of the Yamuna River - an Overview of Flow, Pollution Load and Human Use*, TERI University. Available online at: http://fore.yale.edu/files/Current_Condition_of_Yamuna_River.pdf

Shimamura, T., Ibuka, A., Fushinobu, S., Wakagi, T., Ishiguro, M., and Ishii, Y., et al. (2002). Acyl-intermediate structures of the extended spectrum class A beta-lactamase, Toho-1, in complex with cefotaxime, cephalothin and benzyl penicillin. *J. Biol. Chem.* 277, 46601–46608. doi: 10.1074/jbc.M207884200

Thomas, C. M., and Nielsen, K. M. (2005). Mechanisms of, and barriers to, horizontal gene transfer between bacteria. *Nat. Rev. Microbiol.* 3, 711–721. doi: 10.1038/nrmicro1234

Upadhyay, S., and Joshi, S. R. (2015). TEM mediated extended spectrum cephalosporin resistance in clinical and environmental isolates of Gram negative bacilli: a report from northeast India. *Indian J. Med. Res.* 142, 614–617. doi: 10.4103/0971-5916.171294

Vervoort, J., Baraniak, A., Gazin, M., Sabirova, J., Lammens, C., Kazma, M., et al. (2012). Characterization of two new CTX-M-25-group extended spectrum β-lactamase variants identified in *Escherichia coli* isolates from israel. *PLoS ONE* 7:e46329. doi: 10.1371/journal.pone.0046329

Walsh, F. (2013). The multiple roles of antibiotics and antibiotic resistance in nature. *Front. Microbiol.* 4:255. doi: 10.3389/fmicb.2013.00255

Wattal, C., Goel, N., Oberoi, J. K., Raveendran, R., Datta, S., and Prasad, K. J. (2010). Surveillance of multidrug resistant organisms in a tertiary care hospital in Delhi, India. *J. Assoc. Physicians India* 58, 32–36.

Wellington, E. M. H., Boxall, A. B. A., Cross, P., Feil, E. J., Gaze, W. H., Hawkey, P. M., et al. (2013). The role of the natural environment in the emergence of antibiotic resistance in Gram-negative bacteria. *Lancet Infec. Dis.* 13, 155–165. doi: 10.1016/S1473-3099(12)70317-1

Woodford, N., Carattoli, A., Karisik, E., Underwood, A., and Ellington, M. J. (2009). Complete nucleotide sequences of plasmids pEK204, pEK499, and pEK516, encoding CTX-M enzymes in three major *Escherichia coli* lineages from the United Kingdom, all belonging to the international O25:H4-ST131 clone. *Antimicrob. Agents Chemother.* 53, 4472–4482. doi: 10.1128/AAC.00688-09

Zhang, Z., Guo, X., and Zhang, Q. (2009). Prevalence characterization of extended spectrum β-lactamases among *Escherichia coli* isolates collected in Zhengzhou. *J. Clin. Lab. Anal.* 23, 404–407. doi: 10.1002/jcla.20351

Zhou, Y., Xu, Y., Xu, J., Zhang, X., Xu, S., and Du, Q. (2015). Combined toxic effects of heavy metals and antibiotics on a pseudomonas fluorescens strain zy2 isolated from swine wastewater. *Int. J. Mol. Sci.* 16, 2839–2850. doi: 10.3390/ijms16022839

21

Antibiotic Resistance in the Food Chain: A Developing Country-Perspective

Luria Leslie Founou [1], Raspail Carrel Founou [1,2] and Sabiha Yusuf Essack [1]*

[1] Antimicrobial Research Unit, Department of Pharmacy, School of Health Sciences, University of KwaZulu-Natal, Durban, South Africa, [2] Department of Microbiology, Centre of Expertise and Biological Diagnostic of Cameroon, Yaoundé, Cameroon

***Correspondence:**
Luria Leslie Founou
luriafounou@gmail.com

Antibiotics are now "endangered species" facing extinction due to the worldwide emergence of antibiotic resistance (ABR). Food animals are considered as key reservoirs of antibiotic-resistant bacteria with the use of antibiotics in the food production industry having contributed to the actual global challenge of ABR. There are no geographic boundaries to impede the worldwide spread of ABR. If preventive and containment measures are not applied locally, nationally and regionally, the limited interventions in one country, continent and for instance, in the developing world, could compromise the efficacy and endanger ABR containment policies implemented in other parts of the world, the best-managed high-resource countries included. Multifaceted, comprehensive, and integrated measures complying with the One Health approach are imperative to ensure food safety and security, effectively combat infectious diseases, curb the emergence and spread of ABR, and preserve the efficacy of antibiotics for future generations. Countries should follow the World Health Organization, World Organization for Animal Health, and the Food and Agriculture Organization of the United Nations recommendations to implement national action plans encompassing human, (food) animal, and environmental sectors to improve policies, interventions and activities that address the prevention and containment of ABR from farm-to-fork. This review covers (i) the origin of antibiotic resistance, (ii) pathways by which bacteria spread to humans from farm-to-fork, (iii) differences in levels of antibiotic resistance between developed and developing countries, and (iv) prevention and containment measures of antibiotic resistance in the food chain.

Keywords: antibiotic resistance, zoonotic transmission, food chain, developing country, one health approach, global action plan, prevention, containment measures

INTRODUCTION

Antibiotics are natural, synthetic, or semi-synthetic substances which interfere that the growth of or kill microorganisms, specifically bacteria, and are used to treat or prevent infections in humans and animals (O'Neill, 2015a; WHO, 2015a). Their development is one of the greatest accomplishments of modern medicine, their availability being vital to medical practices in communities and hospitals globally (O'Neill, 2015a; WHO, 2015a). Antibiotics are now an "endangered species" facing extinction due to the worldwide emergence of antibiotic resistance (ABR) and the void in the development of new therapeutic substances (O'Neill, 2015a; WHO, 2015a). An increasing number of treatment failures have been reported in patients with infections caused by multi-, extensive-, and pan-drug resistant bacteria. Once antibiotics normally used against bacteria are no longer effective, it becomes necessary to use others, so-called "reserve" or "last resort" options that are often more expensive and/or toxic preparations (O'Neill, 2015a).

Antibiotic use is the key factor in the selection of resistant bacteria, with community and hospital settings forming the principal ecological niches of emergence in human health (O'Neill, 2015a; WHO, 2015a). However, it is the use of antibiotics in animals that has contributed to the magnitude of the global challenge of ABR (FAO, 2015). In the intensification of food animal production and aquaculture, antibiotics are administered not only as therapy, but also as metaphylactics, where the identification of disease symptoms in one animal prompts the treatment for the whole flock or herd, and as prophylactics where, sub-therapeutic doses are administered to counteract the adverse effect of stress responses that generally lead to infectious diseases (FAO, 2015). In addition, the extensive use of antibiotics as growth promoters for the rapid growth of food animals and fish exacerbates the emergence and spread of ABR (FAO, 2015). The emergence of ABR in the food chain is considered a cross-sectoral problem, as (i) antibiotics are widely used in aquaculture, livestock production, and crop culture (Acar and Moulin, 2006; FAO, 2015), (ii) antibiotic-resistant bacteria and antibiotic-resistant genes (ARGs) can easily spread at each stage of the food production chain (da Costa et al., 2013; FAO, 2015), and (iii) can cause infections in humans (Chang et al., 2015; WHO, 2015a). The emergence of ABR along the food chain is thus a major global public health issue, with several studies having reported food animals and products being colonized and/or infected and contaminated by antibiotic-resistant strains, such as methicillin-resistant *Staphylococcus aureus* (MRSA) (Price et al., 2012), antibiotic-resistant *Campylobacter* spp. (Ewnetu and Mihret, 2010), and extended spectrum-beta-lactamase (ESBL) producing-*Enterobacteriaceae* (viz. *Salmonella* spp., *Shigella* spp., *Escherichia coli*, *Klebsiella* spp., etc.; Fischer et al., 2012; Al Bayssari et al., 2015). The situation has been recently worsened with the emergence of antibiotic-resistant bacteria having significant pandemic potential, such as carbapenem-resistant *Enterobacteriaceae* (CRE) (harboring a VIM-1 carbapenemase resistant to the beta-lactam antibiotics family plus additional co-resistance; Fischer et al., 2012) and colistin-resistant *E. coli* (harboring mcr-1 gene and co-resistance genes; Liu et al., 2016), as well as emerging livestock associated-methicillin resistant *S. aureus* (LA-MRSA; Price et al., 2012), in German, Chinese, and Dutch pigs, respectively. In fact, these resistant strains recognized as having an animal origin, are associated with multiple hosts adaptability (Ewers et al., 2012; Price et al., 2012; Fernandes et al., 2016; Liu et al., 2016), virulence mechanisms (Ewers et al., 2012; Price et al., 2012) and high genetic exchanges (Price et al., 2012; Liu et al., 2016), are serious threats to the world as they could lead to the emergence of new and more resistant, virulent and mobile strains, unknown from the human immune system (Wulf and Voss, 2008). This phenomenon termed "superburg" is one of the main concern feared by the international scientific community as it could result in pandemic situations caused by as resistant and virulent bacteria (Wulf and Voss, 2008; Ewers et al., 2012).

Antibiotic-resistant bacteria may reach humans (i) indirectly along the food chain through consumption of contaminated food or food derived products, and (ii) following direct contact with colonized/infected animals or biological substances such as blood, urine, feces, saliva, and semen among others (Chang et al., 2015). Given the direct interaction of humans with the animal-ecosystem interface, it is essential to prevent the zoonotic transmission of antibiotic-resistant bacteria and ARGs from food animals-associated reservoirs to humans. The Food and Agriculture Organization of the United Nations (FAO), the World Organization for Animal Health (OIE), and the World Health Organization (WHO) endorsed the One Health approach, affirming that healthy animals contribute to healthy people and environments (FAO, 2015; WHO, 2015a). In keeping with this, supranational programs and systems for monitoring antimicrobial resistance in animals and foodborne (viz. originating from food or food products) pathogens, namely, the Global Foodborne Infections Network, the WHO's Advisory Group on Integrated Surveillance of Antimicrobial Resistance and the Codex Alimentarius Commission, have been established. The WHO's Global Action Plan (WHO, 2015a) and FAO's Action Plan on Antimicrobial Resistance (FAO, 2016) were recently published to address this worldwide threat.

Several programs monitoring antibiotic use and ABR in food animals, foodstuff, and humans, have been successfully implemented in high resource settings such as the European Union (EU), Denmark, Netherlands, Sweden, Japan and United States (US) (The Japanese Veterinary Antimicrobial Resistance Monitoring System in the Field of Animal Hygiene (JVARM), 2013; DANMAP, 2014; FDA, 2014; NethMap-MARAN, 2015; SWEDRES-SVARM, 2015; EFSA and ECDC, 2016). A number of low- and middle-income countries (LMICs) have also initiated efforts to contain ABR, albeit with a focus on human health. India introduced and has begun to implement national guidelines for antibiotic use in 2013. China launched a National Antibiotic Restraining Policy to reduce antibiotic consumption in the country, Thailand implemented a national strategy for emerging diseases, including ABR, and a policy for rational drug use in 2011, as well as an ABR Containment Program for 2012–2016. South Africa developed and implemented a National Framework of Antimicrobial Resistance for 2014–2024.

The majority of LMICs are however still far behind high-resource settings in terms of curbing the spread of ABR generally, and via the food chain specifically. This despite that substantial risk factors for communicable diseases and extensive animal-occupational exposure exist in LMICs. The true burden of ABR in food animals is only partially documented and its threat via the food chain is under-estimated in low resource settings. Given the expansion of the human population, globalization of trade in animals and food products, international travels and host movements, ABR can easily spread globally via the food chain (Holmes et al., 2016). If preventive and containment measures are not applied locally, nationally, regionally and internationally, the limited interventions in one country or continent, for instance, in the developing world, can compromise the efficacy and endanger the policies of containment of ABR implemented in other parts of the world, the best-managed high-resource countries included. ABR is therefore a global problem, requiring integrated, multi-sectoral, and global solutions, as there are no geographic boundaries to its worldwide spread.

This review evidences the danger of ABR in the food chain and particularly in developing countries as a serious global public health threat. First, it assesses and summarizes background information on the emergence of ABR. Second it highlights transmission routes of ABR along the food chain; third, it compares the current status of ABR in food animals in developed vs. developing countries and finally, it delineates prevention and containment measures of ABR from farm-to-fork.

EMERGENCE OF ANTIBIOTIC RESISTANCE

Antibiotic use has always been associated with the development of resistance. Indeed, whenever an antibiotic is consumed, it eliminates susceptible bacterial cells, leaving behind or selecting those unusual strains that continue to grow in its presence through a Darwinian selection process. Those resistant variants then multiply, becoming the predominant bacterial population, and transmit their genetic resistance characteristics to offspring (Apata, 2009; Holmes et al., 2016). Such phenomenon can occur in saprophytic, commensal and pathogenic bacteria in humans, animals. and the environment.

Food animals, fish, and vegetables are considered large reservoirs of antibiotic-resistant bacteria, as the food production chain is an ecosystem composed of different ecological niches, where large quantities of antibiotics are used and numerous bacteria co-exist (Acar and Moulin, 2006). There are two principal biological pathways involved in the evolution and development of ABR. First, resistance can be mediated by a pre-existing phenotype in natural bacterial populations. During the evolutionary process, bacterial cells accumulate genetic errors in existing genes (in the chromosome or plasmid) and transfer the resistant genes to progeny cells via vertical gene transfer (VGT), leading to an *innate* or *intrinsic* or *natural* resistance (**Figure 1**). The second scenario, called *acquired* resistance, involves genetic exchanges within and between bacterial species (Apata, 2009; Holmes et al., 2016). It implies horizontal gene transfer (HGT) and the acquisition of new resistant genes harbored on mobile genetic elements, such as plasmids, integrons, transposons, insertion sequences, and phage-related elements. Such genetic materials are transferred through conjugation (transfer of DNA from donor to recipient bacterial through cell-to-cell contact and aided by a fertility-factor called pili), transformation (naked-DNA present in the environment is taken-up by the recipient cell), and transduction (a bacteriophage acts as vector and inserts DNA into recipient cell; Apata, 2009; Holmes et al., 2016; **Figure 1**).

HGT leads to new bacterial populations carrying a combination of new resistant genes and mechanisms, resulting in different resistance profiles (Acar and Moulin, 2006). This genetic process has been identified as the main driving force

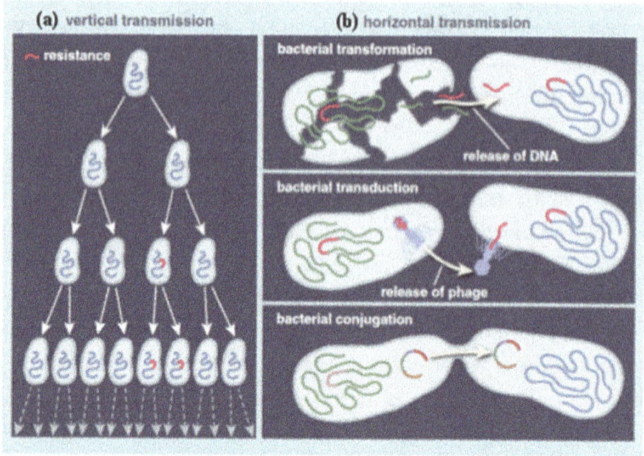

FIGURE 1 | Principal biological pathways involved in the evolution and development of antibiotic resistance. (A) Vertical transmission **(B)** Horizontal transmission. Reprinted by permission from American Scientist (Dantas and Sommer, 2014), Copyright (2014).

behind the spread of ABR, as it allows interspecies transmission, which is especially effective in the bacterial microbiome (gastro-intestinal tract, naso-pharyngeal mucosa, and skin) of animals and humans (Apata, 2009; Holmes et al., 2016). It is further important to note that VGT and HGT may occur concomitantly in a bacterial population (Acar and Moulin, 2006). These two types of mechanisms create a resistant population where selective pressure exerted by antibiotic use will substantially increase their number and risk of spread (Apata, 2009; Holmes et al., 2016). Antibiotic-resistant bacteria may act as reservoir of ARGs for other bacteria, which might be conserved within the bacterial population, even without the related antibiotics (Apata, 2009; Holmes et al., 2016).

TRANSMISSION ROUTES OF ANTIBIOTIC RESISTANCE ALONG THE FOOD CHAIN

The spread of ABR is possible along the food chain through direct or indirect contact. Direct contact occurs following immediate exposure of humans with animals and biological substances (such as blood, urine, feces, milk, saliva, and semen), and enhances the rapid and easy dissemination of resistant bacteria from host-to-host. Occupationally exposed workers such as veterinarians, farmers, abattoir workers and food handlers, as well as those directly in contact with them, are at high risk of being colonized or infected with antibiotic-resistant bacteria (Marshall and Levy, 2011). Although this transmission did not initially appear as a threat at population-health level, it is now acknowledged that exposed workers and their families provide a likely route for the entry of antibiotic-resistant bacteria and ARGs into the community and health care settings, where subsequent exchanges and the acquisition of resistance mechanisms are evident (Marshall and Levy, 2011).

In addition, the human population may be exposed indirectly to antibiotic-resistant bacteria and ARGs via contact with or consumption of contaminated food products (e.g., meat, eggs, milk, and dairy products). This indirect transmission through the food chain is a far-reaching and more complex pathway (**Figure 2**). Recently, numerous reports have described the presence of large quantities of antibiotic-resistant bacteria and ARGs in various food products (ready-to-eat meat, cooked meat, and bulk milk) from various animal sources, such as cattle, poultry, swine, goat, and sheep, and from different stages of food production (Price et al., 2012; Coetzee et al., 2016; Liu et al., 2016). Several studies have further identified similar or clonally related antibiotic-resistant bacteria and ARGs of animal origin in human populations without occupational exposure, providing likely evidence for transfer following the consumption and/or handling of food (Acar and Moulin, 2006; Marshall and Levy, 2011). Farmers, abattoir workers and food handlers as well as consumers are thus the large number of people directly at risk of acquiring antibiotic-resistant bacteria via the food chain. In the developing world, where biosecurity and food safety measures are limited along the farm-to-fork continuum and where humans interact intimately with animals and the environment, the public health risk is likely to be associated with both the direct and indirect transmission of antibiotic-resistant bacteria and ARGs (Padungtod et al., 2008). In contrast, in developed countries, the indirect contamination seems to be more prevalent as antibiotic-resistant bacteria and ARGs emerging on-farms, are maintained throughout the food production and contaminated food products reach the end consumers to create foodborne infections (EFSA and ECDC, 2015).

A large proportion of antibiotics are not transformed into inactive compounds, and retain their activities after renal or biliary excretion (Thanner et al., 2016). The dissemination of active antibiotics, metabolites or degradation products of those antibiotics, termed antibiotic residues, as well as ARGs and antibiotic-resistant bacteria excreted via food animals waste, have established the environment as another important reservoir of ABR (da Costa et al., 2013; Zhu et al., 2013; Woolhouse et al., 2015; Thanner et al., 2016; **Figure 2**). Farm soils, manure, and wastewater have been identified as "hot spots" of ABR pollution, with antibiotic residues being detected across the world (Zhu et al., 2013; Wu et al., 2014; Thanner et al., 2016). Antibiotic residues lead to various adverse effects for human health, such as allergic hypersensitivity reactions, toxic effects, hepatotoxicity, nephropathy, mutagenicity, carcinogenicity, and ABR (Mensah et al., 2014). Although the concern associated with the presence of antibiotic residues in food animals has been mitigated in high resource economies, with <1% of these substances detected in food products in the European Union (EU), it remains a major public health threat in LMICs, with prevalence ranging from 4 to 90% (Mensah et al., 2014). The high prevalence of these residues in various ecological niches in the farm-to-fork continuum exacerbates the issue of ABR in the developing world, as it enhances the pool of antibiotic-resistant bacteria and ARGs in the ecosystem as a result of exposure to sub-inhibitory concentrations of antibiotics and their residues.

HGT has further been documented in environmental niches, such as manure, water and soil, leading to microbial communities containing various levels of antibiotic-resistant bacteria and ARGs (Zhu et al., 2013; Thanner et al., 2016). Several LMICs use animal and human waste, without appropriate treatment, as fertilizer in crop lands and for feeding of fish and shellfish in aquaculture (Zhu et al., 2013). The environmental pollution may therefore lead to the emergence and spread of new antibiotic-resistant bacteria and ARGs in food products, fish,

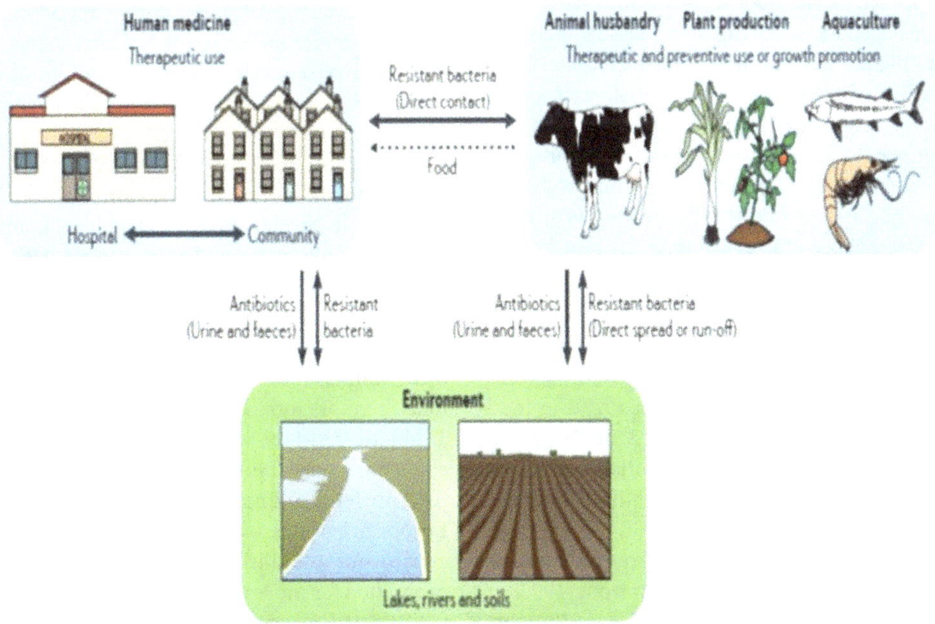

FIGURE 2 | Antibiotic use and different transmission routes of antibiotic resistance in the food chain. Adapted by permission from MacMillan Publishers Ltd: [Nature Reviews Microbiology], (Andersson and Hughes, 2014), Copyright (2014).

shellfish, vegetables, feed and water, which may in turn colonize or infect animals and humans, thereby enhancing the public health risks associated with the presence of ABR in the food chain (Acar and Moulin, 2006; Thanner et al., 2016). The key issues regarding these reservoirs are (i) identifying the different ecological niches and pathways associated with the presence of ABR in the food chain, and, (ii) understanding the public health implications for the human population when the transfer of these antibiotic-resistant bacteria and ARGs from these intermingled reservoirs occurs. It further reveals knowledge gaps regarding the magnitude and dynamic nature of the spread of antibiotic-resistant bacteria and/or ARGs within and between different ecological niches in the farm-to-fork continuum, which deserves to be considered when assessing the transmission of ABR along the food chain (Acar and Moulin, 2006; Woolhouse et al., 2015). Substantial metagenomics studies ascertaining the bacterial resistome, the HGT between antibiotic-resistant bacteria present in the above niches, as well as providing phylogenetic evidence and transmission dynamics within and between populations, are vital to determine the evolutionary origins of bacterial lineages, and may provide new perspectives on understanding the implications of ABR in the food chain (Woolhouse et al., 2015).

CURRENT STATUS OF ANTIBIOTIC RESISTANCE IN THE FOOD CHAIN

Different types of antibiotic-resistant bacteria have increasingly been identified in food animals, products, and feeds as well as in humans (exposed or not). Such antibiotic-resistant bacteria are either (i) indicator or commensal, (ii) foodborne, or (iii) emergent organisms. ARGs emerging in commensal bacteria are likely spread to foodborne ones and vice versa, while the numerous genetic exchanges occurring between different ecological niches lead to new resistant bacteria or genes or combination thereof. Antibiotic-resistant bacteria and ARGs of animal origin are globally reported, with the prevalence differing greatly between geographic locations and differentially resourced settings. MRSA and ESBL-producing *Enterobacteriaceae* (e.g., *Salmonella* spp., *E. coli*, *Shigella* spp., *K. pneumoniae*, *Enterobacter* spp., etc.) are among the best-known examples.

Developed Countries

In high-resource developed countries, an assortment of systems and programs to monitor antibiotic use, as well as ABR in food animals, food products, and humans have been implemented (**Table 1**). Such initiatives have led to the substantial decrease of antibiotic consumption and rates of resistance in these settings. In Norway for instance, The NORM/NORM-VET reported a very low annual antibiotic use of 5.927 tons in terrestrial animals in 2014, representing a total decrease of 38% from 1995 to 2014 (NORM/NORM-VET, 2015). The 2014's DANMAP report revealed a decrease of 2% compare to 2013, with 114 tons of active compounds consumed in livestock (DANMAP, 2014). Similarly, in the Netherlands, 207 tons of antibiotics were consumed in 2014, showing a reduction of 4.4% from 2013, and an overall decrease of 58.1% over the period 2009–2014 (NethMap-MARAN, 2015). In the European Union (EU), antibiotics were banned for growth-promotion in 2006, while the United States (US) implemented legislation based on a voluntary cessation of antibiotic use for growth-promotion as well as re-labeling of antibiotics.

Transmission of antibiotic-resistant bacteria via direct contact from animals to exposed workers, and indirectly following consumption of contaminated food products (broiler meat, beef, pork, milk, etc.), is well-documented in these countries (**Table 2**; DANMAP, 2014; NORM/NORM-VET, 2015; EFSA and ECDC, 2016). In the EU, a new legislation on monitoring of ABR in animals and food was implemented to ensure the comparison of similar and high-quality data in 2013 (EFSA and ECDC, 2016). As a result, harmonized data from the 28 EU member states were collated by the EFSA and ECDC to provide continent-specific estimates of ABR in food animals and products. The 2014's EFSA/ECDC EU Summary report on ABR in zoonotic bacteria revealed increased prevalence of multi-drug resistant (MDR) *S. Infantis* (more than 70% in broiler meats), MDR-*E. coli* (55% in broiler meats) and MRSA (26.5% in all food animals) in the EU (EFSA and ECDC, 2016). These bacteria are recognized as a serious public health threat due to their resistance to several antibiotics, often critically important for human health, thereby limiting the choice of effective antibiotic agents available for treatment.

In a country-specific context, the NORM/NORM-VET detected high levels of ESBL-producing *E. coli* from broilers (36%) and broiler meat samples (30%) in Norway, whereas rates of vancomycin resistant *Enterococcus* spp. were quite low (7%) in 2014 (NORM/NORM-VET, 2015). Meanwhile, monitoring of ABR in food animals in the Netherlands by MARAN revealed a 12% prevalence of ESBL-producing *Salmonella* spp. and 43% of fluoroquinolone-resistant *Salmonella* spp. in poultry. It also showed diverse levels of ESBL/AmpC- producing *E. coli* in food animals and products, these being 67% in broilers, 18% in pigs, 9% in dairy cows, 51% in turkey meat, and 67% in poultry meat (NethMap-MARAN, 2015). The DANMAP reported low rates of MDR-*Salmonella* spp. (7%) in pigs and ESBL-producing *E. coli* (9%) in broiler meat in Denmark, confirming the country as an example in terms of containing ABR (DANMAP, 2014). Transmission of antibiotic-resistant bacteria along the food chain has nevertheless been demonstrated in the country, with a 28% prevalence of ESBL-producing *E. coli* from imported broiler meat samples (DANMAP, 2014). This evidence strongly suggests that there are no geographic borders to curtail the spread of antibiotic-resistant bacteria, and that their emergence in the food chain threatens the world equally. In US, the epidemiology of ABR in food animals appears to be notably different than in European countries, where the substantial ABR research has been carried out and antibiotic use for growth promotion has been prohibited for more than a decade. Antibiotic use in food animals is estimated to account 70% of the country's annual antibiotic consumption (FDA, 2014). The report from the NARMS, over the period 2012–2013, identified MDR-*E. coli* in turkey (62%), chicken (62%), and swine (22%) as well as MDR-non-typhoidal

TABLE 1 | Examples of programs for surveillance and containment of antibiotic resistance.

Monitoring programs	Country	Target population	Target bacteria	References
Danish Integrated Antimicrobial Resistance Monitoring and Research Programme (DANMAP)	Denmark	Humans, animals, and food products	*Salmonella* spp. *Campylobacter* spp. *Enterococcus* spp. *Escherichia coli* *Klebsiella pneumonia* *P. aeruginosa* *Streptococcus* spp. *Staphylococcus aureus*	DANMAP, 2014
Norwegian Surveillance System for Antimicrobial Drug Resistance (NORM/NORM-VET)	Norway	Humans, animals, and food products	*Escherichia coli* *Enterococcus* spp. *Salmonella* spp. *Campylobacter* spp. *Yersinia enterocolitica* *Shigella* spp.	NORM/NORM-VET, 2015
Swedish Veterinary Antimicrobial Resistance Monitoring (SVARM)	Sweden	Animals and food products	*Salmonella* spp. *Campylobacter* spp. *Staphylococcus aureus* *Staphylococcus pseudointermidius* *Enterobacteriaceae* *Enterococcus* spp.	SWEDRES-SVARM, 2015
European Antimicrobial Resistance Surveillance Network (EARS-Net)	Multinational[a]	Humans	*Streptococcus pneumoniae* *Staphylococcus aureus* *Enterococcus* spp. *Escherichia coli* *Klebsiella pneumoniae* *P. aeruginosa*	ECDC, 2015
European Surveillance of Antimicrobial Consumption Network (ESAC-Net)	Multinational[b]	Humans	*Streptococcus pneumoniae* *Staphylococcus aureus* *Enterococcus* spp. *Escherichia coli* *Klebsiella pneumoniae* *P. aeruginosa*	ECDC, 2014
Monitoring and analysis of food-borne diseases in Europe (EFSA)	Multinational[c]	Humans, animals and food products	*Salmonella* spp. *Campylobacter* spp. *Escherichia coli* *Staphylococcus aureus*	EFSA and ECDC, 2016
Monitoring of Antimicrobial Resistance and Antibiotic Usage in Animals in the Netherlands (MARAN)	Netherlands	Animals and food products	*Salmonella* spp. *Campylobacter* spp. *Escherichia coli* *Enterococcus* spp.	NethMap-MARAN, 2015
National Antimicrobial Resistance Monitoring System (NARMS)	United States	Humans, animals and food products	*Salmonella* spp. *Campylobacter* spp. *Enterococcus* spp. *Shigella spp.* *Escherichia coli* *Vibrio spp.* other than *V. cholera*	FDA, 2014

(Continued)

TABLE 1 | Continued

Monitoring programs	Country	Target population	Target bacteria	References
Canadian Integrated Program for Antimicrobial Resistance Surveillance (CIPARS)	Canada	Humans, animals and food products	*Salmonella* spp. *Campylobacter* spp. *Enterococcus* spp. *Escherichia coli*	Government of Canada, 2014
L'Observatoire National de l'Epidémiologie de la Résistance Bactérienne aux Antibiotiques (ONERBA)	France	Humans and Animals	*Enterobacteriaceae and non-fermenters* *Staphylococcus aureus* *Streptococcus* spp. *Enterococcus* spp.	ONERBA, 2015
The Japanese Veterinary Antimicrobial Resistance Monitoring System in the Field of Animal Hygiene (JVARM)	Japan	Animals	*Salmonella* spp. *Campylobacter* spp. *Enterococcus* spp. *Escherichia coli*	The Japanese Veterinary Antimicrobial Resistance Monitoring System in the Field of Animal Hygiene (JVARM), 2013
Japanese Nosocomial Infections Surveillance (JANIS)	Japan	Humans	*Enterobacteriaceae and non-fermenters* *Staphylococcus* spp. *Streptococcus* spp. *Enterococcus* spp.	JANIS, 2016
The Finnish Veterinary Antimicrobial Resistance Monitoring and Consumption of Antimicrobial Agents report (FINRES-VET)	Finland	Animals and food products	*Escherichia coli* *Enterococcus* spp. *Salmonella* spp. *Campylobacter* spp. *Staphylococcus aureus* *Staphylococcus pseudointermidius*	FINRES-Vet, 2007-2009
Pilot Surveillance Program for Antimicrobial Resistance in Bacteria of Animal Origin	Australia	Animals	*Campylobacter* spp. *Escherichia coli* *Enterococcus* spp.	The department, 2007
Colombian Integrated Program for Antimicrobial Resistance Surveillance (COIPARS)	Colombia	Humans, Food animals, and products	*Salmonella* spp. *Campylobacter* spp. *Escherichia coli*	COIPARS, 2011
Pilot Integrated Food Chain Surveillance System	Mexico	food animals and products	*Salmonella* spp. *Campylobacter* spp.	Zaidi et al., 2008, 2012

[a] *33 European countries.*
[b] *34 European countries.*
[c] *28 European countries.*

Salmonella in turkey (34%) and ground beef (20%). Several studies have further reported human colonization and outbreak situations associated with antibiotic-resistant bacteria and ARGs of food animal origins (FDA, 2014).

Notwithstanding the difference in rates of ABR demonstrated in the food chain in developed countries, it is important to mention that most have national programs to monitor antibiotic use and ABR from humans, animals, and food products (**Table 1**). In response to the data generated from these programs, these countries have adopted a set of policies and control measures to contain ABR while preserving their productivity. Denmark has taken major initiatives to address the challenge of ABR over the last 20 years, and actions taken by the Danish government have been acknowledged as a worldwide model (O'Neill, 2015b). The DANMAP, a system for monitoring the impact of withdrawal of antibiotic growth-promoters on the development of ABR in food animals and humans was established in the country to measure the effect of interventions and inform future policies (DANMAP, 2014). From the ban of avoparcin in 1995 up to 2008, poultry production has increased slightly and overall antibiotic consumption decreased by 90%, from 5 to 0.5 tons (used exclusively for therapy)

TABLE 2 | Prevalence of antibiotic-resistant bacteria isolated from food animals and products in developed and developing countries.

Country	Isolation year	Origin/type of specimens	Antibiotic-resistant bacteria	Prevalence (%)	References
DEVELOPED COUNTRIES					
European Union	2014	Broiler meat	MDR-*Salmonella Infantis*	>70	EFSA and ECDC, 2016
		Broiler meat	MDR-*E. coli*	55	
Norway	2014	Broiler	ESBL-producing *E. coli*	36	NORM/NORM-VET, 2015
		Broiler meat	ESBL-producing *E. coli*	30	
		Broiler	Vancomycin resistant *Enterococcus* spp.	7	
Netherlands	2014	Poultry	ESBL-producing *Salmonella* spp.	12	NethMap-MARAN, 2015
		Poultry	Fluoroquinolone-resistant *Salmonella* spp.	43	
		Pig	ESBL/AmpC-*E.coli*	18	
		Dairy cow	ESBL/AmpC-*E.coli*	9	
		Turkey meat	ESBL/AmpC-*E.coli*	51	
		Poultry meat	ESBL/AmpC-*E.coli*	67	
Denmark	2014	Pigs	MDR-*Salmonella* spp.	7	DANMAP, 2014
		Broiler meat	ESBL-producing *E. coli*	9	
United States	2012–2013	Turkey	MDR-*E. coli*	62	FDA, 2014
		Turkey	MDR-non-typhoidal *Salmonella*	34	
		Chicken	MDR-*E. coli*	62	
		Pig	MDR-*E. coli*	22	
		Ground beef	MDR-non-typhoidal *Salmonella*	20	
DEVELOPING COUNTRIES					
China	2015	Pig	Plasmid mediated colistin resistant *E. coli*	21	Liu et al., 2016
		Raw meat	Plasmid mediated colistin resistant *E. coli*	15	
Thailand	2007	Poultry	ESBL-producing *S. Typhimurium*	77.3	Padungtod et al., 2008
		Pig	ESBL-producing *S. Typhimurium*	40.4	
	2012–2013	Pig	ESBL-producing *E. coli*	77	Boonyasiri et al., 2014
		Pork	ESBL-producing *E. coli*	61	
		Pork	MDR-*A. baumannii* and *P. aeruginosa*	40	
		Poultry	ESBL-producing *E. coli*	40	
		Poultry meat	ESBL-producing *E. coli*	50	
Vietnam	2007	Poultry	MDR-*E. coli*	91.5	Usui et al., 2014
Indonesia	2007	Poultry	MDR-*Enterococcus faecalis*	84.5	
Brazil	2000–2016	Pigs	Plasmid mediated colistin resistant *E. coli*	1.8	Fernandes et al., 2016
		Chicken	Plasmid mediated colistin resistant *E. coli*	5	
Egypt	2010	Meat and dairy products	MDR-Shiga-toxin-producing *E. coli* O157:H7	57.4	Ahmed and Shimamoto, 2015a
	2010	Meat and dairy products	MDR-*Shigella spp.*	89	Ahmed and Shimamoto, 2015b
Algeria	2005–2006	Broilers	MDR- *Salmonella spp.*	51	Elgroud et al., 2009
Tunisia	2010–2011	Raw meat	MDR-*Enterococcus spp.*	24.5	Klibi et al., 2013
		Raw meat	LA-MRSA ST398	0.6	Chairat et al., 2015
South Africa	2014	Cattle	MDR-*E. coli*	100	Iweriebor et al., 2015
	2015	Poultry	Plasmid mediated colistin-resistant *E. coli*	79	Coetzee et al., 2016

MDR, Multi-drug resistant.

in 2008 (DANMAP, 2014). The prevalence of vancomycin resistant *Enterococcus faecium* substantially declined in pig and poultry production between 1996 and 2008 (DANMAP, 2014). Several developed countries have also recently responded to and followed the recommendations of the WHO, OIE, and FAO tripartite alliance to strengthen the containment of ABR, with the development and implementation of their national action plans.

Developing Countries

In contrast with developed countries, the majority of LMICs have minimal or no programs or systems to monitor antibiotic use or ABR in food animals, food products, and humans, its true burden being only partially documented, and reliant on point-prevalence rather than long-term studies. Moreover, antibiotics are extensively used in agriculture for growth-promotion, and the danger of ABR in the food chain is further neglected and under-estimated (Eagar et al., 2012; Van Boeckel et al., 2014). For example, two-third of the 1500 tons of antibiotics sold for animal use over a 3 years' period (2002–2004) in South Africa were for growth-promotion purposes and included WHO-banned substances (Eagar et al., 2012). A recent modeling study suggests that up to a third of the global increase (67%) in antibiotic consumption in food animals, over the period 2010-2030, will be attributable to LMICs (Van Boeckel et al., 2015). For Brazil, Russia, India, China, and South Africa, this increase is projected to reach 99%, up to seven times the estimated population growth of these countries (Van Boeckel et al., 2015). By 2030, antibiotic use in food animals is estimated to be 51,851 tons in Asia alone, representing more than 80% of the global antibiotic consumption in food animals in 2010 (Van Boeckel et al., 2015). In 2007, China was the largest antibiotic producer and consumer, with 210,000 tons produced, with 46% being used in livestock production. The country was also the world's pig and poultry producer in 2014, with 56.7 and 17.5 million tons, respectively (Liu et al., 2016). The increase in agriculture and food production in LMICs parallels what developed countries experienced over the last 100 years when income rose (Collignon and Voss, 2015). The damaging consequences of this intensification in food production has resulted in several sub-optimal practices, such as over-crowding of animals, large quantities of antibiotics consumed, and often poor hygienic measures and farming practices (Collignon and Voss, 2015). The incidence of ABR is thus undoubtedly worse in developing countries, where humans interact intimately with animals and the environment, infectious diseases rates are higher, regulations on antibiotic use, and the development, implementation, and monitoring of ABR prevention and containment measures are rare and frequently non-existent.

Several studies have documented new resistance mechanisms and elevated rates of antibiotic-resistant bacteria in Asian and African developing nations (**Table 2**). A recent Chinese routine surveillance study revealed a highly mobile and transferable plasmid-mediated colistin-resistance gene, called mcr-1, in commensal *E. coli* isolated from pigs (21%) and raw meat (15%; (Liu et al., 2016)). The study also revealed that 1% of clinical isolates from hospitalized Chinese patients harbored this new resistant gene (Liu et al., 2016). It is thought that this gene originated from animals and spread into humans via the food chain (Liu et al., 2016). Plasmid mediated mcr-1 colistin-resistant *E. coli* were also detected in chicken (14/515) and pigs (2/515) in Brazil (Fernandes et al., 2016). This finding is of great concern, as although not frequently used in human medicine, colistin remains a drug of last resort, with the global emergence of extensively-drug resistant Gram negative bacteria.

In Thailand, high levels of ESBL-producing *Salmonella Typhimurium* in poultry (77.3%) and pigs (40.4%) were reported, with an overall 86% prevalence of MDR (Padungtod et al., 2008). In the same country, Boonyasiri et al. (2014) identified elevated prevalence of ESBL-producing *E. coli* in the food chain during the years 2012–2013, these being 77% in pigs, 40% in poultry, 77% in farmers, 76% in food handlers, 61% in pork, and 50% in chicken. The same study further reported 40% of MDR-*Acinetobacter baumannii* and *Pseudomonas aeruginosa* in pork (Boonyasiri et al., 2014). MDR-*E. coli* strains were also detected in chicken fecal samples in Vietnam (91.5%) and Indonesia (62.8%) with isolates being concomitantly resistant to up to 10 antibiotics (Usui et al., 2014). In Africa, there is a paucity of research and consequently data on antibiotic-resistant bacteria and ARGs in food animals and food products. However, high level of MDR-bacteria isolated from various food animals have been documented in several African countries. Ahmed and Shimamoto (2015a,b) reported MDR-Shiga-toxin-producing *E. coli* O157:H7 (57.4%) and MDR-*Shigella* spp. (89%) from food products (meat and dairy products) in Egypt, while a maximum prevalence (100%) of MDR-*E. coli* has been identified in rectal samples of cattle in South Africa (Iweriebor et al., 2015). MDR-*Enterococcus* spp. (24.5%) (Klibi et al., 2013) and MDR-*Salmonella spp.* (51%) (Elgroud et al., 2009) were isolated from meat samples and broilers in Tunisia and Algeria, respectively. A recent nation-wide surveillance in poultry settings described substantial increases in colistin-resistance in *E. coli* strains in 2015 in South Africa. Accordingly, the emergence of mcr-1 was confirmed in 79% of colistin-resistant strains isolated (Coetzee et al., 2016). Clinical isolates of colistin-resistant *E. coli* from hospitalized ($n = 3$) and outpatients ($n = 6$) were further detected in the same study (Coetzee et al., 2016). Carbapenemase producing-*P. aeruginosa* and *A. baumannii* have further been recently identified in food animals in Lebanon, confirming the serious threat associated with the emergence of ABR in the food chain (Al Bayssari et al., 2015).

The majority of developing countries are substantive exporters of food animals and food products. Brazil is the world's largest exporter of chicken meat (Fernandes et al., 2016) and Thailand exports not <70% of its poultry production (Boonyasiri et al., 2014). This means that antibiotic-resistant bacteria and/or ARGs emerging in these countries and other LMICs will easily spread across the world via the food chain (Boonyasiri et al., 2014; Fernandes et al., 2016; Holmes et al., 2016). Grami et al. (2016) recently reported high prevalence of plasmid mediated mcr-1 *E. coli* in fecal samples of chicken imported from European countries in Tunisia. This is also of grave concern as antibiotic-resistant bacteria and ARGs emerging in food animals and products in developed nations could endanger safety, public health in already overburdened health care settings of developing countries, where prevention and containment of ABR are limited and where high levels of ABR prevail (**Table 2**). This confirms that globalization of trade in food animals and products are major determinants of the worldwide dissemination of ABR from farm-to-fork.

Additionally, travelers visiting developing countries from developed nations may be colonized or infected by antibiotic-resistant bacteria and/or ARGs, and in turn become vectors of transmission in their home countries. Dutch travelers to North Africa (Tunisia), South America (Peru, Bolivia, and Colombia), and Asia (Thailand, China, Vietnam, Laos, and Cambodia) were recently reported to be colonized by colistin-resistant *E. coli* strains harboring mcr-1 gene (Coetzee et al., 2016). Likewise, the prevalence of ESBL-producing *Enterobacteriaceae,* colonization in Swedish, Dutch, and Australian tourists, increased from 2.4–8.6 to 30–49% following travel to India, Southeast Asia, and China (Boonyasiri et al., 2014). Travelers from developed nations seeking healthcare in LMICs, generally to avoid high costs, long delays or due to legal or cultural restrictions in their home countries, have also been involved in the spread of ABR (Chen and Wilson, 2013). A recent study confirmed that recent international travel was an independent risk factor for septicemia after trans-rectal prostate biopsy (Chen and Wilson, 2013). Several authors further documented the implication of travelers, including medical tourists, in the global spread of ABR (Coetzee et al., 2016; Fernandes et al., 2016; Holmes et al., 2016). The travelers likely acquired antibiotic-resistant bacteria and/or ARGs following the consumption of contaminated foods, water and/or contact with the environment in developing countries (Coetzee et al., 2016; Fernandes et al., 2016).

The variations observed between countries, with an important north-to-south gradient, reveal that the spread of antibiotic-resistant bacteria in the food chain is likely to be higher in LMICs than in developed countries (**Table 2**). There is clear evidence that ABR is a global public health problem, which appears to be worse in developing countries, although it threatens the world equally. Despite the fact that some governments, notably China, India, Thailand, Brazil, Malaysia, and South Africa have taken significantly actions and policies toward the rationalization of antibiotic use and containment of ABR in humans, such initiatives still lag far behind in food animals. Having good data on antibiotic consumption and trends of antibiotic-resistant bacteria and ARGs in food animals, food products and humans, as well as political commitment, are imperative to better understand and manage the concern of ABR via the food chain in developing countries.

PREVENTION AND CONTAINMENT MEASURES OF ANTIBIOTIC RESISTANCE FROM FARM-TO-FORK

Emergence and spread of antibiotic-resistant bacteria and ARGs in the food chain, has given rise to severe health and socio-economic repercussions globally. Resistant foodborne infections are amongst the main public health issues associated with the threat of ABR in the food chain. This global concern equally affects developed and developing countries, and may cause outbreaks and pandemic situations (Padungtod et al., 2008). The problem is more serious in the developing world, where resistant infections significantly increase morbidity and mortality rates, whereas in developed countries, these infections will enhance therapeutic costs (Harbarth et al., 2015). The majority of developing countries are not implementing adequate measures to prevent and curb the spread of ABR from farm-to-fork, thus, posing a significant threat for global public health. Combating ABR effectively at a global scale means tackling it in the developing world first, whether in the food chain or not. The One Health approach was endorsed to address the threat of ABR by supranational entities, following the coalition between the WHO, FAO, and OIE referred as the "Tripartite Alliance." The WHO, in collaboration with its Tripartite partners, published the Global Action Plan on Antimicrobial Resistance in 2015, an attempt to counteract effectively this worldwide concern (WHO, 2015a). The FAO similarly launched its Antimicrobial Resistance Strategy in September 2016 to support the implementation of the WHO's Global Action plan in the food and agricultural sectors (FAO, 2016). Noting that ABR in the food chain is a serious global threat which is considerably neglected/under-estimated in developing countries, this section consequently proposes solutions for an effective containment of ABR from farm-to-fork, albeit relatively applicable in both developed and developing nations. The five strategic objectives of the WHO's Global Action Plan, namely (i) heighten awareness and understanding on antibiotic use and antibiotic resistance, (ii) strengthen knowledge via surveillance and research, (iii) reduce infectious diseases, (iv) optimize rational antibiotic use, and (v) mobilize resources, research and development, have been used as framework to set out integrated prevention and containment measures of ABR in the food chain (WHO, 2015a, **Table 3**).

Heightening Awareness and Understanding of Antibiotic Resistance

Public Awareness Campaigns on Antibiotic Use and Antibiotic Resistance

Heightening national awareness campaigns on antibiotic use, ABR, and food safety are important to address this global challenge from farm-to-fork, as knowledge leads to prevention. Well-designed and simple key messages that target populations and engage all-stakeholders (viz. farm, and abattoir workers, food handlers, consumers, veterinarians, pharmacists, food production industries, healthcare workers) are essential for successful awareness campaigns (Harbarth et al., 2015). Strengthened awareness through mass and social media continuously repeating key messages may contribute to effectively lessen antibiotic consumption and ABR rates (Harbarth et al., 2015). The choice of indicators and targets are crucial in monitoring the impact of such campaigns (Harbarth et al., 2015).

Global awareness campaigns on antibiotic use and ABR have been increasingly advocated, with sustainable communication measures having been implemented at international level, e.g., the "European antibiotic awareness day" in EU, the "get smart:

TABLE 3 | Summary of prevention and containment measures of antibiotic resistance from farm-to-fork.

Measures	World Health Organization's Global Action Plan Strategic Objectives				
	Increase awareness	**Strengthen surveillance**	**Reduce infectious diseases**	**Optimize rational antibiotic use**	**Mobilize resources, strengthen research and development**
Basic	National awareness campaigns on antibiotic usage and ABR	Integrated food chain surveillance systems	Implement biosecurity measures	Prohibit the growth-promotion use of antibiotics	Political will
	Food safety awareness campaigns	Establish reference laboratory		Prohibit unrestricted access of antibiotics	
	Achieve effective "culture change"	Harmonized-laboratory methods	Institute massive immunization campaigns	Establish guidelines for veterinary use of antibiotics	Sustainable commitment involving all stakeholders
		Reinforced education and fostered excellence			Assess and manage food safety risk
Moderate	Cross-disciplinary research	Research on total bacterial resistome and mobilome	Organic farming practices	Develop methods to verify judicious antibiotic use	Institute sustainable collaboration (North-to-South, South-to-South, Private-to-Publi)
	Provide assistance, support and training to occupationally exposed workers		Well-controlled extensive farming practices	Institute veterinary oversight	
			Reinforce veterinary legislation and enforcement policies		Leverage resources
Advanced	Evaluate the impact of the educational programs	State-of-the-art methods	Predictive microbiology	Institute Incentives/disincentives	Pre-, pro-, and syn-biotics
			Diagnostic tool based-nanoscale materials	Implement legal regulatory framework	Phage-related therapies
					Genetically modified food animals
					Nano-antibiotics

know when antibiotics work" in US, and the first "World Antibiotic Awareness Week" held in November 2015. Although challenging, awareness or educational campaigns are relatively successful, with some good examples reported across the world (Harbarth et al., 2015). Farmers, abattoir workers, food handlers, and veterinarians are not the only ones affected by the threat of ABR in the food chain, but all categories of the general population must be involved and educated.

Food Safety Awareness Campaigns

Food safety is a scientific discipline aiming to ensure safe food and prevent foodborne diseases throughout all stages of the food production chain including handling, transport, storage, and preparation. Food safety awareness campaigns are essential to improved consumer's and food handlers' knowledge to prevent foodborne infectious diseases and hazards (including antibiotic residues, ARGs, and antibiotic-resistant bacteria). Some basic food safety measures, such as convenient hand-washing with water and soap several times during the day (especially before and after meal preparation, after usage of toilets), effective vegetable-washing, adequate cooking temperatures, and food storage are important to reduce the spread of antibiotic-resistant bacteria and the prevalence of ABR- foodborne infections. In this regard, the WHO has summarized these practices into a simple and strong tool called "five keys to safer food" to help ensure food safety from farm-to-fork (Mwamakamba et al., 2012). It is the responsibility of stakeholders involved along the food chain, including food production industries, agricultural practitioners, food handlers, and consumers to ensure safe food using the adequate food safety measures, as depicted by the WHO, albeit governments have the central role in providing an adequate framework to implement food safety-associated health promotion programs. Several countries in Africa and Asia have implemented food safety education programs using the WHO five keys to safer foods (Prabhakar et al., 2010; Mensah et al., 2012; Mwamakamba et al., 2012).

Behavior Change, Education, and Training

Behind these sensitization efforts, human behavior, whether through inter alia individualism, lack of education, culture or social beliefs, is an important factor that needs to be considered when educating/creating an awareness on antibiotic use and ABR, as new knowledge is not immediately translated into new practices. For a successful intervention, it is important to implement cross-disciplinary research involving anthropologists, sociologists, psychologists, and ethnographers to investigate the target groups' perception and knowledge beforehand. This will enable the most efficient strategies to be developed to modify behaviors, and achieve and enact effective "culture change" (Prabhakar et al., 2010; Mensah et al., 2012; Mwamakamba et al., 2012; Harbarth et al., 2015).

Reinforced education and fostering excellence in both private and public veterinarians about conservative prescription of antibiotics, the emergence of ABR and the One Health approach have a crucial role to play in containing ABR from farm-to-fork. The OIE provides guidelines on initial veterinary education, highlighting the basis for an organized profession with high-quality professionals (OIE, 2016). It is also essential to provide assistance, support and training to occupationally exposed workers (viz. to farmers, abattoir and food workers), as well as guidance on rational antibiotic use and good agricultural practices, according to their education level. Such initiative must be supported at a global level, and adapted at the local level through leadership from relevant ministers, industries, agricultural practitioners, and veterinarians. Monitoring strategies must also be developed to evaluate the impact of the educational programs.

Strengthening Surveillance and Research

Integrated Food Chain Surveillance Systems

An essential step toward addressing the public health threat of ABR is to determine the resistance burden from different ecological niches in the entire food chain (farm, abattoir, market, etc.). This is more evident in developing countries, where data on ABR, antibiotic use and foodborne illnesses is scarce. Integrated food chain surveillance systems, conducting sustainable research (long-term epidemiological and molecular studies) from farm-to-fork, endorsing the One Health approach and the Codex Alimentarius Commission guidelines, and reporting a combination of passive, active, and outbreak data sources are needed to fill the data gaps, as well as to assess the impact of public awareness campaigns on rational antibiotic use and ABR (Prabhakar et al., 2010; FAO and WHO, 2011; Acar and Moulin, 2013). The generated information from such surveillance could inform decision-makers, evidence-based policies, and help to allocate appropriate resources for preventing and containing ABR via the food chain. These systems further need to establish harmonized laboratory methods and provide specifications for the target populations, samples, settings and bacteria, in keeping with the WHO's AGISAR, in order to compare results nationally and internationally.

The NARMS, DANMAP, and MARAN are well-known integrated food chain surveillance systems that have been established in developed countries to undertake research along the food chain, combine data from various sources and use strong multi-sectorial partnerships with other entities (DANMAP, 2014; FDA, 2014; NethMap-MARAN, 2015). Colombia is a notable developing country example, having successfully piloted an integrated surveillance system to monitor trends in antibiotic resistance on poultry farms, abattoirs and retail markets in order to develop adequate ABR prevention and containment measures (Donado-Godoy et al., 2015). The pilot Colombian Integrated Program for Antimicrobial Resistance Surveillance (COIPARS) was able to meet animal health and welfare requests of food producers, and address public health concerns associated with the antibiotic use in food animals and ensure food safety. The COIPARS is regarded as a model in Latin America by the International Molecular Subtyping Network for Foodborne Disease Surveillance (PulseNet International) and the WHO Global Foodborne Infections Network (Donado-Godoy et al., 2015). The WHO AGISAR has further used COIPARS as a guide to harmonize methods for monitoring of ABR and antibiotic use in food animals in the Americas (Donado-Godoy et al., 2015).

Similarly, Mexico implemented a pilot on integrated food chain surveillance system to prevent and contain *Salmonella* spp., *Campylobacter* spp., and *E. coli* from farm-to-fork in four regions and ascertained its cost-effectiveness. Samples were collected from sick and healthy humans, locally produced retail chicken, pork, beef, and their intestines at slaughterhouses, with a sample size representative of the regional consumption of each retail meat using standardized laboratory protocols (Zaidi et al., 2008, 2015; Donado-Godoy et al., 2015). Within a 3 years-period, and with a limited financial investment, the Mexican's integrated food chain surveillance system was able to yield meaningful epidemiological data on emerging public health threats, identified effectively strains of greatest public health threat, as well as the main food animal reservoirs, showing that these systems are technically and economically feasible in developing countries (Zaidi et al., 2008, 2012, 2015).

Reference Laboratory and Harmonized-Laboratory Methods

National reference laboratories are essential to provide harmonized, high quality, and precise information when assessing ABR bacteria (indicator, foodborne, and emerging bacteria) with the potential to threaten food safety. The majority of developed countries have well-designed reference laboratories that focus their activities on humans as well as animals, while few LMICs have established national reference laboratories, with those that do mainly focusing on humans. National reference laboratories in which bacteria are tested for antibiotic susceptibility exist in 6 out 47 and 6 out of 21 countries of the WHO African and Eastern Mediterranean Regions respectively (WHO, 2015b). Reorientation of the research strategy to include food animals, food derived products, and humans is vital to contain the spread of ABR from farm-to-fork in developing countries (de Balogh et al., 2013).

Research on the Total Bacterial Resistome

Given that food animals are key and persistent reservoirs of ABR, basic food chain surveillance programs focus primarily on foodborne or indicator bacteria. Effectively curbing the emergence and spread of ABR needs to consider the role of commensal flora in the emergence of resistance. Antibiotic use affects and selects largely resistant bacteria in commensal flora, which may subsequently transmit their ARGs to the pathogenic ones (Andremont, 2003). The commensal genetic pool is so huge that it involves several pathways of transferring resistance, including mutations and complex resistance mechanisms (HGT) that are either expressed or silent within subdominant species, and are able to move freely between species (Andremont, 2003). Assessing the whole bacterial resistome and mobilome through food surveillance systems will enable the detection of emerging antibiotic-resistant bacteria and ARGs from farm-to-fork. This is important to inform issues that are often ignored by basic food chain surveillance programs, these being to detect early outbreaks and undertake timely correct actions. This is obviously more feasible in developed and well-resourced countries.

State-of-the-Art Methods

Detecting antibiotic-resistant bacteria and ARGs is based on culturing, antimicrobial susceptibility testing (AST), and polymerase chain reaction (PCR). Although AST and PCR-based methods are excellent for phenotyping resistance profiling and detecting ARGs respectively, both require bacterial culture and do not enable the discovery of distantly related or unknown elements that may be present, and which are particularly crucial in the farm-to-fork continuum. Whole genome sequencing enables the detection and exploration of complete bacterial genome, with a view to identify new genetic traits. Metagenomics also allows the analysis of the whole genome and identification of unknown genetic elements, regardless of the cultural characteristics of the bacteria (Allen, 2014; Thanner et al., 2016). Single nucleotide polymorphisms, novel resistance genes and unforeseen aspects of ARG ecology may be identified through the use of whole genome sequencing and functional metagenomics, respectively (Allen, 2014; Thanner et al., 2016). Plasmid sequence analysis and reconstruction may also be performed using whole genome sequencing and metagenomics. Microarray expression analysis provide useful insights into expressing profiles of bacteria under antibiotic pressure, while recent transcriptomics and meta-transcriptomics tools identifying functional genes are also an important advancement in detecting new genetic elements (Thanner et al., 2016). State-of-the-art tools may be very useful to understand transmission dynamics of resistance gene expression through the different ecological niches prevailing in the food chain (Thanner et al., 2016). Again, these are more feasible in developed and well-resourced countries.

Reducing the Burden of Infectious Diseases

Immunization and Biosecurity

Unprecedented global food demands result in farmers' reliance on antibiotics to produce large quantities of animal protein at low cost although. Evidence exits that improving animal welfare and health have the potential to diminish this over-dependence on antibiotics without affecting productivity and costs. The use of vaccines is recommended as method of preventing infections in animals and should significantly reduce antibiotic consumption while increasing the productivity. Although already available against some viral, parasitical, and bacterial infections (**Table 4**) in food animals, their routine use is generally limited due to few incentives promoting them and the absence of disincentives prohibiting antibiotic consumption in the food production industry (Woolhouse et al., 2015). Mass vaccination campaigns should be implemented as in humans to ensure animal health, as the greater the use of vaccines, the lesser the incidence of infections (Woolhouse et al., 2015). Vaccines can effectively protect animals against bacterial infections, but may require regular "updates" to ensure their continuous efficacy (O'Neill, 2015b).

Biosecurity measures in food and agriculture should further significantly reduce or eliminate ABR-bacteria from farm-to-fork, and thereby, lower the burden of infectious diseases. Biosecurity refers to a holistic concept used to define a set of ongoing measures taken to reduce the risk of the emergence/introduction and dissemination of diseases at herd-, region-, and country-levels (FAO, 2003; FAO and WHO, 2011). It uses "One Health" as a framework, and benefits from this integrated approach by encompassing various concepts, such as good agricultural practices, good hygiene practices, good veterinary practices, hazard analysis, and critical control points (HACCP)-based procedures and microbiological risk assessment and management (FAO, 2003; FAO and WHO, 2011). When animals are healthy, antibiotics are not needed to treat them. However, when ABR occurs, and effective barriers (e.g., good agricultural practices, good hygiene practices, and HACCP-based measures) are present, subsequent transmission will be impeded, with food safety, food security, and public health being ensured. Biosecurity should then play a fundamental role in any disease control program as it expands beyond agricultural production to human and environmental health (Nahar et al., 2014; Postma et al., 2016).

Farming Practices

Well-controlled extensive farming practices using small chemical substances and that favor animal health and welfare to limit the development of infectious diseases and reduce antibiotic use (e.g., all-in-all-out, extensive free-range systems), should be promoted and implemented rather than intensive farming practices. Organic farm systems have recently received considerable interest to meet the global food demand in an effort to reduce the extensive use of antibiotics (Prabhakar et al., 2010). In comparing the occurrence of ABR in food animals in conventional and organic farms, Österberg et al. (2016) reported a significant lower prevalence of ABR-*E. coli* isolated from organic pig farms than from conventional ones in four European countries (Österberg et al., 2016). This suggests that organic farms could be valuable agricultural alternatives to reduce the burden of ABR, although further research is needed to ascertain the consequences related to such practices and improve the productivity. Sweden, the first country that implemented a total ban of antibiotic growth-promoters in food production industry in 1986, is one of the world's references for containment of ABR in the food chain through well-implemented and adequate farming practices (O'Neill, 2015b). Following the 1986's ban, to facilitate the passage to new farming practices, Swedish authorities developed guidelines on management, hygiene, medication, and feed to improve animal health and prevent infectious diseases. Swedish efforts were considerably focused on problem-oriented research and provided extensive support for farmers (O'Neill, 2015b). This led to decrease of sales of antibiotics used in food animals

TABLE 4 | List of some available veterinary bacterial vaccines.

Target animal	Target pathogen	Brand name	Characteristics	References
Pig	*Lawsonia intracellularis*	Enterisol Ileitis	Live oral vaccine	Guedes and Gebhart, 2003
Fish	*Yersinia ruckeri*	AquaVac ERM	Killed oral vaccine	Meeusen et al., 2007
Fish	*Aeromonas salmonicida*	AquaVac Furuvac	Killed oral vaccine	
Fish	*Vibrio anguillarum*	AquaVac Vibrio	Killed oral vaccine	
Chicken	*Salmonella spp.*	Megan Vac1 MeganEgg	Live vaccine	Babu et al., 2004
Cattle	*Brucella abortus*	RB-51	Rifampin-resistant mutant	Moriyon et al., 2004
Pig	*Actinobacillus pleuropneumoniae*	PleuroStar APP	Recombinant proteins	Van Overbeke et al., 2001
Chicken	*Mycoplasma gallisepticum*	Vaxsafe MG	Live vaccine for eye drop administration	Barbour et al., 2000
Chicken	*Mycoplasma synoviae*	Vaxsafe MS	Live vaccine for eye drop administration	Meeusen et al., 2007
Turkeys	*Bordetella avium*	Art Vax	Live for spray inhalation or drinking water	
Sheep	*Chlamydophila abortus*	Ovilis Enzovax	Live vaccine for intramuscular or sub-cutaneous injection	
Pig	*Actinobacillus pleuropneumoniae*	Porcilis APP	Outer membrane proteins	

from 45 tons to around 15 tons of active substances by 2009 (O'Neill, 2015b). In contrast, up to a third of the projected 67% global increase in antibiotic consumption in food animals will be attributable to shifting agricultural practices in LMICs, where extensive farming systems will be substituted by large-scale intensive farming (Van Boeckel et al., 2015). This suggests that LMICs should follow the Swedish experience for sustainable agriculture independent of antibiotics although data relative to such initiatives was limited.

Rapid Infection Diagnostics

There are significant advantages of rapid diagnostic tools, such as culturing, PCR, microarray, and whole genome sequencing, being more readily available to quickly identify bacterial infections, resistance patterns, and determine appropriate treatment in animals and humans (Woolhouse et al., 2015). Chromogenic tests and Matrix-assisted laser desorption/ionization time-of-flight have been proposed, as they allow not only rapid bacterial identification and but also effective resistance profiling. These tools may be suitable for LMICs where diagnostic tool must be relatively economical, rapid, easy to use, and requires less logistic infrastructure (Holmes et al., 2016).

Several mathematical models, such as Predictive Microbial Modeling Lab (PMM-Lab), Pathogen Modeling Program (PMP), Geeraerd and Van Impe Inactivation Model Fitting Tool (GInaFiT), and Combined dataBase (ComBase) Predictor, that predict the bacterial behaviors in various stages of production (e.g., processing, storage, and distribution) have recently received significant interest in the food production industry (Plaza-Rodríguez et al., 2015). Predictive microbiology generates substantive quantitative data and useful estimates that can assist in decision-making during food production process, HACCP-based procedures and food safety risk analysis and management (Plaza-Rodríguez et al., 2015; Thanner et al., 2016). Predictive microbiology could be valuable to reduce antibiotic use and infectious diseases, and contain ABR. However, it must be optimized to encompass important factors, such as the total bacterial resistome, microbial loads, biological mechanisms, and cross-species transmission, with outcomes not only being lethality, but also incidence of diseases, level of pathogenicity and prevalence of antibiotic-resistant bacteria and ARGs (Plaza-Rodríguez et al., 2015; Thanner et al., 2016).

The Artificial Neural Network (ANN) is an advanced mathematical model capable of performing large and simultaneous computations for data processing and knowledge representation. It is able to combine data of different nature collected from various sources, populations and protocols, thereby forming an integrated diagnostic system. Several studies have demonstrated that ANNs could be built and trained to recognize bacterial resistance patterns, and to generate adequate conclusion in terms of ABR profiles (Budak and Übeyli, 2011; Lechowicz et al., 2013). Budak and Übeyli (2011) used ANN to predict the resistance profiles of *Salmonella spp.* to Ampicillin, Chloramphenicol, and Trimethoprim-sulfamethoxazole, and reported overall accuracies of more than 95% (Budak and Übeyli, 2011).

Modern methods, such as Fourier Transform Infrared Spectroscopy (FTIR) and Attenuated Total Reflection-based (ATR)-FTIR, that detect the presence and measure the infrared spectra of intact microbial cells have also been proposed for rapid bacterial strains detection in the food production chain (Rebuffo-Scheer et al., 2007; Lechowicz et al., 2013). The combination of infrared spectroscopy with ANN also allows the rapid identification of bacteria and determination of resistance patterns. Lechowicz et al. (2013) demonstrated that the Multi-Layer Perception network built using the ANN-based FTIR method was able to successfully detect uro-pathogenic *E. coli*, and to classify strains susceptible and resistant to cephalothin with more than 90% of accuracy. Although these tools require sufficient skills, they present an adequate level of accuracies to differentiate bacteria and determine resistance patterns, and could be used routinely for laboratory diagnostics (Rebuffo-Scheer et al., 2007; Lechowicz et al., 2013).

Nanoscale materials have also emerged as an innovative approach to enable rapid, sensitive and cost-effective diagnosis, and to adequately determine bacterial resistance profiles. Antibody-conjugated nanoparticles have reported to be able to identify highly pathogenic *E. coli* O157:H7 within 20 min. A rapid diagnostic tool, using gold nano-wire arrays in conjunction with a linker arm coated to specific *E. coli* antibodies, has recently been developed to detect urinary tract infections (Huh and Kwon, 2011). On-going research using magnetic nanoparticles, such as dextrancoated super-magnetic iron oxide nanoparticles attached with con-A conjugated nano-sensors, is assessing bacterial metabolic activity and antibiotic susceptibility in opaque media, including blood and milk, without any sample preparation. The intention is to achieve fast and reliable diagnostic assays for bacterial infections adapted to the food production chain, although this is not as yet commercially available (Huh and Kwon, 2011).

Rapid diagnostics will allow agricultural practitioners to identify early infection in animals, to separate those that are infected from others, prevent the spread of infection to the whole herd or flock, and thereby reduce antibiotic use (FAO, 2015; O'Neill, 2015b). Technical and financial barriers, as well as resistance to the adoption of innovative ideas are slowing the implementation of such measures around the world, particularly in developing countries.

Optimizing Rational Antibiotic Use

Ban on Antibiotic Use

The burden of ABR has reached and surpassed the pace of development of new antibacterial agents entering clinical use, and has led to a radical re-evaluation of antibiotic use. Given the growing global concern about the spread of antibiotic-resistant bacteria from animals to humans, there is a significant interest in phasing out antibiotics in the food production industry. LMICs should determine their annual antibiotic consumption in food animals and prohibit the growth-promotion use of any antibiotic substances which the WHO considers to be "critically, highly and important antimicrobials in human medicine," as well as those not currently approved for veterinary use (WHO, 2011; OIE, 2015; O'Neill, 2015b). Avoparcin, was the first antibiotic growth-promoter banned in 1995 in Denmark, followed by virginiamycin in 1998 and a complete ban of antibiotics in 2000 (DANMAP, 2014). The effects of the ban were noticeable as the country experienced significant reduction in antibiotic use and ABR, without affecting the pig and poultry productions which continued to thrive albeit with a small drop in productivity at the inception of the ban and until biosecurity efforts were enhanced. Danish farmers increased their pig production by 47% over the period 1992–2008, preserving the standing of country as among the greatest exporters of pork worldwide, with 90% of their pig production being exported (O'Neill, 2015b). Denmark thus illustrated that very productive and sustainable food production is possible alongside low antibiotic use (O'Neill, 2015b). The majority of developing nations are still far behind a total ban of antibiotics for growth-promotion purposes. Considerable efforts are thus needed by way of an incremental process encompassing cultural, political, and socio-economic contexts while taking cognizance of the urgency and gravity of the ABR concern.

Prohibit Unrestricted Access of Antibiotics

As ARGs are generally carried on mobile genetic elements and all antibiotic families have the potential to select, to a certain degree, cross-resistance to other families. The unrestricted access of antibiotics to farmers should thus be prohibited unless under veterinary prescription or oversight. Meaningful veterinary oversight should further be mandatory when classes of antibiotics currently approved for dual use (both animal and human health) to treat or prevent infectious diseases are prescribed. It is also important to develop methods to verify judicious antibiotic use, establish goals for measuring progress and guidelines for consuming veterinary antibiotics (O'Neill, 2015b; OIE, 2016). In 2009, Dutch government implemented a registration process for veterinary prescription of antibiotics. As a result, between 2007 and 2012, Dutch antibiotic sales in food animals decreased by 56% without any loss in terms of productivity and profits. Dutch farmers have changed their farming practices from over-reliance on antibiotics to improved animal health and welfare (O'Neill, 2015b). To the best of our knowledge, such measures have not been significantly implemented in food animals and aquaculture in LMICs, where regulatory framework and legislation implementation are further limited.

Legislative Regulation and Enforcement Policies

The OIE recommended reinforcing veterinary legislation and enforcement policies to ensure compliance with the law and regulations promoting responsible and prudent use of Veterinary Critically Important Antimicrobial Agents (VCIA), Veterinary Highly Important Antimicrobial Agents (VHIA), and Veterinary Important Antimicrobial Agents (VIA) (OIE, 2015, 2016). When antibiotics are justifiably required, it is essential to follow the established principles and criteria for antibiotic use, according to the OIE "List of Antimicrobial Agents of Veterinary Importance." Achieving a balance between minimizing antibiotic use in food production industry, while meeting the unprecedented rise of worldwide food demands, is a fundamental food security/food safety challenge that must be considered when defining target goals for reducing antibiotic use. It is therefore important that every country involves stakeholders from various sectors (governments, industries, experts, practitioners, and international entities) to set an ambitious but realistic and achievable targets to reduce antibiotic consumption (O'Neill, 2016). Developing countries should examine and adapt the Danish, Dutch, and Swedish experiences as well as acquire scientific expertise from these countries in order to reduce their antibiotic consumption in food animals and aquaculture while preserving their productivity. It is further essential to promote and ensure sustainable agriculture not over-reliant on antibiotics in the developing world to reach the United Nations Sustainable Development Goals by 2030. Sustainable support from developed countries, funding agencies and international entities is essential to reduce antibiotic use and ABR in food animals and aquaculture in LMICs.

Sustainable Investment and Development of New Medicines

Political Will

The human and economic burden associated with containing ABR are trivial compared to the cost of complacency or inaction. ABR will account for more than 10 million deaths by 2050, with a cumulative global economic loss of US $100 trillion over the 35 next years if not addressed substantively (O'Neill, 2015a). ABR should be considered a national priority to retain the attention, ensure sustainable investment and allocate resources to successfully contain it. Governments should translate surveillance estimates into policies leading to implementing long-term interventions and activities in animal husbandry systems and agriculture to ensure animal welfare and health, and to contain ABR at local, national, regional, and international levels. More public and private partnerships are also needed to assess the problem in its broader context and find lasting solutions. Active political will is thus indispensable to enact sustainable engagement, investment, research, and alternatives to antibiotics in the food production industry (O'Neill, 2015b; Woolhouse et al., 2015).

Sustainable Engagement

The need to address and fill the gaps in ABR knowledge have never been more imperative. Sustainable engagement of inter alia policy makers, agricultural practitioners, veterinarians, antibiotic providers, industries, food suppliers, the public, and others who may contribute to long-term solutions is an essential component to effectively contain ABR via the food chain. Multi-sectorial and coordinated efforts should cohesively identify and target research priorities as well as increase research funding to effectively overcome this global challenge (Woolhouse et al., 2015; O'Neill, 2016).

Leverage Resources

Addressing the issue of ABR globally requires greater efforts in developing countries, where interventions may be restricted as a result of inadequate resources. It is thus important to approach to donor funding agencies and supranational entities to improve prevention and containment of ABR via the food chain. An example is the Fleming Funds with its £265 million allocated by the UK government to help improve surveillance in LMICs (O'Neill, 2016). The World Bank's International Development Association (IDA) is another funding mechanism through which LMICs could request support to strengthen surveillance programs, built laboratory-capacity, and prevent and contain ABR. More international support to LMICs are however still needed.

Alternatives to Antibiotics for Food Animals

The global scientific community recognizes the urgent need to reinvigorate the therapeutic pipeline with new antibiotics. The community is further aware of the need for effective and adequate alternative solutions to antibiotics in food animals as an essential strategy to circumvent the challenge of ABR. The range of these potential alternatives is, for the most part, similar to those already documented in human medicine and may include prebiotics, probiotics, synbiotics (viz. mixing of prebiotics and probiotics), substances targeting bacterial communication (quorum sensing), phage enzymes, phage-related therapies and the use of genetically modified food animals (already resistant to infection; Woolhouse et al., 2015).

Synthetic biology (SB) provides a novel approach to discover new antibiotics, and to exploit and improve existing drugs. It uses the genomic data generated by state-of-art technology to identify biological machineries of various bacteria predicted to be able to produce antibiotics. Synthetic bacteria with beneficial functionalities are designed and new antibiotics bio-synthesized with novel antibacterial activity under artificial and engineered control systems (Takano and Breitling, 2014). SB offers an exciting prospect to expand the therapeutic arsenal, as it could generate libraries of novel, predicted and different drug variants with broader activities and better pharmacokinetics (Takano and Breitling, 2014).

Nano-antibiotics, either having antimicrobial activity by themselves or as novel nano-sized drug delivery platforms, are also part of the most interesting alternatives to antibiotics. Unlike other antibiotic substances and proposed strategies, nano-antibiotics exert their activity through several pathways, such as (i) a combination of numerous mechanisms to inhibit bacteria (e.g., nitric oxide-releasing nanoparticles, chitosan-, and metal-containing nanoparticles) (ii) encapsulating several antibiotics within the same nanoparticles, (iii) reduced uptake and increased drug efflux, and (iv) site specific action releasing high concentration of antibiotics at the site of infection (Huh and Kwon, 2011; Pelgrift and Friedman, 2013). Nano-antibiotics offer several advantages, not only in overcoming ABR and reducing acute adverse effects (although toxicity upon long-term exposure is yet uncertain) but they also remain stable on long-term storage and are cost-effective preparations compared with antibiotic synthesis (Huh and Kwon, 2011; Pelgrift and Friedman, 2013). Considerable investments in research are still needed before any of the above possibilities become commercially available on a global scale and can effectively replace antibiotics.

CONCLUSION

ABR is a global public health challenge with severe health and socio-economics repercussions that is significantly influenced by antibiotic use in food animals. Combating ABR effectively at a global scale means addressing it equally in the developed and developing world. Multifaceted, comprehensive and integrated strategies, as advocated by the WHO Global Action Plan and FAO Action Plan in line with the One Health approach, are urgently required to (i) prevent the transmission of ABR and infectious diseases from farm-to-fork, (ii) circumvent potential pandemic situations, and (iii) preserve the efficacy of antibiotics and assure food safety, food security, and global health. Countries should therefore follow WHO, OIE, and FAO recommendations to implement national action plans encompassing human, (food) animal, and environmental sectors to improve policies, interventions and activities that address the prevention and containment of ABR from farm-to-fork.

AUTHOR CONTRIBUTIONS

LF co-conceptualized the study, searched the literature, extracted and collated data, and drafted the manuscript. RF extracted and collated data and contribute to the writing of the manuscript. SE co-conceptualized the study, provided substantial revision of the manuscript. All authors read and approved the final manuscript.

FUNDING

This work was supported by the Antimicrobial Research Unit (ARU) and College of Health Sciences (CHS) of the University of KwaZulu-Natal.

REFERENCES

Acar, J. F., and Moulin, G. (2006). Antimicrobial resistance at farm level. *Rev. Sci. Tech.* 25, 775–792. doi: 10.20506/rst.25.2.1695

Acar, J. F., and Moulin, G. (2013). Integrating animal health surveillance and food safety: the issue of antimicrobial resistance. *Rev. Sci. Tech.* 32, 383–392. doi: 10.20506/rst.32.2.2230

Ahmed, A. M., and Shimamoto, T. (2015a). Molecular analysis of multidrug resistance in Shiga toxin-producing *Escherichia coli* O157:H7 isolated from meat and dairy products. *Int. J. Food Microbiol.* 193, 68–73. doi: 10.1016/j.ijfoodmicro.2014.10.014

Ahmed, A. M., and Shimamoto, T. (2015b). Molecular characterization of multidrug-resistant *Shigella* spp. of food origin. *Int. J. Food Microbiol.* 194, 78–82. doi: 10.1016/j.ijfoodmicro.2014.11.013

Al Bayssari, C., Dabboussi, F., Hamze, M., and Rolain, J.-M. (2015). Emergence of carbapenemase-producing *Pseudomonas aeruginosa* and *Acinetobacter baumannii* in livestock animals in Lebanon. *J. Antimicrob. Chemother.* 70, 950–951. doi: 10.1093/jac/dku469

Allen, H. K. (2014). Antibiotic resistance gene discovery in food-producing animals. *Curr. Opin. Microbiol.* 19, 25–29. doi: 10.1016/j.mib.2014.06.001

Andersson, D. I., and Hughes, D. (2014). Microbiological effects of sub-lethal levels of antibiotics. *Nat. Rev. Microbiol.* 12. 465–478. doi: 10.1038/nrmicro3270

Andremont, A. (2003). Commensal flora may play key role in spreading antibiotic resistance. *Am. Soc. Microbiol. News* 69, 601–607.

Apata, D. F. (2009). Antibiotic resistance in poultry. *Int. J. Poult. Sci.* 8, 404–408. doi: 10.3923/ijps.2009.404.408

Babu, U., Dalloul, R. A., Okamura, M., Lillehoj, H. S., Xie, H., Raybourne, R. B., et al. (2004). Salmonella enteritidis clearance and immune responses in chickens following Salmonella vaccination and challenge. *Vet. Immunol. Immunopathol.* 101, 251–257. doi: 10.1016/j.vetimm.2004.05.002

Barbour, E. K., Hamadeh, S. K., and Eidt, A. (2000). Infection and immunity in broiler chicken breeders vaccinated with a temperature-sensitive mutant of Mycoplasma gallisepticum and impact on performance of offspring. *Poult. Sci.* 79, 1730–1735. doi: 10.1093/ps/79.12.1730

Boonyasiri, A., Tangkoskul, T., Seenama, C., Saiyarin, J., Tiengrim, S., and Thamlikitku, V. (2014). Prevalence of antibiotic-resistant bacteria in healthy adults, foods, food animals, and the environment in selected areas in Thailand. *Pathog. Glob. Health* 108, 235–245. doi: 10.1179/2047773214Y.0000000148

Budak, F., and Übeyli, E. D. (2011). Detection of resistivity for antibiotics by probabilistic neural networks. *J. Med. Syst.* 35, 87–91. doi: 10.1007/s10916-009-9344-z

Chairat, S., Gharsa, H., Lozano, C., Gómez-Sanz, E., Gómez, P., Zarazaga, M. et al. (2015). Characterization of staphylococcus aureus from raw meat samples in tunisia: detection of clonal lineage ST398 from the african continent. *Foodborne Pathog. Dis.* 12, 686–692. doi: 10.1089/fpd.2015.1958

Chang, Q., Wang, W., Regev-Yochay, G., Lipsitch, M., and Hanage, W. P. (2015). Antibiotics in agriculture and the risk to human health: how worried should we be? *Evol. Appl.* 8, 240–245. doi: 10.1111/eva.12185

Chen, L. H., and Wilson, M. E. (2013). The Globalization of healthcare: implications of medical tourism for the infectious disease clinician. *Clin. Infect. Dis.* 57, 1752–1759. doi: 10.1093/cid/cit540

Coetzee, J., Corcoran, C., Prentice, E., Moodley, M., Mendelson, M., Poirel, L., et al. (2016). Emergence of plasmid-mediated colistin resistance (MCR-1) among *Escherichia coli* isolated from South African patients. *S. Afr. Med. J.* 106, 449–450. doi: 10.7196/SAMJ.2016.v106i5.10710

Collignon, P., and Voss, A. (2015). China, what antibiotics and what volumes are used in food production animals? *Antimicrob. Resist. Infect. Control* 4, 16. doi: 10.1186/s13756-015-0056-5

Colombian Integrated Program for Antimicrobial Resistance Surveillance (COIPARS) (2011). *Consolidation Pilot Project Integrated Surveillance of Antimicrobial Resistance in Colombia.* Available online at: http://coiparsamr.wix.com/coipars#! (Accessed October 20, 2016).

da Costa, P. M., Loureiro, L., and Matos, A. J. F. (2013). Transfer of multi-drug resistant bacteria between intermingled ecological niches: the interface between humans, animals and the environment. *Int. J. Environ. Res. Public Health* 10, 278–294. doi: 10.3390/ijerph10010278

DANMAP (2014). *Use of Antimicrobial Agents and Occurrence of Antimicrobial Resistance in Bacteria from Food Animals, Food and Humans in Denmark.* ISSN 1600-2032. Available online at: www.danmap.org (Accessed July 14, 2016).

Dantas, G., and Sommer, M. (2014). How to fight back against antibiotic resistance. *Am. Sci.* 102, 42–51. doi: 10.1511/2014.106.42

de Balogh, K., Halliday, J., and Lubroth, J. (2013). Integrating the surveillance of animal health, foodborne pathogens and foodborne diseases in developing and in-transition countries. *Rev. Sci. Tech.* 32, 539–548. doi: 10.20506/rst.32.2.2241

Donado-Godoy, P., Castellanos, R., Leon, M., Arevalo, A., Clavijo, V., Bernal, J., et al. (2015). The establishment of the Colombian Integrated Program for Antimicrobial Resistance Surveillance (COIPARS): a pilot project on poultry farms, slaughterhouses and retail market. *Zoonoses Public Health* 62, 58–69. doi: 10.1111/zph.12192

Eagar, H., Swan, G., and van Vuuren, M. (2012). A survey of antimicrobial usage in animals in South Africa with specific reference to food animals. *J. S. Afr. Vet. Assoc.* 83:16. doi: 10.4102/jsava.v83i1.16

Elgroud, R., Zerdoumi, F., Benazzouz, M., Bouzitouna-Bentchouala, C., Granier, S. A., Fremy, S., et al. (2009). Characteristics of Salmonella contamination of broilers and slaughterhouses in the region of Constantine (Algeria). *Zoonoses Public Health* 56, 84–93. doi: 10.1111/j.1863-2378.2008.01164.x

European Centre for Disease Prevention and Control (ECDC) (2014). *Surveillance of Antimicrobial Consumption in Europe 2012.* Stockholm: ECDC.

European Centre for Disease Prevention and Control (ECDC). (2015). *Antimicrobial Resistance Surveillance in Europe 2014.* Stockholm: ECDC.

European Food Safety Authority (EFSA) and European Centre for Disease Prevention and Control (ECDC) (2015). The European Union Summary Report on Trends and sources of zoonoses zoonotic agents and food-borne outbreaks in 2013. *EFSA J.* 13:3991. doi: 10.2903/j.efsa.2015.3991

European Food Safety Authority (EFSA) and European Centre for Disease Prevention and Control (ECDC). (2016). The European Union summary report on antimicrobial resistance in zoonotic and indicator bacteria from humans, animals and food in 2014. *EFSA J.* 14:4380. doi: 10.2903/j.efsa.2016.4380

Ewers, C., Bethe, A., Semmler, T., Guenther, S., and Wieler, L. H. (2012). Extended-spectrum beta-lactamase-producing and AmpC-producing *Escherichia coli* from livestock and companion animals, and their putative impact on public health: a global perspective. *Clin. Microbiol. Infect.* 18, 646–655. doi: 10.1111/j.1469-0691.2012.03850.x

Ewnetu, D., and Mihret, A. (2010). Prevalence and antimicrobial resistance of Campylobacter isolates from humans and chickens in Bahir Dar, Ethiopia. *Foodborne Pathog. Dis.* 7, 667–670. doi: 10.1089/fpd.2009.0433

Fernandes, M. R., Moura, Q., Sartori, L., Silva, K. C., Cunba, M. P., Esposito, F., et al. (2016). Silent dissemination of colistin-resistant *Escherichia coli* in South

America could contribute to the global spread of the mcr-1 gene. *Euro. Surveill.* 21, pii=30214. doi: 10.2807/1560-7917.ES.2016.21.17.30214

FINRES-Vet (2007-2009). *Finnish Veterinary Antimicrobial Resistance Monitoring and Consumption of Antimicrobial Agents.* Helsinki: Finnish Food Safety Authority Evira.

Fischer, J., Rodriguez, I., Schmoger, S., Friese, A., Roesler, U., Helmuth, R., et al. (2012). Escherichia coli producing VIM-1 carbapenemase isolated on a pig farm. *J. Antimicrob. Chemother.* 67, 1793–1795. doi: 10.1093/jac/dks108

Food and Agriculture Organization of the United Nations (FAO). (2003). *Biosecurity in Food and Agriculture.* Rome: Food and Agriculture Organization of the United Nations.

Food and Agriculture Organization of the United Nations (FAO) (2015). *Status Report on Antimicrobial Resistance.* Rome: Food and Agriculture Organization of the United Nations.

Food and Agriculture Organization of the United Nations (FAO) (2016). *The FAO Action Plan on Antimicrobial Resistance 2016-2020.* Rome: Food and Agriculture Organization of the United Nations.

Food and Agriculture Organization of the United Nations (FAO) and World Health Organization (WHO) (2011). *Guidelines for Risk Analysis of Foodborne Antimicrobial Resistance (CAC/GL 77-2011).* Available online at: http://www.fao.org/input/download/standards/11776/CXG_077e.pdf (Accessed July 4, 2016).

Food and Drug Administration of the United States (FDA). (2014). *National Antimicrobial Resistance Monitoring System Integrated report 2012-2013: Enteric Bacteria.* Available online at: http://www.fda.gov/AnimalVeterinary/SafetyHealth/AntimicrobialResistance/NationalAntimicrobialResistanceMonitoringSystem/ucm059103.htm (Accessed August 26, 2016).

Government of Canada (2014). *Canadian Integrated Program for Antimicrobial Resistance Surveillance (CIPARS) 2012 Annual Report.* Public Health Agency of Canada, Guelph, ON.

Grami, R., Mansour, W., Mehri, W., Bouallegue, O., Boujaafar, N., Madec, J., et al. (2016). Impact of food animal trade on the spread of mcr-1-mediated colistin resistance, Tunisia, July 2015. *Euro. Surveill.* 21:pii=30144. doi: 10.2807/1560-7917.ES.2016.21.8.30144

Guedes, R. M., and Gebhart, C. J. (2003). Onset and duration of fecal shedding, cell-mediated and humoral immune responses in pigs after challenge with a pathogenic isolate or attenuated vaccine strain of *Lawsonia intracellularis. Vet. Microbiol.* 91, 135–145. doi: 10.1016/S0378-1135(02)00301-2

Harbarth, S., Balkhy, H. H., Goossens, H., Jarlier, V., Kluytmans, J., Laxminarayan, R., et al. (2015). Antimicrobial resistance: one world, one fight!. *Antimicrob. Resist. Infect. Control* 4:49. doi: 10.1186/s13756-015-0091-2

Holmes, A. H., Moore, L. S., Sundsfjord, A., Steinbakk, M., Regmi, S., Karley, A., et al. (2016). Understanding the mechanisms and drivers of antimicrobial resistance. *Lancet* 387, 176–187. doi: 10.1016/S0140-6736(15)00473-0

Huh, A. J., and Kwon, Y. J. (2011). "Nanoantibiotics": a new paradigm for treating infectious diseases using nanomaterials in the antibiotic-resistant era. *J. Control. Release* 156, 128–145. doi: 10.1016/j.jconrel.2011.07.002

Iweriebor, B. C., Iwu, C. J., Obi, L. C., Nwodo, U. U., and Okoh, A. I. (2015). Multiple antibiotic resistances among Shiga toxin producing *Escherichia coli* O157 in feces of dairy cattle farms in Eastern Cape of South Africa. *BMC Microbiol.* 15:123. doi: 10.1186/s12866-015-0553-y

Japan Nosocomial Infections Surveillance (JANIS). (2016). *Annual Open Report 2013.* Available online at: http://www.nih-janis.jp/english/report/index.html (Accessed October 23, 2016).

Klibi, N., Said, L. B., Jouini, A., Slama, K. B., Lopez, M., Sallem, R. B., et al. (2013). Species distribution, antibiotic resistance and virulence traits in enterococci from meat in Tunisia. *Meat. Sci.* 93, 675–680. doi: 10.1016/j.meatsci.2012.11.020

Lechowicz, L., Urbaniak, M., and Adamus-Bialele, W. (2013). The use of infrared spectroscopy and artificial neural network for detection of uropathogenic *E. coli* strains susceptibility to cephalothin. *Acta Biochim. Polonica* 60, 713–718.

Liu, Y.-Y., Wang, Y., Walsh, T. R., Yi, L.-X., Zhang, R., Spencer, J., et al. (2016). Emergence of plasmid-mediated colistin resistance mechanism mcr-1 in animals and human beings in China: a microbiological and molecular biological study. *Lancet Infect. Dis.* 16, 161–168. doi: 10.1016/S1473-3099(15)00424-7

Marshall, B. M., and Levy, S. B. (2011). Food animals and antimicrobials: impacts on human health. *Clin. Microbiol. Rev.* 24, 718–733. doi: 10.1128/CMR.00002-11

Meeusen, E. N., Walker, J., Peters, A., Pastoret, P.-P., and Jungersen, G. (2007). Current status of veterinary vaccines. *Clin. Microbiol. Rev.* 20, 489–510. doi: 10.1128/CMR.00005-07

Mensah, P., Mwamakamba, L., Kariuki, S., Fonkoua, M. C., and Aidara-Kane, A. (2012). Strengthening foodborne diseases surveillance in the WHO African region: a essential need for disease control and food safety surveillance. *Afr. J. Food Agric. Nutr. Dev.* 12, 6336–6353.

Mensah, S. E., Koudande, O. D., Sanders, P., Laurentie, M., Mensah, G. A., and Abiola, F. A. (2014). Antimicrobial residues in foods of animal origin in Africa: public health risks. *Rev. Sci. Tech.* 33, 987–996.

Moriyon, I., Grillo, M. J., Monreal, D., Gonzalez, D., Marin, C., Lopez-Goni, I., et al. (2004). Rough vaccines in animal brucellosis: structural and genetic basis and present status. *Vet. Res.* 35, 1–38. doi: 10.1051/vetres:2003037

Mwamakamba, L., Mensah, P., Fontannaz-Aujoulat, F., Hlabana, M., Maiga, F., Bangoura, F., et al. (2012). The WHO five keys to safer food: a tool for food safety health promotion. *Afr. J. Food Agric. Nutr. Dev.* 16, 6245–6259.

Nahar, A., Siddiquee, M., Nahar, S., Anwar, K. S., Ali, S., and Islam, S. (2014). Multi-drug resistance *Proteus mirabilis* isolated from chicken droppings in commercial poultry farms: biosecurity concern and emerging public health threat in Bangladesh. *J. Biosaf. Health Educ.* 2:120. doi: 10.4172/2332-0893.1000120

NethMap-MARAN (2015). *Monitoring of Antimicrobial Resistance and Antibiotic Usage in Animals in the Netherlands in 2014.* Lelystad: Central Veterinary Institute of Wageningen University and Research Centre in collaboration with the Food and Consumer Product Safety Authority (NVWA), the National Institute for Public Health and the Environment (RIVM) and the Netherlands Veterinary Medicines Authority (SDa).

NORM/NORM-VET (2015). *Usage of Antimicrobial Agents and Occurrence of Antimicrobial Resistance in Norway.* Tromsø; Oslo. ISSN: 1502-2307 (print) / 1890-9965 (electronic). Available online at: www.vetinst.no (Accessed July 15, 2016).

Observatoire National de l'Epidémiologie de la Résistance Bactérienne aux Antibiotiques (ONERBA). (2015). *Annual Report 2013-2014.* Available online at: http://www.onerba.org/spip.php?rubrique19 (Accessed October 18, 2016).

O'Neill, J. (2015a). *Tackling a Global Health Crisis: Initial Steps.* London: Wellcome Trust. Available online at: http://www.amr-review.org

O'Neill, J. (2015b). *Antimicrobials in Agriculture and the Environment: Reducing Unnecessary Use and Waste.* London: Wellcome Trust. Available online at: www.amr-review.org

O'Neill, J. (2016). *Tackling Drug Resistance Globally: Final Report.* London: Wellcome Trust. Available online at: www.amr-review.org

Österberg, J., Wingstrand, A., Jensen, A. N., Kerouanton, A., and Cobin, V. (2016). Antibiotic resistance in *E. coli* from pigs in organic and conventional farming in four *European countries. PLoS ONE* 11:e0157049. doi: 10.1371/journal.pone.0157049

Padungtod, P., Kadohira, M., and Hill, G. (2008). Livestock production and foodborne diseases from food animals in Thailand. *J. Vet. Med. Sci.* 70, 873–879. doi: 10.1292/jvms.70.873

Pelgrift, R. Y., and Friedman, A. J. (2013). Nanotechnology as a therapeutic tool to combat microbial resistance. *Adv. Drug Delivery Rev.* 65, 1803–1815. doi: 10.1016/j.addr.2013.07.011

Plaza-Rodríguez, C., Thoens, C., Falenski, A., Weiser, A. A., Appel, B., Kaesbohrer, A., et al. (2015). A strategy to establish food safety model repositories. *Int. J. Food Microbiol.* 204, 81–90. doi: 10.1016/j.ijfoodmicro.2015.03.010

Postma, M., Backhams, A., Collineau, L., Loesken, S., Sjolund, M., Belloc, C., et al. (2016). Evaluation of the relationship between the biosecurity status, production parameters, herd characteristics and antimicrobial usage in farrow-to-finish pig production in four European countries. *Porcine Health Manag.* 2:9. doi: 10.1186/s40813-016-0028-z

Prabhakar, S. V. R. K., Sano, D., and Srivastava, N. (2010). "Food safety in the Asia-Pacific Region: current status, policy perspectives and a way forward," in *Sustainable Consumption and Production in the Asia-Pacific Region: Effective Responses in a Resource Constrained World White Paper III* (Hayama: Institute for Global Environmental Strategies), 215–298.

Price, L. B., Stegger, M., Hasman, H., Aziz, M., Larsen, J., Andersen, P. S., et al. (2012). *Staphylococcus aureus* CC398: host adaptation and emergence of methicillin resistance in livestock. *MBio* 3, e00305–e00311. doi: 10.1128/mBio.00305-11

Rebuffo-Scheer, C. A., Schmitt, J., and Scherer, S. (2007). Differentiation of Listeria monocytogenes serovars by using artificial neural network analysis of fourier-transformed infrare spectra. *Appl. Environ. Microbiol.* 73, 1036–1040. doi: 10.1128/AEM.02004-06

SWEDRES-SVARM (2015). *Consumption of Antibiotics and Occurrence of Antibiotic Resistance in SWEDEN.* Solna; Uppsala.

Takano, E., and Breitling, R. (2014). *Antimicrobial Resistance – A New Drug Perspective Using Synthetic Biology.* Houston, TX: Emerging and Persistent Infectious Diseases (EPID): Focus on Antimicrobial Resistance.

Thanner, S., Drissner, D., and Walsh, F. (2016). Antimicrobial resistance in agriculture. *MBio* 7, e02227–e02215. doi: 10.1128/mBio.02227-15

The department (2007). *Pilot Surveillance Program for Antimicrobial Resistance in Bacteria of Animal Origin.* Australian Government Department of Agriculture Canberra. Available online at: http://www.agriculture.gov.au/animal/health/amr/antimicrobial-resistance-bacteria-animal-origin#acknowledgements. (Accessed October 23, 2016).

The Japanese Veterinary Antimicrobial Resistance Monitoring System in the Field of Animal Hygiene (JVARM). (2013). *A Report on the Japanese Veterinary Antimicrobial Resistance Monitoring System 2008 to 2011.* National Veterinary Assay Laboratory, Ministry of Agriculture, Forestry and Fisheries, Tokyo.

Usui, M., Ozawa, S., Onozato, H., Kuge, R., Obata, Y., Uemae, T., et al. (2014). Antimicrobial susceptibility of indicator bacteria isolated from chickens in Southeast Asian countries (Vietnam, Indonesia and Thailand). *J. Vet. Med. Sci.* 76, 685–692. doi: 10.1292/jvms.13-0423

Van Boeckel, T. P., Brower, C., Gilbert, M., Grenfell, B. T., Levin, S. A., Robinson, T. P., et al. (2015). Global trends in antimicrobial use in food animals. *Proc. Natl. Acad. Sci. U.S.A.* 112, 5649–5654. doi: 10.1073/pnas.1503141112

Van Boeckel, T. P., Gandra, S., Ashok, A., Caudron, Q., Grenfell, B. T., and Levin, S. A. (2014). Global antibiotic consumption 2000 to 2010: an analysis of national pharmaceutical sales data. *Lancet Infect. Dis.* 14, 742–750. doi: 10.1016/S1473-3099(14)70780-7

Van Overbeke, I., Chiers, K., Ducatelle, R., and Haesebrouck, F. (2001). Effect of endobronchial challenge with *Actinobacillus pleuropneumoniae* serotype 9 of pigs vaccinated with a vaccine containing Apx toxins and transferrin-binding proteins. *J. Vet. Med. B Infect. Dis. Vet. Public Health* 48, 15–20. doi: 10.1046/j.1439-0450.2001.00419.x

Woolhouse, M., Ward, M., van Bunnik, B., and Farrar, J. (2015). Antimicrobial resistance in humans, livestock and the wider environment. *Philos. Trans. R. Soc. B* 370, 20140083. doi: 10.1098/rstb.2014.0083

World Health Organization (WHO) (2011). *Critically Important Antimicrobials for Human Medicine.* Geneva: World Health Organization.

World Health Organization (WHO) (2015a). *Global Action Plan on Antimicrobial Resistance.* Geneva: World Health Organization.

World Health Organization (WHO) (2015b). *Worldwide Country Situation Analysis: Response to Antimicrobial Resistance.* Geneva: World Health Organization.

World Organization for Animal Health (OIE) (2015). *List of Antimicrobial Agents of Veterinary Importance.* Paris: World Organization for Animal Health.

World Organization for Animal Health (OIE) (2016). *Terrestrial Animal Health Code.* Paris: World Organization for Animal Health.

Wu, X. L., Xiang, L., Yan, Q. Y., Jiang, Y. N., Li, Y. W., Huang, X. P., et al. (2014). Distribution and risk assessment of quinolone antibiotics in the soils from organic vegetable farms of a subtropical city, Southern China. *Sci. Total Environ.* 487, 399–406. doi: 10.1016/j.scitotenv.2014.04.015

Wulf, M., and Voss, A. (2008). MRSA in livestock animals - an epidemic waiting to happen? *Clin. Microbiol. Infect.* 14, 519–521. doi: 10.1111/j.1469-0691.2008.01970.x

Zaidi, M. B., Calva, J. J., Estrada-Garcia, M. T., Leon, V., Vazquez, G., Figueroa, G., et al. (2008). Integrated food chain surveillance system for *Salmonella* spp. in Mexico. *Emerg. Infect. Dis.* 14, 429–435. doi: 10.3201/eid1403.071057

Zaidi, M. B., McDermott, P. F., Campos, F. D., Chim, R., Leon, M., Vazquez, G., et al. (2012). Antimicrobial-resistant campylobacter in the food chain in Mexico. *Foodborne Pathog. Dis.* 9, 841–847. doi: 10.1089/fpd.2012.1127

Zaidi, M. B., Dreser, A., and Figueroa, I. M. (2015). A collaborative initiative for the containment of antimicrobial resistance in Mexico. *Zoonoses Public Health* 62, 52–57. doi: 10.1111/zph.12166

Zhu, Y.-G., Johnson, T. A., Su, J.-Q., Qiao, M., Guo, G.-X., Stedtfeld, R. D., et al. (2013). Diverse and abundant antibiotic resistance genes in chinese swine farms. *Proc. Natl. Acad. Sci. U.S.A.* 110, 3435–3440. doi: 10.1073/pnas.1222743110

Permissions

All chapters in this book were first published by Frontiers; hereby published with permission under the Creative Commons Attribution License or equivalent. Every chapter published in this book has been scrutinized by our experts. Their significance has been extensively debated. The topics covered herein carry significant findings which will fuel the growth of the discipline. They may even be implemented as practical applications or may be referred to as a beginning point for another development.

The contributors of this book come from diverse backgrounds, making this book a truly international effort. This book will bring forth new frontiers with its revolutionizing research information and detailed analysis of the nascent developments around the world.

We would like to thank all the contributing authors for lending their expertise to make the book truly unique. They have played a crucial role in the development of this book. Without their invaluable contributions this book wouldn't have been possible. They have made vital efforts to compile up to date information on the varied aspects of this subject to make this book a valuable addition to the collection of many professionals and students.

This book was conceptualized with the vision of imparting up-to-date information and advanced data in this field. To ensure the same, a matchless editorial board was set up. Every individual on the board went through rigorous rounds of assessment to prove their worth. After which they invested a large part of their time researching and compiling the most relevant data for our readers.

The editorial board has been involved in producing this book since its inception. They have spent rigorous hours researching and exploring the diverse topics which have resulted in the successful publishing of this book. They have passed on their knowledge of decades through this book. To expedite this challenging task, the publisher supported the team at every step. A small team of assistant editors was also appointed to further simplify the editing procedure and attain best results for the readers.

Apart from the editorial board, the designing team has also invested a significant amount of their time in understanding the subject and creating the most relevant covers. They scrutinized every image to scout for the most suitable representation of the subject and create an appropriate cover for the book.

The publishing team has been an ardent support to the editorial, designing and production team. Their endless efforts to recruit the best for this project, has resulted in the accomplishment of this book. They are a veteran in the field of academics and their pool of knowledge is as vast as their experience in printing. Their expertise and guidance has proved useful at every step. Their uncompromising quality standards have made this book an exceptional effort. Their encouragement from time to time has been an inspiration for everyone.

The publisher and the editorial board hope that this book will prove to be a valuable piece of knowledge for researchers, students, practitioners and scholars across the globe.

List of Contributors

Anna Johnning
Department of Infectious Diseases, Institute of Biomedicine, University of Gothenburg, Gothenburg, Sweden
Department of Mathematical Sciences, Chalmers University of Technology, Gothenburg, Sweden

Erik Kristiansson
Department of Mathematical Sciences, Chalmers University of Technology, Gothenburg, Sweden

Jerker Fick
Department of Chemistry, Umeå University, Umeå, Sweden

Birgitta Weijdegård and D. G. Joakim Larsson
Department of Infectious Diseases, Institute of Biomedicine, University of Gothenburg, Gothenburg, Sweden

Inna Lysnyansky
Mycoplasma Unit, Division of Avian and Aquatic Diseases, Kimron Veterinary Institute, Beit Dagan, Israel

Roger D. Ayling
Department of Bacteriology, Animal and Plant Health Agency, Addlestone, UK

Jasna Kovač, NežaČ adež and Sonja Smole Možina
Department of Food Science and Technology, Biotechnical Faculty, University of Ljubljana, Ljubljana, Slovenia

Beatrix Stessl and Martin Wagner
Department for Farm Animals and Veterinary Public Health, Institute of Milk Hygiene, Milk Technology and Food Science, University of Veterinary Medicine, Vienna, Austria

Kerstin Stingl
National Reference Laboratory for Campylobacter, Department of Biological Safety, Federal Institute for Risk Assessment, Berlin, Germany

Igor Gruntar and Matjaž Ocepek
Institute of Microbiology and Parasitology, Veterinary Faculty, University of Ljubljana, Ljubljana, Slovenia

Marija Trkov
Department for Public Health Microbiology Ljubljana, Centre for Medical Microbiology, National Laboratory of Health, Environment and Food, Ljubljana, Slovenia

Yafei Li, Baoyi Feng, Zhenling Zeng, Bingxu Zhang and Huanzhong Ding
Laboratory of Veterinary Pharmacology, College of Veterinary Medicine, South China Agricultural University, Guangzhou, China

Xiaoyan Gu
Centre for Veterinary Drug Residues, College of Veterinary Medicine, South China Agricultural University, Guangzhou, China

Dawei Yang
China Institute of Veterinary Drug Control, Beijing, China

Catarina M. Marinho, Tiago Santos and Alexandre Gonçalves
Department of Genetics and Biotechnology, School of Life and Environment Sciences, University of Trás-os-Montes and Alto Douro, Vila Real, Portugal
Functional Genomics and Proteomics Unit, University of Trás-os-Montes and Alto Douro, Vila Real, Portugal

Patrícia Poeta
Veterinary Science Department, University of Trás-os-Montes and Alto Douro, Vila Real, Portugal
UCIBIO-REQUIMTE, Faculty of Science and Technology, University Nova of Lisbon, Lisbon, Portugal

Gilberto Igrejas
Department of Genetics and Biotechnology, School of Life and Environment Sciences, University of Trás-os-Montes and Alto Douro, Vila Real, Portugal
Functional Genomics and Proteomics Unit, University of Trás-os-Montes and Alto Douro, Vila Real, Portugal
UCIBIO-REQUIMTE, Faculty of Science and Technology, University Nova of Lisbon, Lisbon, Portugal

Boris Shaskolskiy, Ekaterina Dementieva, Arvo Leinsoo and Dmitry Gryadunov
Laboratory for Molecular Diagnostics Technologies, Engelhardt Institute of Molecular Biology, Russian Academy of Sciences, Moscow, Russia

Anastassia Runina, Denis Vorobyev, Xenia Plakhova, Alexey Kubanov and Dmitrii Deryabin
State Research Center of Dermatovenerology and Cosmetology of the Russian Ministry of Health, Moscow, Russia

Qiu-E. Yang, Jian Sun, Liang Li, Hui Deng, Bao-Tao Liu, Liang-Xing Fang and Xiao-Ping Liao
Laboratory of Veterinary Pharmacology, College of Veterinary Medicine, South China Agricultural University, Guangzhou, China

Ya-Hong Liu
Laboratory of Veterinary Pharmacology, College of Veterinary Medicine, South China Agricultural University, Guangzhou, China
Jiangsu Co-Innovation Centre for Prevention and Control of Important Animal Infectious Diseases and Zoonoses, Yangzhou, China

Zhen Xu, Hermine V. Mkrtchyan and Ronald R. Cutler
School of Biological and Chemical Sciences, Queen Mary University of London, London, UK

Ethan R. Wyrsch and Steven P. Djordjevic
The ithree Institute, University of Technology Sydney, Sydney, NSW, Australia

Piklu Roy Chowdhury
The ithree Institute, University of Technology Sydney, Sydney, NSW, Australia
NSW Department of Primary Industries, Elizabeth Macarthur Agricultural Institute, Sydney, NSW, Australia

Toni A. Chapman and Jeffrey M. Hammond
NSW Department of Primary Industries, Elizabeth Macarthur Agricultural Institute, Sydney, NSW, Australia

Ian G. Charles
Institute of Food Research, Norwich Research Park, Norwich, UK

Wen-Hui Zhang, Xiang-Yan Lin, Liang Xu, Xi-Xi Gu, Ling Yang, Wan Li, Si-Qi Ren,Ya-Hong Liu, Zhen-Ling Zeng and Hong-Xia Jiang
National Risk Assessment Laboratory for Antimicrobial Resistance of Animal Original Bacteria, College of Veterinary Medicine, South China Agricultural University, Guangzhou, China

Hanifa Ziane, Soumia Bektache and Mohamed Tazir
Service de Microbiologie Médicale, Centre Hospitalo-Universitaire Mustapha Bacha, Faculté de Médecine, Algiers, Algeria

Vera Manageiro
National Reference Laboratory of Antibiotic Resistances and Healthcare Associated Infections, Department of Infectious Diseases, National Institute of Health Doutor Ricardo Jorge, Lisbon, Portugal
Centre for the Studies of Animal Science, Institute of Agrarian and Agri-Food Sciences and Technologies, University of Oporto, Oporto, Portugal

Eugénia Ferreira, Inês B. Moura and Manuela Caniça
National Reference Laboratory of Antibiotic Resistances and Healthcare Associated Infections, Department of Infectious Diseases, National Institute of Health Doutor Ricardo Jorge, Lisbon, Portugal

Shahper N. Khan and Asad U. Khan
Interdisciplinary Biotechnology Unit, Aligarh Muslim University, Aligarh, India

Christian J. H. von Wintersdorff and Nathan D. Mills
Department of Medical Microbiology, NUTRIM School for Nutrition and Translational Research in Metabolism, Maastricht University Medical Center, Maastricht, Netherlands

John Penders and Petra F. G. Wolffs
Department of Medical Microbiology, NUTRIM School for Nutrition and Translational Research in Metabolism, Maastricht University Medical Center, Maastricht, Netherlands
Department of Medical Microbiology, Caphri School for Public Health and Primary Care, Maastricht University Medical Center, Maastricht, Netherlands

Julius M. van Niekerk, Snehali Majumder and Lieke B. van Alphen
Department of Medical Microbiology, Caphri School for Public Health and Primary Care, Maastricht University Medical Center, Maastricht, Netherlands

Paul H. M. Savelkoul
Department of Medical Microbiology, NUTRIM School for Nutrition and Translational Research in Metabolism, Maastricht University Medical Center, Maastricht, Netherlands
Department of Medical Microbiology, Caphri School for Public Health and Primary Care, Maastricht University Medical Center, Maastricht, Netherlands
Department of Medical Microbiology and Infection Control, VU University Medical Center, Amsterdam, Netherlands

Zengping Xu, Baochen Yang, Liyun Pang and Tianjun Liu
Tianjin Key Laboratory of Biomedical Material, Institute of Biomedical Engineering, Peking Union Medical College - Chinese Academy of Medical Sciences, Tianjin, China

Yuxiang Gao
Department of Materials Chemistry, Nankai University, Tianjin, China

Shuai Meng
Tianjin Key Laboratory of Biomedical Material, Institute of Biomedical Engineering, Peking Union Medical College - Chinese Academy of Medical Sciences, Tianjin, China
Tianjin Medical University Cancer Institute and Hospital, Tianjin, China

Chen Wang
Tianjin Medical University Cancer Institute and Hospital, Tianjin, China

Christine Parrott
Centre for Population Health Research, School of Health and Social Development, Deakin University, Geelong, VIC, Australia
Young People's Health Service, Department of Adolescent Medicine, The Royal Children's Hospital, Parkville, VIC, Australia

Gillian Wood
Perinatal Medicine, Mercy Hospital for Women, Heidelberg, VIC, Australia
Department of Microbiology, Dorevitch Pathology, Heidelberg, VIC, Australia

Ekaterina Bogatyreva and Catherine M. Bennett
Centre for Population Health Research, School of Health and Social Development, Deakin University, Geelong, VIC, Australia

Geoffrey W. Coombs
School of Veterinary and Life Sciences, Murdoch University, Murdoch, WA, Australia
Path West Laboratory Medicine - Fiona Stanley Hospital, Murdoch, WA, Australia

Paul D. R. Johnson
Department of Infectious Diseases, Austin Health, Heidelberg, VIC, Australia

Alexandra Badura, Judith C. Holzer, Gebhard Feierl and Andrea J. Grisold
Institute of Hygiene, Microbiology and Environmental Medicine, Medical University of Graz, Graz, Austria

Gudrun Pregartner
Institute for Medical Informatics, Statistics and Documentation, Medical University of Graz, Graz, Austria

Bushra Jamil and Muhammad Imran
Microbiology and Public Health Group, Department of Biosciences, COMSATS Institute of Information Technology, Islamabad, Pakistan

Huma Habib
Center for Micro and Nano Devices, COMSATS Institute of Information Technology, Islamabad, Pakistan

Shahid A. Abbasi
Department of Pathology, Al-Sayed Hospital, Rawalpindi, Pakistan

Ayesha Ihsan
Industrial Biotechnology Division, National Institute of Biotechnology and Genetic Engineering, Faisalabad, Pakistan

Habib Nasir
School of Natural Sciences, National University of Sciences and Technology, Islamabad, Pakistan

Xiuhua Kuang
MOA Laboratory for Risk Assessment of Quality and Safety of Livestock and Poultry Products, Huazhong Agricultural University, Wuhan, China
Hubei Collaborative Innovation Center for Animal Nutrition and Feed Safety, Huazhong Agricultural University, Wuhan, China

Haihong Hao and Zonghui Yuan
MOA Laboratory for Risk Assessment of Quality and Safety of Livestock and Poultry Products, Huazhong Agricultural University, Wuhan, China
Hubei Collaborative Innovation Center for Animal Nutrition and Feed Safety, Huazhong Agricultural University, Wuhan, China
National Reference Laboratory of Veterinary Drug Residues and MOA Key Laboratory for Detection of Veterinary Drug Residues, Huazhong Agricultural University, Wuhan, China

Menghong Dai and Yulian Wang
Hubei Collaborative Innovation Center for Animal Nutrition and Feed Safety, Huazhong Agricultural University, Wuhan, China
National Reference Laboratory of Veterinary Drug Residues and MOA Key Laboratory for Detection of Veterinary Drug Residues, Huazhong Agricultural University, Wuhan, China

Ijaz Ahmad
National Reference Laboratory of Veterinary Drug Residues and MOA Key Laboratory for Detection of Veterinary Drug Residues, Huazhong Agricultural University, Wuhan, China

Zhenli Liu
MOA Laboratory for Risk Assessment of Quality and Safety of Livestock and Poultry Products, Huazhong Agricultural University, Wuhan, China
National Reference Laboratory of Veterinary Drug Residues and MOA Key Laboratory for Detection of Veterinary Drug Residues, Huazhong Agricultural University, Wuhan, China

Ying Huang and Lu Zhang
Department of Food Science and Technology, The Ohio State University, Columbus, OH, USA

Laura Tiu
South Centers, The Ohio State University, Piketon, OH, USA

Hua H. Wang
Department of Food Science and Technology, The Ohio State University, Columbus, OH, USA
Department of Microbiology, The Ohio State University, Columbus, OH, USA
School of Biological Sciences, Fudan University, Yangpu, Shanghai, China

Mudsser Azam and Qazi M. R. Haq
Microbiology Research Laboratory, Department of Biosciences, Jamia Millia Islamia, New Delhi, India

Arif T. Jan
Molecular Biology Laboratory, School of Biotechnology, Yeungnam University, Gyeongsan, South Korea

Luria Leslie Founou and Sabiha Yusuf Essack
Antimicrobial Research Unit, Department of Pharmacy, School of Health Sciences, University of KwaZulu-Natal, Durban, South Africa

Raspail Carrel Founou
Antimicrobial Research Unit, Department of Pharmacy, School of Health Sciences, University of KwaZulu-Natal, Durban, South Africa
Department of Microbiology, Centre of Expertise and Biological Diagnostic of Cameroon, Yaoundé, Cameroon

Index

www.ingramcontent.com/pod-product-compliance
Lightning Source LLC
LaVergne TN
LVHW060537210926
848485LV00005B/1219